Dietary Supplements

FORENSIC
SCIENCE AND MEDICINE

Steven B. Karch, MD, Series Editor

DIETARY SUPPLEMENTS

TOXICOLOGY
and
CLINICAL PHARMACOLOGY

Edited by

Melanie Johns Cupp, PharmD, BCPS
and
Timothy S. Tracy, PhD

West Virginia University
Morgantown, WV

HUMANA PRESS ✳ TOTOWA, NEW JERSEY

© 2003 Humana Press Inc.
999 Riverview Drive, Suite 208
Totowa, New Jersey 07512

www.humanapress.com

Production Editor: Robin B. Weisberg
Cover design by Patricia F. Cleary

For additional copies, pricing for bulk purchases, and/or information about other Humana titles, contact Humana at the above address or at any of the following numbers: Tel.: 973-256-1699; Fax: 973-256-8341; E-mail: humana@humanapr.com or visit our website: http://humanapress.com

This publication is printed on acid-free paper. ∞
ANSI Z39.48-1984 (American National Standards Institute) Permanence of Paper for Printed Library Materials.

Printed in the United States of America. 10 9 8 7 6 5 4 3 2 1

Library of Congress Cataloging-in-Publication Data

Dietary supplements : toxicology and clinical pharmacology / edited by Melanie Johns Cupp and Timothy S. Tracy.
    p. ; cm.— (Forensic science and medicine)
  Includes bibliographical references and index.
  ISBN 1-58829-014-X (alk. paper) 1-59259-303-8 (e-book)
  1. Dietary supplements —Physiological effect. 2. Dietary supplements—Toxicology. I. Cupp, Melanie Johns. II. Tracy, Timothy S. III. Series.
  [DNLM: 1. Dietary Supplements, adverse effects. 2. Pharmacology, Clinical. QU 145.5 D5648 2003]
RM258.5 .D545 2003
615'.1—dc21   2002027544

Preface

Sales of dietary supplements have skyrocketed over the past few years. Despite widespread interest in and use of these products, information about the safety and efficacy of dietary supplements in humans is generally sparse compared with the information available about prescription drugs. Herbalists and laypersons have used herbs for centuries, but most nonherbal dietary supplements came into vogue only within the past few decades, further limiting the information available about these products. The companion volume, *Toxicology and Clinical Pharmacology of Herbal Products* addressed herbal dietary supplements, whereas *Dietary Supplements: Toxicology and Clinical Pharmacology* focuses on nonherbal dietary supplements. Supplements were chosen for inclusion based on their popularity, toxicity, and the quantity and quality of information available. Some supplements described here are no longer available as dietary supplements (e.g., gamma-hydroxybutyric acid and related substances, L-tryptophan), but are available through various channels, either legal or illegal. Others are advertised as dietary supplements, although the Food and Drug Administration does not view them as such (e.g., hydrazine sulfate).

The aim of this book is to present, in both comprehensive and summary formats, objective information on nonherbal dietary supplements from the most reliable sources, with an emphasis on information not readily available elsewhere (i.e., detailed descriptions of case reports of adverse effects, pharmacokinetics, and chemical and biofluid analysis). It is not designed to be a prescriber's handbook; the intended audience is both forensic and health care professionals, particularly researchers and clinicians interested in more detailed information than is available in most "herbal" or "natural product" references.

Although information about dietary supplements is widely available on the Internet, it is usually provided by product distributors and is designed to sell products rather than provide objective information about product efficacy and toxicity. Even reviews of dietary supplements in journals, newsletters, books, and electronic databases can be biased or incorrect. In compiling information to be included in *Dietary Supplements: Toxicology and Clinical Pharmacology,* emphasis was placed on original studies published in reputable, peer-reviewed journals. Older studies as well as more current literature were utilized for completeness. Where appropriate, information was obtained from meta-analyses, systematic reviews, or other high-quality reviews such as those written by recognized experts. Case reports of adverse effects and interactions, although anecdotal in nature, were used to identify and describe uncommon, but potentially serious, adverse events that may not have been noted in controlled studies because of small sample size or short duration. The detail in which studies in this section is described is a function of the popularity of the supplement, the extent to which study results conflict with each other and with advertised efficacy claims, the attention recent supplement studies have received in both lay and medical news, and other factors described in the text.

This volume begins with an updated discussion of the legal aspects of dietary supplements. Each of the following supplement monographs includes a review of the product's history, current promoted uses, sources and chemical composition, and descriptions of available products, which are kept general owing to the myriad of ever-changing products on the market. Product quality is also discussed in this section. For those supplements that are endogenous to humans, the physiologic role is then described. The pharmacologic effects of the products, divided into in vitro/animal data and clinical studies, are reviewed. The in vitro/animal data included were chosen to provide an explanation for the product's clinical effects in humans and to show the rationale for clinical studies. It should be noted that because of the nature of dietary supplement claims (*see* Part I, Legal/Regulatory Aspects), some promoted product uses might not have been studied in humans; conversely, known pharmacologic and therapeutic effects might not be promoted commercially. As a result, in most chapters there is a mismatch between the information in the Current Promoted Uses and Clinical Studies sections.

The Pharmacokinetics section covers absorption, tissue distribution, elimination, and body fluid concentrations. Such pharmacokinetic information is not usually included in other sources and may be useful in forensic investigations, or in the clinical setting when the product is used in patients with renal or hepatic insufficiency. A section on Adverse Effects and Toxicity follows, which includes detailed information on case reports of adverse reactions to the supplement. The Interactions section discusses interactions between the supplement and drugs or foods, as well as the effects of drugs on endogenous levels of the supplement if it is an endogenous compound. The Reproduction section is generally limited, owing to lack of information. Methods of Chemical and Biofluid Analysis are included for forensic professionals and for those investigating the product in clinical studies. Each monograph ends with a discussion of Regulatory Status of the product. The amount of information included in each of these sections varies according to availability.

At the end of each monograph is a summary presenting key information in bulleted form. A table at the end of the book summarizes supplement toxicities and adverse effects, drug interactions, and use in special populations (e.g., pregnancy and lactation, renal and hepatic impairment). The source of this information (animal data, in vitro effects, clinical trials, case reports, and theoretical concerns) are given. This section is intended for quick reference, and readers should refer to the chapter for more detailed discussion.

Adverse reactions to dietary supplements appear to be uncommon compared with those attributed to prescription drugs. This may be a function of health care and forensic professionals' unfamiliarity with a product's pharmacology and toxicology or assumption that a product is "natural" and therefore safe. Thus, an adverse reaction may go unrecognized or be attributed to a prescription medication. It is hoped that the information in *Dietary Supplements: Toxicology and Clinical Pharmacology* will be used to solve clinical or forensic problems involving dietary supplements, to promote dialog between health care professionals and patients, and to stimulate intellectual curiosity about these products, fostering further research on their therapeutic and adverse effects.

Melanie Johns Cupp

Contents

CONTENTS OF THE COMPANION VOLUME

Toxicology and Clinical Pharmacology of Herbal Products

PART I
Legal/Regulatory Aspects of Dietary Supplements

Chapter 1

Legal/Regulatory Aspects of Dietary Supplements

Melanie Johns Cupp

A discussion of the regulation of dietary supplements is best appreciated in the context of the regulation of drugs. A drug is defined, at least from a legal standpoint, as an article intended for the diagnosis, cure, mitigation, treatment, or prevention of a disease. Notice that a drug is defined based on its *intended (labeled) use*, not on whether it is of synthetic or natural origin. For example, the drugs digoxin, penicillin, and morphine all come from natural sources, but are regulated as drugs because they are labeled for the treatment of diseases. Another important point is that even if the consumer uses a product to treat a disease, the product is not a drug unless labeled for such use by the manufacturer. For example, if a consumer purchases an industrial lubricant at a hardware store and applies it topically to treat arthritis, the consumer's use of the product does not make it a drug (Abood & Brushwood, 1997).

Under the Dietary Supplement Health and Education Act of 1994 (DSHEA), dietary supplements are defined as vitamins, minerals, herbs, botanicals, amino acids, or dietary substances for use by man to supplement the diet by increasing the total dietary intake. Concentrates, metabolites, constituents, extracts, or combinations of the former are also considered dietary supplements (Abood & Brushwood, 1997). Only products for ingestion can be marketed as dietary supplements (FDA, 1995). Products labeled for use by other routes (buccal, parenteral, topical, transdermal, sublingual) cannot be marketed as dietary supplements. Note that if a dietary supplement is labeled for the treatment or prevention of disease, it becomes a drug, and must be proven safe and effective prior to marketing. The Food, Drug, and Cosmetic Act (FDCA) requires that a drug be proven safe and effective for its labeled use prior to marketing. Dietary supplements are not drugs, and therefore are not subject to the usual FDA drug approval process (Abood & Brushwood, 1997); however, manufacturers are responsible for the safety of their products. Although dietary supplements that were marketed prior to October 15, 1994 are permitted to stay on the market, any new dietary supplement is allowed to enter the market only after a 75-d period during which the FDA has the

From: *Forensic Science: Dietary Supplements: Toxicology and Clinical Pharmacology*
Edited by: M. J. Cupp and T. S. Tracy © Humana Press Inc., Totowa, New Jersey

opportunity to review the manufacturer's data supporting safety of the supplement (USP, 2001d).

A precursor to the DSHEA was the Nutrition Labeling and Education Act (NLEA) of 1990, which amended the FDCA and prohibited health claims for foods or dietary supplements unless a petition containing evidence supporting the claim was submitted. DSHEA was passed in response to industry and consumer concern that the NLEA would allow the FDA to remove many supplements from the market (Abood & Brushwood, 1997). Congress reportedly received more mail in 1993 protesting the FDA's restriction of supplement availability than any other issue since the Vietnam War. Obviously, the U.S. public is very interested in self-medication with these products (Vance, 1997).

The DSHEA can be regarded as a compromise between patient autonomy and paternalistic oversight by the FDA. DSHEA also frees supplement manufacturers and distributors from the financial burden of proving their products are safe and effective. Because the cost of drug development may be more than $200 million per drug and usually takes more than 10 yr, pharmaceutical manufacturers are unlikely to make the financial commitment necessary to amass safety and efficacy data for a supplement for which patent protection does not apply (Vance, 1997). Thus, the DSHEA allows consumers access to supplements, but without the consumer protection provided by the FDA drug approval process. It has been suggested that the dollar value provided by the pharmaceutical manufacturers regarding the expense of developing a new drug are inflated, and that one or two properly designed clinical trials involving large numbers of patients could be quickly and inexpensively performed and would answer safety and efficacy questions about supplements (Marwick, 1995). The Nutraceutical Research & Education Act (NREA) (HR 3001), introduced in October 1999 by Representative Frank Pallone (D-NJ) would provide 10 yr of health claim exclusivity to supplement manufacturers who justify the health claim by conducting an FDA-approved study. Such an act would foster research by the supplement industry and help ensure products' safety and efficacy (F-D-C reports, 2000f).

DSHEA requires that dietary supplement labels be truthful and not misleading (USP, 2001d). Despite that dietary supplements are not held to the same safety and efficacy standards as drugs, the DSHEA currently allows supplement labeling to carry claims about the product's ability to affect the structure or function of the human body or to promote general well-being (Kurtzweil, 1999). For example, a glucosamine product can claim to promote joint flexibility and support comfortable joint function, but it cannot claim to treat or prevent osteoarthritis, which would qualify as a disease claim. Implied disease claims, such as, "Prevents bone fragility in postmenopausal women," are not allowed. Implied disease claims made through the name of the product (e.g., "CancerCure") or through pictures, vignettes, or symbols (e.g., EKG tracings) are also not allowed. Health maintenance claims such as, "Maintains a healthy circulatory system" and claims regarding common, minor symptoms associated with life stages are also allowed. This would include claims that the product is useful for PMS symptoms or hot flashes (Anonymous, 2000a). For consumers, structure/function claims might be difficult to distinguish from disease treatment/prevention claims. For example, would most consumers understand that "Supports cardiovascular health" is not synonymous with "Prevents coronary artery disease?" Study in this area is ongoing.

This concept of the structure/function claim is particularly controversial in regard to pregnancy. Under DSHEA, minor pregnancy-related problems such as morning sickness and leg swelling are considered common conditions associated with a life stage, not with diseases. Because supplements are not required to undergo fetal toxicity studies, the consumer watchdog Public Citizen Health Research Group opposes the labeling of supplements for use to treat pregnancy-related conditions. For example, vitamin A, a common ingredient in dietary supplements, is known to be teratogenic in high doses (F-D-C reports, 2000c). Regardless of the risks to the fetus, this group, as well as the Teratology Society, opposes labeling for pregnancy-related conditions because pregnancy-related problems could be symptoms of a serious disorder that requires medical attention. For example, leg swelling could be a symptom of pre-eclampsia (F-D-C reports, 2000c, 2000d). Public Citizen also argues that if a condition is uncomfortable enough for a pregnant woman to seek treatment, the condition is serious enough to be considered a disease. Another opponent of supplement labeling for pregnancy-related conditions is Philip Landrigan, MD, chairman of the Mount Sinai Medical Center Department of Community Medicine, who is concerned that products labeled for the treatment of pregnancy-related conditions are potentially harmful to both the pregnant woman and her fetus (F-D-C reports, 2000c). The March of Dimes also points out that changes that occur during pregnancy can represent normal physiologic adaptations or a disease process, and that medical evaluation is necessary to distinguish the two (F-D-C reports, 2000d).

The March of Dimes proposes that all dietary supplements bear the following statement: "Women of childbearing age should consult with a physician before taking this product because dietary supplements are exempt from many aspects of Food and Drug Administration oversight." Products shown to prevent vitamin or mineral deficiency states during pregnancy would be exempt from carrying this warning. The American Academy of Pediatrics also favors a warning for all supplements. Both the Public Citizen Health Research Group and epidemiologist Juliette Kendrick, MD, of the Centers for Disease Control and Prevention (CDC) feel that although a warning label is needed, instruction to consult a health care professional before using the product may not be enough to protect the public health. For example, the physician or "health care professional" might not be aware of the risks of the dietary supplement in pregnancy, or might not be qualified (i.e., acupuncturist, herbalist, massage therapist) to give such advice. Because of these potential problems, Public Citizen Health Research Group Director Sidney Wolfe, MD, recommends that all supplements carry the statement "Do not use if you are pregnant" (F-D-C reports, 2000d). The trade associations Council for Responsible Nutrition (CRN), Consumer Healthcare Products Association (CHPA), and the American Herbal Products Association (AHPA) oppose such broad warnings. CRN proposes that the FDA provide a guidance document outlining data the FDA would consider necessary to support a claim for a pregnancy related symptom. CHPA has called on its members to include, "If pregnant or nursing, ask a health professional" or equivalent statement on all dietary supplements. Vitamin and mineral supplements in doses recognized by authoritative bodies to be safe and important for use during pregnancy would be exempt (F-D-C reports, 2000b), as would products marketed for use by postmenopausal women, men, or children (F-D-C reports, 2000g). Some CHPA members already use a similar label statement. AHPA feels blanket disclaimers such as the one proposed by CHPA are inappropriate in light of the availability of pregnancy-related information for some supplements. AHPA is also concerned that the presence of a disclaimer for all supplements would minimize the importance of the statement on those supplements that are known to be harmful. In lieu of a general statement for all supplements, AHPA advocates use of a warning on those supplements that are unsafe for pregnant or nursing women. AHPA currently requires its members to include pregnancy warnings on approximately 200 of the 644 products in its *Botanical Safety Handbook* (F-D-C reports, 2000b). Until such concerns can be addressed, the FDA is asking dietary supplement manufacturers not to make any pregnancy-related claims on their products, and is urging pregnant women to consult their physicians before using any dietary supplement (Anonymous, 2000b). According to the CRN, manufacturers are not currently planning on making label statements about morning sickness or pregnancy-associated edema (F-D-C reports, 2000b).

In addition to pregnancy, other natural states or processes recognized by the FDA include menopause, aging, menses, and adolescence. Accordingly, dietary supplements may be labeled for use for conditions associated with these life stages, including hot flashes, common symptoms associated with the menstrual cycle, mild memory problems or hair loss associated with aging, and nonycstic acne. No prior FDA approval is needed in order for a supplement manufacturer to make these or other structure/function claims; however, the manufacturer must notify the FDA of the statement being made no later than 30 d after first marketing the supplement. Another type of claim that manufacturers can make is one that relates the benefits of the product to a nutrient deficiency disease (e.g., scurvy), provided that the manufacturer also discloses the prevalence of the deficiency in the United States (FDA, 2000).

A type of supplement claim that requires pre-marketing FDA notification is a health claim. A health claim characterizes the relationship of a nutrient in a dietary supplement to a disease. For example, a claim regarding the association between adequate calcium intake and osteoporosis prevention would be a health claim. (For comparison, a claim that "calcium builds strong bones" is a structure/function claim). To make a health claim, the manufacturer must demonstrate that the use of the supplement at levels necessary to justify the claim is safe, and that there is "significant scientific agreement" among experts that the claim is justified based on the available scientific evidence. Unless the FDA issues a regulation modifying or prohibiting the claim, or a federal district court finds that statutory requirements have not been met, the claim may be used 120 d after submission (FDA, 2000).

The significant scientific agreement (SSA) standard is used by the FDA to determine if a health claim is justified. However, a federal appeals court ruled in January 1999 (*Pearson v Shalala*) that this standard must be more clearly defined. They also concluded that the FDA's decision to deny four specific dietary supplement health claims was a violation of the First Amendment (F-D-C reports, 1999a). These four health claims related dietary fiber and antioxidant vitamins to cancer prevention, omega-3 fatty acids to prevention of heart disease, and folic acid to prevention of neural tube defects. The FDA had rejected these claims because research has shown a relationship only between consumption of foods containing these dietary components and disease-risk reduction, rather than consumption of the dietary supplement itself. The Court suggested that such uncertainty concerning the supplements efficacy in disease-risk reduction could be communicated to consumers by use of a disclaimer explaining that risk reduction has been shown only with dietary consumption of the substance. In October 2000, the FDA announced that it would permit the use of a health claim if the scientific evidence supporting the claim outweighs the evidence against the claim, the claim is appropriately qualified, all statements in the claim are consistent with the scientific evidence, and consumer health and safety are not threatened. Of the four claims at issue in *Pearson v Shalala*, the FDA allowed only the claim for antioxidant vitamins. Although the FDA determined that the claims for folic acid and omega-3 fatty acids did not meet the SSA standard, the agency drafted examples of "qualified" claims for folic acid and omega-3 fatty acids that would be allowed on product labeling. Based on the available scientific evidence regarding dietary fiber and colon cancer risk, the FDA concluded that a "qualified" claim would not compensate for the lack of evidence meeting the SSA standard (Degnan, 2000). A group of supplement manufacturers later challenged the FDA's decision regarding folic acid. A federal judge granted the companies' request for a preliminary injunction preventing the FDA from taking action against the claim that "0.8 mg of folic acid in a dietary supplement is more effective in reducing the risk of neural tube defects than a lower amount in foods in common form." The judge ruled that the FDA's refusal to allow the claim violated the manufacturers' First Ammendment rights (Anonymous, 2001c). In response to a subsequent action (*Whitaker v Shalala*), the FDA has also allowed the claim that "as part of a well-balanced diet that is low in saturated fat and cholesterol, folic acid, vitamin B6, and vitamin B12 may reduce the risk of vascular disease." Immediately adjacent and directly beneath this claim, the disclaimer, "FDA evaluated the above claim and found that, although it is known that diets low in saturated fat and cholesterol reduce the risk of heart disease and other vascular diseases, the evidence in support of the above claim is inconclusive" must appear (Anonymous 2001a).

The FDA responded to the Court's charge to clarify the phrase "significant scientific agreement" by publishing draft guidance in December 1999 characterizing "significant scientific agreement" as lying somewhere between unanimous agreement and "emerging science." Bruce Chassy, PhD, a food science expert from the University of Illinois who has served on the FDA's Food Advisory Committee, suggested creation of a separate category of dietary supplement claims based on emerging science. He defined emerging science as "science that we do not know will endure, which has not met the highest standards." Chassy felt there may be hundreds or thousands of products that could be marketed pursuant to an "emerging science" standard. Chassy also suggested establishing a panel to review the available scientific data pertaining to product claims. Chassy's rationale for creation of the new category was that establishing such a category would be preferable to lowering the SSA standard. Industry trade group CRN favors establishing different categories of claims based on the quality of supporting evidence, with claims supported by SSA representing the highest level in their proposed hierarchy of claims (F-D-C reports, 2000a).

Creating different categories of products based on level of scientific evidence does not address safety issues, however. CRN, as well as an attorney who represented the *Pearson v Shalala* plaintiffs, have stated that safety should focus only on the ingredients themselves, and should not be taken into account when considering the appropriateness of a health claim. One exception would be a health claim that recommends doses in excess of those allowed by law. It has also been suggested that once a product is marketed, disclaimers could be added to products if adverse effects are discovered postmarketing, much in the same way that drug product prescribing information is altered if postmarketing experience reveals an adverse effect or drug interaction. Concerns expressed about such postmarketing safety-related labeling changes include: the amount of FDA resources needed to continuously review new information and recommend labeling changes, whether a labeling change regarding safety will actually change consumers' use of the product once it has been marketed, and whether consumers' will actually take note of new safety-related labeling information (F-D-C reports, 2000a).

Note that supplement health claims characterize the relationship of a nutrient in a dietary supplement to a disease, implying disease prevention. The CHPA would like to see the FDA allow health claims that relate supplement ingredients to treatment of disease as well. CHPA suggests that the FDA establish criteria by which a supplement claim could meet the definition of a "disease treatment-related health claim." An example would be the use of a calcium supplement to support healing of a bone fracture. CHPA supports establishing different supplement categories based on safety and efficacy data. For example, although use of calcium to help heal fractures might be considered almost unquestionable in regard to safety and efficacy, the use of red yeast rice extract as an adjunct to the treatment of hyperlipidemia or the use of St. John's wort to treat depression pose risks that might outweigh the benefit for certain users. The American Urological Association Health Policy Council Chair Logan Holtgrewe, MD, takes exception to the idea of disease claims for dietary supplements because use of such products to self-medicate could delay treatment. For example, bladder and prostate symptoms always arise from disease, and may even be symptoms of cancer. Holtgrewe favors FDA control of any product marketed for the treatment of disease (F-D-C reports, 2000e).

Even if the FDA allows a claim, regardless of whether it is a health claim or a structure/function claim, herbal product labels must bear the following disclaimer: "This statement has not been evaluated by the Food and Drug Administration. This product is not intended to diagnose, treat, cure, or prevent any disease." It has been argued that the use of this disclaimer may serve as a source of confusion for consumers, rather than helping them make a decision regarding use of the product (F-D-C reports, 1999b). In the future, more federal court rulings may lead to changes in the type of information seen on herbal labels.

One recent labeling change was the result of a rule that went into effect on March 23, 1999. The FDA now requires an information panel titled "Supplement Facts" to appear on the label of dietary supplements. It is similar to the "Nutrition Facts" panel required on foods and includes the common or usual name of the herb, or in certain cases the herb's botanical name; the part of the plant used to make the product (e.g., root, stem, leaf); manufacturer's suggested serving size; and amount per serving. If the product contains nutrients (e.g., iron, calcium, vitamins), these must appear on the panel just as they would on a "Nutrition Facts" label on a food, with the percent of the recommended daily value listed. For "proprietary blends," the total weight of the blend must be listed, but the weights of the individual ingredients do not have to be listed; however, each component of the blend must be listed in order of predominance by weight. Products labeled prior to March 23, 1999 may remain on shelves until stocks are depleted (Anonymous, 1999a).

The "Supplement Facts" box is perceived by at least one industry insider as detrimental because it allows consumers to compare products based on quantity of ingredients without regard to potential quality differences among supplements sold by different manufacturers. This makes setting high prices for brand-name supplements difficult; consumers might not be willing to pay a higher price for a brand-name product if a less expensive product contains the same ingredients. Manufacturers such as Warner-Lambert and Whitehall Robins, which have traditionally produced prescription and over-the-counter pharmaceuticals, have begun producing dietary supplements. Although these manufacturers stress in their advertising the quality and science behind their relatively high-priced products, consumers have not bought their message that their products are worth the higher price, and the "Supplement Facts" panel is being blamed (F-D-C reports, 2000f).

The FDA has not yet extensively addressed product quality; however, the United States Pharmacopeial Convention has long been interested in the purity and potency of dietary supplements. The United States Pharmacopeia (USP) was first published in 1820, and has always included standards for botanicals; however, with the advent of modern medicinal chemistry, many of these were replaced by monographs for synthetic drugs. With the passage of the DSHEA, setting standards for botanicals has become important once again (USP, 1999). In fact, DSHEA recognizes the USP as the official reference standard for dietary supplements (USP, 2001a).

Herbs are complex because they are not uniform by nature and contain many different chemicals that can vary depending on soil, climate, season, cultivar, and part of the plant used. Confusing the issue is that for many herbs, the specific active ingredient is unknown, and the effects of an herb might manifest via a combined effect of several different ingredients. In the absence of better data, "marker compounds" are designated that are used to standardize the product. Marker compounds are chemicals most likely to be responsible for therapeutic effect. USP has played an important role in designating marker compounds for various herbs (USP, 1999).

The USP publishes both "USP" and "NF" monographs. The USP and NF are designated as *the* official compendia by the Food, Drug, and Cosmetic Act as well as by state pharmacy practice acts (Valentino, 1983). The difference between a USP (United States Pharamopeia) and an NF (National Formulary) monograph is that USP monographs include only items with FDA-approved or USP-accepted uses; otherwise, the item is included in the NF. The USP and NF are now published in the same book. The current USP edition is the 26th, and the current NF edition is the 21st, so the book is referred to as the "USP26–NF21." The USP26-NF21 contains more than 10 botanical monographs, including ones for feverfew, ginger, ginkgo, ginseng, St. John's wort, saw palmetto, chamomile, cranberry, garlic, licorice, and valerian. These monographs include specifications for identity, purity, packaging, and labeling. In developing the botanical monographs, US and international information is evaluated, including chemical information, historical literature, expert opinion, anecdotal writings, case reports, and clinical trials. The resulting monographs must be supported by good science, so the level of evidence is considered. The USP Committee of Revision and its advisory panels make the final decision on the information included in each monograph (USP, 1999). Although currently no monographs for nonbotanical dietary supplements are included in the USP–NF, recently recognized problems with glucosamine/chondroitin product quality suggests that monographs for such products are needed (American

Nutraceutical Association, 2000). Currently, the USP–NF contains more than 900 standards for nutritional products and dietary supplements (USP, 2001b).

The USP Dietary Supplement Verification Program began in 2002. If a product meets USP's standards for product potency and purity, and the manufacturer follows good manufacturing practices for dietary supplements, the USP will allow the manufacturer to use a special verification mark on the product label certifying that the product meets USP standards (USP, 2001a). The verification program does not address product efficacy or safety; however, products with known safety problems will not be eligible for the program (USP, 2001d). Once a product receives the verification mark, USP will periodically test verified supplements to ensure continued quality. The program is voluntary, and the onus is on the manufacturers to contact USP regarding program participation (USP, 2001c).

When reading an herbal product label, one must be aware that the use of the word "standardized" does not mean that the product meets USP–NF standards. "Standardized" simply means that the manufacturer is claiming that a certain concentration of one or more ingredients is consistent among batches. However, use of "NF" on the label means that the product meets the NF standard for purity, strength of marker compound, and labeling. It does *not* mean that the product meets a safety or efficacy standard (Anonymous, 1999b).

Another function provided by the USP is the Drug Product Problem Reporting Program (DPPR), which records health care providers' observations of poor product quality, unclear labeling, defective packaging, therapeutic ineffectiveness, suspected counterfeiting, and product tampering to manufacturers, labelers, the FDA and the USP Committee of Revisions. Problems with dietary supplements can be reported to this free service by calling 1-800-638-6725. More than 50 reports regarding herbal products, including efficacy concerns and serious adverse effects, have been reported to the DPPR (USP, 1999). Health care professionals may also contact the FDA's MedWatch program at 1-800-FDA-1088 with reports of serious adverse effects involving dietary supplements or drugs.

The Institute of Medicine, part of the National Academy of Sciences, recently developed a guideline for the FDA for the evaluation of supplement safety. Glucosamine, chromium picolinate, melatonin, and shark cartilage will be among the first products reviewed (Anonymous, 2002).

Regulation of supplements varies among countries around the globe. For example, in the United Kingdom, any substance not granted a license as a medicinal product by the Medicines Control Agency is treated as a food, and by law cannot carry a health claim or medical advice on the label, although many do (Marwick, 1995). Similarly, botanicals are sold as dietary supplements in the Netherlands. In Germany, herbal monographs called the German Commission E monographs are prepared by an interdisciplinary committee using historical information; chemical data; experimental, pharmacological, clinical, and toxicological studies; epidemiological data; case reports; and unpublished manufacturers' data. If an herb has an approved monograph, it can be marketed. References are not published in the monographs. Unlike the USP–NF, potency and purity standards are not included. In other Western European countries, herbal products are treated as drugs, and are generally sold in pharmacies as licensed prescription and nonprescription drugs, with registrations based on quality, safety, and efficacy. The European Scientific Cooperative on Phytotherapy (ESCP) has produced 50 monographs since 1997. Like the German Commission E monographs, the ESCP monographs address therapeutics, and do not set product quality standards. Both German Commission E monographs and the ESCP monographs include information such as indications, dosage, side effects, contraindications, and recommended duration of use (Blumenthal, 1998). Note though, that regulation of non-herbal dietary supplements is not addressed by the German Commission E monographs or by the ESCP monographs.

The German monograph system is not without precedent in the United States. Non-prescription drugs that were on the market prior to 1962 (e.g., pseudoephedrine, acetaminophen, aspirin) are marketed despite not having endured the FDA approval process as it presently exists. Such products can be marketed if they meet the standards set forth in monographs developed by FDA advisory committees in the 1970s and 1980s. These monographs delineate which ingredients may be used in nonprescription products; which combinations of active ingredients may be used together; labeling requirements; and quality testing procedures. A general section applies to all nonprescription drugs, and sets forth acceptable inactive ingredients, manufacturing processes, drug registration, container specifications, and labeling requirements required of all nonprescription drugs (e.g., "Keep this and all drugs out of reach of children") (Gilbertson, 1986). Drugs that were judged safe and effective, and thus for which monographs are available, are called category I drugs. Drugs deemed unsafe or ineffective are called category II drugs, and category III drugs are those for which data is insufficient to make a determination. This system has been criticized because it relies on data supplied by manufacturers; thus, potentially safe and effective drugs may be placed in category III simply because no manufacturer felt it worthwhile financially to compile and submit the necessary data (Tyler, 1994). Clearly, there are drawbacks to such a monograph system.

As with older nonprescription drugs, perhaps dietary supplements will one day be marketed in the United States pursuant to monographs prepared by FDA advisory committees, and formulated to meet USP–NF standards. Properly designed clinical trials using adequate numbers of patients and sound statistical methods, funded by government or the private sector, would add to our knowledge base about these products. Until then, patients and health care professionals must use caution in the "wild west" world of dietary supplements.

1.1. SUMMARY

- The DSHEA of 1994 allows dietary supplements to carry claims concerning their ability to affect the structure or function of the human body, or claims about a nutrient's relationship to a disease (i.e., health claim).
- Dietary supplements cannot be promoted for the treatment or prevention of disease.
- Unlike drugs, dietary supplements do not have to be proven safe and effective for their labeled use prior to marketing.
- Supplement labels must include a "Supplement Facts" panel, similar to the "Nutrition Facts" label required on foods.
- The use of the word "standardized" on a supplement label means only that the manufacturer is claiming consistency from batch to batch, not that the product meets a statutory standard.
- Current areas of debate concerning supplements include labeling of supplements in regard to use in pregnancy and lactation, and creation of different categories of products based on quality of safety and efficacy data.

REFERENCES

Abood RR, Brushwood DB. Pharmacy practice and the law. Gaithersburg, MD: Aspen Publishers, Inc., 1997.

American Nutraceutical Association. Dietary supplements containing glucosamine and chondroitin sulfate found in University of Maryland College of Pharmacy study to contain significantly less ingredients when compared to label claims. Available from: http://www.ana.jana.org/press.html. Accessed 2000 July 24.

Anonymous. Dietary supplements now labeled with more information. HHS News. March 23, 1999. Available from URL:http://www.fda.gov/bbs/topics/NEWS/NEW00678.html. Accessed 1999a March 30.

Anonymous. [No title]. Pharmacist's letter 1999b;15(3):13.

Anonymous. FDA finalizes rules for claims on dietary supplements. FDA Talk Paper. Food and Drug Administration. U.S. Department of Health and Human Services. Public Health Service. Rockville, MD. Available from: URL: http://vm.cfsan.fda.gov/~lrd/tpdsclm.html. Accessed 2000a January 18.

Anonymous. FDA statement concerning structure/function rule and pregnancy claims. HHS Statement. U.S. Department of Health and Human Services. Available from: URL: http://www.fda.gov/bbs/topics/NEWS/NEWW00715.html. Accessed 2000b February 22.

Anonymous. FDA agrees to disclaimer on B6, B12 and folic acid. Natural Medicine Law Newsletter 2001a;4(5).

Anonymous. Pharmacy fax monitor. Totowa, NJ: Healthcare News Monitor, Inc. February 14, 2001b.

Anonymous. Pharmacy fax monitor. Totowa, NJ: Healthcare News Monitor Inc. July 24, 2002.

Blumenthal M. The complete German Commission E monographs. Therapeutic guide to herbal medicines. Austin, TX: American Botanical Council, 1998.

Degnan FH. FDA's recent steps to implement *Pearson v Shalala*. JANA 2000;3(3):3–5.

FDA. Dietary Supplement Health and Education Act of 1994. U.S. Food and Drug Administration. Center for Food Safety and Applied Nutition. December 1, 1995. Available from: http://www.cfsan.fda.gov/~dms/dietsupp.html. Accessed 2001 November 15.

F-D-C Reports. FDA clarification of health claims "scientific agreement" standard ordered. "The Tan Sheet" 1999a;7(4):3–4.

F-D-C reports. Health claims with disclaimers may convey "incompatible" message-attorney. "The Tan Sheet" 1999b;7(8):4–5.

F-D-C Reports. Emerging science-based supplement health claims category proposed. "The Tan Sheet" 2000a;8(15):3–4.

F-D-C Reports. "Evidence-based" pregnancy claim strategy raised by Levitt. "The Tan Sheet" 2000b; 8(14):4.

F-D-C reports. Morning sickness, edema of pregnancy are diseases-Public Citizen. "The Tan Sheet" 2000c;8(6):19.

F-D-C reports. Pregnancy does not fit within DSHEA Framework-March of Dimes. "The Tan Sheet" 2000d;8(14):5.

F-D-C reports. Supplement/disease claim continuum suggested by CHPA. "The Tan Sheet" 2000e;8(15):4–5.

F-D-C reports. "Supplement Facts" box, S-F claims final reg has hurt industry-Israelsen. "The Tan Sheet" 2000f;8(14):13–4.

F-D-C reports. Supplements pregnancy warning statement petition pending from CHPA. "The Tan Sheet" 2000g;8(13):3.

Food and Drug Administration (FDA). Department of Health and Human Services. Regulations on statements made for dietary supplements concerning the effect of the product on the structure or function of the body. Final rule. 21 CFR Part 101. Feb 7, 2000.

Gilbertson WE. The FDA's OTC drug review. Handbook of nonprescription drugs, 8th edition. Washington, DC: American Pharmaceutical Association; 1986. pp. 1–8.

Kurtzweil P. FDA Consumer: an FDA guide to dietary supplements. U.S. Food and Drug Administration Publication No. (FDA) 99-2323. Available from: URL:http://vm.cfsan.fda.gov/~dms/fdsupp.html. Accessed 1999 April 6.

Marwick C. Growing use of medicinal botanicals forces assessment by drug regulators. JAMA 1995;273:607–9.

Tyler VE. Herbs of choice. Binghamton, NY: Pharmaceutical Products Press, 1994.

USP. Botanicals: the dilemmas involved in developing standards for natural products. USP Quality Review 1999; April (65).

USP. USP Announces launch of dietary supplement verification program. News release. Rockville, MD: United States Pharmacopeial Convention. 2001a.

USP. USP dietary supplement verification program. Rockville, MD: United States Pharmacopeial Convention. 2001b.

USP. USP dietary supplement verification program frequently asked questions. Rockville, MD: United States Pharmacopeial Convention. 2001c.

USP. USP dietary supplement verification program regulatory issues. Rockville, MD: United States Pharmacopeial Convention. 2001d.

Valentino JG. USP—the cornerstone of pharmacy practice. Presentation to the National Council of State Pharamceutical Association Executives. New Orleans, LA. April 1983.

Vance DA. An ancient heritage beckons pharmacists. Int J Pharmaceutical Compounding 1997;1(1):22–4.

PART II
MONOGRAPHS

Chapter 1

Androstenedione and Other Over-the-Counter Steroids

Jason L. Duncan, Melanie Johns Cupp, and Timothy S. Tracy

1.1. HISTORY

Androstenedione first appeared in early 1997 in body-building magazines, where it was advertised as a natural anabolic agent. It has become an attractive, legal alternative to anabolic steroids for professional and recreational athletes, particularly those engaged in "power" sports who wish to increase muscle mass and endurance (Anonymous, 1998; Anonymous, 1998, Uralets and Gillette, 1999).

The focus of this chapter is androstenedione. Dehydroepiandrosterone (DHEA) is covered in a subsequent chapter. Other over-the-counter steroids available in the United States are mentioned in this chapter, but only in passing owing to a paucity of information.

1.2. CHEMICAL STRUCTURE

See Fig. 1-1 for chemical structures of androstenedione and the structural analogs 19-norandrosterone, 19-norandrostenedione, 19-norandrostenediol, 5-androstenediol, and 4-androstenediol.

1.3. CURRENT PROMOTED USES

Androstenedione is marketed as a nonprescription "prohormone" that will "boost testosterone," enhancing muscle strength and mass (Ballantyne et al., 2000). Advertisements often cite the German patent application for androstendione as proof of androstendione's efficacy, although this document presents no evaluable data (Brown et al., 2000b). Androstenedione is also promoted as an alternative to sildenafil (Viagra®) (Kachhi and Henderson, 2000).

From: *Forensic Science: Dietary Supplements: Toxicology and Clinical Pharmacology*
Edited by: M. J. Cupp and T. S. Tracy © Humana Press Inc., Totowa, New Jersey

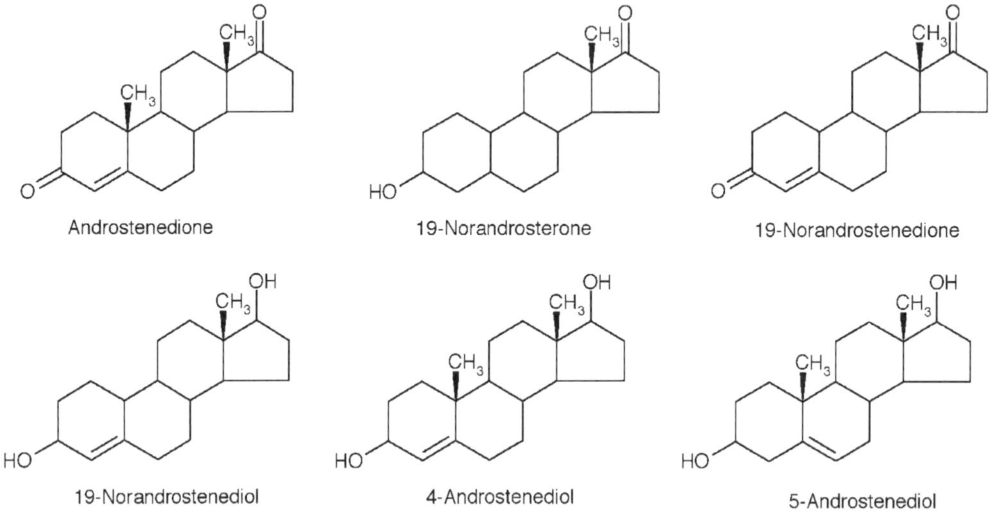

Fig. 1. Chemical structure of (top row) androstenedione, 19-norandrosterone, and 19-norandrostenedione, as well as (bottom row) 10-norandrostendiaol, 4-androstenediol, and 5-androstenediol

1.4. SOURCES AND CHEMICAL COMPOSITION

Androstenedione's chemical name is 4-androsten-3,17-dione (Uralets and Gillette, 1999). Endogenous androstenedione is synthesized in the adrenal gland, primarily from DHEA, and to a lesser extent from 17-hydroxyprogesterone (Goldifien, 1998a). The testes and ovaries also produce androstenedione from 17-hydroxyprogesterone and DHEA (Ballantyne et al., 2000). Androstenedione is produced chiefly by the adrenals (Goldifien, 1998b), although in adult males, the testes and adrenals contribute almost equally to the production of androstenedione (Vermeulen, 1976). Additional androstenedione is formed in peripheral tissues from DHEA and dehydroepiandrosterone sulfate (DHEA-S) (Longcope, 1996). Androstenedione marketed as a dietary supplement is of synthetic origin (Ballantyne et al., 2000) and is derived from diosgenin, a chemical in wild yams (King et al., 1999; Brown et al., 2000b; Catlin et al., 2000).

1.5. PRODUCTS AVAILABLE

Androstenedione is available in tablet, capsule, sublingual tablet, and nasal spray forms. A commonly promoted combination product is Andro-6® (Experimental and Applied Sciences, Golden, CO), which contains androstenedine 100 mg, DHEA 50 mg, indole-3-carbinol 100 mg, saw palmetto 180 mg, chrysin 208 mg, and *Tribulus terrestris* 250 mg per capsule. The additional ingredients are included in the product because they are thought to either increase testosterone levels or promote conversion of androstenedione to testosterone rather than to other steroids. For example, DHEA (discussed in detail in a subsequent chapter) may increase testosterone in women, although it has not been shown to increase testosterone concentrations in men. Indole-3-carbinol, from cruciferous vegetables, enhances elimination of estrogens by enhancing their oxidative metabolism and excretion. Chrysin, a flavonoid from *Passiflora caerulea*, inhibits aromatization of estrogen precursors in vitro. Saw palmetto inhibits 5α-reductase, thus theoretically promoting conversion of ingested androstenedione and DHEA to testosterone while minimizing their conversion to estrogens and dihydrotestosterone. *Tribulus terrestris* is purported to increase testosterone concentrations by increasing serum luteinizing hormone (LH), but evidence is lacking. Andro-6 has been assayed for purity and content (Brown et al., 2000b). Andro-6 was discontinued by the manufacturer, but was still available through some Internet sites as of fall 2002.

Other examples of androstendione products advertised on the Internet include Andro 250 (androstenedione 250 mg per capsule), GEN ANDRO*GEN (androstenedione 50 mg and 100 mg capsules), and Androplex 700 (androstenedione 50 mg, *Tribulus terrestris* 250 mg, and DHEA 50 mg per capsule).

The potency and purity of androstenedione products vary among brands. Beginning in 1997, the UCLA Olympic Analytical Laboratory noted an increase in athletes testing positive for 19-norandrosterone, the major metabolite of the anabolic steroid nandrolone. This was a surprising finding: nandrolone fell out of favor with athletes in the 1980s because its metabolite is detectable in the urine for weeks. Although 19-norandrosterone of endogenous origin may be detectable in the urine, International Olympic Committee cutoffs were changed to reflect this in 1998. Because of reports that use of androstenedione could cause positive urine drug screens for 19-norandrosterone, the Olympic Analytical Laboratory tested the potency and purity of androstenedione 100 mg capsules (six brands), 50 mg capsules (two brands), and 250 mg capsules (one brand) purchased from stores. The investigators discovered that one brand contained no androstenedione or other steroids, although its labeled content was androstenedione 50 mg per capsule. The other product labeled as containing androstenedione 50 mg per capsule contained a mean of only 35 mg per capsule. Of the six brands purporting to contain androstenedione 100 mg per capsule, the mean amount of androstenedione per capsule ranged from 85 to 103 mg; three products were within ±10% of the labeled amount, and three contained less than 90% of the labeled amount. Most alarming was a product purporting to contain androstenedione 250 mg per capsule that was found to contain 168 mg of androstenedione and 10 mg of testosterone. One brand (Sports One® Klein Laboratories, Wallingford, CT) was found to contain, on average, 7.6 µg of norandrostenedione per capsule. 19-Norandrosterone was found in the urine samples of all 24 subjects administered this product but was not found in urine samples collected before product administration. The source of 19-norandrosterone was thought to be metabolism of 19-norandrostenedione. It is important to note that this product, although contaminated with 19-norandrostenedione, was very pure based on Food and Drug Administration (FDA) and U.S. Pharmacopeia (USP) standards for pharmaceuticals. Nevertheless, ingestion of this product would cause the user to test positive for nandrolone (Catlin et al., 2000).

An independent laboratory (Integrated Biomolecule, Tuscon, AZ) verified that androstenedione marketed by Experimental and Applied Sciences (Golden, CO) was approximately 99% pure via high-performance liquid chromatography (HPLC) (Brown et al., 2000a). In another study, HPLC analysis of 13 androstenedione 100 mg capsules (Sports One®, Klein Laboratories, Wallingford, CT) revealed an androstenedione content ranging from 83.9 to 113.9 mg (mean 99.8 mg; Leder et al., 2000).

Androstenediol and norandrostenedione are commonly available in capsule form. Examples of such products include Androdiol 100 mg capsules and Norandro 50 mg capsules (Uralets and Gillette, 1999). Other steroid products advertised on the Internet include 4Diol 250® (4-androstenediol 250 mg per capsule), Androdiol Select 300 (4-androstenediol 300 mg per capsule), 5Diol 250 (5-androstenediol 250 mg per capsule), GEN Androdiol™ (4-androstenediol 100 mg), Androsol Sports Skin Tonic™ (4-androstenediol 50 mg per 7 sprays), Andro Spray (4-androstenediol 400 mg per 10 sprays to the skin), Norandro Spray (19-norandrostenediol 200 mg per 10 sprays to the skin), Norandrodiol Select 300 (19-norandrostenediol 150 mg per capsule), and 3-Andro Xtreme (4-androstenediol 100 mg, 5-androstenediol 100 mg, 19-norandrostenedione 100 mg, caffeine 200 mg, ephedra extract 400 mg, L-phenylalanine 100 mg, and L-tyrosine 100 mg per capsule). Androsat-6 Popper is a buccal tablet containing 4-androstenediol 125 mg, 5-androstenediol 5 mg, 4-androstenedione 5 mg, 5-androstenedione 5 mg, 19-norandrostenedione 5 mg, and 19-norandrostenediol 5 mg.

1.6. PHYSIOLOGIC ROLE

Androstenedione itself is only a weak androgen (Mahesh and Greenblatt, 1962). In the testes, ovaries, and adrenal glands, androstenedione is converted to testosterone via the action of 17-β-hydroxysteroid dehydrogenase. Androstenedione can also be converted to estrone and then to estradiol via aromatization (King et al., 1999; Ballantyne et al., 2000). Some androstenedione is present in the bloodstream. This circulating androstenedione can be converted to testosterone and estrogens peripherally (Labrie et al., 1998; King et al., 1999). The rationale behind androstenedione supplementation is that peripheral conversion of androstenedione to testosterone will result in enhanced muscle size and strength (Ballantyne et al., 2000). Studies have been undertaken to determine whether significant amounts of testosterone can be produced from exogenously administered androstenedione.

1.7. CLINICAL STUDIES

A study conducted by King and colleagues (1999) involved 30 healthy, normotestosterogenic men between the ages of 19 and 29. The study subjects were not taking any nutritional supplements and had not engaged in a resistance training program within the past year. Twenty of these subjects performed 8 wks of whole-body resistance training and were randomized to either androstenedione 100 mg or placebo (rice flour) taken three times daily during weeks 1, 2, 4, 5, 7, and 8. This method of supplementation was recommended by the manufacturer and was meant to mimic the cyclic fashion in which athletes use anabolic steroids. A dose of 300 mg was chosen because it exceeded the dose commonly recommended by manufacturers. The androstenedione product used was derived from wild yams and was provided by Experimental and Applied Sciences in capsule form.

The main outcome measures were change in serum testosterone and estrogen concentrations, muscle strength, muscle fiber cross-sectional area, body composition, blood lipids, and liver transaminase activity. Statistical analysis was performed using two-way ANOVA with the Bonferroni correction for multiple comparisons. Serum-free and total testosterone concentrations were not affected by short- or long-term androstenedione administration. Serum estradiol concentrations were higher in the androstenedione group at wks 2, 5, and 8 compared with baseline ($p < 0.05$) and were higher than the placebo group at weeks 2 and 5 ($p < 0.05$). The serum estrone concentration was also higher in the androstenedione group at weeks 2 and 5 compared with baseline ($p < 0.05$). Serum high-density lipoprotein (HDL) was decreased by 12% compared with baseline at wks 2, 5, and 8 ($p < 0.05$) in the androstenedione group. Liver transaminases (γ-glutamyltransferase, aspartate aminotransferase, and alanine aminotransferase) were unaffected. Effects of androstenedione and placebo on resistance training, muscle strength, muscle histochemistry, and body composition were similar.

Ten additional subjects (mean age 23 yrs) were randomized to receive either a single dose of androstenedione 100 mg or placebo in a double-blind fashion. The additional study was conducted to measure the effect of androstenedione on hormone levels. The dose was based on a previous study (Mahesh and Greenblatt, 1962) showing that androstenedione 100 mg increased blood testosterone levels four- to sevenfold in women. After a 1-wk washout, subjects were crossed over to the other treatment. Blood samples for measurement of serum androstendione, free and total testosterone, LH, and follicle-stimulating hormone (FSH) were taken before and every 30 minutes after ingestion for 6 hours. Statisical analysis was performed in a manner analogous to the resistance training portion of the study. Serum androstenedione concentration increased 175% during the first 60 minutes after ingestion and was 325–350% of baseline between 90 and 270 min after ingestion. Between 270 and 360 min after ingestion, androstenedione levels decreased, but remained above baseline. Other hormones were not affected.

Forty male subjects, aged 40–60 yrs (mean age 48.1 yrs) with weight training experience were randomized to receive androstenedione 50 mg twice daily, DHEA 50 mg twice daily, or placebo for 3 months. At baseline and at weeks 6 and 12, body composition, hormone profile, prostate-specific antigen (PSA), glucose, insulin, lipids, alanine aminotransferase (ALT), well-being, libido, strength, and aerobic capacity were measured. Patients were instructed to maintain their normal diet. Two-way ANOVA was used to analyze the data, along with the Scheffe test for identification of specific pairwise differences. Baseline vs postsupplementation data were analyzed using *t*-tests. Pearson product moment correlation was performed to identify significant correlations between variables. Statistical significance was accepted at the $p < 0.05$ level. Androstenedione had no effect on any variable studied (Wallace et al., 1999).

In a Canadian study (Ballantyne et al., 2000) designed to examine the effect of androstenedione on hormone levels and resistance training, 10 males (mean age 24 yr) with a history of resistance training but no history of anabolic steroid use were given androstenedione 100 mg (Sports One, Klein Laboratories) twice daily for 2 d. In the week prior to beginning androstenedione supplementation, blood samples for determination of baseline concentrations of total and free testosterone, LH, estradiol, and androstenedione were taken every 3 h for 12 h. An additional blood sample was drawn at 8:30 AM the following day. The next week, androstenedione was administered. On day 2 of androstenedione supplementation, blood samples were taken as at baseline. An additional blood sample was taken 24 h after ingestion of the last capsule. At least 2 wk later, subjects performed resistance training after being randomly assigned to placebo, 2 capsules twice daily for 2 d, or androstenedione 100 mg twice daily for 2 d. There was a 2-wk washout between treatments, and both the study subjects and the investigators were blinded to the treatment. The capsules were ingested at 9 AM and 3 PM, and the training sessions took place between 4 PM and 5:30 PM. Blood samples for measurement of hormone concentrations and hematocrit were taken before and after exercise.

Two-way ANOVA with the Tukey *post hoc* test was used to analyze the data, with statistical significance set at $p = 0.05$. Plasma androstenedione levels increased two- to three-fold with androstenedione supplementation. Levels were significantly higher than after placebo supplementation 3, 6, 9, and 12 h after the third dose ($p < 0.05$). LH levels were approximately 70% higher with androstenedione supplementation. This difference was statistically significant just prior to the third dose, 3 h after the third dose, and 3 and 12 h after the fourth dose. Testosterone levels were not affected to a statistically significant extent, but they increased slightly in the morning with androstenedione supplementation and decreased in the afternoon such that levels were lower than with placebo. Estradiol levels were higher than with placebo at all time points, but this difference was not significantly significant. With exercise, estradiol increased significantly compared with placebo ($p < 0.05$). These results are similar to those of King and colleagues (1999) in that androstenedione administration did not increase testosterone levels.

A study conducted by Rasmussen and associates (2000) was designed to determine whether 5 d of oral androstenedione (Ultimate Nutrition, Farmington, CT; 50 mg/capsule; minimum purity, 99.5%) 100 mg/d had an anabolic effect in young, healthy, eugonadal men. Six subjects participated. Hormone levels and effects on muscle protein kinetics were measured before and after treatment. Anabolic effect was measured using a three-compartment model involving infusion of L-phenylalanine, blood sampling from the femoral artery and vein, and muscle biopsies. Plasma hormone levels were determined by radioimmunoassay (RIA). Plasma testosterone and LH concentrations did not change from baseline in the androstenedione group in this short-term study; however, plasma androstenedione and estradiol concentrations were significantly increased ($p < 0.05$, *t*-test), with androstenedione levels increasing threefold 4 h after ingestion. Compared with control subjects, androstenedione did not affect muscle protein synthesis and breakdown or phenylalanine net balance across the leg. It appears that androstenedione at a dose of 100 mg/d for 7 d does not increase plasma testosterone concentrations and has no anabolic effect in young, eugonadal men.

Brown and colleagues (2000b) studied the effects of Andro-6, an androstenedione-containing combination product (*see* Products Available section for detailed product description). Thirty male subjects (age 19–29 yr) with no history of supplement use or resistance training participated in the study. Ten men were randomly assigned to receive a single dose of Andro-6 or placebo in a double-blind fashion on two occasions separated by a 1-wk washout. Every 30 min for 6 h after ingestion, blood samples were taken for determination of serum androstenedione, free testosterone, total testosterone, estradiol, LH, and FSH. In addition, 20 men were randomly assigned to receive Andro-6 or placebo three times daily in a double-blind fashion. The supplement was administered for three 2-wk periods separated by a 1-wk washout. This pattern of ingestion was chosen to mimic the manufacturer's dosing recommendations and is thought to decrease the risk of side effects such as gynecomastia and lipid abnormalities. Subjects performed resistance on training 3 nonconsecutive days each wk for 8 wk. Strength testing and body composition were tested at baseline and after wk 4 and 8. At baseline and after wk 2, 5, and 8, blood samples were drawn for analysis of serum free and total testosterone, androstenedione, estrone, estradiol, estriol, lipids, and liver function tests (LFTs). Glucose tolerance testing and muscle biopsies were performed at baseline and after training. Statistical significance was accepted at $p < 0.05$ and was determined using two-way ANOVA with the Newman-Keuls multiple comparisons test.

In the 10 subjects who received a single dose of Andro-6, androstenedione concentrations increased within 150 min, peaked 300 min after ingestion, and remained higher than baseline or placebo period levels at 360 min after ingestion ($p < 0.05$). Estradiol increased after both placebo and Andro-6 administration compared with baseline ($p < 0.05$), but estradiol levels did not differ between placebo and androstenedione administration periods. In the patients who received supplementation for 8 wk, androstenedione concentrations were higher at wk 2, wk 5, and wk 8 compared with baseline $p < 0.05$), and estradiol concentrations were higher at wk 2, 5, and 8 compared with both baseline and placebo ($p < 0.05$). Other hormones were not affected. Andro-6 did not affect resistance training, muscle strength, muscle histochemistry (percent of type I fibers and cross-sectional area of type II fibers), or body composition. Similar to the findings of King et al. (1999), HDL had decreased by 12% from baseline by wk 2 and remained depressed for the remainder of the study ($p < 0.05$). Other lipids, LFTs, and glucose tolerance were unaltered by Andro-6. In addition to demonstrating that Andro-6 was unable to increase serum testosterone concentrations despite an increase in androstenedione concentrations, this study also suggests that the other ingredients in Andro-6 (*see* Products Available) did not exert their purported effects in the doses used in this study. For example, DHEA did not increase testosterone concentrations, and *Tribulus terrestris* did not alter hypothalamic-pituitary function, as evidenced by the lack of effect on LH.

Brown and colleagues (2000a) also investigated the effects of androstenedione ingestion in healthy 30–56-yr-old men. Subjects who were taking or who had previously taken nutritional supplements were excluded. Subjects were randomized to receive 100 mg of androstenedione (Experimental and Applied Sciences) or placebo three times daily for 28 d in a double-blind fashion. Compliance was assessed using pill counts and a patient diary. Subjects were instructed to maintain their usual diet and activity level throughout the study. Serum androstenedione, dihydrotestosterone, free and total testosterone, estradiol, PSA, liver enzymes, protein, albumin, globulin, blood chemistries, glucose, and lipids were measured at baseline and each week throughout the supplementation period. Data were analyzed using a three-way (wk, supplement, decade of life) repeated measures ANOVA with the Newman-Keuls test multiple comparisons test.

As in previous studies, androstenedione supplementation was found to cause a decrease in serum HDL concentrations of approximately 10% ($p < 0.05$). The investigators also found that ingestion of androstenedione did not increase serum total testosterone but did increase serum estradiol, dihydrotestosterone, and androstenedione concentrations compared with baseline ($p < 0.05$). Contrary to the findings of previous studies (King et al., 1999; Brown et al., 2000b) that used lower doses, in this study, free testosterone was noted to increase in the androstenedione group compared with baseline ($p < 0.05$). Notably, baseline serum free testosterone concentrations were lower in the subjects in this study, who were older than the subjects in the previous studies. This finding suggests that supplementation with androstenedione 300 mg/d is able to increase testosterone serum concentrations in men with low serum free test-osterone levels. The mechanism behind the increase in free testosterone levels may involve competition between dihydrotestosterone and testosterone for sex hormone-binding globulin, or a decrease in sex hormone-binding globulin levels, as demon-strated by Leder and associates (2000).

In a study by Leder et al. (2000), 42 healthy men between the ages of 20 and 40 were randomized to receive oral androstenedione capsules (Sports One, Klein Labo-ratories) 100 mg/d, 300 mg/d, or no androstenedione (control group) for 7 d. Although subjects were randomized to one of the three groups, the study was not blinded. Baseline characteristics were similar among the three groups except for body mass index ($p = 0.005$, Kruskal-Wallis test). The primary outcome measures were area under the curve (AUC) for each steroid hormone on days 1 and 7 of the study. Serum testosterone, andros-tenedione, estrone, and estradiol levels were measured 0, 15, 30, 45, 60, 90, 120, 180, 240, 360, and 480 min after administration on days 1 and 7. On days 2 and 6, these measurements were taken just prior to dosing. Hematocrit and serum sex hormone-binding globulin were obtained on days 1 and 7. LFTs, LH, FSH, creatinine, and total cholesterol were obtained daily. A mixed model analysis of covariance (ANCOVA) was used to analyze the data. Compared with the control group and the 100-mg androstenedione group, the change in testosterone AUC from baseline was significant for the 300-mg/d group ($p < 0.001$), but there was no difference in change from baseline in the 100-mg/d group compared with the control group ($p = 0.48$). Four of the 14 subjects in the 300-mg group had serum testosterone levels that exceeded the upper limit of normal. In both the 100- and 300-mg groups, androstenedione, estrone, and estradiol levels increased significantly from baseline compared with the control group. Sex hormone-binding globulin decreased in both androstenedione groups. These data suggest that oral androstenedione 300 mg/d increases serum testosterone and estradiol concentrations in certain populations of healthy men. Like the investigation by Brown and colleagues (2000a), this study included "older" men, who might experience the largest increase in testosterone levels with androstenedione supplementation; how-ever, subgroup analysis was not performed (Leder et al., 2000).

Broeder and colleagues (2000) studied the physiologic and hormonal effects of oral androstenediol 100 mg twice daily, androstenedione 100 mg twice daily, and placebo in 72 men 35–65 yr of age participating in a 12-wk high-intensity training program. Fifty men completed this double-blind study. Participants were not consum-ing any androgenic substances and had normal total testosterone, PSA, hemoglobin, hematocrit, liver function, renal function, and cardiac function. Subjects were ran-domly assigned to one of the three treatment groups. Before and after treatment, sub-jects completed a health history survey, mood survey, sexual function questionnaire, 3-d diet history, physical activity questionnaire, pulmonary function test, ECG, echocardiogram, cardiac stress test with measurement of VO_2max, body composition testing, bone density measurement, strength assessment, and measurement of serum lipid, estrone, estradiol, total testosterone, free testosterone, androstetnedione, LH, FSH, and DHEA-S levels. Data were analyzed using ANOVA. Statistical significance was accepted at the p 0.05 level. The treatment groups were similar in baseline characteristics; however, the androstendiol group had significantly higher total cholesterol, LDL, and apolipoprotein B levels compared with the other groups ($p < 0.02$); therefore, ANCOVA was used to control for these differences in lipids.

At the end of the 12-wk treatment period, the androstendione group exhibited a significant (183%) increase in serum androstenedione levels (p 0.03) compared with baseline. Androstenedione levels were also higher in the androstenedione group than in the placebo group (p 0.01) or the androstenediol group (p 0.004). Androstenedione levels were 62% higher in the androstenediol group compared with baseline (p 0.03) and were also higher compared with the placebo group (p 0.01). DHEA-S, estrone, and estradiol levels were higher in the androstenedione group and in the androstenediol group compared with baseline (p 0.03) and with the placebo group (p 0.01). DHEA-S levels were higher in the androstenediol group than in the androstenedione group (p 0.004).

After 1 mo of treatment, free testosterone had increased in the androstenedione group, but this did not differ significantly from placebo. By month 2, free testosterone levels in the androstenedione group had decreased but were higher than those of the placebo group ($p = 0.05$), because levels decreased in the placebo group as well. Free testosterone levels decreased even further by month 3 such that the androstenediol group had a significantly higher free testosterone level compared with the androstenedione group ($p < 0.05$). This decrease in free testosterone levels is probably the result of downregulation of testosterone production, as evidenced by a decrease in LH levels. Cardiac lipid profile risk [(LDL-HDL)/(apolipoprotein A/apolipoprotein B)] was higher in the androstenedione group compared with the placebo group ($p = 0.05$). The investigators concluded that supplementation with androstenedione or androstenediol does not improve the results of resistance training but that it downregulates testosterone production, increases DHEAS levels, increases levels of the aromatization products estradiol and estrone, and increases the risk of coronary artery disease.

A placebo-controlled, double-blind, 4-wk study examined the effects of Androstat 6 Popper (*see* Products Available section for description) on body composition, exercise performance (30-second cycle sprint and vertical leap), serum lipids, LFTs, kidney function, and testosterone, estradiol, and LH levels (Ziegenfuss and Kerrigan, 1999). Fourteen eugonadal men, mean age 23.7 yr, were given placebo or Androstat 6 Popper 150 mg three times daily. Data were analyzed using repeated measures ANOVA. There were statistically significant increases in body mass, fat-free body mass, vertical leap, total body water, and extracellular fluid volume in the Androstat 6 Popper group. In contrast to previous studies of androstenedione and androstenediol, HDL increased. The investigators also claim that they had previously documented increases in testosterone levels with another product containing mainly 4-androstenediol, but testosterone levels did not increase in this study. Studies of longer duration are needed to determine whether the benefits in exercise performance documented in this study would be maintained with long-term use.

In summary, an androstenedione dose of at least 300 mg is necessary to increase serum testosterone in healthy males. Studies to date do not support androstenedione's ability to increase strength or enlarge muscle mass. Low dose, small sample size, low bioavailability, downregulation of hormone production by feedback mechanisms, weak androgenic effect of androstenedione, and use in men with normal baseline hormone levels are possible reasons for lack of effect of androstenedione in these studies. Androstenediol 200 mg/d also does not appear to have ergogenic or anabolic effects. Although one small study using androstenediol 375 mg/d suggests that this supplement may have ergogenic and anabolic effects without significant side effects (Ziegenfuss and Kerrigan, 1999), more study of the safety and efficacy of this supplement is needed.

1.8. PHARMACOKINETICS

Androstenedione is primarily bound to serum proteins. The percentage bound to albumin is 19.4%, and that bound to sex hormone-binding globulin is 78.8%. Unbound androstenedione is found in the blood at a concentration of 1.73%. The clearance of endogenous androstenedione is approximately 2000 L/d in women (Longcope, 1998).

First-pass metabolism inactivates most of the given dose of androstenedione and 4-androstenediol, converting them to the inactive steroids androsterone and etiocholanolone. Other urinary metabolites of androstenedione include testosterone, epitestosterone, 5α-androstanediol, 5β-androstanediol, and 11-hydroxyandrosterone. An unidentified metabolite, perhaps hydroxyandrostenedione, is also excreted in the urine. Very little unchanged androstenedione is detectable in the urine (Uralets and Gillette, 1999). Approximately 8% of an administered androstenedione dose is converted to dihydrotestosterone in the prostate, skin, and adipose tissue by the action of 5α-reductase (Brown et al., 2000a). Other enzymes involved in the metabolism of androstenedione include 17β-hydroxylase, which converts it to testosterone, and aromatase, which biotransforms it to estradiol, estrone, and estriol (King et al., 1999; Leder et al., 2000). These enzymes are found in skeletal muscle, fat, blood, and other tissues (King et al., 1999; Leder et al., 2000). Muscle and fat appear to contribute equally to the aromatization of androstenedione to estrone (King et al., 1999).

4-Androstenediol, like androstenedione, is metabolized to testosterone; however, it is a more effective testosterone booster than androstenedione. Urinary metabolites of 4-androstenediol are the same as those of androstenedione, with the exception of 3α- and 3β-hydroxyandrostene-17-one, which are detectable in the urine after administration of 4-androstenediol but not after administration of androstenedione. The difference in urinary metabolites between androstenedione and 4-androstenediol is a reflection of their differing metabolic pathways. These two metabolites are intermediates in the metabolism of 4-androstenediol to testosterone. This intermediate step slows first-pass metabolism, allowing more testosterone to enter the bloodstream (Uralets and Gillette, 1999).

19-Norandrosterone has been detected in the urine of subjects administered androstenedione. The product administered was found to contain small quantities (mean, 0.0076% or 7.6 μg per 100-mg capsule) of 19-norandrostenedione, another over-the-counter steroid. Administration of 19-norandrostenedione alone also resulted in detection of norandrosterone, as well as 19-noretiocholanolone, in the urine. Urine concentrations resulting from administration of 10 μg of pure 19-norandrostenedione resulted in 19-norandrosterone concentrations that were of the same order of magnitude as those produced by the contaminated androstenedione capsules. This finding suggests that norandrosterone is a metabolite of 19-norandrostenedione, but not of androstenedione (Catlin et al., 2000).

In a study in which young males were given androstenedione 100 mg twice daily for 2 d, the exogenous androstenedione was completely cleared 24 h after the last dose was taken (Ballantyne et al., 2000).

1.9. ADVERSE EFFECTS AND TOXICITY

Androstenedione has been shown to reduce serum HDL cholesterol (King et al, 1999). Anecdotal reports of headache, blurred vision, eye twitching, aggressive behavior, mood swings, sunburn, increased libido in female users, decreased libido in male users, hair loss, facial hair growth, acne, gynecomastia, decrease in testicular size, prostatitis, dizziness, nausea, insomnia, and difficulty concentrating can be found on Internet bulletin boards (Androstenedine, 2001). Premature closure of epiphyseal growth plates in preadolescents and adolescents is of concern (DeCree, 1999) but is not documented.

There is a published report of a man developing priapism after taking androstenedione (Kachhi, 2000). Prior to presenting to the emergency room (ER) with a spontaneous, painful erection of 30 hr duration, the patient, a 30-yr-old black man, had reportedly ingested androstenedione every day for 1 wk. Over the past year, he had taken androstenedione sporadically and during this time experienced an episode of priapism after use of androstenedione that had resolved spontaneously. Physical exam and history were otherwise unremarkable, and other causes of priapism were ruled out. The patient was treated with aspiration and saline irrigation of the corpora cavernosa, followed by intracavernosal injection of the α-agonist phenylephrine.

Elevated serum androstenedione levels are associated with pancreatic cancer and with prostate cancer in some, but not all, studies (King et al., 1999).

1.10. INTERACTIONS

Finasteride inhibits 5α-reductase, the enzyme necessary for the metabolism of androstenedione. This could cause increased androstenedione levels following androstenedione administration. In one study, in which the epithelium and stroma of human prostate tissue was treated with finasteride 75 nmols and androstenedione 220 nmols, 5α-reductase was inhibited by 69% in the epithelium and by 52% in the stroma. This inhibition was dose-dependent and competitive (Weisser and Krieg, 1998). These results suggest that use of androstenedione in men taking finasteride might lead to increased androstenedione levels.

1.11. REPRODUCTION

No teratogenicity data are available. Androstenedione should not be taken during pregnancy or lactation. One study involving the infusion of androstenedione to pregnant monkeys at 0.3 mg/kg/h resulted in premature labor and delivery and elevated corticotropin-releasing hormone (CRH) (Giussani et al., 1998).

1.12. CHEMICAL AND BIOFLUID ANALYSIS

See Products Available section for a discussion of androstenedione interference with drugs of abuse testing in athletes.

Androstenedione concentrations have been measured by a number of analytical methodologies including gas chromatography/mass spectrometry (GC/MS), RIA, and liquid chromatography/mass spectrometry (LC/MS) (Wudy et al., 1992, 1995; Boschi et al., 1994; Hill et al., 1996). Antibody-based systems such as RIA have the advantage of being extremely sensitive and relatively rapid, but they can suffer from lack of specificity (antibody crossreacts with other hormones, producing falsely high levels) or requiring the use of radioactive substances (which create disposal issues). GC/MS and LC/MS methods have been demonstrated to be both sensitive and specific for the measurement of androstenedione.

Wudy and colleagues (1992) report a sensitive and specific method of measuring androstenedione and five additional steroids (testosterone, 17α-hydroxyprogesterone, 5α-androstane-3α,17β-diol, 5α-dihydrotestosterone, and dehydroepiandrosterone) in human plasma using GC/MS. This method has been shown to be satisfactory for measuring endogenous levels of androstenedione and thus more than adequate for measuring levels achieved following oral dosing of the compound. Plasma (1–2 mL) is mixed with internal standard ([7,7-^{2}H$_2$]androst-4-ene-3,17-dione), in an ethanolic solution at a concentration expected for androstenedione in vivo and allowed to stand for 30 min at 37°C. The steroid is then extracted twice with 2–4 mL (depending on the initial plasma volume) of a mixture of dichloromethane-isooctane (1:2 v/v); the resulting organic layers are combined and then extracted to dryness under a stream of nitrogen. The dried extracts are reconstituted in 5 mL of cyclohexane/ethanol (9:1 v/v) and passed through a Sephadex LH-20 mini column (50 × 5 mm i.d.) with the first 1 mL going to waste and the next 4 mL collected and evaporated to dryness. To facilitate analysis, the samples are derivatized by adding 100 µL acetonitrile and 20 µL of heptafluorobutyric anhydride to the dried residue; they are then allowed to stand for 1 h at room temperature. The excess reagent is then removed under a stream of nitrogen, and the residue is dissolved in 50 µL cyclohexane for injection onto the GC/MS. GC is performed on an OV-1 fused silica column (25 m × 0.15 mm; 0.1-µm film thickness) using helium as the carrier gas at a column head pressure of 1.8 bar.

The initial column temperature is set to 50°C and after 6 min is increased to 230°C at a rate of 30°C per min. This temperature is maintained for 2 min, and then raised to 290°C at a rate of 3°C per min. The mass selective detector is run in selected ion monitoring mode, and the energy of the electron beam is set to 70 eV. The ion source temperature is 250°C. Androstenedione is monitored at an *m/z* of 482 and the internal standard [7,7-^{2}H$_2$]androst-4-ene-3,17-dione at an *m/z* of 484. Coefficients of variation for accuracy and precision of the assay are less than 10%, and the assay limit of sensitivity is 10 pg of androstenedione injected on a column, more than adequate to measure concentrations in both adults and children of either sex.

An alternative method reported by Uralets and Gillette (1999) may be used to detect not only androstenedione, but also 19-norandrostenedione and androstenediol. However, this method measures urinary excretion and requires deconjugation of the steroids from glucuronic acid. Briefly, a steroid internal standard (ISTD)/enzyme mixture is prepared containing 300 µL of 5α-androstan-17-one (1 mg/mL), 150 µL of 4-chlorotestosterone (1 mg/mL), and 25 mL of β-glucuronidase to a 475 mL solution of acetate buffer (pH 5.2). Next, 1 mL of the ISTD/enzyme mixture is added to 4 mL of urine and allowed to incubate for 3 h at 52°C. The tubes are then centrifuged and the liquid applied to a C18 solid phase extraction column that has been preconditioned with 3 mL of methanol and 3 mL of water. The column is washed with 2 mL of 30% acetonitrile/water (v/v). The column is then dried under vacuum for 15 min and the steroids subsequently eluted with 3 mL methanol; the resulting eluate is evaporated to dryness. The dried residue is derivatized with 75 µL *n*-methyl-*N*-(trimethylsilyl)trifluoroacetamide (MSTFA)/ammonium iodide/dithioerythritol (1000:2:3, v/w/w) for 15 min at 70°C. One microliter of this solution is then injected into the gas chromatograph. GC/MS is used for analyte separation and quantitation. Chromatography is achieved using an HP-1 fused silica column (17 m × 0.2 mm i.d., 0.11-µm film thickness) using helium as the carrier gas flowing at 40 cm/s. The injector temperature is set to 270°C and the transfer line temperature to 280°C. The oven temperature is programmed as follows: 180°C (0.3 min), increased to 231°C at 3°C/min, then to 310°C at 30°C/min and then held at that temperature for 1.07 min. The injection split ratio is set to 1:10. The analytes of interest and relevant metabolites are eluted in approximately 18 min.

1.13. Regulatory Status

Owing to the Dietary Supplement Health and Education Act of 1994, the FDA is unable to rule on the safety and efficacy of androstenedione. The Anabolic Steroid Control Act of 1990 classifies testosterone and a number of its derivatives as Schedule III drugs under the Controlled Substance Act. However, the provisions of this Act do not apply to androstenedione because, although it is structurally and pharmacologically related to testosterone, it has not been shown to promote muscle growth. Although there is no restriction on the sale of androstenedione in the United States, androstenedione is banned by the National Football League (NFL), the International Olympic Committee (IOC), the National Collegiate Athletic Association (NCAA 2002;Yesalis, 1999), and the National Basketball Association (NBA; Zurer, 1998; NBA, 2000; Office of the Attorney General, State of California, 2001). Androstenedione is illegal in Canada (Blum, 1998). Androstenediol, norandrostenedione, and norandrostenediol are also banned by the NCAA (NCAA, 2002). The DEA is currently reviewing steroid dietary supplements to determine whether they promote muscle growth and should be scheduled (Sapienza, 2000). In 2001, California's Attorney General filed suit against several androstenedione manufacturers and distributors, contending that androstenedione is an anabolic steroid capable of causing reproductive harm and therefore supplements should carry a warning about the potential for adverse effects. The basis for this suit is the Safe Drinking Water Toxic Enforcement Act of 1986, which provides that California residents be warned prior to exposure to chemicals that cause cancer or adverse reproductive effects (Office of the Attorney General, State of California, 2001).

1.14. SUMMARY

- Androstenedione is a weak androgen and testosterone precursor marketed as an athletic performance enhancer and sexual tonic.
- An androstenedione dose of at least 300 mg is necessary to increase serum testosterone in healthy males. Studies of androstenedione have failed to confirm its purported ability to increase strength or improve athletic performance.
- Adverse effects associated with androstenedione use are mostly anecdotal and are androgenic in females and largely estrogenic in males. Decreased HDL was a consistent finding in several controlled studies.
- Although androstenedione is sold as a dietary supplement in the United States, its use is banned by several amateur and professional sports organizations.
- Androstenediol and 19-norandrostenedione are related over-the-counter steroids. Their effects have been less studied. 19-Norandrostenedione can also be found as an unlabeled ingredient in androstenedione products. 19-Norandrostenedione can be metabolized to 19-norandrosterone, a nandrolone metabolite, thus causing users to test positive for nandrolone use.

REFERENCES

Androstenedione. Available from: URL: http://www.nutritionalsupplements.com. Accessed June 13, 2001.

Anonymous. Creatine and androstenedione—two "dietary supplements." Med Lett Drugs Ther 1998;40:105–6.

Ballantyne CS, Phillips SM, MacDonald JR, Tarnopolsky MA, MacDougall JD. The acute effects of androstenedione supplementation in healthy young males. Can J Appl Physiol 2000;25:68–78.

Birchard K. Body-building supplement fails to strengthen and may harm health. Lancet 1999;353:1943.

Blum R. Decision on androstenedione months away. Associated Press. New York. October 30, 1998. Available from: URL: http://www.augustasports.com/stories/10098/oth_LS0234-9000.shtml. Accessed on January 24, 2001.

Boschi S, De Iasio R, Mesini P, et al. Measurement of steroid hormones in plasma by isocratic high performance liquid chromatography coupled to radioimmunoassay. Clin Chim Acta 1994;231:107–13.

Broeder CE, Quindry J, Brittingham K, et al. The andro project: physiological and hormonal influences of androstenedione supplementation in men 35 to 65 years old participating in a high-intensity resistance training program. Arch Intern Med 2000;160:3093–104.

Brown GA, Vukovich MD, Martini ER, et al. Endocrine responses to chronic androstenedione intake in 30- to 56-year-old men. J Clin Endocrinol Metab 2000a;85:4074–80.

Brown GA, Vukovich MD, Reifenrath TA, et al. Effects of anabolic precursors on serum testosterone concentrations and adaptations to resistance training in young men. Int J Sport Nutr Exerc Metab 2000b;10:340–59.

Catlin DH, Leder BZ, Aherns B, et al. Trace contamination of over-the-counter and positive urine test results for a nandrolone metabolite. JAMA 2000;284:2618–21.

DeCree C. Androstenedione and dehydroepiandrosterone for athletes. Lancet 1999;354:779–80.

Giussani DA, Winter JA, Jenkins SL, et al. Changes in fetal plasma corticotropin-releasing hormone during androstenedione-induced labor in the Rhesus monkey: lack of an effect on the fetal hypothalamo-pituitary-adrenal axis. Endocrinology 1998;139:2803–10.

Goldfien A. Adrenocroticosteroids and adrenocortical antagonists. In: Katzung BG (ed.) Basic and clinical pharmacology. 7th ed. Stamford, CT: Appleton and Lange; 1998a.

Goldifien A. The gonadal hormones and inhibitors. In Katzung BG (ed.) Basic and clinical pharmacology, 7th ed. Stamford, CT: Appleton and Lange; 1998b.

Hill M, Hampl R, Petrik R, Starka L. Concentration of the endogenous antiandrogen epitestosterone and androgenic C19-steroids in hyperplastic prostatic tissue. Prostate 1996;28:347–51.

Kachhi PN, Henderson SO. Priapism after androstenedione intake for athletic performance enhancement. Ann Emerg Med 2000;35:391–3.

King DS, Sharp RL, Vukovich MD, et al. Effect of oral androstenedione on serum testosterone and adaptations to resistance training in young men. JAMA 1999;281:2020–8.

Kochakian CD, Murlin JR. The relationship of synthetic male hormone androstenedione to the protein and energy metabolism of castrated dogs and the protein metabolism of a normal dog. Am J Physiol 1936;117:642–57.

Labrie F, Belanger A, Luu-The V, et al. DHEA and the intracrine formation of androgens and estrogens in peripheral target tissues: its role in aging. Steroids 1998;63:322–8.

Leder BZ, Longcope C, Catlin DH, et al. Oral androstenedione administration and serum testosterone concentrations in young men. JAMA 2000;283:779–82.

Longcope C. Androgen metabolism and the menopause. Semin Reprod Endocrinol 1998;16:111–15.

Longcope C. Dehydroepiandrostereone metabolism. J Endocrinol 1996;150(suppl):S125–7.

Mahesh VB, Greenblatt RB. The in vivo conversion of dehydroepiandrosterone and androstenedione to testosterone in the human. Acta Endocrinol 1962;41:400–6.

NBA (National Basketball Association) News. NBA committee adds andro as banned substance, upsets union, New York, March 20, 2000. Available from: URL: www.webcraawler-sports.excite.com/nba/news/ando. Accessed Jan 24, 2001.

NCAA. 2002–2003 NCAA Banned Drug Classes. Available from: URL:http://www.ncaa.org. Accessed Sept 3, 2002.

Office of the Attorney General, State of California. Attorney General Lockyer seeks consumer warnings on popular bodybuilding "andro" supplements as required by California's Proposition 65. Available from: http://www.caag.state.ca.us/newsalerts/2001/01-081.htm. Accessed December 21, 2001.

Rasmussen BB, Volpe E, Gore DC, Wolfe RR. Androstenedione does not stimulate muscle protein anabolism in young healthy men. J Clin Endocrinol Metab 2000;85:55–9.

Rouse JE, Spoerke D. Androstenedione. AltMedDex. Micromedex, Inc.

Sapienza, F. Presentation at National Association of State Controlled Substances Authorities (NASCSA). 16th Annual Education Conference, Louisville, KY, Nov. 1, 2000.

Uralets VP, Gillette PA. Over-the-counter anabolic steroids 4-androsten-3,17-dione; 4-androsten-3β, 17β-diol; and 19-nor-4-androsten-3,17-dione: excretion studies in men. J Anal Toxicol 1999; 23:357-66.

Vermeulen A. Plasma levels and secretion rate of steroids with anabolic activity in man. Environ Qual Saf 1976;(5 suppl):171–80.

Wallace MB, Lim J, Cutler A, Bucci L. Effects of dehyroepiandrosterone vs androstenedione supplmentation in men. Med Sci Sports Exerc 1999;31:1788–92.

Weisser H, Krieg M. In vitro inhibition of androstenedione 5-alpha-reduction by finasteride in epithelium and stroma of human benign prostatic hyperplasia. J Steroid Biochem Mol Biol 1998; 67:49–55.

Wudy SA, Wachter UA, Homoki J, Teller WM. 17β-Hydroxyprogesterone, 4-androstenedione, and testosterone profiled by routine stable isotope dilution/gas chromatography-mass spectrometry in plasma of children. Pediatr Res 1995;38:76-80.

Wudy SA, Wachter UA, Homoki J, Teller WM, Shackleton CHL. Androgen metabolism assessment by routine gas chromatography mass spectrometry profiling of plasma steroids: part 1, unconjugated steroids. Steroids 1992;57:319–24.

Yesalis CE. Medical, legal, and societal implications of androstenedione use. JAMA 1999;281:2043–44.

Ziegenfuss TN, Kerrigan DJ. Safety and efficacy of prohormone administration in men. Abstract presented at the American Society of Exercise Physiologists 2nd Annual Meeting, 1999.

Zurer P. Androstenedione: out of the park or out in left field? Sci Insights 1998;76:39.

Chapter 2

Chitosan

Kimberly Novak, Melanie Johns Cupp,
and Timothy S. Tracy

2.1. HISTORY

Chitosan was purportedly first discovered in 1859 by Rouget while he was experimenting with chemical and thermal manipulation of the natural fiber chitin (Au Natural Herbals, 2001). Since then, chitosan has been used as a pharmaceutical excipient in sustained release dosage forms, as an immunostimulant, and to promote wound healing (Colombo and Sciutto, 1996). Chitosan's ability to bind to a variety of substances including acids, lipophilic substances, and minerals (Jing et al., 1997) has enabled it to be used for water purification for more than 30 yr. Chitosan has been sold in Europe and Japan for the past 20 yr as a nonprescription product to inhibit fat absorption (Au Natural Herbals, 2001). Chitosan was first marketed as a dietary supplement in the United States in the late 1990s.

2.2. CHEMICAL STRUCTURE

See Fig. 2-1 for the chemical structure of chitosan.

2.3. CURRENT PROMOTED USES

Because of its ability to inhibit fat absorption, chitosan is promoted primarily for use in obesity and hyperlipidemia.

2.4. SOURCES AND CHEMICAL COMPOSITION

Chitosan is a fiber product that is obtained from deacetylated chitin. Chitin is a naturally occurring substance found in the shells of crustaceans, invertebrates, and fungi (Sciutto and Colombo, 1995). Chitin is a linear polysaccharide comprised of N-acetyl-D-glucosamine chains [$\beta(1–4)$-2-acetamide-2-deoxy-D-glucose]. It is similar to

From: *Forensic Science: Dietary Supplements: Toxicology and Clinical Pharmacology*
Edited by: M. J. Cupp and T. S. Tracy © Humana Press Inc., Totowa, New Jersey

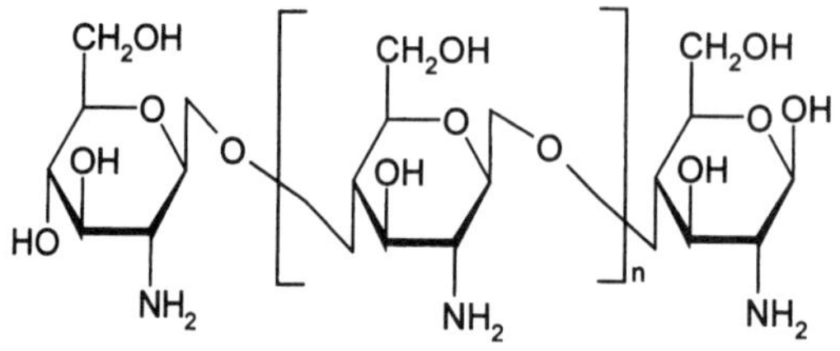

Fig. 1. Chemical structure of chitosan.

unramified cellulose and is insoluble in water. After deacetylation with sodium hydroxide, the resulting chitosan becomes soluble in acid, such as is present in the stomach. Once solubilized, the chitosan forms a gel-like substance that binds lipids in the gastrointestinal tract, resulting in their fecal elimination (Macchi, 1996).

A new form of chitosan has been extracted and purified. This electrostatically charged chitosan is poorly absorbed systemically but is able to bind lipids and prevent their digestion. The positively charged amino groups on the chitosan molecule bind to the negatively charged carboxylic groups of free fatty acids. This electromagnetic bond seems to be stronger than those observed in other dietary fibers. Additionally, hydrophobic bonds are also formed between chitosan and neutral fats such as cholesterol and triglycerides (Macchi, 1996).

2.5. PRODUCTS AVAILABLE

Chitosan is available in dietary supplements sold under several proprietary names. Products may be combined with a starch excipient. Additionally, chitosan may be found in combination with other substances, such as appetite suppressants, stimulants, chromium picolinate, carnitine, or amino acids in products marketed for weight loss (Candlish, 1999).

2.6. ANIMAL DATA

Muzzarelli (1999) reviewed animal data pertinent to chitosan's therapeutic effects. In hypercholesterolemic, apolipoprotein E-deficient mice, which develop high blood cholesterol levels and atherosclerosis without scientific manipulation, 20 wk of dietary chitosan resulted in a 52% reduction in serum cholesterol. Additionally, the area of plaque in the aortic arch was 50% lower in treated mice compared with control mice. On the other hand, the chitosan-fed mice experienced increased growth, with an overall 65% weight gain; the control mice experienced growth retardation.

In dogs given 2 wk of oral chitosan, total cholesterol levels decreased to 77% of baseline by day 7 of therapy and then to 54% of baseline by day 14. Levels returned to baseline on day 28. Other dogs treated with chitin or celluloses experienced no reduction in cholesterol (Muzzarelli, 1999).

Another study examined the hyperglycemic and hypolidemic effects of chitosan in normal and diabetic mice. Diabetic mice consisted of obese mice with hyperinsulinemia (KK-Ay) and lean mice with hypoinsulinemia [neonatal streptozocin-induced diabetic mice (NSZ)]. After 4 wk of a 5% chitosan diet, no change in body weight was observed in any of the mice groups. In the normal mice, decreased levels of blood glucose, cholesterol, and triglycerides were observed. In NSZ mice, significant reductions in blood glucose and cholesterol were also observed; however, no reductions were observed in the KK-Ay mice.

2.7. CLINICAL STUDIES

Several studies have examined the effects of the new electrostatically charged, polycationic chitosan on lipids and body weight (Giustina and Ventura, 1995; Sciutto and Colombo, 1995; Colombo and Sciutto, 1996; Veneroni et al., 1996; Macchi, 1996;). An additional study with findings not supporting chitosan's efficacy in reducing weight and serum lipids does not identify the product as being the new electostatically charged form (Pittler et al., 1999). Most of the chitosan studies examined the effects of a hypocaloric diet (1000–1100 kcal/d) plus chitosan (1 gm twice daily before main meals) vs the same hypocaloric diet plus placebo in mildly obese (10–25% overweight) subjects (Giustina and Ventura, 1995; Sciutto and Colombo, 1995; Colombo and Sciutto, 1996; Veneroni et al., 1996). These double-blind, placebo-controlled trials show statistically significant reductions in body weight, percent overweight, total and LDL cholesterol, and triglycerides and an increase in HDL in all treatment groups compared to baseline; however, between-group comparisons favor the groups receiving chitosan (Colombo and Sciutto, 1996; Giustina and Ventura, 1995; Sciutto and Colombo, 1995; Veneroni et al., 1996). Three studies also examined chitosan's effects on systolic and diastolic blood pressure and found that both diastolic (Giustina and Ventura, 1995; Sciutto and Colombo, 1995; Macchi, 1996) and systolic (Sciutto and Colombo, 1995; Macchi, 1996) blood pressure were reduced with chitosan. One of these studies examined the effect on respiratory rate and found it to be reduced in both treatment groups, with a statistically greater effect in the chitosan group (Giustina and Ventura, 1995).

One double-blind, placebo-controlled study of 30 moderately obese (25% overweight) subjects examined the effects of chitosan 1 g twice daily before main meals plus a hypocaloric diet (1200 kcal/d), placebo plus a hypocaloric diet, and chitosan plus an unrestricted diet. The chitosan plus hypocaloric diet and chitosan plus unrestricted diet groups showed a statistically significant decease in body weight, body mass index (BMI), body fat, and skinfold thickness compared with baseline ($p < 0.0001$, Wilcoxon matched pairs, signed rank test). The diet plus placebo group also showed a statistically significant decrease in weight ($p < 0.0001$), BMI, body fat, and skinfold thickness ($p < 0.001$). The decrease was greatest in the chitosan plus hypocaloric diet group. Additionally, these reductions were greater in the chitosan plus unrestricted diet group than in the placebo plus hypocaloric diet group. For example, the average weight loss was 4 kg ($p < 0.0001$) in the chitosan plus hypocaloric diet group, 2.6 kg ($p < 0.0001$) in the placebo plus hypocaloric diet group, and 2.8 kg ($p < 0.0001$) in the chitosan plus unrestricted diet group.

Statistically significant reductions in total cholesterol and triglycerides were seen in all groups, with the greatest reductions observed in the chitosan groups. The average reduction in total cholesterol was 26 mg/dL ($p < 0.0001$) in the chitosan plus hypocaloric diet group, 15 mg/dL ($p < 0.01$) in the placebo plus hypocaloric diet group, and 28 mg/dL ($p < 0.0001$) in the chitosan plus unrestricted diet group. The average reduction in triglycerides was 27 mg/dL ($p < 0.01$) in the chitosan plus hypocaloric diet group, 26 mg/dL ($p < 0.0001$) in the placebo plus hypocaloric diet group, and 27 mg/dL ($p < 0.0001$) in the chitosan plus unrestricted diet group. A statistically significant increase in HDL cholesterol (11 mg/dl, $p < 0.001$) was seen only in the chitosan plus unrestricted diet group.

Statistically significant reductions in systolic blood pressure (6 mmHg, $p < 0.01$ and 11 mmgHg, $p < 0.0001$) and diastolic blood pressure (7 mmHg, $p < 0.001$ and 9 mmHg, $p < 0.001$) were seen in the chitosan plus hypocaloric diet and in the chitosan plus unrestricted diet groups, respectively, but not in the placebo plus hypocaloric diet group. Heart rate did not change significantly during the study (Macchi, 1996).

A randomized, double blind, placebo-controlled study examined the effect of chitosan vs placebo in 34 overweight subjects maintaining their normal diet. After 4 wk of treatment, weight, BMI, blood pressure, total cholesterol, and triglycerides were not different in subjects receiving chitosan compared with those receiving placebo. For example, baseline and 4-wk weights in the chitosan group were 71.8 ± 8.4 kg and 72.6 ± 8.6 kg, respectively; values in the placebo group were 76.4 ± 9.5 kg and 77.9 ± 10.8 kg (NS). Baseline and 4-wk total cholesterols in the chitosan group were 5.77 ± 0.87 mmol/l and 5.32 ± 0.93 mmol/L, respectively; values in the placebo group were 5.36 ± 0.92 mmol/L and 5.64 ± 1.31 mmol/L (NS). Similar patterns were seen in the other outcome measures (Pittler et al., 1999).

A discussion in a metaanalysis conducted by two authors from the previous study criticizes the studies of chitosan in conjunction with a hypocaloric diet. Although the metaanalysis of the included studies (Giustina and Ventura, 1995; Sciutto and Colombo, 1995; Colombo and Sciutto, 1996; Macchi, 1996; Veneroni ct al., 1996) indicated that the weighted mean difference between chitosan and placebo groups is 3.28 kg (95% CI, 1.5–5.1), the authors suggest that some other mechanism might be involved in the weight loss in those studies. This is postulated because the extra 3.28 kg weight loss in the chitosan groups would require a fecal fat loss of more than 100 g/d. This amount of fat would not normally be consumed from a hypocaloric diet of 1000–1200 kcal/d. Further criticism reveals that the articles were not cited in searchable databases, but rather were provided from one manufacturer and appeared in the same journal, although the journal is peer-reviewed and of accepted standing in its field (Ernst and Pittler, 1998).

Chitosan has also been studied in the treatment of the sequelae of chronic renal failure in hemodialysis patients. In an unblinded study (Jing et al., 1997), 40 hemodialysis patients were administered 10 tablets containing chitosan (Kitosan Shokuhin Kogyo) 45 mg three times daily for 12 wk. The chitosan used in the study had a molecular weight of 27,000 daltons and was 89% deacetylated. At baseline and every 4 wk thereafter, the patients' blood pressure, weight, serum creatinine, blood urea nitrogen (BUN), lipids, hemoglobin, and electrolytes were measured. Means for the outcome measures were compared with those of a control group that did not receive chitosan. Data analysis was performed using repeated t-tests. Statistical significance was accepted at the $p < 0.05$ level. At weeks 8 and 12, total cholesterol and lipoprotein were significantly lower in the treatment group. At weeks 4, 8, and 12, hemoglobin was higher and BUN and creatinine were significantly lower in the treatment group. Subjective improvements in sleep, appetite, physical strength, halitosis, and itching were noted. Because chitosan is not capable of binding to creatinine in vitro, it was hypothesized that the effects of chitosan on creatinine and hemoglobin were secondary to its binding "uremic toxins" in the gastrointestinal tract, leading to improvement in residual renal function. Symptom improvement could also be attributed to binding of these toxins and nitrogenous wastes in the gut. Placebo-controlled trials are needed to confirm the results of this study and to assess the long-term safety and pharmacokinetics of chitosan in this population.

2.8. PHARMACOKINETICS

Experimental evidence suggests that chitosan is partially digested and absorbed owing to the acidic environment of the stomach, enzymes present in saliva and gastric juice, and bacterial enzymes in the large intestine. Oral intake of 1 g/day of chitosan increases the serum concentration of *N*-acetyl-D-glucosamine. Serum levels remain high 48 h after ingestion (Muzzarelli, 1999).

2.9. ADVERSE EFFECTS AND TOXICITY

Chitosan is generally considered to be nontoxic, and, unlike medication used to treat hyperlipidemia, chitosan has no activity on enzymes involved in cholesterol biosynthesis (Muzzarelli, 1999). In clinical studies, very few adverse effects have been reported. Adverse effects have been mild and transient and have consisted of mild nausea (Giustina and Ventura, 1995; Sciutto and Colombo, 1995; Veneroni et al., 1996), flatulence (Colombo and Sciutto, 1996), throat irritation, itching (Jing et al., 1997), constipation rarely requiring laxatives (Macchi, 1996), and soft fatty stool (Veneroni et al., 1996). Adverse effects did not occur more frequently in patients receiving chitosan than in those receiving placebo (Giustina and Ventura, 1995; Sciutto and Coluombo, 1995; Colombo and Sciutto, 1996; Veneroni et al., 1996).

2.10. INTERACTIONS

Theoretically, there has been concern that chitosan could bind fat-soluble vitamins and deprive the body of these essential nutrients. It has been suggested that vitamin supplements should be taken at a separate time from chitosan in order to avoid any potential interaction (Muzzarelli, 1999). Absorption of vitamins E (Muzzarelli, 1999; Pittler et al., 1999), D, and A and β-carotene is not altered by chitosan intake (Pittler et al., 1999). One study found that vitamin K levels were significantly higher after 4 wk of treatment with chitosan but were not outside the normal range (Pittler et al., 1999). Theoretically, this could lead to a decrease in the efficacy of warfarin.

It was also once thought that chitosan might interfere with intestinal absorption of trace metal ions such as iron and zinc (Muzzarelli, 1999) and mineral salts (Colombo and Sciutto, 1996). Studies have shown, however, that absorption of these substances is not inhibited by chitosan administration (Giustina and Ventura, 1995; Sciutto and Colombo, 1995; Colombo and Sciutto, 1996; 1999; Veneroni et al., 1996; Muzzarelli, Pittler et al., 1999).

2.11. REPRODUCTION

Chitosan's effects on fertility, pregnancy, and lactation are not known.

2.12. CHEMICAL AND BIOFLUID ANALYSIS

Chitosan is a mixture of chitooligosaccharides that to our knowledge have not been measured in human tissue (e.g., blood or urine). Lopatin and colleagues (1985) described a technique involving liquid chromatography-mass spectrometry (LC-MS) for characterizing *N*-acetylchitooligosaccharide derivatives that may be adaptable to measuring concentrations in blood, if desired. However, some modifications of the method will be needed since it was developed for use in analyzing crab shells.

The initial step involves hydrolysis of the shell to release the chitosan. Chitosan (10 g) is dissolved in 0.5% acetic acid (1000 mL), and then 30 mg of lyophically dried chitinases complex (from *Streptomyces kurssanovii*) is added to the solution. The mixture is then partially purified by metal-ion affinity chromatography. The solution is stirred for 4 h at 45°C, an additional 40 mg of enzyme complex is added and allowed to mix for an additional 16 h at 37°C. This is followed by heating to denature the enzymes. Finally, once cool, the solution is filtered through a Diasorb C-16 (1 × 10 cm) column, and the filtrate is lyophilized to dryness. (It should be noted that this hydrolysis step may not be necessary when measuring concentrations in human blood or urine.) The lyophilized residue is then dissolved in 50 mL of water; 10 mL of methanol and 20 mL of acetic anhydride are added to acetylate the chitooligosaccharides. The reaction is allowed to proceed for 16 h, and then the residue is concentrated under vacuum until the acetic acid odor disappears. The resulting residue [*N*-acetylchitooligosaccharides (GlcNAc$_{2-7}$)] is dissolved in 30 mL of water, and 2 g of Amberlit MB-3 resin is added and stirred for 15 min. The solution is then dried to a powder.

The sample is initially fractionated on a Sephadex G-25 sf (3 × 70 cm) column with water as the mobile phase and a flow rate of 225 mL/h. Ten mL fractions (10 mL) are collected, concentrated and identified by reversed-phase chromatography.

For the chromatographic separation, a LiChrospher 100 RP-18 column (4 × 250 mm) is used. Water (0.5 mL/min) is used as the mobile phase and detection is via an ultraviolet (UV) detector set at 206 nm. The samples are readily separated with a maximum run time of 60 min for GlcNAc$_7$. For positive peak identification, mass spectra are obtained on a time/flow biochemical mass spectrometer with plasma desorption by fission products of californium-252. The *N*-acetylchitooligosaccharides are dissolved in 0.1% trifluoroacetic acid and then dried prior to introduction into the mass spectrometer. Once the peak identities have been conclusively verified, it may be possible to omit the mass spectrometric detection and simply quantitate the samples via the LC-UV chromatography step.

As an alternative method, Chang and associates (1979) have developed an indirect method for quantitating chitooligosaccharides using an amino acid analyzer. The preparative stages of this assay are also somewhat complex, as with the LC method just described. Also, this method has not been used to quantitate the oligosaccharides in biologic tissues.

2.13. REGULATORY STATUS

Chitosan is regulated as a dietary supplement in the United States and is not approved for use as a drug by the Food and Drug Administration. It is marketed as a food additive or supplement in Japan, England, Italy, and Portugal (Muzzarelli, 1999).

2.14. SUMMARY

• Chitosan is a glucosamine polymer derived from shellfish that, among other properties, is capable of adsorbing lipophilic and acidic substances.
• Chitosan appears to be modestly effective in improving body composition, decreasing serum lipids, and decreasing blood pressure in mild-to-moderately overweight patients.
• Chitosan may be useful in treating anemia, pruritis, weakness, and fatigue associated with chronic renal failure in hemodialysis patients by removing nitrogenous wastes and uremic toxins.
• Chitosan is partially digested in the gastrointestinal tract and can be absorbed systemically.
• Gastrointestinal complaints are the most common adverse effects associated with chitosan.
• Theoretically, chitosan might interfere with the action of warfarin by increasing vitamin K levels, but no interactions have thus far been reported.

REFERENCES

Au Natural Herbals. Chitosan history. Available from: URL: http://www.chitosan-weight-loss.net/history.html. Accessed November 22, 2001.

Candlish JK What you need to know: over the counter slimming products—their rationality and legality. Singapore Med J 1999;40:550–2.

Chang JJ, Hash JH. The use of an amino acid analyzer for the rapid identification and quantitative determination of chitosan oligosaccharides. Anal Biochem 1979;95:563–67.

Colombo P, Sciutto AM. Nutritional aspects of chitosan employment in hypocaloric diet. Acta Toxicol Ther 1996;17:278–302.

Ernst E, Pittler MH. Chitosan as a treatment for body weight reduction? A meta-analysis. Perfusion 1998;11:461–5.

Giustina A, Ventura P. Weight-reducing regimens in obese subjects: effects of a new dietary fiber integrator. Acta Toxicol Ther 1995;16:199–214.

Jing S, Li L, Ji D, Takiguchi Y, Yamaguchi T. Effect of chitosan on renal function in patients with chronic renal failure. J Pharm Pharmacol 1997;49:721–3.

Lopatin SA, Ilyin MM, Pustobaev VN, et al. Mass-spectrometric analysis of N-acetyl-chitooligosaccharides prepared through enzymatic hydrolysis of chitosan. Anal Biochem 1995;227:285–288.

Macchi G. A new approach to treatment of obesity: chitosan's effects on body weight reduction and plasma cholesterol's levels. Acta Toxicol Ther 1996;17:303–20.

Muzzarelli RAA. Clinical and biochemical evaluation of chitosan for hypercholesterolemia and overweight control. EXS 1999;87:293–304.

Pittler MH, Abbott NC Harkness, Ernst E. Randomized, double-blind trial of chitosan for body weight reduction. Eur J Clin Nutr 1999;53:379–81.

Sciutto AM, Colombo P. Lipid-lowering effect of chitosan dietary integrator and hypocaloric diet in obese subjects. Acta Toxicol Ther 1995;16:215–30.

Veneroni G, Veneroni F, Contos S, et al. Effect of a new chitosan dietary integrator and hypocaloric diet on hyperlipidemia and overweight in obese patients. Acta Toxicol Ther 1996;17:53–70.

Chapter 3

Chromium Picolinate

Aleshia R. Haslacker, Melanie Johns Cupp, and Timothy S. Tracy

3.1. HISTORY

Chromium supplements have been advertised to the general public since at least the early 1990s. Chromium was the second most frequently mentioned ingredient in a study of health and bodybuilding magazines purchased during the summer of 1991 (Philen et al., 1992).

3.2. CHEMICAL STRUCTURE

See Fig. 3-1 for chemical structure of chromium picolinate.

3.3. CURRENT PROMOTED USES

Chromium is a cofactor for insulin; therefore, chromium may play a significant role in the metabolism of glucose, lipids, and amino acids (Kaats et al., 1996). Chromium picolinate has several proposed uses, including improving insulin sensitivity, improving lipid levels, lowering glucose levels in patients with diabetes, raising glucose levels in patients with hypoglycemia, reducing body fat, improving body composition, and increasing muscle mass (Kaats et al., 1996; Allen, 2000). Adequate intake (AI) for chromium is 20–30 µg/d in normal individuals, 30 µg/d in pregnant women and 45 µg/ d in lactating women, as recommended by the Institute of Medicine (2002). On the Internet, chromium picolinate is promoted for all its proposed uses, with the most common being to "burn fat," to increase muscle mass, and to improve blood glucose levels.

3.4. SOURCES AND CHEMICAL COMPOSITION

Chromium is an essential trace mineral that is used by the human body in several nutritional processes. Chromium can occur in multiple oxidative states, ranging from 2– to 6+ (Cerulli et al., 1998). The two most common oxidative states are 3+ (trivalent

From: *Forensic Science: Dietary Supplements: Toxicology and Clinical Pharmacology*
Edited by: M. J. Cupp and T. S. Tracy © Humana Press Inc., Totowa, New Jersey

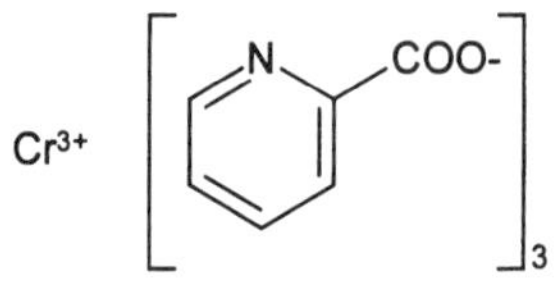

Fig. 1. Chemical structure of chromium picolinate.

form) and 6+ (hexavalent form). The hexavalent form of chromium is found in several industrial products and occupational work areas. Some of these include dye manufacturing, leather tanning, chrome plating, welding, chromate pigment production, and tobacco smoke (Gargas et al., 1994; Cerulli et al., 1998). The trivalent form of chromium is found naturally in food sources, including brewer's yeast, beer, oysters, liver, cheese, potatoes, seafood, whole grains, milk, cereals, spices, fresh vegetables, and vitamin supplements (Gargas et al., 1994; Martin and Fuller, 1998; Allen, 2000). Picolinic acid is a metal chelator synthesized from tryptophan in mammalian kidney cells and brewer's yeast. Picolinic acid is combined with trivalent chromium to allow for greater bioavailability and utilization of trivalent chromium (Press et al., 1990). The trivalent form of chromium and picolinic acid, when combined, is known as chromium picolinate.

3.5. Products Available

Chromium picolinate is commercially available in tablets, capsules, liquids, injectable solutions, tinctures, and lozenges. Some of the names of these products are Chromemate® capsules, Dr. Powers Colloidal Mineral Source liquid, Sundown® Chromium Picolinate tablets, and chromium picolinate solution (Allen, 2000). Popular outlets commonly sell chromium picolinate 200 µg and 300 µg as single-entity products. These stores also sell herbal combination products containing chromium picolinate, such as Hydroxycut™ and Metabolife356®.

3.6. Animal Data

Experiments in rats have shown that animals fed chromium-deficient diets had higher serum cholesterol levels and greater formation of aortic plaques than rats whose diets included chromium chloride. A similar study was performed in rabbits. These animals were fed high-cholesterol diets in order to induce atherosclerotic plaques and were then injected with potassium chromate. The potassium chromate injection initiated a regression of the plaques (Press et al., 1990).

3.7. Clinical Studies

Clinical studies have been performed for different uses of chromium picolinate. Some representative studies are described below.

3.7.1. Lipid Levels

Press and colleagues (1990) studied the effects of chromium picolinate on lipid levels in 32 volunteers 25–80 yr of age with total cholesterol levels of 220–320 mg/dL.

None had a history of hypothyroidism, renal failure, liver disease, diabetes mellitus, bleeding disorders, multiple allergies, known familial lipid disorder, alcohol or drug abuse, or pregnancy. None of the study subjects were taking β-blockers, thiazide diuretics, steroids, chromium supplements, or any investigational drugs. They were asked not to change their diets or exercise routines for the duration of the study. The volunteers were randomized to receive either chromium picolinate 200 μg or placebo for 42 d. After a 14-d wash-out, subjects were crossed over to the alternate treatment for 42 d. Heart rate, blood pressure, weight, temperature, total cholesterol, low-density lipoprotein (LDL) cholesterol, high-density lipoprotein (HDL) cholesterol, triglycerides, apolipoprotein A-1, and apolipoprotein B were measured at the beginning, after 3 wk, and at the end of each treatment period. Paired t-tests were used to analyze the data.

In the group that received chromium picolinate, total cholesterol ($p = 0.007$), LDL-cholesterol ($p = 0.015$), and apolipoprotein B ($p = 0.003$) were significantly lower than baseline after the first treatment phase. Apolipoprotein A-1 (the main protein of the HDL fraction) level was significantly higher than baseline ($p = 0.047$) during this treatment period. No significant changes were seen in this group when it was crossed over to placebo, suggesting a carryover effect of chromium picolinate. The "placebo first" group, however, had statistically significant decreases in total cholesterol ($p = 0.009$) and LDL cholesterol ($p = 0.003$) and an increase in apolipoprotein A-1 levels ($p = 0.007$) during the second treatment period. This study suggests that chromium picolinate has a beneficial effect on serum lipids in humans.

3.7.2. Body Composition and Strength

Of the published studies of chromium's effects on body composition and strength, only three (Evans, 1989; Kaats et al., 1996, 1998) demonstrate benefit from chromium. In the study by Kaats and colleagues (1996), "body composition improvement" (BCI) was the primary outcome measure. BCI was calculated by adding increases in fat-free mass and loss of body fat as positive changes, whereas increases in body fat and decreases in fat-free mass were added as negative changes. The investigators felt that BCI was a more sensitive measure of change in body composition than percent body fat and also that it was a more accurate reflection of body composition than percent fat, weight, or body mass index (BMI); however, this measurement has not been previously validated. Another problem with this study was that the dose of chromium was not well controlled; subjects were asked to consume "at least" two servings of a protein/carbohydrate supplement drink that contained 0, 100, or 200 μg of chromium per serving. Other weaknesses of this study included no control for potential differences between groups in exercise and diet and the large number of dropouts ($n = 65$). The relatively large sample size ($n = 219$) was a strength of this study.

These investigators subsequently performed a study differing from their previous study in that the daily chromium intake was better controlled, with subjects ingesting either chromium picolinate 400 μg or a placebo capsule daily for 90-d (Kaats et al., 1998). As before, subjects were not instructed in a particular exercise program; however, unlike the previous study (Kaats et al., 1996), in which the subjects were recruited using a television commercial, the subjects in this study ($n = 122$) were health club members and friends and family of health club members. Efforts were made to control for caloric intake and physical activity by having subjects record these variables. All subjects also wore a pedometer to better assess activity. Measures included body composition (body fat percent, fat mass, and fat-free-mass) measured using dual-energy radiography and weight.

The only statistically significant difference between groups at the end of the study was greater reduction in fat mass in the chromium group ($p = 0.023$, t-test for independent samples). Controlling for differences in activity and caloric intake, the chromium group experienced a greater reduction in percent body fat ($p = 0.03$, ANCOVA) and fat mass ($p = 0.01$, ANCOVA) than the placebo group. Using a different statistical maneuver, in which t-tests were used after corrections for differences in energy expenditure and caloric intake were made, the treatment group exhibited greater reductions in weight ($p < 0.001$), percent body fat ($p < 0.001$), and fat mass ($p < 0.001$).

Five studies comparing chromium with placebo plus exercise measured body composition using skinfold thickness (Hasten et al., 1992; Clancy et al., 1994; Hallmark et al., 1996Lukasi et al.,1996), hydrodensitometry (Clancy et al., 1994; Hallmark et al., 1996), body circumference (Clancy et al., 1994; Trent and Thieding-Cancel, 1995), whole body muscle mass (Lukasi et al.,1996), and dual-energy radiography (Lukasi et al.,1996). No benefit from chromium was noted. Strength was not affected in any of the studies in which it was an outcome measure (Hasten et al., 1992; Clancy et al., 1994; Hallmark et al., 1996; Lukaski et al., 1996). The sample sizes were smaller than in the Kaats studies (1996, 1998).

Eighteen healthy men aged 56–69 yr were randomized in double-blind fashion to receive chromium 500 μg twice daily as chromium picolinate (Nutrition 21, San Diego, CA) or placebo while participating in 12 weeks of resistance training (Campbell et al., 1999). Subjects were mildly overweight. For 5 d during weeks 1, 7, and 13, subjects consumed a controlled diet and were asked to maintain their normal diet during the remainder of the study. Body composition was measured using hydrodensitometry, skinfold thickness, and body circumference, and whole body muscle mass was assessed using creatinine excretion. Although strength, muscle size, power, and body composition improved in both groups, there were no significant differences between groups. The investigators suggested that any benefit of chromium picolinate was minimal. In a recent small ($n = 19$), 8-wk, randomized, double-blind, placebo-controlled study, this same dose of chromium had no significant benefit on lipids, insulin sensitivity, or body composition in healthy older (63–77 yr of age) men and women of normal body weight (Amato et al., 2000).

3.7.3. Diabetes

The pharmacologic effects of chromium picolinate have been investigated in type 2 diabetes patients (Anderson et al., 1997). In this study, 180 type 2 diabetic patients, aged 35–65 yr, with fasting blood glucose levels of 130–275 mg/dL, 2-h blood glucose levels of 169–300 mg/dL, and HbA$_{1c}$ values of 8–12% were enrolled in the study. These patients were of normal height, weight, and BMI and had had diabetes for less than 10 yr. Twenty-two of the subjects were taking no medication for treatment of diabetes. Nine patients were taking insulin, and several were on more than one medication. Patients were randomized to receive either placebo, chromium picolinate 100 μg twice daily, or chromium picolinate 500 μg twice daily for 4 mo. A fasting blood sample and a blood sample after a 2-h 75 g glucose challenge were taken at baseline, at 2 mo, and at 4 mo. Data were analyzed using three-factor repeated measures. Patients receiving either dose of chromium picolinate (100 or 500 µg twice daily) had significant reductions in HbA_{1c}, fasting insulin values and 2-h insulin values after 4 mo of treatment. Patients receiving chromium picolinate 500 µg twice daily also showed significant decreases in fasting glucose and two-hour glucose levels ($p < 0.0001$) after 2 and 4 mo of treatment.

This study was excluded from a subsequent meta-analysis of studies of chromium picolinate for management of glycemic control, in part because the subjects may have been chromium-deficient. This meta-analysis concluded that chromium picolinate has no effect on glucose or insulin concentrations in nondiabetic persons, and that more study is needed to clarify its effect in patients with diabetes (Althuis et al., 2002).

Corticosteroids can reduce insulin sensitivity. This adverse effect may be secondary to the increased urinary chromium loss documented to occur with these agents. Administration of chromium 600 µg/d as chromium picolinate to three patients with corticosteroid-induced diabetes resulted in a clinically significant decrease in fasting plasma glucose (from 250 to 150 mg/dL), as well as a decrease in the need for antidiabetic medications. A double-blind controlled study is needed to confirm these results (Ravina et al., 1999).

3.8. PHARMACOKINETICS

In a pharmacokinetic study of eight volunteers, the estimated amount of chromium (III) absorbed after a 400-µg dose of chromium picolinate was 1.5–5.2%. The peak urinary chromium concentration was 3.58–19.13 µg chromium/g creatinine (Gargas et al., 1994). Chromium (III) kinetics can be described by either a 3-compartment or a 10-compartment kinetic model (Stearns et al., 1995a). Both models give similar results, but the 3-compartment model is more straightforward; therefore, the 3-compartment model is discussed. After absorption, chromium (III) is proposed to distribute rapidly into three compartments. The first compartment is considered the fast eliminating compartment. Forty percent of the ingested chromium distributes into this compartment and is eliminated with a half-life of 7 h. Chromium is also thought to be eliminated from the second compartment with a half-life of 15 d. Fifty percent of the ingested chromium distributes into this compartment. The third compartment is considered to be a slow eliminating compartment. The elimination half-life is 3 yr, and 10% of ingested chromium is thought to distribute to this compartment. The elimination rate constants for the first, second, and third compartments are 876 yr^{-1}, 16.9 yr^{-1}, and 0.231 yr^{-1} respectively (Gargas et al., 1994).

In one study rats were given a single injection of chromium chloride hexahydrate. Four days later the rats showed accumulations of chromium (III) in the spleen, kidney, testes, and epididymis (Hopkins, 1965). A similar study, performed in rabbits, demonstrated that after three weeks of daily $Cr(NO_3)_3 \cdot 9H_2O$ intraperitoneal injections, levels of chromium (III) in the liver were eightfold higher than in controls, and after an additional 3 wk of injections, liver levels of chromium were 68-fold higher than controls. However, after 6 wk, blood chromium (III) levels were sixfold higher for the chromium (III)-treated animals compared with controls. These data suggest that blood concentrations are not directly correlative with chromium (III) accumulation in tissues and that after continuous, long-term use, tissue accumulation of chromium (III) can occur (Tandon et al., 1978).

3.9. ADVERSE EFFECTS AND TOXICITY

Although no adverse effects were reported in most studies performed to evaluate the potential uses of chromium picolinate, none of these studies evaluated adverse effects systematically; therefore, these studies may have missed actual adverse effects associated with chromium picolinate. Clinical studies need to be performed to determine the short-term and long-term adverse effects associated with the use of chromium picolinate. Mild gastrointestinal disturbances are generally the primary adverse effects described (Huszonek, 1993). Case reports describing chromium picolinate-associated toxicities have since been published.

A 29-yr-old man who had been taking Humulin-N® 9 U/d since age 20 for type 2 diabetes experienced a hypoglycemic episode after beginning a regimen of chromium 200 µg (as the picolinate salt) twice weekly and 300 µg three times weekly to enhance his body-building efforts. Although this patient's blood glucose levels normally ranged from 90 to 120 mg/dL, a blood glucose of approximately 30 mg/dL was noted by emergency medical personnel. Accompanying symptoms included mental status changes, weakness, and incoordination. After the patient had been evaluated by a neurologist and an occupational medicine specialist and had undergone neuropsychiatric evaluation, the patient's family physician discovered the patient had been taking chromium picolinate. The family physician discontinued the patient's insulin and increased his chromium dose to 1000 µg/d. The patient's blood glucose ranged from 90 to 140 mg/dL on this dose, but after 6 mo of therapy, he again experienced a hypoglycemic episode. Chromium picolinate was discontinued, and glyburide was substituted with no further reports of hypoglycemia, although duration of follow-up was not specified (Bunner and McGinnis, 1998). It should be noted that the patient's first episode of hypoglycemia occurred after a particularly physically demanding day, and his decreased requirement for exogenous insulin may have been due, at least in part, to increased body-building efforts.

A 35-yr-old man took chromium picolinate 200–400 µg on three separate occasions, and each time, he experienced progressively worse central nervous system symptoms. The patient reported that 1 h after taking chromium picolinate 200 µg, he experienced a brief sensation that he described as "feeling funny." Three months later, the patient took chromium picolinate 400 µg and reported "disruption" or "short-circuiting" of his thought process within 1 h. Several months later, approximately 90 min after taking chromium picolinate 400 µg, he felt as though his thought processes were slowed, and he had to concentrate very hard while driving to work, having even to slow down and pull off the road. He recovered within 2 h. The patient was not taking any medications, had no medical illness, and did not abuse controlled substances. He was undergoing psychotherapy for marital difficulties but had no acute stresses associated with these central nervous system symptoms. Blood glucose was not checked (Huszonek, 1993).

Dermatologic reactions have been associated with chromium picolinate ingestion. In one case (Young et al., 1999), a 32-yr-old man presented with a confluent, red, pustular exanthum of his trunk and proximal extremities 4 d after beginning supplementation with chromium picolinate 1 mg/d. The eruption was most serious in the antecubital and popliteal fossae. Other symptoms included sore throat and malaise. Findings on physical exam included fever (37.4°C), tender cervical lymphadenopathy, and mild redness of the throat. A 2-wk prednisone taper was prescribed, and the eruption resolved within 1 wk, followed by desquamation of the affected areas. Acute generalized exanthematous pustulosis (AGEP), a type IV delayed hypersensitivity reaction, was diagnosed after ruling out bacterial and fungal infections. Patch tests performed using chromium picolinate and potassium dichromate were negative, a finding that occurs in approximately 50% of cases of AGEP.

Fowler (2000) described red scaly patches that appeared on the lower legs, ankles, hands, and wrists of a 35-yr-old man after several weeks' ingestion of various vitamin and mineral supplements. Reactions to patch testing with potassium dichromate were 2+ at 48 and 96 h, with accompanying flare of dermatitis at affected sites. The patient had a history of an allergic reaction to a leather watch band. This was thought to be the source of his sensitization to chromium, since most leather is tanned with chromates.

A 49-yr-old woman took chromium picolinate 600 µg/d for 6 wk for weight reduction. Her only other medications were antihypertensives. Five mo later, she presented with a serum creatinine (SCr) of 5.9 mg/dL and blood urea nitrogen (BUN) of 74 mg/dL. Renal function tests performed 2 yr previously had been normal. Urinalysis revealed protein 30 mg/dL, trace blood, 0–1leukocytes per high power field, and 24-h protein 782 mg. Renal biopsy revealed chronic intersitial nephritis. Prednisone 60 mg/d was prescribed, and after 2 mo, her SCr had decreased to 3.8 mg/L (Wasser et al., 1997a). Although hexavalent chromium, an oxidant, has caused acute tubular necrosis in occupational exposures, this is the first case report of renal failure associated with trivalent chromium (McCarty, 1997). Although McCarty (1997) maintains that trivalent chromium is not a nephrotoxin and is poorly absorbed, the picolinic acid salt crosses biologic membranes and achieves high blood concentrations. In addition, hexavalent chromium is converted intracellularly to trivalent chromium, so it cannot be assumed to be inoccuous (Wasser et al., 1997b).

Another subsequent report involved a 33-yr-old woman who presented to the hospital with weight loss, anemia, thrombocytopenia, hemolysis, liver dysfunction, and renal failure after taking chromium picolinate 1200–2400 µg daily for 4–5 mo. She had a 1–2 wk history of severe fatigue and malaise, which had worsened over the previous 3 d. She complained of fever, chills, abdominal pain, nausea, and vomiting. She had just recently been diagnosed with schizophrenia and depression and was being treated with paroxetine and monthly fluphenazine injections until 2 wk prior to admission. She had also lost approximately 10 pounds within the 2 wk prior to admission and a total of 25 pounds over the previous 3 mo. She was diagnosed with an eating disorder while in the hospital. Plasma chromium concentration obtained on day 2 of her admission was 4.6 µg/mL (normal 0.1–2.1 µg/mL). On admission, alkaline phosphatase was 131 IU/L, AST was 1274 IU/L, ALT was 992 IU/L, and bilirubin was (3.7 mg/dL). Her BUN and serum creatinine were elevated at 152 mg/dL and 5.3 mg/dL, respectively, and her urine output was low (100–200 mL/d). She also had a serum chromium level of 4.6 µg/mL. Urinalysis revealed brown, cloudy urine containing muddy brown casts, red blood cells, white blood cells, 2+ bacteria, protein greater than 300 mg/dL, glucose 100 mg/dL, urobilinogen 1 EU/L, nitrates, and leukocytes. Urine pH was 5. The urine culture grew *Citrobacter koseri*; she was treated with ofloxacin for 7 d.

This patient required hemodialysis for 2 wk. An abdominal/renal ultrasound was performed and revealed enlarged kidneys consistent with an acute infiltrative process. Upon discharge 26 d later, the patient's alkaline phosphatase was 116 IU/mL, AST was 17 IU/mL, bilirubin was 0.6 mg/dL, BUN was 40 mg/dL, serum creatinine was 1.3 mg/dL, and urine output was 4000 mL/d . However, her serum chromium level, which was last drawn on day 12, was still elevated at 5.3 μg/mL. The final diagnosis was hemolysis, acute liver failure, and renal failure secondary to chromium toxicity. Reversal of all presenting symptoms had occurred at 1-yr follow-up (Cerulli et al., 1998).

Another case report (Martin and Fuller, 1998) described a 24-yr-old, 67-kg woman who took chromium picolinate 1200 μg (Ultra Chromium Slim Plus and Fat Inhibitor®) for 6 d. She presented to the hospital with dehydration, a 4-d history of diffuse muscle weakness, pain, and bilateral leg cramping. She had muscular hypertrophy with normal tone and complained of mild discomfort upon palpation of her quadriceps. The patient also had increased creatine kinase levels (22,260 U/L), liver enzymes (ALT 158 U/L and AST 697 U/L), and lactate dehydrogenase (1914 U/L). Glucose was 65 mg/dL. Her BUN and serum creatinine were normal at 14 mg/dL and 0.9 mg/dL, respectively. Urinalysis revealed a clear yellow specimen with myoglobin less than 27 μg/L. The sample was negative for protein and drugs. The patient was treated with cyclobenzaprine 10 mg, ibuprofen 800 mg, lactated Ringer's solution, and Tylenol #3®. She was discharged after 4 d with a creatine kinase of 9952 U/L, lactase dehydrogenase of 1801 U/L, ALT of 129 U/L, and AST of 86 U/L. This patient's diagnosis was chromium picolinate-induced rhabdomyolysis. The mechanism by which chromium picolinate may have induced rhabdomyolysis in unknown. However, the authors of this case report suggested that chromium picolinate's effects on glucose metabolism, amino acid uptake, and lean body mass may be possible explanations. Doses above the recommended dietary allowance should not be used pending further safety data.

The hexavalent form of chromium is a known carcinogen in both humans and animals (Stearns et al., 1995b). The trivalent form of chromium is considered "not classifiable as to carcinogenic potential" by the International Agency for Research on Cancer (Stearns et al., 1995a). Stearns and colleagues (1995b) examined the ability of chromium picolinate to cause chromosomal damage in Chinese hamster ovary cells. This study examined soluble and particulate forms of chromium picolinate. Chromium picolinate in solution at doses of 0.050, 0.10, 0.50, and 1.0 mM produced chromosomal damage 3- to 18-fold more than control. Chromium picolinate at particulate doses of 8.0 μg/cm^2 (equivalent to a 0.10 mM soublized dose) and 40 μg/cm^2 produced chromosomal damage 4- to 16-fold greater than controls. Further evaluation of this study demonstrated that picolinic acid was the harmful component of this particular formulation (Stearns et al., 1995b), but there is additional evidence supporting the carcinogenic effect of chromium (III). Many experts believe that chromium (III) is also responsible for chromium (IV)-induced cancers (Stearns et al., 1995a). Although chromium (IV) is believed to be 100 times more toxic than chromium (III) (Cerulli, et al., 1998), chromium (IV) is reduced to chromium (III) once it enters the cells. Because chromium (III) is slowly excreted from cells, accumulation occurs (Stearns et al., 1995a). Chromium (III) can then be reduced to chromium (II), which is susceptible to oxidation. The oxidized species can in turn generate hydroxyl radicals, which can damage DNA. Hydroxyl radicals can also be formed via interaction between chromium (III) and hydrogen peroxide. These reactions have been demonstrated in vitro at physiologically plausible chromium (III) concentrations (Speetjens et al., 2000).

3.10. INTERACTIONS

There are currently no reported drug interactions associated with the use of chromium picolinate. This may reflect the lack of large clinical studies and drug interaction studies.

3.11. REPRODUCTION

Although it is an essential mineral, there is insufficient information to assess whether doses of chromium above the recommended adequate intake for pregnant women (30 µg/d) have any harmful effects. It should not be taken at doses above the upper intake limit during pregnancy. Supplementation with the picolinate salt should be avoided during pregnancy.

3.12. BIOFLUID ANALYSIS

Chromium and picolinic acid (the resulting acid from cleavage of the ester bond) are measured by separate technologies and thus must be conducted as separate assays. Chromium has been measured in urine samples using atomic absorption spectrometry (Veillon et al., 1982). In this method, standard stock solutions are prepared using demineralized water and isothermally distilled hydrochloric acid (or high-purity HCl from commercial sources). Dilutions to the appropriate concentrations are made with 1 *M* HCl. A 25-µL aliquot of patient sample or calibration curve stock solution is then placed in the instrument and the furnace program is started. The furnace program is set for the following sequence:

Step 1. Ramp to 100°C over 15 s and hold for 20 s.
Step 2. Ramp to 130°C over 10 s and hold for 20 s.
Step 3. Ramp to 1200°C over 15 s and hold for 60 s.
Step 4. Ramp to 2700°C immediately and hold for 4 s (to atomize the sample).
Step 5. Hold at 2700°C for an additional 4 s to clean out the system.

The source for the instrument is a chromium hollow cathode discharge tube (25 mA) with a tungsten-halogen lamp as a background corrector. The wavelength is 357.9 nm, and the slit is set at 0.7 nm.

The picolinic acid portion resulting from the molecule can be measured by high-performance liquid chromatography (HPLC). Following the method of Dazzi and associates (2001), samples are first spiked with methyl-DL-tryptophan (internal standard) and then subjected to protein precipitation with cold 2% perchloric acid. Samples are then centrifuged for 5 min at 13,000g, and the resulting pellet is discarded. The supernatant is then neutralized with 0.4 *M* KOH, filtered through a 0.45-μm filter, and analyzed on the HPLC system. Analytes are separated using a SymmetryShield (150 × 3.9 mm) column and detected with an ultraviolet detector set at a wavelength of 265 nm. The mobile phase consists of 2% methanol/1 m*M* tetrabutylammonium hydrogen sulfate/30 m*M* phosphate, pH 8.0 flowing at a rate of 1 mL/min. All components of interest are eluted in 15 min. If multiple samples are to be analyzed, the column can be washed by switching to a wash solution of 50% methanol/phosphate buffer, pH 8.0, for an additional 15 min and then reequilibrating with the original mobile phase for an additional 15 min. It may be necessary to decrease the flow rate during the early stages of the wash because of excessive column backpressure owing to the methanol concentrations in the wash solution.

An additional method for measurement of picolinic acid has also been reported using either liquid chromatography-mass spectrometry or gas chromatography-mass spectrometry with outstanding sensitivity (Naritsin et al., 1995). This method may be useful if extremely low concentrations of picolinic acid are to be measured.

3.13. REGULATORY STATUS

Chromium picolinate is regulated under the Dietary Health Supplement Act as a dietary supplement.

3.14. SUMMARY

- Chromium picolinate plays a role in the metabolism of fats, carbohydrates, and proteins, but its therapeutic utility in persons with diabetes or hyperlipidemia and normal chromium levels remains to be seen. Its effects on body composition, if any, are probably small.
- Chomium picolinate can accumulate intracellularly, where chromium (III) can exist for years.
- There is evidence that chromium picolinate is a carcinogen.
- Chromium picolinate is well tolerated in clinical trials. Case reports associating its use with nephrotoxicity, rhabdomyolysis, and cognitive impairment have been published.

REFERENCES

Allen LV. Handbook of Nonprescription Drugs, 12th ed. Washington, DC: American Pharmaceutical Association, 2000.

Althius MD, Jordan NE, Ludington, EA, Wittes JT. Glucose and insulin responses to dietary chromium supplements: a meta-analysis. Am J Clin Nutr 2002;76:148–55.

Amato P, Morales AJ, Yen SS. Effects of chromium picolinate supplementation on insulin sensitivity, serum lipids, and body composition in healthy, nonobese, older men and women. J Gerontol A Biol Sci Med Sci 2000;55:7260–3.

Anderson RA, Cheng N, Bryden NA, et al. Elevated intakes of supplemental chromium improve glucose and insulin variables in individuals with Type 2 Diabetes. Diabetes 1997;46:1786–91.

Bunner SP, McGinnis R. Chromium-induced hypoglycemia [letter]. Pschosomatics 1998;39:298–9.

Campbell WW, Joseph LJO, Davey SL, et al. Effects of resistance training and chromium picolinate on body composition and skeletal muscle in older men. J Appl Physiol 1999;86:29–39.

Cerulli J, Grabe DW, Gauthier I, Malone M, McGoldrick MD. Chromium picolinate toxicity. Ann Pharmacother 1998;32:428–31.

Clancy SP, Clarkson PM, DeCheke ME, et al. Effects of chromium picolinate supplementation on body composition, strength, and urinary chromium loss in football players. Int J Sports Med 1994;4:142–53.

Dazzi C, Candiano G, Massazza S, Ponzetto A, Varesio L. New high-performance liquid chromatographic method for the detection of picolinic acid in biological fluids. J Chromatogr B Biomed Sci Appl 2001;751:61–68.

Evans GW. The effect of chromium picolinate on insulin controlled parameters in humans. Int J Biosocial Med Res 1989;11:163–80.

Fowler JF. Systemic contact dermatitis caused by oral chromium picolinate. Cutis 2000;65:116.

Gargas ML, Norton RL, Paustenbach DJ, Finley BL. Urinary excretion of chromium by humans following ingestion of chromium picolinate. Drug Metab Dispos 1994;22:522–9.

Hallmark MA, Reynolds TH, DeSouza CA, et al. Effects of chromium and resistive training on muscle strength and body composition. Med Sci Sports Exerc 1996;28:139–44.

Hasten DL, Rome EP, Franks DB, Hegsted M. Effect of chromium picolinate on beginning weight training students. Int J Sport Nutr 1992;2:343–50.

Hopkins LL. Distribution in the rat of physiological amounts of Cr (III) with time. Am J Physiol 1965;209:731–5.

Huszonek J. Over-the-counter chromium picolinate [letter]. Am J Psychiatry 1993;150:1560–1.

Institute of Medicine. Dietary reference intakes for vitamin A, vitamin K, arsenic, boron, chromium, copper, iodine, iron, manganese, molybdenum, nickel, silicon, vanadium, and zinc. 2002. Available from: URL: http://www.nap.edu/books/0309072794/html/. Accessed 1-21-0002.

Kaats GR, Blum K, Fisher JA, Adelman JA. Effects of chromium picolinate supplementation on body composition: a randomized, double-masked, placebo-controlled study. Curr Ther Res 1996;57:747–56.

Kaats GR, Blum K, Pulin D, Keith SC, Wood R. A randomized, double-masked, placebo-controlled study of the effects of chromium picolinate supplementation on body composition: a replication and extension of a previous study. Curr Ther Res 1998;59:379–88.

Lukaski HC, Bolonchuk WW, Siders WA, Milne DB. Chromium supplementation and resistance training: effects on body composition, strength, and trace element status of men. Am J Clin Nutr 1996;63:954–65.

Martin WR, Fuller RE. Suspected chromium picolinate-induced rhabdomyolysis. Pharmacotherapy 1998;18:860–2.

McCarty MF. Over-the-counter chromium and renal failure [letter]. Ann Intern Med 1997;127:654–5.

Naritsin DB, Boni RL, Markey SP. Pentafluorobenzylation method for quantification of acidic tryptophan metabolites using electron capture negative ion mass spectrometry. Anal Chem 1995;67:863–70.

Philen RM, Ortiz DU, Auerbach SB, Falk H. Survey of advertising for nutritional supplements in health and bodybuilding magazines. JAMA 1992;268:1008–11.

Press RI, Geller J, Evans GW. The effect of chromium picolinate on serum cholesterol and apolipoprotein fractions in human subjects. West J Med 1990;152:41–5.

Ravina A, Slezak L, Mirsky N, Bryden NA, Anderson RA. Reversal of corticosteroids-induced diabetes mellitus with supplemental chromium. Diabet Med 1999;16:164–7.

Speetjens JK, Collins RA, Vincent JB, Woski SA. The nutritional supplement chromium (III) tris(picolinate) cleaves DNA. Chem Res Toxicol 1999;12:483–7.

Stearns DM, Belbruno JJ, Wetterhahn KE. A prediction of chromium(III) accumulation in humans form chromium dietary supplements. FASEB J 1995a;9:1650–7.

Stearns DM, Wise JP, Patierno SR, Wetterhahn KE. Chromium(III) picolinate produces chromosome damage in Chinese hamster ovary cells. FASEB J 1995b;9:1643–9.

Tandon SK, Saxena DK, Gaur JS, Chandra SV. Comparative toxicity of trivalent and hexavalent chromium: alterations in blood and liver. Environ Res 1978;15:90–9.

Trent LK, Thieding-Cancel D. Effects of chromium picolinate on body composition. J Sports Med Phys Fitness 1995;35:273–80.

Veillon C, Patterson KY, Bryden NA. Chromium in urine as measured by atomic absorption spectrometry. Clin Chem 1982;28:2309–11.

Wasser WG, Feldman NS, D'Agati VD. Chronic renal failure after ingestion of over-the-counter chromium picolinate [letter]. Ann Intern Med 1997a;126:410.

Wasser WG, Yusuf SA, D'Agati VD. In response [letter]. Ann Intern Med 1997b;127:656.

Young PC, Turiansky GW, Bonner MW, Benson PM. Acute generalized exanthematous pustulosis indued by chromium picolinate. J Am Acad Dermatol 1999;41:820–3.

Chapter 4

Coenzyme Q10 (Ubiquinone, Ubidecarenone)

Melanie Johns Cupp and Timothy S. Tracy

4.1. HISTORY

Moore and colleagues identified coenzyme Q10 in 1940 (Greenberg and Frishman, 1988). In 1957, coenzyme Q10 was isolated from beef heart by Dr. Frederick Crane. Karl Folkers, a scientist at Merck Sharpe and Dohme, elucidated its chemical formula the following year. In 1972, Dr. Folkers and an Italian researcher identified a deficiency of coenzyme Q10 in human heart disease (Sinatra, 1999). Based on data from only a small number of patients, the Japanese government approved coenzyme Q10 for the treatment of congestive heart failure in 1974 (Khatta et al., 2000). In 1978 a Nobel Prize was awarded for the discovery of coenzyme Q10's role in energy transport. The 1980s saw an increase in the number of clinical studies of coenzyme Q10 (Sinatra, 1999). From 1977 through 1991, Dr. Folkers and other researchers published *Biomedical and Clinical Aspects of Coenzyme Q*, a work of six volumes in which much often-cited coenzyme Q10 research was published. Coenzyme Q10 capsules were advertised to health care professionals by Doctor's Mutual Service Company of California in the late 1980s. Promotion of coenzyme Q10 to consumers in the U.S. began in the late 1990s.

4.2. CHEMICAL STRUCTURE

The chemical structure of coenzyme Q10 (ubiquinone) can be seen in Fig. 4-1.

4.3. CURRENT PROMOTED USES

Depressed coenzyme Q10 levels have been documented in cardiovascular disease (Overvad et al., 1999), and supplementation has attracted the interest of cardiologists for the treatment of a variety of cardiovascular disorders. In fact, coenzyme Q10

From: *Forensic Science: Dietary Supplements: Toxicology and Clinical Pharmacology*
Edited by: M. J. Cupp and T. S. Tracy © Humana Press Inc., Totowa, New Jersey

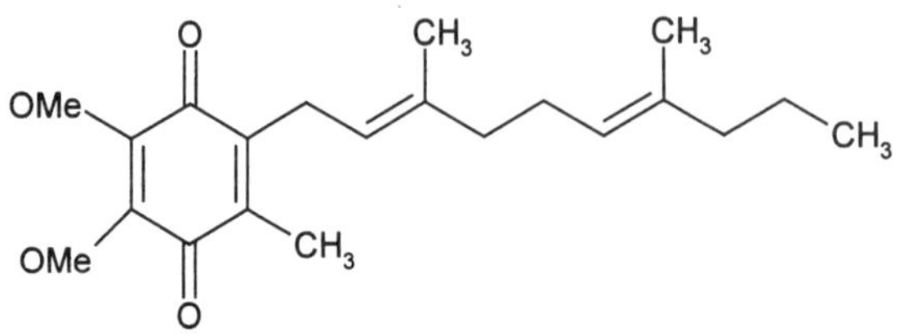

Fig. 1. Chemical structure of coenzyme Q10.

is on formulary in at least one hospital in the United States (Sinatra, 1999). Although dietary intake and biosynthesis of coenzyme Q10 appear to meet the daily requirement for coenzyme Q10 in otherwise healthy persons (Overvad et al., 1999), coenzyme Q10 supplements are promoted to consumers as a means of improving heart function, lipid levels, energy efficiency, body composition, athletic performance, and immune function.

4.4. SOURCES AND CHEMICAL COMPOSITION

Coenzyme Q10 is a fat-soluble quinone (Greenberg and Frishman, 1990). It is ubiquitous in foods, and the average dietary intake is 5–10 mg/d (Sinatra, 1999). Assuming a normal diet, 60% of plasma coenzyme Q10 is of endogenous origin (Palomaki et al., 1998). Coenzyme Q10 is biosynthesized in all human cells from tyrosine and acetyl CoA; the quinone ring is synthesized from tyrosine; and the side chain originates from acetyl CoA, using the same biosynthetic pathway as cholesterol (Bargossi et al., 1994). Vitamin B6, vitamin C, vitamin B2, folic acid, vitamin B12, nicotinamide, pantothenic acid, 5,6,2,8-tetrahydrobiopterin, and trace elements are all cofactors in its synthesis (Folkers and Simonsen, 1995). Commercially available products are purportedly produced by the fermentation of beets and sugar cane by particular yeast strains (Fuke et al., 2000). In human tissues, except the brain and lungs, coenzyme Q10 is found chiefly in its reduced form, ubiquinol, which acts as an antioxidant (Palomaki et al., 1998). Coenzyme Q10 is found mainly in the mitochondria (Greenberg and Frishman, 1990).

4.5. PRODUCTS AVAILABLE

Popular formulations include powder-filled capsules, tablets, and (more commonly) softgels containing coenzyme Q10 suspended in soybean oil or vitamin E. In vitro dissolution of these products has generally been found to be poor. The Tishcon Corporation, the manufacturer of Q-Gel®, has performed studies demonstrating that their product has superior bioavailability compared with tablets, capsules, and other softgels (Chopra et al., 1998). This product was used in several clinical studies reviewed here. Coenzyme Q10 is also found in several topical antiaging cosmetic formulations.

The independent laboratory ConsumerLab.com has tested the potency and purity of 29 brands of coenzyme Q10 products commonly available through catalogs, retail stores, multilevel marketing companies, and the Internet. Only one of the products tested failed to meet ConsumerLab.com's standards because it contained only 17% of the labeled amount of coenzyme Q10 (ConsumerLab.com, 2002). A list of coenzyme Q10 products that passed testing, as well as details about testing methodology, is available at the web site www.consumerlabs.com.

4.6. Physiologic Role

Coenzyme Q10 is involved in mitochondrial electron transport and thus is vital to cellular respiration. It has membrane-stabilizing activity and acts as an antioxidant (Greenberg and Frishman, 1990). The mechanism of coenzyme Q10's antioxidant effects may be direct as well as indirect; it may act directly by scavenging free radicals (molecules with an unpaired electron that makes the molecule highly reactive) or indirectly by regenerating oxidized α-tocopherol. If this second mechanism is important, plasma α-tocopherol concentrations may be a rate-limiting factor in the antioxidant action of coenzyme Q10 (Kaikkonen et al., 1997). Because coenzyme Q10 acts as a free radical scavenger, it may prevent atherosclerosis by virtue of its ability to inhibit oxidation of low-density lipoproteins (LDLs) (Mortensen et al., 1997; Palomaki et al, 1998; Khatta et al., 2000).

4.7. In Vitro Effects and Animal Data

The ability of various concentrations of coenzyme Q10 to scavenge superoxide ($O^{2-}\cdot$) and hydroxyl (OH·) radicals in vitro was measured using electron spin resonance spectroscopy (Zhou et al., 1999). The hydroxyl radicals were generated using the Fenton reaction, and the superoxide radicals were generated using the xanthine/ xanthine oxidase system. Coenzyme Q10 was shown to scavenge the hydroxyl radicals in a dose-dependent manner, but it was ineffective in scavenging superoxide radicals. Coenzyme Q10's ability to scavenge free radicals results in its antioxidant, anti-ischemic, and membrane-stabilizing activities (Greenberg and Frishman, 1988).

The effects of intravenous administration of a water-soluble, liposomal coenzyme Q10 on serum and myocardial coenzyme Q10 concentrations, as well as recovery of function, aerobic efficiency, and oxidant stress were studied in adult male Sprague-Dawley rats after an ischemia/reperfusion injury (Niibori et al., 1998). Recovery of function was defined by developed left ventricular pressure (DP) determined using an intraventricular balloon and by coronary flow measured using a digital flow meter. Aerobic efficiency was defined as DP/MVO2, where MVO2 = oxygen consumed per minute per gram of myocardium. Creatine kinase (CK) activity was used as a measure of oxidant stress.

Coenzyme Q10 10 mg/kg or placebo was administered 15, 30, and 60 min prior to removal of the hearts. The hearts were then perfused and subjected to ischemia for 25 min, followed by reperfusion for 40 min. All statistical analysis was performed using ANOVA, and statistical significance was accepted if $p < 0.05$. Pre-ischemic serum coenzyme Q10 levels in control rats and in rats treated at 15, 30, and 60 minutes were all statistically different from each other ($p < 0.03$, ANOVA). Pre-ischemic myocardial coenzyme Q10 levels in rats treated at 30 min differed significantly from both the control rats and the rats treated 15 min prior to heart removal ($p < 0.03$). DP at the end of reperfusion was significantly better for the treatment rats in the 30-min group compared with the control rats or the rats in the 15-min- group ($p < 0.03$). Myocardial efficiency in the rats in the 30-min group was better than all other groups ($p < 0.001$). CK levels were higher in all treatment groups compared with controls ($p < 0.04$), reflecting less diminishment of CK activity after reperfusion, or perhaps increased cell damage. The investigators concluded that serum and myocardial levels of coenzyme Q10 can be increased with intravenous administration of a liposomal formulation; that myocardial levels correlate better than serum levels with protection from ischemia/reperfusion injury; and that intravenous coenzyme Q10 administration prior to an ischemic insult improves myocardial function and efficiency and decreases oxidative injury.

The effect of coenzyme Q10 supplementation on hypertensive rats has been studied (Iwamoto et al., 1974). Thirty-five rats were divided into three groups. One group served as a control group, and the other two groups were unilaterally nephrectomized. Normal saline and deoxycorticosterone 25 mg/kg were administered to the nephrectomized rats to induce hypertension. One of the two nephrectomized groups was administered coenzyme Q10 50 mg/kg for 4 wk, followed by 100 mg/kg for 2 wk. Systolic blood pressure was measured weekly. Leukocyte, heart, kidney, and liver mitochondrial succinate dehydrogenase-coenzyme Q10 reductase activity, an indicator of coenzyme Q10, was measured at the end of the 6-week study. The untreated hypertensive rats had lower leukocyte succinate dehydrogenase-coenzyme Q10 reductase activity than control rats ($p < 0.05$), but this deficiency was not noted in the treated hypertensive rats. Similarly, liver and kidney succinate dehydrogenase-coenzyme Q10 reductase activity was higher in the treated hypertensive rats ($p < 0.01$) than in the control group or in the untreated rats. The mean weight of the hearts of the untreated hypertensive rats was greater ($p < 0.05$) than that of control rats, whereas heart enlargement was not noted in treated rats. The investigators hypothesized that hypertension causes an increased need for coenzyme Q10 that can be met through supplementation but not biosynthesis. Although other investigators reported that coenzyme Q10 reduced blood pressure in rats with hypertension induced by saline and deosycorticosterone, these investigators (Iwamoto et al., 1974) did not report the effect of coenzyme Q10 supplementation on blood pressure.

Other animal and in vitro findings deserve brief mention. Coenzyme Q10 has been shown to protect against doxorubicin-associated myocardial damage in isolated animal hearts (Ohhara et al., 1981), and incubation of human sperm with coenzyme Q10 increased motility in sperm with impaired motility, but not in sperm with normal motility (Lewin and Lavon, 1997).

4.8. CLINICAL STUDIES

There have been literally hundreds of investigations of coenzyme Q10 in humans, including studies of the relationship between coenzyme Q10 levels and human disease. A representative sample of trials of oral coenzyme Q10 supplementation has been chosen for review here.

4.8.1. Heart Failure

Decreased coenzyme Q10 concentrations in both the blood and myocardium of patients with heart failure were noted in studies performed in the 1970s and 1980s. This deficiency may worsen the compromised contractility of myocardial cells, and in fact the degree of deficiency correlates with the severity of heart failure clinically. Patients in New York Heart Association (NYHA) functional class III or IV have significantly lower blood levels of coenzyme Q10 than patients with functional class I or II. It should be noted, however, that some patients with class III or IV failure have normal levels, and patients with the most severe organ congestion do not always have the lowest coenzyme Q10 levels (Langsjoen et al., 1985). The failing heart also demonstrates oxidative stress, which could theoretically be ameliorated by coenzyme Q10's antioxidant effects.

Many studies of both oral and parenteral coenzyme Q10 supplementation in heart failure have been performed and exhibit conflicting results. Studies showing benefit have generally used doses of 100 or 150 mg/d. Problems with these studies include inadequate numbers of study subjects to detect changes in mortality or other clinical endpoints, lack of blinding, use of subjective endpoints, measurement of ejection fraction using echocardiography rather than radionuclide ventriculography, inclusion of minimally symptomatic patients, and use of inappropriate statistics (Khatta et al., 2000). Measurement of plasma coenzyme Q10 levels is important, particularly in studies showing no benefit, to demonstrate bioavailability of the product used (Sinatra, 1999); however, because coenzyme Q10 is primarily found intracellularly, some authors maintain that a lack of change in plasma levels with supplementation does not necessarily indicate poor bioavailability (Taggart et al., 1996). Because the treatment of heart failure has changed significantly over the years and now includes the use of β-blockers, findings of older studies or studies that included patients not treated according to contemporary medical standards may not be applicable to current practice. The result of several representative published studies follow.

Langsjoen and associates (1985) studied the effect of coenzyme Q10 supplementation in patients with stable NYHA functional class III or IV cardiomyopathy in a small double-blind study. Exclusion criteria were ischemic heart disease, alcoholism, or life-threatening illness. After a 4-wk stabilization period, 19 patients were randomized to conezyme Q10 100 mg/d or placebo for 12 wk and then crossed over to the alternate therapy for 12 wk. Conventional therapy was continued. The two groups were comparable in gender, age, chest X-ray findings, and medications. Chest X-ray and electrocardiogram (ECG) were performed at baseline and at weeks 16 and 28. Ejection fraction, stroke volume determined by impedence cardiograph, complete blood cell count (CBC), erythrocyte sedimentation rate, plasma protein and immunoglobuin concentrations, coenzyme Q10 blood levels, vitals, weight, and clinical status were assessed at baseline and at weeks 4, 16, and 28. Compliance was determined based on pill counts and patient interviews.

In the group that received coenzyme Q10 first, coenzyme Q10 blood levels were higher after 12 wk of supplementation compared with baseline ($p < 0.001$). Stroke volume was also higher after 12 wk of therapy. Twelve weeks after crossing over to placebo, coenzyme Q10 levels and stroke volume had decreased such that there were no statistically significant differences from baseline. Ejection fraction data were analyzed using ANOVA, *t*-test, and linear regression. Normal distribution of each dataset was confirmed. Contingency tables were analyzed with Chi-squared and Fisher's exact tests, as appropriate. Ejection fraction was significantly higher after 12 wk of coenzyme Q10 supplementation than after 12 wk of placebo ($p < 0.0001$). In the group randomized to receive coenzyme Q10 for the first 12 wk, there appeared to be some residual effect of coenzyme Q10 on ejection fraction during the subsequent placebo crossover, which diminished as coenzyme Q10 levels decreased. In the patients randomized to receive placebo for the first 12 wk, coenzyme Q10 levels did not increase significantly compared with baseline; however, after crossover to coenzyme Q10, blood levels were significantly higher after 12 wk of therapy ($p < 0.001$). The combination endpoint of cardiac size, pulmonary vascular markings, and ECG changes improved with coenzyme Q10 supplementation ($p < 0.01$). Eighteen of the 19 study patients reported subjective improvement with coenzyme Q10, primarily in regard to tolerance of physical activity. There were no statistically significant changes in vitals, CBC, erythrocyte sedimentation rate, plasma protein, or immunoglobulin concentration.

The statistically significant improvement in several endpoints in this small study was impressive. Although the method of determination of ejection fraction tended to overstimate ejection fraction compared with radionuclide scanning, the relative change in ejection fraction compared with baseline was valid. Inclusion of patients with baseline coenzyme Q10 deficiency as well as patients with normal levels may have affected the results, but owing to the small sample size, no conclusions can be made regarding the differential effect of supplementation on these two groups.

Morisco and colleagues (1993) performed a multicenter, double-blind, parallel study designed to assess the effects of coenzyme Q10 on mortality, life-threatening events, and hospitalization in patients with NYHA functional class III or IV. Patients with a history of myocardial infarction within the previous 3 months, unstable angina, need for cardiac revascularization, aortic or mitral valve stenosis requiring surgery, renal failure (serum creatine > 2 mg/dL), liver disease, or hematologic disorders were excluded. Six hundred forty-one patients were enrolled in the study. Patients were stratified based on gender, age, NYHA class, and cardiovascular drug therapy and were randomized to placebo or coenzyme Q10 2 mg/kg/d (50 mg two or three times daily). The two groups were similar in baseline characteristics. Follow-up was arranged after 3, 6, and 12 mo of therapy. At each visit, NYHA class was assessed, and patients were asked about hospitalization since the last visit, pulmonary edema, cardiac asthma, medication use, compliance, and adverse effects. An ECG was also obtained. Physicians and patients were also asked to rate the overall effects of treatment on a scale of 1 to 3. Statistical analysis was not described. Sixteen patients in the coenzyme Q10 group died, and 23 patients dropped out. Twenty-one patients in the placebo group died, and 18 dropped out. These differences were not statistically significant.

There was a progressive and statistically significant decrease in NYHA class in the coenzyme Q10 group at months 3, 6, and 12. No change occurred in the placebo group. There was also a progressive increase in both the patient and physician overall treatment scores in the coenzyme Q10 group, but not in the placebo group. The incidence of both pulmonary edema and cardiac asthma was significantly less in the coenzyme Q10 group ($p < 0.001$). The incidence of arrhythmias was higher in the placebo group ($p < 0.05$). Forty percent of patients in the placebo group and 20% of patients in the coenzyme Q10 group required hospitalization during the study ($p < 0.01$). Limitations of this study include inadequate sample size to detect a statistically significant decrease in mortality in the coenzyme Q10 group.

In a placebo-controlled double-blind randomized crossover study, the efficacy of coenzyme Q10 in congestive heart failure (CHF) was investigated in 30 patients aged 18–75 yr recruited from a heart transplant unit (Watson et al., 1999b). Patients had had heart failure for 41 ± 35 mo owing to ischemic or idiopathic dilated cardiomyopathy. Ejection fraction had been less than 35% for at least 3 mo. NYHA class was not specified. All were stable on the maximum angiotensin-converting enzyme (ACE) inhibitor dose that could be tolerated. Other medications included digoxin ($n = 24$), furosemide ($n = 28$), and hydralazine and/or nitrates ($n = 25$). Exclusion criteria were pregnancy, valvular heart disease, renal or hepatic disease, a history of alcohol or drug use, or echocardiography inadequate to document ejection fraction. Patients were randomized to receive coenzyme Q10 (Health World Limited, Brisbane, Australia) 33 mg three times daily for 12 wk, or placebo. After a 1-wk washout, patients were switched to the alternative therapy. Other medications were altered if clinically necessary. Echocardiography was performed after each 12-wk treatment phase and was evaluated by sonographers blinded to treatment. Swan-Ganz catheterization was also performed at baseline and at the end of each treatment. Quality of life (well-being and functional capacity) was assessed using the Minnesota "Living with Heart Failure" questionnaire. Plasma coenzyme Q10 levels, blood chemistry, liver function tests, and blood count were measured at baseline and after each treatment.

Despite an increase in coenzyme Q10 levels from 903 ± 345 nmol/L at baseline to 2029 ± 856 nmol/L, using multivariate ANOVA, after treatment the coenzyme Q10 group did not differ statistically from the placebo group in ejection fraction, cardiac volumes, cardiac index, wedge pressure, or systemic vascular resistance. Quality of life scores did not differ after coenzyme Q10 vs. placebo using Friedman two-way ANOVA. Coenzyme Q10 was well tolerated, and there were no changes in any blood tests performed. Reasons for the negative results of this study include selection of patients with end-stage disease, potential for failure to replenish myocardial coenzyme Q10 stores despite a twofold increase in plasma levels, and unavoidable changes in other medications that might have affected results. Although this study was relatively small, it possessed adequate power to detect an increase in ejection fraction of 5%.

A randomized, double-blind, placebo-controlled trial (Khatta et al., 2000) performed by clinicians at the University of Maryland School of Medicine examined the effects of coenzyme Q10 200 mg/d (PharmaNord, Sadlmadervej, Denmark) on ejection fraction measured by radionuclide ventriculography and peak oxygen consumption measured with a graded symptom-limited exercise test using the Naughton protocol. Inclusion criteria were NYHA class III or IV disease, ejection fraction less than 40%, and maximal oxygen consumption less than 17mL/kg or less than 50% predicted. These criteria were chosen to select patients having the greatest potential for improvement. For comparision, the investigators explained that a maximal oxygen consumption of less than 14 mL/min is one criterion for heart transplant, and the mean peak oxygen consumption of the patients enrolled in this study was 13.1 mL/min. Medications had remained stable for at least 1 mo prior to enrollment. Patients who had previously taken coenzyme Q10 were excluded. Fifty-five patients were randomized to receive coenyzme Q10 200 mg or placebo for 6 mo, at which time oxygen consumption and ejection fraction were again measured. Nine patients (4 placebo) did not complete the study, for reasons including death ($n = 3$), conditions that prevented them from exercising ($n = 4$), error in enrollment criteria ($n = 1$), and study withdraw due to unstated reasons ($n = 1$).

Serum coenzyme Q10 concentrations were measured at baseline and were found to be similar in both groups. With supplementation, levels increased from a mean of 0.95 μg/mL to 2.2 μg/mL at 6 mo in the treatment group. This was significantly different from the placebo group ($p < 0.001$, unpaired t-test). Maximal oxygen consumption did not improve significantly in either group, and the difference between the two groups was not significant. Exercise duration did not change significantly in either group. Coenzyme Q10 supplementation also did not improve ejection fraction. The sample size in this study may have been inadequate to detect significant differences.

4.8.2. Heart Surgery

Because oxygen free radicals play an important role in myocardial reperfusion injury, the ability of coenzyme Q10 to protect the myocardium against ischemia and reperfusion injury during open heart surgery has been studied. Based on the efficacy of coenzyme Q10 in preventing acute ischemic injury in animal models, Tanaka and colleagues (1982) performed a randomized study of coenzyme Q10 in 50 patients undergoing open heart surgery for treatment of valvular heart disease. Patients with heart failure or hypertension were excluded. Patients were randomized to receive no treatment or coenzyme Q10 30–60 mg beginning 6 d prior to surgery. All patients were taking digitalis and/or diuretics. All surgeries and postoperative care were performed by the same surgeons, who were blinded as to which patients had received coenzyme Q10. There was a lower incidence of low cardiac output in the coenzyme Q10 group ($p < 0.05$, Chi-squared test).

In an unblinded study (Chello et al., 1994), 40 patients scheduled for nonemergent coronary bypass surgery were randomized to coenzyme Q10 50 mg or no treatment (control group) three times daily for 7 d prior to surgery. All patients had stable angina and were taking β-blockers, nitrates, and/or calcium channel blockers. Coenzyme Q10 plasma levels were measured at baseline and after 7 d of treatment. Blood samples were also taken before, during, and after surgery for analysis of oxygen, oxygen saturation, carbon dioxide, pH, creatine kinase myocardial isoenzyme (CK-MB), and measures of oxidative stress (malondialdehyde and conjugated dienes). Postoperatively, hemodynamic monitoring was perfomed every 4 h for 24 h. Cardiac rhythm was monitored via Holter monitoring for 48 h postoperatively. ANOVA for repeated measures with Scheffe's multiple-comparison test was used to identify significant within-group changes over time. Between-group comparisons were made using the Mann-Whitney U test. Linear regression analysis was used to identify associations between variables. Fisher's exact test and t-tests were used when appropriate. The two groups of patients were similar in age, gender, NYHA class, medications, total bypass time, cross-clamp time, and number of grafts.

Baseline plasma coenzyme Q10 levels did not differ between patients in the control and coenzyme Q10 treatment group; however, levels were higher in the treatment group compared with the control group at day 7 ($p < 0.001$). During reperfusion, there was a significant increase in conjugated diene levels in the arterial blood 15 min after release of the aortic cross-clamp in the control group, but not in the treatment group. Arterial malondialdehyde and CK-MB levels increased in both groups during reperfusion, but levels were significantly higher in the control group ($p < 0.001$). There was a significant correlation between plasma malondialdehyde and CK-MB levels ($p < 0.01$). Postoperative hemodynamic variables did not differ between groups, although the control group required significantly higher dopamine doses than did the coenzyme Q10 group ($p < 0.001$). The incidence of serious ventricular arrhythmias was higher than in the control group ($p < 0.05$). Although this study was uncontrolled, the findings suggest that pretreatment with coenzyme Q10 protects the myocardium from oxidative damage during bypass surgery.

In a double-blind study (Chen et al., 1994), patients were randomized to no treatment or coenzyme Q10 (Eisai Pharmaceutical Corp., Tokyo, Japan) 150–200 mg/d for 5–7 d prior to surgery for valvular heart disease ($n = 17$) congenital heart disease ($n = 3$), coronary artery disease ($n = 1$), or Marfan's syndrome ($n = 1$). A total of 1000 mg of coenzyme Q10 was administered to each patient. All surgeries were performed by the same surgeon. The two groups were comparable in regard to demographics and preoperative cardiothoracic ratio. NYHA functional class, ventricular function, ischemic time, cardiopulmonary bypass time, and degree of systemic hypothermia were similar between groups. Hemodynamic and ultrastructural studies were used to assess myocardial preservation. Hemodynamic measurements included arterial pressure, pulse pressure, heart rate, and frequency of low cardiac output. "Low cardiac output" was defined as the need for dopamine 6 µg/kg/min or more for more than 12 h to maintain blood pressure above 90 mmHg after optimizing filling pressure. Biopsies were obtained from the right atria and left and right ventricles before arortic cross-clamping and at the end of ischemia. The biopsy specimens were examined with electron microscopy and were graded on a scale of 0 to 4 based on mitochondrial ischemic injury. Data were analyzed using nonpaired *t*-tests, paired *t*-tests, or Chi-square test analysis, as appropriate. Statistical significance was accepted if the p value was 0.05 or less.

Postoperative pulse pressure was higher in the coenzyme Q10 group ($p < 0.005$), suggesting better cardiac function in this group. Patients who did not receive coenzyme Q10 were more likely to have low cardiac output, but the difference between groups did not reach statistical significance. There was also a trend toward higher left atrial pressure in the patients who did not receive coenzyme Q10. In both groups, postoperative ischemic grade was higher than baseline in the right atrium and both ventricles. In the coenzyme Q10 group, postoperative left ventriular ischemic grade was lower than the postoperative right atrium ischemic grade ($p < 0.0005$), suggesting poorer preservation of atrial than ventricular myocardium. The investigators concluded that treatment with coenzyme Q10 prior to cardiac surgery favorably affects cardiac function and benefits the ventricular myocardium more than the atrial myocardium.

Because previous investigations had shown that supplementation with coenzyme Q10 improves cardiac function, reduces cardiac enzyme release, and preserves ventricular architecture when administered the week prior to heart surgery, Taggart and colleagues (1996) designed a study to evaluate the efficacy of a shorter course of preoperative coenzyme Q10. In this double-blind, placebo-controlled trial, 20 patients undergoing elective cardiac bypass were randomized to receive coenzyme Q10 300 mg in soy bean oil in a gelatin capsule (Pharma Nord UK) or identical placebo at 6 PM the evening before and 6 AM on the morning prior to surgery. The two patient groups were similar with respect to age, ejection fraction, number of grafts, and time of ischemia. Patients with unstable symptoms, concomitant medical illnesses, ejection fraction less than 30%, and those requiring additional procedures (e.g., endarterectomy) were excluded. The same surgeon performed all surgeries. Outcome measures were clinical events, ECG changes, and cardiac enzymes. Coenzyme Q10, troponin, and CK-MB levels were measured before surgery and at 1, 6, 24, 72, and 120 h after reperfusion. Serial ECGs were performed before and 1, 24, and 72 h postoperatively.

There was no difference in plasma levels of coenzyme Q10 levels before surgery between the placebo and coenzyme Q10 groups. Coenzyme Q10 levels decreased in both groups postoperatively, with the placebo group experiencing a greater drop. This difference was not statistically significant (two-way ANOVA). The increase in biochemical markers of myocardial injury was not statistically significant between the two groups (two-way ANOVA). Although ECG changes were common in both groups, no perioperative infarct was diagnosed in any patient. All patients survived, and none had a clinically significant decrease in cardiac output. Two patients in the placebo group and three in the coenzyme Q10 group developed atrial fibrillation requiring digoxin. No adverse effects from coenzyme Q10 were reported.

The investigators concluded that short-term coenzyme Q10 supplementation does not protect against myocardial ischemia in patients with well-preserved ventricular function undergoing coronary bypass requiring relatively short ischemic times. Perhaps patients with longer ischemic times, poor ventricular function, or lower baseline coenzyme Q10 levels would have benefited. The investigators indicate that the study results cannot be applied to patients undergoing valve replacement surgery, who generally experience greater myocardial trauma, and in whom a week of preoperative coenzyme Q10 supplementation has been shown to be beneficial in previous studies. Although coenzyme Q10 supplementation did not increase plasma coenzyme Q10 levels in this study, the investigators suggest that this may reflect the intracellular storage of coenzyme Q10 in the liver and myocardium.

Chello and associates (1996) subsequently examined the efficacy of prophylactic coenzyme Q10 in decreasing reperfusion injury in patients undergoing aoritic crossclamping during elective vascular surgery for aortoiliac obstructive disease or repair of an infrarenal abdominal aortic aneurysm. Patients with recent myocardial infarction, angina, congestive heart failure, or diabetes were excluded. Thirty patients were randomized to receive coenzyme Q10 50 mg or placebo three times daily beginning 7 d prior to surgery. Baseline echocardiogram revealed good ejection fraction in all patients, and pulmonary disease was absent based on chest X-ray and pulmonary function tests. The two groups were similar in age, gender predominance, baseline electocardiogram, nature of vascular disease, and mean aortic cross-clamping time. Coenzyme Q10 plasma levels were measured at baseline and after 7 d of supplementation. Blood samples were also taken from the radial artery and inferior vena cava catheters just prior to anesthesia induction, 5 and 30 min after aortic cross-clamping, and 5 and 30 min after reperfusion for measurement of plasma malondialdehyde, conjugated dienes, CK, and lactate dehydrogenase (LDH).

Baseline coenzyme Q10 plasma levels were similar between the two groups. After 7 d of supplementation, plasma levels were significantly higher in the treatment group compared with the placebo group ($p < 0.01$). Inferior vena cava malondialdehyde levels were significantly higher in the placebo group than in the treatment group 30 min after reperfusion ($p < 0.01$). Arterial levels of conjugated dienes increased from baseline during reperfusion in the coenzyme Q10 group, but this increase was barely significant ($p = 0.04$). Inferior vena cava levels of conjugated dienes increased in both the placebo and coenzyme Q10 groups but was less significant in the latter ($p < 0.01$ vs $p = 0.03$). Compared with the placebo group, coenzyme Q10 significantly reduced release of CK and LDH 30 minutes after release of the aortic cross-clamp ($p < 0.01$). Coenzyme Q10 supplementation had no effect on hemodynamics. The investigators concluded that prophylactic coenzyme Q10 administration may decrease oxidative damage during vascular surgery requiring aortic cross-clamping.

4.8.3. Hypertension

Based on studies demonstrating a deficiency of coenzyme Q10 in hypertensive rats and humans, Yamagami et al. (1976) studied the effect on coenzyme Q10 on blood pressure in 11 patients with a leukocyte coenzyme Q10 deficiency. These same researchers had previously studied coenzyme Q10 30–45 mg/d for 2–16 wk in 17 patients with essential hypertension and noted a decrease in blood pressure in only 4 patients. For this reason, only patients with a leukocyte coenzyme Q10 deficiency were enolled in this open-label study. None of these patients were taking antihypertensives. The coenzyme Q10 dosage was 30–75 mg/d for 3 d to 5 mo. Blood pressure and leukocyte coenzyme Q10 concentrations were measured every 1–2 wk. Statistical analysis was not described. Results for the five patients for whom complete data were available were presented. Four patients showed a significant decrease in systolic blood pressure ($p < 0.05$ to $p < 0.001$). Three of these patients also demonstrated a significant decrease in diastolic blood pressure ($p < 0.05$ to $p < 0.01$). The systolic blood pressure of a patient who was treated for only 8 d increased ($p < 0.01$).

Subsequent studies also showed a deficiency of coenzyme Q10 in patients with hypertension and demonstrated improvement in blood pressure as well as normalization of cardiac output with supplementation. In an open study performed in the early 1990s (Langsjoen et al., 1994), coenzyme Q10 was added to standard antihypertensive therapy in 109 cardiology patients with a diagnosis of essential hypertension for at least 1 yr. Most patients also had CHF, with the majority having NYHA class I or II failure. The dose of coenzyme Q10 was individualized to maintain a coenzyme Q10 level of 2 µg/mL. Doses ranged from 75–360 mg/d (mean 225 mg/d). The supplement was administered to most patients in tablet form and chewed with fatty food (e.g., peanut butter) once or twice daily. Physical exams and blood pressure measurements were performed regularly, and echocardiograms were performed when appropriate.

Mean NYHA class improved significantly ($p < 0.001$) from 2.40 to 1.36, with 66% of subjects improving by one functional class. Use of digoxin, diuretics, β-blockers, calcium channel blockers, ACE inhibitors, and antiarrhythmics decreased with coenzyme Q10. Mean systolic blood pressure decreased from 159 to 147 mmHg ($p < 0.001$), and mean diastolic pressure decreased from 94 to 85 mmHg ($p < 0.001$). Over half of the patients were able to discontinue one or more antihypertensive drugs. Of the 25 patients who were able to maintain normal blood pressure on coenzyme Q10 alone, blood pressure decreased from 151 mmHg on one or more antihypertensive medications to 139 mmHg on coenzyme Q10 alone ($p < 0.005$). Approximately 40% of patients had a baseline echocardiogram and at least one subsequent echocardiogram. Left ventricular end-diastolic volume increased ($p < 0.001$), left ventricular wall thickness decreased ($p < 0.001$), and diastolic function as measured by mitral valve inflow slope improved ($p < 0.001$). Results of studies of coenzyme Q10 for hypertension, although promising, need confirmed in large, double-blind placebo-controlled studies.

4.8.4. Cancer

Lockwood and colleagues (1994) studied supplementation of coenzyme Q10 90 mg plus 20 vitamins, minerals, and fatty acids in 32 women with breast cancer. The basis of the study was previous studies demonstrating a coenzyme Q10 deficiency in cancer patients (possibly related to deficiencies of the multitude of cofactors required for coenzyme Q10 synthesis); research on the function of coenzyme Q10 in the immunologic and hematopoietic systems; clinical and preclinical data suggesting a role of coenzyme Q10 in the prevention and treatment of cancer; and studies suggesting a role for other vitamins and nutrients in cancer prevention and treatment. This open study included only "high-risk" patients, although this term was not defined. Patients ranged in age from 32 to 81 yr. All patients had metastases to the lymph nodes, and some had distant metastases. Patients were treated using "standard" therapy (i.e., surgery, chemotherapy, radiation, and tamoxifen for estrogen receptor-positive disease). Patients were evaluated every 3 mo for disease recurrence, and mammograms, bone scans, chest or spine X-rays, and biopsies were performed if indicated. Blood pressure, body weight, analgesic use, and quality of life were assessed. Blood samples for analysis of coenzyme Q10 were taken at 0, 3, and 12 mo. Additionally, in approximately one-third of patients, blood cell counts and blood levels of calcium, magnesium, selenium, manganese, zinc, copper, lithium, vitamin E, pyridoxine, and β-carotene were also measured. Wilcoxan's test was used for data analysis.

Mean coenzyme Q10 levels were significantly higher after 3 and 12 mo of therapy compared with baseline ($p < 0.01$), but there was no statistically significant difference between coenzyme Q10 levels at 12 vs 3 mo of therapy. No patient died during 18 mo of follow-up, although the expected mortality was four patients based on statistical prognostic data for breast cancer patients. Six patients achieved partial remission, and all patients improved clinically. No patient experienced weight loss, the use of analgesics was reduced, and quality of life was improved. After an additional 6 mo of follow-up, no patient had died, and two patients had achieved complete remission associated with an increased coenzyme Q10 dose (300–390 mg/d). Conclusions are difficult to draw given the lack of a control group and the multitude of nutrients administered.

4.8.5. Doxorubicin-Induced Cardiotoxicity

Doxorubicin is a cancer chemotherapeutic agent known to cause arrhythmias and heart failure. The mechanism is unknown, but it is proposed to involve inhibition of coenzyme Q10. In vitro and in vivo animal studies suggest a protective effect from coenzyme Q10 administration. In an open-label study, Cortes and colleagues (1978) investigated the ability of coenzyme Q10 to protect cardiac function in patients receiving doxorubicin. Serial systolic time intervals (STIs; the ratio of the preejection period to left ventricular ejection time) were used as a noninvasive measurement of ventricular function. Coenzyme Q10 50 mg/d was administered to 30 patients receiving a doxorubicin-containing chemotherapy regimen. STIs were determined every 4 wk. Serial STIs were also determined in a control group of 63 patients receiving the same chemotherapy regimen. Only patients receiving a total doxorubicin dose of at least 200 mg/m^2 and followed for at least 5 mo were considered evaluable for cardiotoxicity.

The two groups of patients were similar in baseline characteristics, except that the patients in the coenzyme Q10 group were older. Only 10 of the control patients and 8 of the coenzyme Q10 patients were evaluable. Eight of the 10 evaluable control patients experienced an increase in STI with increasing cumulative doxorubicin dose. In addition, the mean STI of the 10 patients increased with increasing dose. Two patients who had received chest irradiation and were taking digoxin prior to beginning chemotherapy developed CHF. The mean STI in the eight evaluable coenzyme Q10 patients decreased with increasing doxorubicin dose. Only two patients experienced a gradual increase in STI, and one developed CHF. The investigators concluded that coenzyme Q10 might protect against doxoribicin-associated cardiotoxicity and that the results should be confirmed in a prospective randomized study of longer duration.

4.8.6. Hyperlipidemia

High lipoprotein(a) levels have been associated with an increased risk of premature coronary artery disease in certain populations. Conventional antilipemics are largely ineffective in lowering lipoprotein(a) levels. The effect of coenzyme Q10 supplementation on lipoprotein(a) levels in patients with coronary artery disease (CAD) was studied based on the hypothesis that coenzyme Q10 may be present in lipoprotein(a) and may inhibit platelet aggregation. Singh and Niaz (1999), randomized 51 patients with CAD and a lipoprotein(a) concentration of 20–50 mg/dL to receive coenzyme Q10 (Q-Gel) 60 mg twice daily or placebo. The placebo capsules contained low-dose B-complex vitamins (thiamine mononitrate 3 mg, riboflavin 3 mg, pyridoxine hydrochloride 1 mg, and nicotinamide 25 mg). The placebo and coenzyme Q10 capsules were not identical, so in an effort to maintain blinding, patients were instructed not to compare their capsules with those of other patients or to show them to their doctors. The capsules were dispensed in identical containers, and compliance was determined using pill counts. Subjects were recruited from patients admitted to a coronary care unit for treatment of acute myocardial infarction, unstable angina, or angina pectoris. The two treatment groups did not differ in age, weight, body mass index, gender, diagnosis, or drug therapy. The percentage of patients who smoked and who had a prior history of CAD was slightly higher in the coenzyme Q10 group. Blood was drawn for measurement of total cholesterol, lipoproteins, glucose, and measures of oxidative stress (malondialdehyde, lipid peroxides, and diene conjugates) at baseline and after 4 wk of treatment.

Compared with baseline, coenzyme Q10 supplementation was associated with a significant increase in HDL and diene conjugates ($p < 0.05$, two-tailed t-test) and a reduction in fasting blood glucose, malondialdehyde, and lipoprotein(a) ($p < 0.01$, two-tailed t-test). Total cholesterol and LDL were unaffected. The 31% decrease in lipoprotein(a) levels was clinically significant. The investigators concluded that coenzyme Q10 administered as Q-Gel 120 mg/d can significantly decrease elevated lipoprotein(a) levels in patients with CAD and can also reduce fasting blood glucose.

Although in vitro studies and small uncontrolled human studies using 90 mg/d of coenzyme Q10 for 2 wk or 300 mg/d for 11 d demonstrated benefit in improving LDL and very low-density lipoprotein (VLDL) oxidation resistance, a larger ($n = 142$) placebo-controlled study in male smokers failed to demonstrate such benefit (Kaikkonen et al., 1997). The investigators suggest that higher doses of coenzyme Q10 may be necessary to benefit smokers.

4.8.7. Diabetes

Coenzyme Q10 is involved in oxidative reactions such as glycolysis and could theoretically enhance insulin sensitivity. Based on evidence from previous studies as well as their patients' experiences suggesting an effect of coenyzme Q10 on on blood glucose control, investigators from Denmark examined the effect of coenzyme Q10 on glycemic control and insulin requirements in 34 patients with type 1 diabetes. Diagnosis was confirmed by measurement of C-peptide levels. The patients had few diabetic complications: only two had microalbuminuria, none had proliferative retinopathy, and all had normal responses to hypoglycemia. The study began with a 1 month run-in during which subjects were trained to measure and report their blood glucose twice weekly; insulin dosing adjustments were made by diabetologists. Study subjects were then randomized to coenzyme Q10 100 mg (Bioquinon, Pharma Nord, Vejle, Denmark) or placebo to be taken each morning for 3 mo. Subjects continued to measure and report their blood glucose twice weekly, with dosing adjustments made accordingly. Serum coenzyme Q10 levels, lipids, glycosylated hemoglobin (HbA_{1c}), blood pressure, and weight were measured at baseline and at the end of the study. The mean of the blood glucose concentrations measured during the last week of the run-in was compared with the mean of those measured during the last week of the intervention period. The number of hypoglycemic episodes experienced during these same time periods was also compared. Before randomization and after the intervention period, patients rated their physical, psychological, and general well-being using a visual analog scale (VAS).

At baseline, the two groups were similar in body mass index (BMI), insulin requirement, and diabetic control (t-test for unpaired data). Despite an increase from baseline in serum coenzyme Q10 levels in the treatment group ($p < 0.005$, t-test for paired data), coenzyme Q10 supplementation did not improve glycemic control as measured by insulin requirement, mean blood glucose concentrations, or HbA_{1c}. Coenzyme Q10 did not affect lipid concentrations or number of hypoglycemic episodes, and there was no change in patient well-being (Henriksen et al., 1999).

4.8.8. Exercise Capacity

Several double-blind, placebo-controlled studies of coenzyme Q10's effect on exercise performance have been published in the peer-reviewed medical literature. A representative sample is reviewed here.

Because of unsubstantiated claims that coenzyme Q10 levels decrease with age, Porter and colleagues (1995) tested the hypothesis that coenzyme Q10 supplementation might enhance exercise performance in middle-aged men. Porter and colleagues mention that a previous uncontrolled study showed favorable results of supplementation on oxygen consumption in trained, college-aged cyclists (Guerra et al., 1987). An additional study in untrained cyclists in this same age group did not demonstrate a convincing benefit (Zuliani et al., 1989). Although coenzyme Q10 had been studied with favorable results in middle-aged and older cardiac patients, no studies had yet been performed to determine the effect of coenzyme Q10 supplementation on exercise performance in otherwise healthy middle-aged males. The investigators felt that middle-aged men might derive more benefit from coenzyme Q10 than younger men owing to decreased coenzyme Q10 levels.

The study was designed to determine whether coenzyme Q10 supplementation could improve maximal oxygen consumption (VO2max), lactate threshold, and heart rate response to exercise in middle-aged untrained men. Additionally, the investigators examined the effect of coenzyme Q10 supplementation on upper extremity blood flow, oxygen uptake, and lactate release. Inclusion criteria for the Porter study were age between 35 and 60 yr; coenzyme Q10 levels not exceeding 1 µg/mL; VO2max 30–50 mL/kg/min; stable activity level over the past 3 mo; and willingness to maintain the current level of exercise. Exclusion criteria were recent or current use of high-dose B-complex vitamins; cardiovascular or pulmonary disease that would interfere with maximal exercise testing; history of major lower extremity injury; participation in upper body or weight training or endurance training; or biliary tract disease, which might alter coenzyme Q10 bioavailability. Study participants were 15 "middle-aged" (44.7 ± 2 yr) volunteers. Participants with "lower" coenzyme Q10 levels were assigned coenzyme Q10 (Aspen Nutrients, Aspen, CO) 150 mg/d (five 30 mg tablets) with a meal; seven "control" patients were assigned to take a placebo capsule (Cebocap 3, Forest Pharmaceuticals, St. Louis, MO) once each day with a meal. Subjects were blinded as to treatment group and whether their exercise tolerance was expected to improve or deteriorate. Exercise testing consisted of forearm-hand grip testing and cycle ergometry.

Compared with baseline, after 2 mo, coenzyme Q10 levels had increased with supplementation ($p < 0.001$) but did not increase in the placebo group ($p > 0.05$). Neither placebo nor coenzyme Q10 supplementation improved VO2max. There was no significant difference between groups over time in forearm oxygen uptake, forearm blood flow, or forearm lactate release during hand dynamometry. There was also no significant difference in heart rate, lactate threshold, VO2max, or maximal workload during cycle ergometry between groups over time. Although it was not a primary outcome measure, subjective perception of vigor increased in the coenzyme Q10 group ($p < 0.05$). Statistical methods were not well defined. The investigators concluded that 2 mo of coenzyme Q10 supplementation increased coenzyme Q10 levels in middle-aged, untrained men with a corresponding increase in perceived vigor without an increase in objective measures of aerobic capacity.

In a subsequent study, 18 male athletes (triathletes and cyclists) were randomized to receive coenzyme Q10 1 mg/kg/d or placebo for 28 d. Coenzyme Q10 levels were significantly increased from baseline in the treatment group ($p < 0.05$). Subjects perfomed graded cycling exercise tests at baseline and after supplementation. Coenzyme Q10 supplementation did not improve aerobic capacity (Weston et al., 1997).

Overvad and colleagues (1999) reviewed several studies of the effects of coenzyme Q10 supplementation on exercise capacity, including those by Porter and colleagues (1995) and Weston and associates (1997); they concluded that studies performed thus far have not clarified the importance of coenzyme Q10 supplementation in physical activity.

4.8.9. Myopathies

The success of coenzyme Q10 supplementation in an adult with late-onset muscular dystrophy prompted researchers to perform two double-blind trials in children and adults with a variety of muscular dystrophies and neurogenic muscle atrophies. Because there is an association between muscle disease and cardiac disease, these investigators were interested in cardiac function as well as physical performance as an outcome measure (Folkers et al., 1985; Folkers and Simonsen, 1995). The first of these trials was undertaken in 1985 (Folkers et al., 1985). Subjects included patients aged 7–69 years with Duchenne type muscular dystrophy, Becker's muscular dystrophy, limb-girdle muscular dystrophy, myotonic dystrophy, Charcot-Marie-Tooth disease, and Wohlfart-Kugelberg-Welander disease. Eight patients received coenzyme Q10 33 mg three times daily, and four patients received placebo three times daily for 3 mo. Statistical analysis was not described.

Coenzyme Q10 blood levels, which were slightly lower than normal at baseline, increased in all subjects in the coenzyme Q10 group but did not increase in the placebo group. The cardiac function of all coenzyme Q10 patients improved based on stroke volume or cardiac output, whereas none of the placebo patients improved ($p < 0.003$). Seven of eight coenzyme Q10 patients achieved a statisitically significant increase in cardiac output, stroke volume, or both ($p < 0.001$). Half of the patients in the coenzyme Q10 group experienced improved physical well-being, compared with none of the placebo patients. The investigators suggested that, based on their experience in treating patients with cardiomyopathy, continued therapy would be expected to produce continued physical improvement as well as a higher incidence of physical improvement. After the double-blind portion of the study, all patients were given coenzyme Q10 in open-label fashion. The cardiac function of three of the four placebo patients improved when they were crossed over to coenzyme Q10 ($p < 0.001$). Only six of the eight patients who received coenzyme Q10 during the double-blind portion of the study participated in the open-label portion of the study. Five of the six maintained their improved cardiac function, and one responded better than during the double-blind study ($p < 0.001$ vs $p < 0.054$ for months 1–3). The investigators concluded that coenzyme Q10 offers promise in the treatment of otherwise untreatable muscular disorders.

Folkers and Simonsen (1994) later performed a second trial in 15 patients with Duchenne type muscular dystrophy, Becker's muscular dystrophy, limb-girdle muscular dystrophy, myotonic dystrophy, Charcot-Marie-Tooth disease, Welander's disease, fascioscapulohumeral muscular disease, and congenital hypotonia ranging in age from 8 to 74 yr. Stroke volume increased significantly in all eight patients who received coenzyme Q10, and cardiac output increased in six. Both cardiac output and stroke volume increased in one placebo patient. Stroke volume and cardiac output increased in all the patients administered coenzyme Q10 during the subsequent open-label portion of the study. Based on the relatively small increase in coenzyme Q10 levels from baseline in this study, as well as data from heart failure patients, the investigators suggested that future studies should use 300–400 mg of coenzyme Q10.

There are several different disorders resulting from dysfunction of the mitochondria, causing brain and muscle dysfunction, as well as morphologic and biochemical abnormalities. All such patients have high serum lactate levels as a result of impairment of oxidative metabolism. Because previous studies had shown benefit from coenzyme Q10 in select patients with various mitochondrial encephalomyopathies, Bresolin and colleagues (1990) performed a larger, multicenter study. Coenzyme Q10 2 mg/kg/d was administered to 59 patients aged 16–82 yr with chronic progressive ophthalmoplegia (CPEO) and proximal limb weakness, Kearns-Sayre syndrome (KSS), mitochondrial myopathy without ophthalmoplegia, or myoclonus epilepsy with ataxia and ragged red fibers (MERRF syndrome). Serum lactate and pyruvate were measured before and after exercise on a cycle ergometer at baseline and every 2 mo. Triceps muscle biopsies were taken for genetic testing, electron microscopy, and oxidative enzyme analysis. These enzymes were measured in platelets at baseline and every 2 mo, as were coenzyme Q10 levels in serum and platelets.

As part of a complete neurologic evaluation, muscle strength was evaluated at baseline and every 2 mo using the Walton rating scale corrected for the Medical Research Council (MRC) index score. An ECG was obtained at baseline and at month 6. After 6 mo of treatment, patients with at least a 25% decrease in postexercise lactate levels from baseline were termed "responders." These responders were treated for an additional 3 mo with either placebo or coenzyme Q10. During the double-blind phase of the study, serum lactate was measured monthly 5 and 60 min after exercise. Platelet enzymes and serum and platelet coenzyme Q10 levels were measured monthly during this portion of the study. A complete neurologic evaluation, evaluation of muscle strength, and ECG studies were also performed monthly. Statistical analysis was performed using a *t*-test for paired data, linear regression, and Pearson's correlation coefficient.

Fifteen patients dropped out of the open-label portion of the study owing to mental and psychological difficulties that interfered with their ability to participate comfortably in the trial. In the remaining patients, the 5 min postexercise serum lactate level was significantly lower at 6 mo compared with baseline ($p < 0.0001$). There was a significant correlation between serum lactate and pyruvate levels ($p < 0.005$). Platelet mitochondrial succinate dehydrogenase ($p < 0.05$) and succinate cytochrome c reductase ($p < 0.0001$) increased, and citrate synthetase decreased ($p < 0.05$). Coenzyme Q10 levels in platelets ($p < 0.05$) and serum ($p < 0.01$) were higher at 6 mo compared with baseline. The MRC score increased significantly both globally ($p < 0.01$) and in the axial muscle group ($p < 0.05$), the upper limb distal muscles ($p < 0.005$), and the lower limb distal muscles ($p < 0.01$). Improvements were noted in two patients with cerebellar symptoms. No changes in cardiac conduction defects were noted, and no improvement in ptosis or CPEO were seen, perhaps owing to irreversible damage to the affected muscles.

Sixteen "responders" entered the double-blind phase of the trial. Thirteen had CPO with muscle weakness, and one each had MERRF, KSS, and mitochondrial myopathy without CPEO. All responders were found to have ragged red fibers on muscle biopsy. Within the group of responders, statistical analysis showed that the presence of low muscle cytochrome c oxidase activity correlated with low MRC score, which in turn correlated with high postexercise lactate levels. Cytochrome c reductase was also generally low in the nonresponders but did not correlate with MRC score. Ptosis and CPEO were frequently present in the responders, whereas cardiac conduction defects were infrequent. Both ptosis and conduction defects were frequent in the nonresponders, whereas CPOE was slight or lacking. Response to therapy did not correlate with serum or platelet coenzyme Q10 levels or muscle mitochrondrial DNA deletions.

In the responders assigned to coenzyme Q10 during the double-blind phase of the trial, serum lactate levels were significantly lower at month 9 compared with baseline ($p < 0.01$), but there was no additional decrease between months 6 and 9 compared with the decrease from baseline to month 6, suggesting that any improvement from coenzyme Q10 supplementation is maximal after 6 mo of therapy. The placebo-treated responders, who had exhibited a significant difference between baseline serum lactate and serum lactate at month 6 (before crossing over to placebo) ($p < 0.0001$), experienced a worsening of serum lactate after crossing over to placebo (i.e., the difference between baseline and month 9 was not significant in this group). There was a nonsignificant trend toward increased cytochrome c oxidase, succinate dehydrogenase, and succinate cytochrome c reductase activity in platelets of responders treated with coenzyme Q10 between 0, 6, and 9 months. This trend was reversed between months 6 and 9 in the patients crossed over to placebo, but it did not reach statistical significance. Citrate synthetase decreased significantly ($p < 0.05$) between months 0 and 6 in the eight responders continued on coenzyme Q10, but no further decrease was noted with an additional 3 mo of supplementation. In the eight responders randomized to placebo, citrate synthetase increased between months 6 and 9. Regardless of whether the responders were randomized to coenzyme Q10 or placebo for the second phase of the study, coenzyme Q10 levels in serum and platelets did not change. The MRC score of the responders showed a trend toward increased strength in the first 6 mo of the study, with no further change in the second phase of the study, regardless of treatment group.

Small sample size, short duration (3 mo) of the double-blind phase of the study, and high intrinsic variability of the evaluation of muscle strength owing to the subjective nature of the MRC score are possible reasons for the lack of difference between the placebo and coenzyme Q10 groups during the second phase of the study. The investigators concluded that they were unable to identify characteristics that would predict response to coenzyme Q10 in patients with mitochondrial myopathies and that a treatment duration of more than 3 mo may be necessary for response.

In an uncontrolled study (Chan et al., 1998) involving 9 patients with mitochondrial encephalomyopathies, 6 mo (but not 3 mo) of supplemenation with coenzyme Q10 (Zambon Group, Milan, Italy) 50 mg/d had a beneficial effect on mitochondrial function as measured by the venous lactate/pyruvate (L/P) ratio. (The L/P ratio is a measure of the cytosolic redox state and reflects the intracellular NADH/NAD+ ratio.) The four male patients enrolled in the study showed a decrease in the L/P ratio under maximal cycle ergometry workload compared with baseline ($p < 0.005$, paired t-test).

The L/P ratio at rest normalized in all four men, and the L/P ratio with exercise normalized in two of the men and in one of the five women enrolled in the study.

Coenzyme Q10 supplementation was also studied in two patients with mitochondrial myopathy, encephalopathy, lactic acidosis, and stroke-like episodes (MELAS) (Abe et al., 1999). Using noninvasive tissue oximetry of the quadriceps muscle during cycle ergometry, oxygen consumption patterns consistent with mild and severe defects in mitochondrial oxidative phosphorylation (respiration) were documented. With coenzyme Q10 supplementation, the oxygen consumption pattern of the patient with severe disease improved to that consistent with mild disease, and there was a reduction in the sum of the serum lactate and pyruvate content during exercise. The oxygen consumption pattern of the patient with mild disease did not improve with coenzyme Q10 supplementation.

4.8.10. Periodontal Disease

Because previous studies had identified a deficiency of coenzyme Q10 in gingival biopsy tissue from patients with advanced periodontal disease, and because open-label administration of coenzyme Q10 had produced favorable results in seven patients being treated for periodontal disease, a double-blind study of coenzyme Q10 in periodontal disease was undertaken (Wilkinson et al., 1976) Twenty patients with periodontal disease were randomized to receive coenzyme Q10 25 mg or placebo twice daily for 3 wk. Inclusion criteria were measurable periodontal pockets due to inflammation, pseudopocketing, or loss of alveolar bone. Data collected included pocket depth, gingival temperature, crevivular fluid volume, and periodontal health score, which included rating purulent exudate, tooth mobility, swelling, bleeding, redness, pain, and itching on a scale of 1 to 5. Calculus and plaque were similarly scored. Chi-squared analysis was used to analyze data for the number of patients clinically improved in each group. Eighteen of the 20 patients enrolled completed the study (*see Adverse Effects and Toxicity* section for discussion). All 8 of the patients in the coenzyme Q10 group improved from baseline, whereas only 3 of 10 placebo patients improved ($p < 0.01$). Of the three placebo patients who appeared to improve, two were thought to have improved as a result of increased frequency of dental appointments, serving as an impetus for better oral hygiene, and one was improved only marginally.

4.8.11. Photoaging

Topical application of coenzyme Q10 has been shown to penetrate the epidermis, reducing wrinkle depth and UVA-associated oxidative DNA damage and expression of collagenase (Hoppe et al., 1999).

4.8.12. Sperm Function

Coenzyme Q10 is involved in sperm movement and acts as an antioxidant to prevent lipid oxidation in the sperm cell membrane. An uncontrolled study was performed to assess the effects of coenzyme Q10 on sperm motility (Lewin and Lavon, 1997). Seventeen males whose sperm produced low fertilization rates after in vitro intracytoplasmic sperm injection (ICSI) were treated with coenzyme Q10 60 mg/d for a mean of 103 d prior to the following ICSI treatment. A significant increase in fertilization rates was noted after supplementation compared with presupplementation cycles ($p < 0.05$).

4.8.13. Primary Biliary Cirrhosis

Primary biliary cirrhosis is an autoimmune liver disease that causes cholestatic jaundice. Immunosuppressants have limited efficacy in this disorder as well as potentially serious side effects. Ursodeoxycholic acid is a popular treatment, but its clinical efficacy is limited. Fatigue associated with this disorder may be caused by oxidative damage to myocytes and cholestasis is associated with lipid peroxidation of bile duct cells. The use of antioxidants to reduce oxidative damage in primary biliary cirrhosis has been suggested. The effects of two antioxidant preparations, Bio-Antox (selenium, methionine, β-carotene, and vitamins C and E) and Bio-Quinone Q10 (coenzyme Q10 100 mg and α-tocopherol), both from Pharma-Nord UK (Morpeth, Nothumberland, UK), were studied in patients with symptomatic primary biliary cirrhosis (Watson et al., 1999a). Inclusion criteria were liver biopsy compatible with a diagnosis of primary biliary cirrhosis, antimitochondrial antibody titer greater than 1:40 by indirect immunofluoresccence, and liver function tests suggesting cholestasis.

Patients were randomized to receive Bio-Antox four tablets daily (group 1; $n = 11$) or Bio-Antox four tablets daily plus Bio-Quinone Q10 one tablet daily (group 2; $n = 13$) for 3 mo. No patient had had any change in other medications in the previous 3 mo, and no changes were made during the study. The study was not blinded; patients knew they were receiving antioxidants, but they were unaware that there were two treatment arms to the study. Liver function tests, vitamin C levels (a measure of compliance), prothrombin time, and complete blood cell count were measured monthly. At baseline and at month 3, pruritis severity was assessed using a 10-cm VAS, frequency of nocturnal pruritis was rated on a scale of 1 (never) to 6 (more than 4 nights/wk), and fatigue was assessed using the Fisk Fatigue Severity Score (FFSS). The FFSS is a chronic fatigue assessment tool that assesses fatigue in three domains (cognitive, physical, and social fatigue) on a scale of 0 (no problem) to 4 (extreme problem). The FFSS has been previously validated in primary biliary cirrhosis patients. At study completion, patients were asked to to evaluate the improvement of six symptoms (itch, tiredness, dry eyes, dry mouth, bone and joint pain, and abdominal pain) on a scale of 1 (a lot worse) to 5 (a lot better).

Compliance was 100% as assessed using vitamin C levels. No change in any blood test was noted. Compared with baseline, in group 2 there was a statistically significant improvement in nocturnal pruritis and in pruritis measured using the VAS ($p < 0.05$). Overall fatigue score improved posttreatment compared with baseline ($p < 0.05$) in 50% of the 22 patients who completed the study. Sixty-four percent of the patients showed a statistically significant improvement in at least one FFSS domain. Among the group 2 patients, 62% had statistically significant overall improvement, and 77% had a significant improvement in at least one domain. In group 2, physical and social fatigue improved compared with baseline ($p < 0.05$ and $p < 0.01$, respectively), but there was no statistically significant improvement in cognitive fatigue or the overall fatigue score. In group 1, 33 and 44%, respectively, showed statistically significant overall improvement and improvement in at least one domain. As a group, however, there was no statistically significant improvement in overall fatigue score or in any domain. Sixty-four percent of patients evaluated their fatigue as "a lot better," and there was a significant correlation between the ratio of FFSS before and after treatment and subjective fatigue improvement ($r = 0.44$, $p < 0.05$). Improvement in dry eyes, dry mouth, abdominal pain, and bone and joint pain was reported in some patients.

Study limitations include lack of placebo control and blinding, inappropriate mathematical manipulation of ordinal data (i.e., FFSS, pruritis frequency), and limited description of statistical methods used. The investigators called for a double-blind, placebo-controlled crossover study to investigate further the efficacy of Bio-Antox and Bio-Quninone Q10 in improving symptomatology of primary biliary cirrhosis.

4.8.14. Immune Function

Based on studies suggesting that coenzyme Q10 has a role in the body's defense against microorganisms and that lipid-soluble vitamins with free radical scavenging ability (i.e., vitamins E and K) can enhance antibody production, a study was designed to quantify coenzyme Q10's effect on production of antibodies against hepatitis B surface antigen after vaccination (Barbieri et al., 1999). Sixty-three patients, aged 20–66 yr, were randomized, in single-blind fashion, to placebo, coenzyme Q10 90 mg/d, or coenzyme Q10 180 mg/d (Vitamex, Royal Super Co Q10® soft gelatin capsules). The capsules were taken for 90 d, beginning 14 d prior to vaccination. A second vaccine was administered 30 d after the first. Hepatitis B antibody titer was measured at baseline and on days 30, 45, 60, 75, and 90. Complete blood cell count, electrolytes, liver function tests, renal function tests, blood pressure, heart rate, and weight were measured at baseline and at the end of the study. Quantitiative variables were analyzed using ANOVA, and categorical variables were analyzed using Chi-squared analysis.

The three treatment groups were comparable in regard to baseline data and demographics. Coenzyme Q10 180 mg/d produced higher antibody titers than placebo at days 45, 75 ($p < 0.05$), and 90 ($p < 0.01$). The 180 mg/d dose also produced higher titers than 90 mg/d at days 75 and 90 ($p < 0.05$). Coenzyme Q10 90 mg/d did not improve antibody response compared with placebo. Lymphocyte count increased significantly from baseline in all three groups, but it increased more in the placebo group than in the coenzyme Q10 groups ($p < 0.05$). Leukocyte count increased from baseline in the placebo group ($p < 0.001$) but not in the coenzyme Q10 groups, with a significant difference between the placebo and treatment groups ($p < 0.01$). The eosinophil count decreased from baseline in all groups but was statistically significant only in the coenzyme Q10 90 mg/d group ($p < 0.05$). Based on studies of structural analogs of coenzyme Q10, the investigators proposed that the mechanism of coenzyme Q10's attenuation of the increase in lymphocyte and leukocyte counts seen in the placebo group was inhibition of leukotriene production. The investigators also proposed that coenzyme Q10's ability to enhance antibody production is related to its antioxidant effects, which could minimze oxidative stress and cell membrane turnover, thus improving antigen recognition and antibody production.

4.8.15. Chronic Fatigue Syndrome

Because of its role in cellular respiration, clinicians have been prescribing coenzyme Q10 to patients with chronic fatigue syndrome since the late 1980s. In an unpublished study, 16 of 20 female patients requiring bed rest following mild exercise were found to have lower coenzyme Q10 levels than a control group of sedentary females matched for age and weight. Coenzyme Q10 levels decreased further with activity. Supplementation with coenzyme Q10 100 mg daily for 3 mo resulted in improved exercise tolerance, clinical symptoms, and postexercise fatigue in more than 80% of the patients (Werbach, 2000). A large, randomized controlled trial is needed to confirm these results.

4.8.16. Huntington's Disease

Based on animal models of the disease, it has been proposed that the pathogenesis of Huntington's disease involves oxidative damage, defects in electron transport, and activation of the glutamatergic N-methyl-D-aspartate (NMDA) receptor. Thus, a double-blind, placebo-controlled pilot study was designed to assess the effect of coenzyme Q10 300 mg twice daily, remacemide hydrochloride (an investigational NMDA antagonist) 200 mg three times daily, neither, or both on total functional capacity (TFC) after 30 mo of treatment compared with baseline in patients with early Huntington's disease (Huntington Study Group, 2001). Three hundred forty-seven patients were enrolled. This sample size was sufficient to detect a 40% slowing in TFC decline.

There was a nonsignificant, 13% slowing in the rate of TFC decline in the coenzyme Q10 group ($p = 0.15$, two-tailed t-test) compared with no coenzyme Q10. Of the secondary outcome measures, coenzyme Q10 slowed functional decline per the functional assessment checklist of the Unified Huntington's Disease Rating Scale (UHDRS) by 22% ($p = 0.02$) and showed a nonsignificant 18% slowing of the decline in independence measured using the UHDRS independence scale ($p = 0.06$). On measures of cognitive function, coenzyme Q10 benefited the Stroop color naming portion of the UHDRS cognitive assessment ($p = 0.01$) and the Brief Test of Attention ($p = 0.02$). Coenzyme Q10 showed a trend toward benefit in the Stroop word reading portion of the UHDRS cognitive assessment ($p = 0.09$). Any benefit from coenyme Q10 at this dose appears to be small; however, it is possible that the marginal efficacy was caused by limited bioavailability of the coenzyme Q10 preparation used in this study. Blood levels of coenzyme Q10, although assessed at baseline and at months 8 and 30, were not available at the time of publication. A repeat study in this same population using a coenzyme Q10 product with documented bioavailability may be justified.

Based on their results, the investigators have proposed a study of coenzyme Q10 in asymptomatic individuals at risk of Huntington's disease.

4.8.17. Migraine

Mean migraine frequency decreased by over half after 3 mo of treatment with coenzyme Q10 150 mg/d in a recent open-label study (Rozen et al., 2002). No side effects were reported. Thirty-two patients with migraine (with and without aura) were enrolled. A placebo-controlled trial is needed to confirm these promising results. In addition, the study should be of longer duration to evaluate long-term efficacy and safety, and should include a larger sample size to better evaluate safety and to identify patient characteristics that predict response to therapy.

4.9. PHARMACOKINETICS

Coenzyme Q10 is absorbed slowly and incompletely from the small intestine owing to its low water solubility and high molecular weight (Tomono et al., 1986; Kaikkonen et al., 1997). Interindividual variation in absorption has been documented

(Weis et al 1994; Kaikkonen et al., 1997). In one study, peak plasma concentrations occurred at a mean of 6.5 h after oral administration of coenzyme Q10 under fasting conditions. A second peak occurs approximately 24 h after administration of a single dose (Tomono et al., 1986; Greenberg and Frishman, 1990; Weis et al., 1994). Based on data from experiments in guinea pigs, it is thought that this second peak occurs because exogenously administered coenyzme Q10 is transported to the liver by chylomicrons, where it is incorporated into VLDL and secreted into the bloodstream (Tomono et al., 1986; Greenberg and Frishman, 1990). Enterohepatic recirculation has been ruled out as a mechanism for this second peak because it occurs even in guinea pigs whose bile ducts have been cannulated (Tomono et al., 1986).

After leaving the liver, coenzyme Q10 concentrates in the adrenals, spleen, lung, kidney, and heart (Greenberg and Frishman, 1990). The elimination half-life is 33 ± 5 h, and 90% of the steady-state concentration can be expected to be reached in approximately 4 d. After dosing with 100 mg three times daily, a mean steady-state plasma level of 5.4 µg/mL is attained, compared with 0.5–1 µg/mL resulting from endogenous production (Tomono et al., 1986). Although it has been stated that exogenous coenzyme Q10 administration downregulates endogenous production (Kaikkonen et al., 1997; Sinatra, 1999), there was little effect of coenzyme Q10 supplementation on plasma levels of endogenous coenzyme Q10 in one study (Tomono et al., 1986). Elimination is mainly via biliary secretion; 62.5% was found to be excreted in the feces with chronic dosing in healthy volunteers (Greenberg and Frishman, 1990).

A pharmacokinetic study was performed to compare granular and and oil-based coenzyme Q10 formulations in otherwise healthy male smokers in eastern Finland (Kaikkonen et al., 1997). Subjects were recruited using newspaper advertisements. Volunteers were randomized to receive placebo or one of the two coenzyme Q10 formulations (name and manufacturer not specified). After an overnight fast and a standardized breakfast, a single 30-mg dose of coenzyme Q10 was administered. Additional doses were administered after a standardized lunch and dinner. Blood samples for measurement of coenzyme Q10 levels were taken every 2 h for 12 h beginning 2 h after the first dose. Participants were allowed to drink coffee and smoke as desired. The participants continued taking the study supplement or placebo three times daily for 2 mo, and the pharmacokinetic study was repeated. Although a single 30-mg dose of coenzyme Q10 was not sufficient to increase plasma coenzyme Q10 levels, 2 mo of supplementation led to accumulation of coenzyme Q10 in plasma lipids. The bioavailability of the two supplements was similar; however, there was substantial interindividual variation among study participants in coenzyme Q10 bioavailabilty. Both formulations increased plasma coenzyme Q10 levels compared with placebo, but the oil-based formulation increased coenzyme Q10 in serum lipids significantly more than the granular preparation.

Weis and colleagues (1994) compared the bioavailability of four coenzyme Q10 products, including a powder-filled capsule containing coenzyme Q10 100 mg and Emcompress® 400 mg; Bioquinon (coenzyme Q10 100 mg plus soy bean oil 400 mg); a softgel containing coenzyme Q10 100 mg, polysorbate 80 20 mg, lecithin 100 mg, and soybean oil 280 mg; and a softgel containing coenzyme Q10 100 mg polysorbate 80 20 mg, and soybean oil 380 mg. Bioquinon, a coenzyme Q10 suspension in soybean oil without emulsifiers, exhibited the highest bioavailability.

The in vitro dissolution and relative bioavailability of Q-Gel 30 mg softsules (Tishcon, Westbury, NY), a water-soluble coenzyme Q10 product, have been studied (Chopra et al., 1998). This unique water-soluble formulation, containing coenzyme Q10 80 mg in sorbitan monooleate, polysorbate 80, medium chain triglycerides, pro- pylene glycol, d-α-tocopherol, and povidone was compared with softgel capsules con- taining coenzyme Q10 suspension in oil, powder-based tablets, and powder-filled hard capsules. The four products were administered to six subjects each for 3 wk. Coen- zyme Q10 levels were measured weekly and at baseline. Coenzyme Q10 levels increased more than sixfold in the Q-Gel group, whereas levels increased only 2.7- to 3.3-fold in the other groups. In the second part of this study, Q-Gel and the softgel were administered to 12 subjects each for 4 wk. Coenzyme Q10 levels were measured weekly and at baseline. Coenzyme Q10 levels increased over sevenfold compared with baseline for Q-gel, compared with 3.15-fold for the softgels. Levels correspond- ing to a "therapeutic" coenzyme Q10 level (> 2.5 µg/mL) were achieved within 3–4 wk in both studies. The study duration was not sufficient for levels to reach steady state. Using the USP dissolution test, Q-Gel dissolved completely, whereas the other three products did not dissolve at all.

Plasma levels of coenzyme Q10 in male athletes were found to increase from 0.91 ± 0.13 to 1.97 ± 0.27 µg/mL after supplementation with 1 mg/kg/d for 28 d (Weston et al., 1997). Similarly, in a study of diabetic patients, serum levels increased from 0.9 ± 0.2 to 2.0 ± 1.0 µg/mL after supplementation with coenzyme Q10 100 mg/ d in soybean oil (Bioquinon) (Henriksen et al., 1999). In a crossover study (Langsjoen et al., 1985) of patients with NYHA class III and IV cardiomyopathy, supplementa- tion with coenzyme Q10 100 mg/d resulted in an increase in coenzyme Q10 concen- tration from a mean of 0.9 ± 0.14 to 2.46 ± 0.83 µg/mL after 12 wk of supplementation in one group of patients, and from 0.77 ± 0.26 to 1.71 ± 0.58 µg/mL in a similar group. Langsjoen and colleagues have suggested that clinical response in CHF is likely to correlate with a blood level of at least 2 µg/mL (Langsjoen et al., 1985; Chopra et al., 1998). It may take 3 mo to achieve steady-state blood levels (Chopra et al., 1998), so dosage increases should not be made more often than every 12 wk.

4.10. Adverse Effects and Toxicity

Most studies of coenzyme Q10 suggest that it is well tolerated (Tanaka et al., 1982; Langsjoen et al., 1985, 1994; Lockwood et al., 1994; Taggart et al.1996; Chello et al., 1996); however, systematic evaluation of treatment-emergent symptoms was not performed in most studies.

In one study (Shults et al., 1998) in which a coenzyme Q10/vitamin E combina- tion product supplied by Vitaline (Ashland, OR) was utilized, white blood cells were found on urinalysis in two patients with histories of urinary tract infections. One was diagnosed with prostatitis, and the other had a normal repeat urinalysis. Two other subjects taking coenzyme Q10 200 mg four times daily for 4 wks were found to have 3–5 hyaline casts per low-power field (LPF) (normal 0–2). One of the two also had trace protein, and the other had 3–5 granular casts per LPF (normal 0–2). Repeat uri- nalysis after product discontinuation was normal, and there were no biochemical abnormalities suggesting renal dysfunction. The investigators suggested that for patients taking more than 600 mg/d, it would be prudent to monitor renal function until further information is available.

In a study using Q-Gel 60 mg twice daily, adverse effects reported included nausea (36% coenzyme Q10 vs 23% placebo), vomiting (24% vs 9%), epigastric discomfort (16% vs 18%), headache (12% vs 0%), bodyache (8% vs 0%), and hypotension during the first week (24% vs 9%) (Singh and Niaz, 1999).

In a study in which coenzyme Q10 25 mg twice daily was administered to patients with periodontal disease, treatment-emergent symptoms included dizziness and flu-like symptoms (Wilkinson et al., 1976). The investigators did not feel that either patient's complaints were treatment-related, and in fact the patient who reported dizziness was diagnosed with cardiac disease several weeks later.

Clinicians reported that at least three of their patients with type 1 diabetes spontaneously mentioned that after self-medicating with coenzyme Q10, they experienced more frequent hypoglycemic episodes and required a reduction in their insulin dose. A subsequent study by these clinicians using coenzyme Q10 100 mg/d did not confirm the patients' observations. The investigators concluded that coenzyme Q10 can be taken safely by patients with type 1 diabetes (Henriksen et al., 1999).

Asymptomatic elevations of liver function tests, specifically LDH and AST, reportedly have occurred at the 300 mg dosage level (Greenberg et al., 1990). Although several tertiary references and review articles list elevated liver function tests as a consequence of conenzyme Q10 use, this adverse effect is poorly documented.

4.11. INTERACTIONS

An animal study (Lund et al., 1998) suggests that coenzyme Q10 supplementation may be detrimental to patients undergoing radiation therapy for cancer. A human small cell lung cancer line (CPH 054A) was transplanted into nude mice. Once cancer cell growth was established, mice were supplemented intragastically for 4 consecutive days with coenzyme Q10 at a dose of 10, 20, 30, or 40 mg/kg/d in soy oil. Controls received no treatment, or soy oil alone. Three hours after the last dose, half of the tumors in each group were irradiated. Tumor growth was measured before and after treatment in all groups. Neither coenzyme Q10 nor soy oil alone had a significant effect on tumor growth compared with controls. Irradiated tumors in mice that had received coenzyme Q10 at a dose of 40 mg/kg exhibited a significantly lower specific growth delay than those in mice that had not received coenzyme Q10. No radioprotection was conferred by the 10-mg/kg dose, and the effect of 20 mg/kg was "borderline." The mechanism of coenzyme Q10's radioprotectant effect is unknown, but the investigators hypothesized that it does not involve inhibition of the generation of DNA-damaging hydroxyl radicals, which occurs in hydrophilic areas, but rather is confined to lipophilic organelles such as the cell membrane. Although in theory coenzyme Q10 could be used to protect healthy tissues during radiotherapy, the investigators felt their data was sufficient to warn against the use of coenzyme Q10 during radiotherapy because the relative ability of the supplement to protect normal tissue vs neoplastic tissue is unknown. They also stressed that clinical testing is not warranted because the risks of tumor protection outweigh the hypothetical protection of healthy tissue.

Certain cardiovascular medications may decrease endogenous coenzyme Q10 levels. Gemfibrozil (Lopid®) has been shown to reduce circulating levels of coenzyme Q10 (Aberg et al., 1998), as have the 3-hydroxy-3-methyl-glutaryl coenzyme A (HMG Co-A) reductase inhibitors (i.e., statins), including lovastatin (Palomaki et al., 1997), pravastatin, and simvastatin (Watts et al., 1993; Bargossi et al., 1994; Miyake et al., 1999). Conversely, in an open, randomized crossover study in 12 healthy males, neither pravastatin 20 mg/d nor atorvastatin 10 mg/d decreased coenzyme Q10 levels despite decreasing LDL. The lack of effect on coenzyme Q10 may be explained by small sample size, youth (mean age 26 yr) and health of the study subjects, low baseline (mean 0.6 mg/dL) coenzyme Q10 levels, and cultural/dietary differences between these subjects and subjects in previous studies performed abroad (Bleske et al., 2001). The decrease in coenzyme Q10 caused by statins may be owing to the role of HMG Co-A reductase in endogenous coenzyme Q10 production (Palomaki et al., 1998; i.e., conversion of HMG-CoA to mevalonate, a coenzyme Q10 precursor) (Bleske et al., 2001). There is also evidence that the decrease in coenzyme Q10 levels associated with statins is at least partly caused by a decrease in lipoproteins that carry coenzyme Q10 (Human et al., 1997; Miyake et al., 1999); however, cholestyramine does not lower coenzyme Q10 levels despite its effect on cholesterol, and simvastatin dose is inversely proportional to coenzyme Q10 levels even after correcting for differences in plasma cholesterol (Watts et al., 1993).

Theoretically, a drug-induced decrease in coenzyme Q10 might be significant given coenzyme Q10's role as an antioxidant and the role of oxidative stress in coronary artery disease; however, studies have shown that statins have a beneficial effect on cardiovascular morbidity and mortality. It has also been suggested that depression of coenzyme Q10 levels is associated with some of the serious adverse effects of statins such as myopathy, myositis, and rhabdomyolysis (Watts et al., 1993). Although statins are associated with a low serum coenzyme Q10 level and a high blood L/P ratio that may reflect muscle mitochondrial dysfunction (De Pinieux et al., 1996), muscle coenzyme Q10 levels are not decreased with statin treatment despite decreased serum levels (Laaksonen et al., 1995). It should be noted that there is no evidence that coenzyme Q10 supplementation can prevent or treat statin-induced myopathy. Concerns that a statin-induced suppression of coenzyme Q10 levels is associated with an increased risk of cancer have been refuted (Sacks et al., 1999).

Although supplementation with coenzyme Q10 increases plasma coenzyme Q10 concentrations (Bargossi et al., 1994) and LDL coenzyme Q10 content in patients taking statins, supplementation provides little protection against LDL oxidation (Palomaki et al., 1998). In a randomized, double-blind, crossover study, Palomaki et al. (1998) administered lovastatin 20 mg (Lovacol®, Orion, Finland) once daily to 19 patients with CAD and primary hyperlipidemia, with dosage increases to twice daily and three times daily beginning at weeks 2 and 3, respectively. Patients were randomized to receive placebo or coenzyme Q10 (Kino Q10, Leiras, Finland) 60 mg three times daily. After 6 wk of treatment, all subjects were given both lovastatin placebo and coenzyme Q10 placebo for 6 wk. After this placebo washout, all patients were again administered lovastatin and were crossed over to coenzyme Q10 or placebo. No other antilipemics or antioxidants were allowed. Outcome measures were LDL antioxidant (ubiquinol and α-tocopherol) levels and oxidizability of LDL by copper sulfate ex vivo.

Coenzyme Q10 increased LDL ubiquinol concentrations significantly compared with concentrations during lovastatin treatment alone ($p < 0.0001$, two-way RANOVA). Coenzyme Q10 supplementation also increased ubiquinol and α-tocopherol depletion time upon exposure to an oxidizing agent compared with lovastatin plus placebo ($p < 0.0001$, two-way RANOVA). Supplementation with coenzyme Q10 protected LDL from copper sulfate oxidation compared with lovastatin plus placebo ($p < 0.02$, two-way ANOVA), normalizing the time to oxidation to that of the double-placebo group; however, the increase in time to oxidation was only 5%. This finding indicates that a relatively large increase in LDL coenzyme Q10 concentration confers only a small effect on time to oxidation. This may reflect coenzyme Q10's limited role in LDL oxidative defense. Routine coenzyme Q10 supplementation to patients taking statins cannot be recommended at this time.

In addition to statins, some β-blockers have also been shown to decrease coenzyme Q10 levels. Timolol ophthalmic drops, although administered for local effects in the treatment of glaucoma, can have untoward systemic effects, including reduction in heart rate, decreased stroke volume, and increased peripheral vascular resistance. Supplementation with coenzyme Q10 90 mg/d was shown to diminish these cardiovascular side effects without interfering with timolol's effect on intraocular pressure (Takahashi et al., 1989). Timolol's inhibitory effect on the coenzyme Q10-dependent enzyme NADH-oxidase is smaller than that of metoprolol, which is less than that of propranolol. Inhibition of this mitochondrial enzyme, which has an important role in myocardial bioenergetics, may lead to the depression of myocardial contractility caused by β-blockers (Kishi et al., 1977).

Using the activity of leukocyte mitochondrial succinate dehydrogenase-coenzyme Q10 reductase as an indicator of coenzyme Q10 deficiency, it was found that diabetic patients taking tolazamide or phenformin, alone or in combination with other antidiabetic drugs, had a higher incidence of coenzyme Q10 deficiency than collegiate football players ($p < 0.05$ and $p < 0.01$, respectively) (Kishi et al., 1976). There was no difference in the incidence of coenzyme Q10 deficiency between diet-treated, tolbutamide-treated, or glipizide-treated patients and normal controls. Although there was no correlation between fasting blood glucose and coenzyme Q10 deficiency, the investigators suggested that this coenzyme Q10 deficiency might actually worsen diabetic control by inhibiting insulin production. Coenzyme Q10 supplements were not administered to the deficient patients in this study.

There have been several case reports of coenzyme Q10's effect on warfarin. Three patients who experienced a decrease in the international normalized ratio (INR) with coenzyme Q10 supplementation were reported by Spigset (1994). A 68-yr-old man had taken warfarin for 6 yr after experiencing several episodes of pulmonary and cerebral thrombi. Other medications included furosemide 30 mg/d, levothyroxine 150 mg/d, propoxyphene 100 mg/d, and calcipotriol ointment. Two weeks after beginning coenzyme Q10 30 mg/d, INR decreased from approximately 2.5 to 1.31. Coenzyme Q10 was discontinued; the warfarin dose was temporarily increased, and then decreased to the previous dose, with a subsequently stable INR. A second patient, a 72-yr-old man, was prescribed warfarin after treatment for a pulmonary embolism. Over a period of several months, the patient's INR was noted to be erratic, requiring several warfarin dosage modifications. It was later discovered that during periods of decreased INR, the patient had been self-medicating with an unknown dose of coenzyme Q10. Spigset also described a 70-yr-old woman with a history of thromboembolism who, after taking warfarin for several yr, experienced a decrease in INR from the 2–3 range to 1.42 after taking coenzyme Q10 30 mg/d for 2 wk. Coenzyme Q10 was discontinued, and after a temporary increase in warfarin dosage, her INR returned to baseline. Other medications included nifedipine 30 mg/d, metoprolol 50 mg/d, and bendrofluazide 2.5 mg/d. In an additional case reported by Landbo and Almdal (1998), a 72-yr-old woman experienced a decreased response to warfarin while taking coenzyme Q10. Warfarin's anticoagulant effect was restored with coenzyme Q10 discontinuation. The mechanism of the interaction is thought to involve the structural similarity between coenzyme Q10 and vitamin K_2 (Spigset, 1994; Landbo and Almdal, 1998).

Japanese clinicians described two patients in whom coenzyme Q10 30 mg/d was prescribed for treatment of warfarin-associated hair loss (Nagao et al., 1995). Coenzyme Q10 appeared to be effective in stopping hair loss in both patients, with noticeable results within 1 mo. In one patient, hair loss recurred after warfarin discontinuation. The authors postulated that coenzme Q10 might act by improving mitochondrial respiration in hair roots, or by decreasing warfarin's effect. INR transiently decreased in one patient after beginning coenzyme Q10 but then returned to baseline. The authors did not note a change in thromboplastin time after coenzyme Q introduction in the other patient, probably because thromboplastin time is not an appropriate test for warfarin's anticoagulant effect.

4.12. REPRODUCTION

There is insufficient information to determine the safety of coenzyme Q10 in pregnant or lactating women.

4.13. CHEMICAL AND BIOFLUID ANALYSIS

Methods have been developed for the analysis of both the oxidized (ubiquinone-10) and reduced (ubiquinol-10) forms of coenzyme Q10. Because of their electrochemical properties, these methods have generally involved high-performance liquid chromatography (HPLC) with electrochemical detection (Finckh et al., 1999; Podda et al., 1999; Menke et al., 2000). Because of the use of electrochemical detection, these methods are extremely sensitive and selective for the analytes of interest and thus may require minimal volumes of plasma for analysis. Menke and colleagues (2000) report a method that can be used for either 10 or 100 μL of plasma and thus is adaptable for use in the neonate as well as the adult.

Briefly, stock solutions of ubiquinone-9 (internal standard) and ubiquinone-10 are prepared by dissolution in ethanol. Ubiquinol-9 (internal standard) and ubiquinol-10 are prepared by reducing the ubiquinones with sodium dithionite (Lang et al., 1986). All stock solutions are stored under argon at –20°C. For measurement in plasma, a 10-μL microsample is mixed with 50 μL ethanol containing ubiquinol-9 (10 pmol) and ubiquinone-9 (1.5 pmol) as internal standards. Then 50 μL of 2,6-di-tert-butyl-p-cresol (111 mg/100 mL ethanol) is added to prevent lipid autooxidation without reducing the ubiquinones, and the sample is vortex-mixed for 10 s. Hexane (500 μL) is then added, and the sample is vortexed for 2 min and then centrifuged at 1000g for 5 min at 4°C. A 400-μL aliquot of the hexane phase is then removed and evaporated to dryness under argon and reconstituted in 40 µL of reagent alcohol (methanol/ethanol/2-propanol, 100/95/5, v/v) for injection onto the HPLC system. In the case of 100-µL plasma samples, 150 pmol of ubiquinol-9 and 20 pmol ubiquinone-9 are added as internal standards, only 300 µL of the hexane phase is collected, and the sample is reconstituted in 100 µL reagent alcohol.

The chromatographic system consists of a Prontosil 120-3-C18-SH PEEK column (150 × 4 mm, 3-µm particle size) protected by a 10-mm guard column with the same packing. The mobile phase consists of 31.7 mM ammonium formate in methanol/ethanol/2-propanol (800/180/65) at a flow rate of 1.1 mL/min. The electrochemical detection system consists of a conditioning cell followed by an analytical cell, separated by an in-line graphite filter. After chromatographic separation, the components pass the conditioning cell (set to –600 mV), where the ubiquinones are reduced to the corresponding ubiquinols. As the samples pass the analytical cell (electrode 1, –150 mV; electrode 2, +600 mV), all components then undergo oxidation. The signal of electrode 2 is then transferred to the detector. The detection limits of the method are as follows: ubiquinone-9 = 24 fmol/20 µL injection; ubiquinone-10 = 28 fmol/20 µL injection; ubiquinol-9 = 25 fmol/20 µL injection; ubiquinol-10 = 24 fmol/20 µL injection. It is of note that ammonium formate is used as the mobile phase buffer (compared with other methods that use lithium perchlorate), since this buffer is less likely to corrode stainless steel components of the chromatography system, thereby producing metals that can increase background noise and decrease column life. Similarly, a PEEK column is also used to reduce extraneous metals that can increase background noise.

The method of Finckh and colleagues (1999), on which the above method is based, is also viable for measuring ubiquinol-10 and ubiquinone-10. However, it does suffer somewhat from the problems associated with excess metal production owing to deterioration of the stainless steel HPLC components. Podda and colleagues (1999) also report a method for analysis of coenzyme Q10 components, but this method has only been used for tissue and has not been applied to plasma samples.

4.14. REGULATORY STATUS

Coenzyme Q10 is regulated as a dietary supplement in the United States. Q-Gel has been granted Orphan Drug status from the FDA for treatment of mitochondrial cytopathies (Tishcon, 2002) but is not regulated as a drug.

4.15. SUMMARY

• Coenzyme Q10 is important in mitochrondrial energy production and thus has potential therapeutic utility in a wide variety of disorders.
• Bioavailability is a problem with some coenzyme Q10 products.
• Coenzyme Q10 is well tolerated.
• Coenzyme Q10 levels are decreased by several medications, including statins, fibrates, warfarin, β-blockers, and antidiabetic agents. Studies documenting benefit from coenzyme Q10 supplementation in patients taking such medications are lacking.
• Coenzyme Q10 supplementation may interfere with the efficacy of warfarin and radiotherapy.

REFERENCES

Abe K, Matsuo Y, Kadekawa J, Inoue S, Yanagihara T. Effect of coenzyme Q10 (ubiquinone) in patents with mitochondrial myopathy, encephalopathy, lactic acidosis, and stroke-like episodes (MELAS): evaluation by noninvasive tissue oximetry. J Neurol Sci 1999;162:65–8.

Aberg F, Appelkvist EL, Broijersen A, et al. Gemfibrozil-induced decrease in serum ubiquinone and alpha- and gamma-tocopherol levels in men with combined hyperlipidemia. Eur J Clin Invest 1998;28:235–42.

Barbieri B, Lund B, Lundstrom B, Scaglione F. Coenzyme Q10 administration increases antibody titer in hepatitis B vaccinated volunteers—a single blind placebo-controlled and randomized clinical study. Biofactors 1999;9:351–7

Bargossi AM, Battino M, Gaddi A, et al. Exogenous CoQ10 preserves plasma ubiqionone levels in patients treated with 3-hydroxy-3-methylglutaryl coenzyme A reductase inhibitors. Int J Clin Lab Res 1994;24:171–6.

Bleske BE, Willis RA, Anthony M, et al. The effect of pravastatin and atorvastatin on coenzyme Q10. Am Heart J 2001;142:e2. Available from: URL:http://www.mosby.com/ahj.

Bresolin N, Doriguzzi C, Ponzetto C, et al. Ubidecarenone in the treatment of mitochondrial myopathies: a multi-center double-blind trial. J Neurol Sci 1990;100:70–8.

Chan A, Reichmann, Kogel A, Beck A, Gold R. Metabolic changes in patients with mitochondrial myopathies and effects of coenzyme Q10 therapy. J Neurol 1998;245:681–5.

Chello M, Mastroroberto P, Romano R, et al. Protection by coenzyme Q10 from myocardial reperfusion injury during coronary artery bypass grafting. Ann Thorac Surg 1994;58:1427–32.

Chello M, Mastroroberto P, Romano R, et al. Protection by coenzyme Q10 of tissue reperfusion injury during abdominal aortic cross-clamping. J Cardiovasc Surg 1996;37:229–35.

Chen YF, Lin YT, Wu SC. Effectiveness of coenzyme Q10 on myocardial preservation during hypothermic cardioplegic arrest. J Thorac Cardiovasc Surg 1994;107:242–7.

Chopra RK, Goldman R, Sinatra ST, Bhagavan HN. Relative bioavailability of coenzyme Q10 formulations in human subjects. Int J Vitam Nutr Res 1998;68:109–13.

ConsumerLab.com. News. Consumerlab.com tests popular supplement for heart failure. CoQ10 test results released online today. Available from: URL: http://www.consumerlabs.com/news/news_112100.asp. Accessed January 25, 2002.

Cortes EP, Gupta M, Chou C, Amin VC, Folkers K. Adriamycin cardiotoxicity: early detection by systolic time interval and possible prevention by coenzyme Q10. Cancer Treat Rep 1978;62:887–91.

De Pinieux G, Chariot P, Ammi-Said M, et al. Lipid-lowering drugs and mitochondrial function: effects of HMG-CoA reductase inhibitors on serum ubiquinone and blood lactate/pyruvate ratio. Br J Clin Pharmacol 1996;42:333–7.

Finckh B, Kontush A, Commentz J, et al. High-performance liquid chromatography-coulometric electrochemical detection of ubiquinol 10, ubiquinone 10, carotenoids, and tocopherols in neonatal plasma. Methods Enzymol 1999; 299:341–8.

Folkers K, Simonsen R. Two successful double-blind trials with coenzyme Q10 (vitamin Q10) on muscular dystrophies and neurogenic atrophies. Biochimica Biophysica Acta 1995;1271:281–6.

Folkers K, Wolaniuk J, Simonsen R, Morishita M, Vandhanavikit S. Biochemical rationale and the cardiac response of patients with muscle disease to therapy with coenzyme Q10. Proc Natl Acad Sci USA 1985;82:4513–6.

Fuke C, Krikorian SA, Couris RR. Coenzyme Q10: a review of essential functions and clinical trials. US Pharm 2000;25:28, 30, 33–4, 36–8, 41.

Greenberg SM, Frishman WH. Coenzyme Q10: a new drug for myocardial ischemia? Med Clin North Am 1988;72:243–58.

Greenberg S, Frishman WH. Coenzyme Q10: a new drug for cardiovascular disease. J Clin Pharmacol 1990;30:595–608.

Guerra G, Ballardini E, Lippa S, Oradei A, Littarru G. The effect of the administration of ubidecarenone on maximal oxygen consumption and physical performance of a group of young cyclists. Centro Medi Sport 1987;40:359–64.

Henriksen JE, Andersen CB, Hother-Nielsen O, et al. Impact of ubiqinone (coenzyme Q10) treatment on glycaemic control, insulin requirement and well-being in patients with Type I diabetes mellitus. Diabet Med 1999;16:312–8.

Hoppe U, Bergemann J, Diembeck W, et al. Coenzyme Q10, a cutaneous antioxidant and energizer. Biofactors 1999;9:371–8.

Human JA, Ubbink JB, Jerling JJ, et al. The effect of simvastatin on the plasma antioxidant concentrations in patients with hypercholesterolemia. Clin Chim Acta 1997;263:67–77.

Huntington Study Group. A randomized, placebo-controlled trial of coenzyme Q10 and remacemide in Huntington's disease. Neurology 2001;57:397–404.

Iwamoto Y, Yamagami T, Folkers K, Blomqvist CG. Deficiency of coenzyme Q10 in hypertensive rats and reduction of deficiency by treatment with coenzyme Q10. Biochem Biophys Res Commun 1974;58:743–8.

Kaikkonen J, Nyyssonen K, Porkkala-Sarataho E, et al. Effect of oral coenzyme Q10 supplementation on the oxidation resistance of human VLDL+LDL fraction: absorption and antioxidative properties of oil and granule-based preparations. Free Radical Biol Med 1997;22:1195–202.

Khatta M, Alexander BS, Kritchen CM, et al. The effect of coenzyme Q10 in patients with congestive heart failure. Ann Intern Med 2000;132:636–40.

Kishi T, Kishi H, Watanabe T, Folkers K, Bowers CY. Bioenergetics in clinical medicine. XI. Studies on coenzyme Q and diabetes mellitus. J Med 1976;7:307–21.

Kishi T, Watanabe T, Folkers K. Bioenergetics in clinical medicine XV. Inhibition of coenzyme Q10-enzymes by clinically used adrenergic blockers of beta-receptors. Res Commun Chem Pathol Pharmacol 1977;17:157–64.

Laaksonen R, Jokelainen K, Sahi T, Tikkanen MJ, Himberg JJ. Decreases in serum ubiquinone concentrations do not result in reduced levels in muscle tissue during short-term simvastatin treatment in humans. Clin Pharmacol Ther 1995;57:62–6.

Landbo C, Almdal TP. Interaction between warfarin and coenzyme Q10 [Danish]. Ugeskr Laeger 1998;160:3226–7.

Lang JK, Gohil K, Packer L. Simultaneous determination of tocopherols, ubiquinols, and ubiquinones in blood, plasma, tissue homogenates, and subcellular fractions. Anal Biochem 1986; 157:106–116.

Langsjoen P, Langsjoen P, Willis R, Folkers K. Treatment of essential hypertension with coenzyme Q10. Mol Aspects Med 1994;15:265–72S.

Langsjoen PH, Vadhanavikit S, Folkers K. Response of patients in classes III and IV of cardiomyopathy to therapy in a blind and crossover trial with coenzyme Q10. Proc Natl Acad Sci USA 1985;82:4240–4.

Lewin A, Lavon H. The effect of coenzyme Q10 on sperm motility and function. Mol Aspects Med 1997;18(suppl):S213–9.

Lockwood K, Moesgaard S, Hanioka T, Folkers K. Apparent partial remission of breast cancer in 'high risk' patients supplemented with nutritional antioxidants, essential fatty acids and coenzyme Q10. Mol Aspects Med 1994;15(suppl):231–40S.

Lund EL, Quistorff B, Spang-Thomsen M, Kristjansen PEG. Effect of radiation therapy on small-cell lung cancer is reduced by ubiquinone. Folia Microbiol 1998;43:505–6.

Menke T, Niklowitz P, Adam S, et al. Simultaneous detection of ubiquinol-10, ubiquinone-10, and tocopherols in human plasma microsamples and macrosamples as a marker of oxidative damage in neonates and infants. Anal Biochem 2000; 282:209–17.

Miyake Y, Shouzu A, Nishikawa M, et al. Effect of treatment with 3-hydroxy-3-methylglutaryl coenzyme A reductase inhibitors on serum coenzyme Q10 in diabetic patients. Arzneimittleforschung 1999;49:324–9.

Morisco C, Trimarco B, Condorelli M. Effect of coenzyme Q10 therapy in patients with congestive heart failure: a long-term multicenter randomized study. Clin Invest 1993;71:S134–6.

Mortensen SA, Leth A, Agner E, Rohde M. Dose-related decrease of serum coenzyme Q10 during treatment with HMG-CoA reductase inhibitors. Mol Aspects Med 1997;18(suppl):S137–44.

Nagao T, Ibayashi S, Fujii K, Sugimori H, Sadoshima S, Fujishima M. Treatment of warfarin-induced hair loss with ubidecarenone [letter]. Lancet 1995;346:1104–5.

Niibori K, Yokoyama H, Crestanello JA, Whitman GJR. Acute administration of liposomal coenzyme Q10 increases myocardial tissue levels and improves tolerance to ischemia reperfusion injury. J Surg Res 1998;79:141–5.

Ohhara H, Kanaide H, Nakamura M. A protective effect of coenzyme Q10 on the Adriamycin-induced cardiotoxicity in the isolated perfused rat heart. J Mol Cell Cardiol 1981;13:741-52.

Overvad K, Diamant B, Holm L, Holmer G, Mortensen SA, Stender S. Coenzyme Q10 in health and disease. Eur J Clin Nutr 1999;53:764–70.

Palomaki A, Malminiemi K, Metsa-Ketela T. Enhanced oxidizability of ubiquinol and alpha-tocopherol during lovastatin treatment. FEBS Lett 1997;410:254–8.

Palomaki A, Malminiemi K, Solakivi T, Malminiemi O. Ubiquinone supplementation during lovastatin treatment: effect on LDL oxidation ex vivo. J Lipid Res 1998;39:1430–7.

Podda M, Weber C, Traber MG, Milbradt R, Packer L. Sensitive high-performance liquid chromatography techniques for simultaneous determination of tocopherols, tocotrienols, ubiquinols, and ubiquinones in biological samples. Methods Enzymol 1999; 299:330–41.

Porter DA, Costill DL, Zachwieja JJ, et al. The effect of oral coenzyme Q10 on the exercise tolerance of middle-aged, untrained men. Int J Sports Med 1995;16:421–7.

Rozen TD, Oshinsky ML, Gebeline CA, et al. An open-label trial of coenzyme Q10 as a migraine preventive. Cephalalgra 2002;22:137.

Sacks FM, Lewis SJ, Pouleur H, Braunwald E. Reply to: "Care," cancer and coenzyme Q10 [letter]. J Am Coll Cardiol 1999;33:897–9.

Shults CW, Flint Beal M, Fontaine D, Nakano K, Hass RH. Absorption, tolerability, and effects on mitochondrial activity of oral coenzyme Q10 in parkinsonian patients. Neurology 1998;50:93–5.

Sinatra S. Coenzyme Q10-a cardiologist's commentary. Natural Med J 1999;2:9–15.

Singh RB, Niaz MA. Serum concentration of lipoprotein(a) decreases on treatment with hydrosoluble coenzyme Q10 in patients with coronary artery disease: discovery of a new role. Int J Cardiol 1999;68:23–9.

Singh RB, Wander GS, Rastogi A, et al. Randomized, double-blind placebo-controlled trial of coenzyme Q10 in patient with acute myocardial infarction. Cardiovasc Drugs Ther 1998;12:347–53.

Spigset O. Reduced effect of warfarin caused by ubidecarenone [letter]. Lancet 1994;344:1372–3.

Taggart DP, Jenkins M, Hooper J, et al. Effects of short-term supplementation with coenzyme Q10 on myocardial protection during cardiac operations. Ann Thorac Surg 1996;61:829–33.

Takahashi N, Iwasaka T, Sugiura T, et al. Effect of coenzyme Q10 on hemodynamic response to ocular timolol. J Cardiovasc Pharmacol 1989;14:462–8.

Tanaka J, Tominaga R, Yoshitoshi M, et al. Coenzyme Q10: the prophylactic effect on low cardiac output following cardiac valve replacement. Ann Thorac Surg 1982;33:145–51.

Tishcon. Tishcon home page. Available at www.tishcon.com. Acessed January 25, 2002.

Tomono Y, Hasegawa J, Seki T, Motegi K, Morishita N. Pharmacokinetic study of deuterium-labelled coenzyme Q10 in man. Int J Clin Pharmacol Ther Toxicol 1986;24:536–41.

Watson JP, Jones DEJ, James OFW, Cann PA, Bramble MG. Case report: oral antioxidant therapy for the treatment of primary biliary cirrhosis: a pilot study. J Gastroenterol Hepatology 1999a;14:1034–40.

Watson PS, Scalia GM, Galbraith A, et al. Lack of effect of coenzyme Q10 on left ventricular function in patients with congestive heart failure. J Am Coll Cardiol 1999b;33:1549–52.

Watts GF, Castelluccio C, Rice-Evans C, et al. Plasma coenzyme Q (ubiquinone) concentrations in patients treated with simvastatin. J Clin Pharmacol 1993;46:1055–7.

Weis M, Mortensen SA, Rassing MR, et al. Bioavailability of four oral coenzyme Q10 formulations in healthy volunteers Mol Aspects Med 1994;15:273–60S.

Werbach MR. Nutritional stratregies for treating chronic fatigue syndrome. Altern Med Rev 2000;5:93–108.

Weston SB, Zhou S, Weatherby RP, Robson SJ. Does exogenous coenzyme Q10 affect aerobic capacity in endurance athletes? Int J Sport Nutr 1997;7:197–206.

Wilkinson EG, Arnold RM, Folkers K. Bioenergetics in clinical medicine. VI. Adjunctive treatment of periodontal disease with coenzyme Q10. Res Commun Chem Pathol Pharmacol 1976;14:715–9.

Yamagami T, Shibata N, Folkers K. Bioenergetics in clinical medicine. VIII. Administration of coenzyme Q10 to patients with essential hypertension. Res Commun Chem Pathol Pharmacol 1976;14:721–7.

Zhou M, Zhi Q, Tang Y, Yu D, Han J. Effects of coenzyme Q10 on myocardial protection during valve replacement and scavenging free radical activity in vitro. J Cardiovasc Surg 1999;40:355–61.

Zuliani U, Bonetti A, Compana M. The influence of ubiquinone (CoQ10) on the metabolic response to work. J Sports Med Phys Fitness 1989;29:57–62.

Chapter 5

Colloidal Silver

Melanie Johns Cupp and Timothy S. Tracy

5.1. HISTORY

Colloidal silver proteins were marketed as "patent medicines" in the 1880s for treatment of tetanus, rheumatism, and other disorders. In the first part of the 20th century, they were used to treat the common cold and gonorrhea. Marketing of colloidal silver emerged again around 1990 (Fung et al., 1995). In the fall of 2001, reports of bioterrorism attacks using anthrax sent through the U.S. mail prompted the mayor of Howie-in-the-Hills, Florida to officially endorse the use of colloidal silver by townspeople to prevent anthrax (Siegel, 2001).

5.2. CHEMICAL STRUCTURE

Colloidal silver is simply elemental silver and is designated by the chemical symbol Ag.

5.3. CURRENT PROMOTED USES

Colloidal silver is touted as an immunostimulant and antiinflammatory useful in the treatment of over 650 different diseases, primarily infectious disease. It is also promoted as a treatment for cancer, diabetes, allergies, and chronic fatigue syndrome. Despite claims that silver is necessary for the proper functioning of the human body, there is no silver deficiency state and it has no physiologic function (Fung et al., 1995).

5.4. SOURCES AND CHEMICAL COMPOSITION

Colloidal silver is a colloidal suspension of silver protein that may also contain silver chloride and silver iodide (FDA, 1999).

From: *Forensic Science: Dietary Supplements: Toxicology and Clinical Pharmacology*
Edited by: M. J. Cupp and T. S. Tracy © Humana Press Inc., Totowa, New Jersey

5.5. In Vitro Effects

The colloidal silver product CollargolR$_X$® was shown to have activity against *Staphylococus aureus*, *Pseudomonas aeruginosa*, and *Aerobacter aerogenes* in vitro (Bretano et al., 1966).

5.6. Clinical Data

Bretano and colleagues (1996) reported that they had found CollargolR$_X$® in combination with 0.5% silver nitrate useful as a burn dressing that decreases bacterial load without impeding granulation or skin graft "take." There is no information on the efficacy of colloidal silver for any disease when taken internally.

5.7. Adverse Effects and Toxicity

The main toxicity of concern with colloidal silver products is argyria, a permanent blue-gray discoloration of the skin (FDA, 1999). Although silver is deposited throughout the visceral and mucosal tissues, discoloration is noted mainly in sun-exposed areas. This is because the discoloration is caused not by silver itself, but by melanocyte stimulation and sunlight-catalyzed reduction of silver within the dermis, particularly near the sweat glands. The discoloration fades little with time and is resistant to treatment with metal chelators (Gulbranson et al., 2000).

Gulbranson and colleagues (2000) reported the development of a dusky facial coloration and bluish gray color change of the fingernail and thumbnail lunulae in a man who had taken 1 teaspoon of a 200 ppm colloidal silver solution three times daily for 3 yr as an allergy and cold medication. Blood silver levels were 85 µg/L (normal < 5 µg/L). The patient refused nail biopsy. He was advised to discontinue the colloidal silver product. The patient was also advised to avoid sun exposure to minimize the risk of hyperpigmentation. Three months after product discontinuation, there was no improvement in nail discoloration. Despite the patient's adverse experience with colloidal silver, he continued to work as an independent distributor of the product.

5.8. Interactions

It has been proposed that drugs that complex with iron might also complex with colloidal silver, resulting in reduced absorption (e.g., tetracycline, quinolone antibiotics, penicillamine, methyldopa, and thyroxine products). However, no published data exist to confirm this hypothesis.

5.9. Reproduction

Epidemiology studies suggest that increased levels of silver are linked to developmental anomalies of the ear, face, and neck (Fung and Bowen, 1996). Therefore, it is recommended that silver-containing products not be used during pregnancy.

5.10. CHEMICAL AND BIOFLUID ANALYSIS

Information on the determination of silver levels in blood or tissue following administration of silver preparations is scarce. Wan et al. (1991) reported concentrations of silver in blood, urine, and tissues following topical administration of silver sulfadiazine cream. Plasma or urine samples are first diluted fivefold with a Triton X-100 solution (0.5 mL/L aqueous solution of Triton X-100 containing 40 g/L NH_4NO_3). A 20-µL sample volume is then introduced into an atomic absorption spectrophotometer with deuterium lamp background correction and a graphite furnace unit. A silver hollow-cathode lamp with a wavelength of 328.1 nm and a high-density graphite carbon tube are used in the assay. The alternative slit is set at 0.7 µm, the ashing temperature at 700°C, and the atomization temperature at 2100°C. The limit of detection for this assay is 0.4 µg/L and the calibration curve is linear up to 75 µg/L.

Additional methods (Julshamn et al., 1986; Andersen et al., 1986; Boosalis et al., 1987) have been reported for measuring silver concentrations following silver administration, but they appear to require nonstandard instruments and may be less sensitive.

5.11. REGULATORY STATUS

Although colloidal silver is still marketed as a dietary supplement (Gulbranson et al., 2000), the FDA considers a colloidal silver product misbranded if it is marketed for the treatment or prevention of any disease, or if its labeling implies that there is scientific evidence that the product is safe and effective for its intended use. The FDA maintains that adequate directions for use cannot be written that would provide for safe use by consumers; therefore, the products are not appropriate for nonprescription sale, and any colloidal silver product intended for the treatment or prevention of disease would have to be approved as a new drug (FDA, 1999).

5.12. SUMMARY

- There are no data to support the internal use of colloidal silver for the treatment of any condition. It has been used as an external preparation in the treatment of burns.
- Oral consumption of colloidal silver is associated with a permanent blue-gray discoloration of the skin. Additionally, it is deposited in a number of visceral and mucosal tissues.
- Colloidal silver may complex with certain medications that are also known to complex with iron, thus reducing the absorption of these drugs.
- Epidemiology studies have linked increased silver levels to developmental anomalies.

REFERENCES

Andersen KJ, Wikshaland A, Utheim A. Determination of silver in biological samples based on Zeeman effect background and matrix modification. Clin Biochem 1986;19:166–70.

Boosalis MG, McCall JT, Ahrenholz DH, Solem LD, McClain CJ. Serum and urinary silver levels in thermal injury patients. Surgery 1987;101:40–3.

Bretano L, Margraf H, Monafo WW, Moyer CA. Antibacterial efficacy of a colloidal silver complex. Surg Forum 1966;17:76–8.

FDA. FDA issues final rule on OTC drug products containing colloidal silver. FDA Talk Paper, Food and Drug Administration, U.S. Department of Health and Human Services, August 17, 1999. Avaialble from: URL: http://fda/gov/bbs/topics/ANSWERS/ANS00971.html. Accessed November 13, 2001.

Fung MC, Bowen DL. Silver products for medical indications: risk-benefit assessment. J Toxicol Clin Toxicol 1996;34:119–26.

Fung MC, Weintraub M, Bowen DL. Colloidal silver proteins marketed as health supplements [letter]. JAMA 1995;274:1196–7.

Gulbranson SH, Hud JA, Hansen RC. Argyria following use of dietary supplements containing colloidal silver protein. Cutis 2000;66:373–4.

Julshamn K, Andersen KJ, Vik H. Determination of silver biological samples using Zeeman graphite furnace atomic absorption spectrometry. Acta Pharmacol Toxicol Suppl 1986;7:613–15.

Siegel R. Colloidal silver. All Things Considered, National Public Radio (NPR) broadcast, October 23, 2001.

Wan AT, Conyers RAJ, Coombs CJ, Masterton JP. Determination of silver in blood, urine, and tissues of volunteers and burn patients. Clin Chem 1991;37:1683–1687.

Chapter 6

Creatine Monohydrate

Nancy Romanchak, Melanie Johns Cupp,
and Timothy S. Tracy

6.1. HISTORY

The word "creatine," derived from "kreas," which is Greek for flesh, was first used in 1832 by Chevreul, a French scientist who discovered this substance in meat (Balsom et al., 1994; Feldman, 1999). In 1847, Lieberg confirmed that creatine was a constituent of meat. Lieberg also observed that the meat of wild foxes killed during a chase contained 10 times the amount of creatine as that found in captive foxes. From this he concluded that an accumulation of creatine occurs with muscle work (Balsom et al., 1994). Also in the mid-19th century, Heintz and Pettenkofer discovered a substance in the urine that Lieberg later identified as creatinine, a product of creatine degradation (Demant and Rhodes, 1999). In the early 20th century, researchers discovered that only part of an ingested dose of creatine is recovered in the urine, leading them to believe that some was retained in the body. In the early 1900s, it was found that creatine ingestion was able to increase the creatine content in the muscles of cats by up to 70%. In 1923, Hahn and Meyer estimated a total creatine content of 140 g in a 70-kg male, which is similar to current approximations (Balsom et al., 1994). Just a few years later, Fiske and Subbarow discovered a labile phosphorus compound in the resting muscle of cats. This substance, which they named creatine phosphate, disappeared during electrical stimulation of skeletal muscle but increased to previous levels following a recovery period (Demant et al., 1999).

These observations led to the recognition that creatine phosphate and free creatine are key intermediates of skeletal muscle metabolism. Although studies with creatine supplementation began in the late 19th century, it was not until the latter part of the 20th century that exploration into the role of creatine supplementation in exercise performance began (Balsom et al., 1994). Creatine supplementation gained attention after high-profile athletes competing in sprint and power events in the 1992 Olympics claimed their performance had benefited from creatine supplementation (Jacobs, 1999).

From: *Forensic Science: Dietary Supplements: Toxicology and Clinical Pharmacology*
Edited by: M. J. Cupp and T. S. Tracy © Humana Press Inc., Totowa, New Jersey

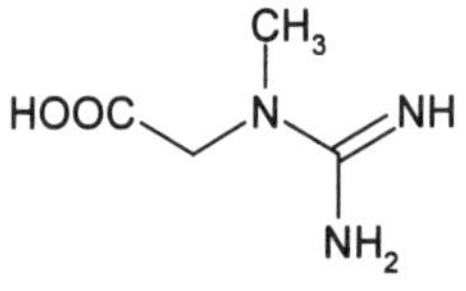

Fig. 1. Chemical structure of creatine.

6.2. CHEMICAL STRUCTURE

See Fig. 6-1 for the chemical structure of creatine.

6.3. CURRENT PROMOTED USES

Creatine monohydrate supplementation is promoted as an ergogenic aid, which refers to a product purported to enhance energy production, utilization, control, and efficiency (Mujika and Padilla, 1997). Creatine is purported to increase power, strength, and muscle mass and to decrease performance time (Demant et al., 1999).

6.4. SOURCES AND CHEMICAL COMPOSITION

Creatine is a nitrogenous molecule that occurs naturally in skeletal and smooth muscle and neural tissue (Clark, 1998). Exogenous (i.e., dietary) sources include fish, fowl, and red meat (Jacobs, 1999). Plants contain, at most, only trace amounts (Balsom et al., 1994). Approximately 1 g of creatine can be obtained from a normal diet, with the remainder being synthesized endogenously. Vegetarians' daily needs are met almost exclusively from endogenous sources due to the low creatine content of their diet (Balsom et al., 1994). Creatine used in supplements is purportedly synthesized by heating an aqueous solution of cyanamide, and sodium sarcosine, an acetic acid derivative, according to industry web sites (Wallack, 2000; Pacific Nutrition 2000).

6.5. PRODUCTS AVAILABLE

Creatine supplements are available as creatine monohydrate, a white powder soluble in warm water (Balsom et al., 1994). Creatine monohydrate is available in a variety of dosage forms, including powders, micronized powders, effervescent tablets, capsules, tablets, liquids, and chewables. Internet retailers claim that micronized powders cause less gastrointestinal distress, diarrhea, and bloating than creatine monohydrate powder in gelatin capsules and that liquid and effervescent formulations also cause less stomach upset. Creatine monohydrate is available alone or in combination with other agents, such as dextrose, ribose, glucose, chromium, α-lipoic acid, glutamine, taurine, and methylsulfonylmethane. The powder is the form most commonly used.

Some popular brands include Basic Nutrition™ Creatine Monohydrate (5 g/tsp powder), Body Fortress™ Creatine Caps (700 mg), Challenge™ Creatine Monohydrate tablets (500 mg), Muscle Link™ Effervescent Creatine Elite™ (5 g/packet), Optimum Nutrition Creatine Liquid Energy (3 g creatine monohydrate and 250 mg methylsulfonylmethane/tbsp liquid), Pro Performance® Pure Creatine Monohydrate

Powder (5 g/tsp powder), Pro Performance® creatine monohydrate chewable tablets (2500 mg), Prolab® Nutrition Creapure™ creatine monohydrate powder (5 g/teaspoon), Twinlab® Creatine Fuel Loading Drink (2500 mg/scoop creatine monohydrate powder plus taurine, L-glutamine, chromium, magnesium, and α-lipoic acid), Twinlab® Creatine Fuel capsules (700 mg) and powder (5 g/tsp), Experimental and Applied Sciences (EAS®) Phosphagen™ Pure Creatine Monohydrate powder (5 g/tsp), Met-Rx® Creatine AC™ [12.4 g creatine monohydrate, 400 mg α-lipoic acid, and 10 g glutamine peptide with glucose per 126 g (3 scoop) serving], Weider™ Pure Creatine Monohydrate capsules (725 mg), and Natrol® 99% Pure Creatine-Creatine Monohydrate powder (5 g/tsp).

In August 2000, the independent laboratory ConsumerLab.com released their results of potency and purity testing of 13 brands of creatine monohydrate commonly available through catalogs, retail stores, multilevel marketing companies, and online. Creatine content as well as product contamination with creatinine and dicyandiamide were measured. Although these contaminants are not known to be harmful, they are not beneficial and are eliminated through the kidney. Eleven (85%) of the products tested met ConsumerLab.com's standards (ConsumerLab.com, 2000). A list of creatine products that passed testing, as well as details about testing methodology, is available at the web site www.consumerlabs.com.

Most manufacturers recommended a loading dose of 20 g/d divided into four doses for 4–7 d, followed by a maintenance dose of 5 g daily. Manufacturers usually recommend that creatine powder be dissolved in fruit juice or sports drinks.

6.6. PHYSIOLOGIC ROLE

Creatine is an important source of chemical energy for muscle contraction. Creatine undergoes rapid phosphorylation to creatine phosphate. Creatine phosphate can then donate a phosphate group to adenosine diphosphate (ADP) to form adenosine triphosphate (ATP), the energy source for muscle contraction. Muscle supplies of ATP and creatine phosphate are limited (Balsom et al., 1994).

6.7. IN VITRO EFFECTS AND ANIMAL DATA

The relationship between muscle isometric tension and creatine phosphate concentration was studied in tetanically stimulated isolated mouse soleus muscle. Tension declined over time. Creatine phosphate concentrations present in cells at the end of the experiment were directly proportional to the isometric tension that the muscle was capable of producing at the end of the experiment. This study demonstrated that the cause of fatigue in isolated mammalian skeletal muscle is depletion of creatine phosphate (Spande et al., 1970).

The importance of creatine in muscle contraction has been demonstrated using other models. Addition of creatine to cell cultures of cardiac or skeletal muscle cells from newborn rats resulted in an increased concentration of intracellular creatine phosphate compared with control cultures. The increase was directly proportional to the concentration of creatine in the culture medium. Increased creatine phosphate was accompanied by a small increase in muscle protein, an increase in the rate of beating of cardiac cells, an increase in the rate of formation of myotubules, and an increase in branching of myotubules. ATP concentration was unchanged. Since the only known pathway for the synthesis of phosphocreatine involves the enzyme creatine phosphokinase (creatine kinase), this study (Seraydarian et al., 1974) also provided evidence that in addition to serving as a storage form of energy, creatine might be involved in a regulatory feedback mechanism ensuring maintenance of the source of energy for muscle contraction. The investigators hypothesized that increased muscle creatine stimulates the mitochondrial creatine kinase, which phosphorylates creatine at the expense of ATP. ADP formed in the mitochondria as a product of this reaction stimulates oxidative phosphorylation, which produces ATP for the resynthesis of creatine phosphate during recovery. Creatine phosphate, in a reaction catalyzed by creatine kinase, provides energy in the form of its phosphate bond to regenerate myosin-bound ATP from ADP for use in muscle contraction. Increased muscle activity increases free creatine, which begins the cycle anew. Thus creatine maintains functional levels of muscle ATP.

Further support for this hypothesis stems from a previous study (Seraydarian et al., 1969) demonstrating that if glycolysis and oxidative phosphorylation are inhibited in cultured cardiac cells, creatine phosphate concentrations are decreased and the cells fail to contract spontaneously despite no change in ATP concentration.

The observation that muscle contraction may cease despite adequate ATP concentrations (Seraydarian et al., 1969) illustrates another important role of creatine, namely, its role as a link between mitochondrial production of ATP and cellular utilization of ATP. Free creatine formed from the breakdown of creatine phosphate by creatine kinase at the M-line region of the myofibril travels to the mitochondria, where it is phosphorylated by a different creatine kinase isoenzyme. Creatine phosphate formed at the mitochondria then travels back to the myosin heads where its potential energy, stored in the phosphate bond, can be utilized for ATP synthesis. This "phosphorylcreatine shuttle" explains the inability to demonstrate experimentally a direct relationship between muscle contraction and intracellular ATP and ADP concentrations (Bessman and Geiger, 1981).

In an investigation designed to study the effect of creatine supplementation on cardiac energy metabolism and creatine concentration in various organs (Horn et al., 1998), 77 Wistar rats consumed a rat chow with creatine supplemented at 0, 1, 3, 5, or 7% of the dietary weight for approximately 40 d. The rats were sacrificed, and the hearts were removed and attached to a perfusion apparatus for the purpose of measuring left ventricular pressure. The concentration of phosphate and high-energy phosphate bonds in the perfused heart was measured via ^{131}P nuclear magnetic resonance (NMR) spectroscopy, and creatine kinase reaction velocity (speed of transfer of phosphate) was measured using ^{131}P magnetization transfer. Total creatine in serum, heart, brain, skeletal muscle, liver, and kidney were measured using high-performance liquid chromatography (HPLC). The five groups of rats were compared using a factorial ANOVA with significant differences between groups identified using Scheffe's F-test.

An analysis of serum creatine levels at the end of the supplementation period showed a dose-dependent increase in serum creatine by 73–202%. The increase in serum creatine did not translate into an increase in mechanical function of the heart (as measured by left ventricular pressure), or cardiac concentrations of ATP, phosphocreatine, inorganic phosphate, creatine kinase reaction velocity, or total creatine. Total creatine content of the liver and kidney increased but remained unchanged in brain and skeletal muscle. The investigators caution that the results of this study cannot be extrapolated to animal models of chronic heart failure and call for investigation of the effects of creatine supplementation in such models. They attributed the disparate effect of creatine supplementation on various organs to differences in baseline creatine content, hypothesizing that the liver and kidney showed increases in creatine content because these organs contain relatively low amounts of creatine, while the brain, skeletal muscle, and heart are high in creatine.

In a study designed to investigate the effect of increasing amounts of dietary creatine monohydrate supplementation on muscle and plasma creatine concentrations in dogs and to characterize the accumulation of creatine in muscle over time, dry crystalline creatine monohydrate at a dose of 0.38–3.05 mmol creatine per kg was administered to 12 adult beagle dogs (Lowe et al., 1998). Muscle biopsies of the biceps femoris analyzed by reverse phase ion-pairing HPLC showed an increase in total creatine in dogs with low initial presupplementation total muscle creatine concentrations (<140 mmol/kg) and a negligible effect on dogs with higher initial total creatine concentrations. Maximal muscle total creatine levels were achieved within 14 d with as little as 0.38 mmol creatine/kg. Little benefit from feeding larger amounts of creatine was found. Plasma creatinine content increased in relation to the amount of creatine ingested and in proportion to plasma creatine. Urinary creatinine excretion also increased (Lowe et al., 1998).

Oral creatine in varying doses was found to be effective in modifying the inflammatory response in rats. It was tested in acute and chronic inflammation and local irritation. No gastrointestinal ulceration occurred at effective doses. Creatine also had analgesic activity (Khanna et al., 1978).

Creatine's effect in an animal model of amyotrophic lateral sclerosis (ALS; Lou Gehrig's disease) has been studied. The pathogenesis of ALS is thought to involve oxidative damage to the mitochondria. The rationale behind creatine supplementation for ALS stems from creatine's role in maintaining and transporting energy. Creatine supplementation in transgenic ALS mice with a mutation affecting expression of the antioxidant superoxide dismutase (G93 transgenic mice) improved motor performance on the rotorod test, extended survival, protected mice from loss of motor neurons and neurons in the substantia nigra, and decreased biochemical evidence of oxidative damage compared with control animals (Klivenyi et al., 1999). Similarly, creatine showed neuroprotective effects in chemically induced Huntington's disease in rats (Matthews et al., 1998). Further study is needed to determine creatine's effect on established or progressive disease and its efficacy in humans.

Creatine monohydrate protected against traumatic brain injury-related tissue damage in mice and rats (Sullivan et al., 2000). In this model, moderate cortical contusion was inflicted, causing severe behavioral deficits, significant cortical tissue loss, disruption of the blood-brain barrier, and loss of hippocampal neurons, thus mimicking human closed-head injury. Mice were pretreated for 1, 3, or 5 d with intraperitoneal creatine monohydrate 3 mg/g body weight in olive oil or olive oil alone, and rats were fed a diet supplemented with 1% creatine monohydrate or control diet for 4 weeks prior to injury. As measured by cortical tissue loss and mitochondrial function, all creatine-treated groups demonstrated less tissue injury compared with controls with the exception of mice treated with creatine for only 1 d. The authors suggest that athletes who take creatine may gain a neuroprotective benefit in the event of head injury.

6.8. CLINICAL STUDIES

6.8.1. Inborn Errors of Metabolism

Creatine supplementation has been studied in humans with good results in the treatment of certain inborn errors of metabolism, such as guanidinoacetate methyltransferase deficiency (Stockler et al., 1996, 1997), that result in creatine deficiency in the brain and symptoms such as developmental delays, mental retardation (van der Knaap et al., 1999; Bianchi et al. 2000), extrapyramidal movement disorders (Stockler et al., 1997; van der Knaap et al., 1999), and epilepsy (van der Knaap et al., 1999). Metabolic diseases resulting in creatine deficiency can also cause muscle fatigue (Tarnopolsky et al., 1997) and visual disturbances (Sipila et al., 1981). In fact, the first therapeutic use of creatine supplementation was in patients with gyrate atrophy of the choroid and retina caused by an inability to produce creatine. In this study (Sipila et al., 1981), seven patients were administered creatine 1.5 g daily for 1 yr. Creatine supplementation not only slowed the progressive loss of visual fields, but also increased the diameter of type II muscle fibers by 43%. Patients also reported increased muscle strength, and one improved his 100-m sprint time. Follow-up results were subsequently published, showing that these benefits could be maintained for up to 5 yr (Vannas-Sulonen et al., 1985). Creatine supplementation was also shown to improve skeletal muscle function and subjective muscle complaints in a double-blind, placebo-controlled crossover study in nine patients with McArdle's disease (myophosphorylase deficiency) (Vorgerd et al., 2000).

6.8.2. Enhancement of Athletic Performance

By far the most common promoted use of creatine is to enhance athletic performance. A cross-sectional survey of health club members in eastern Virginia revealed that 35% of survey respondents used creatine (Sheppard et al., 2000). The rationale for creatine supplementation in sports is related to the limited supply of muscle creatine phosphate and ATP (as mentioned in the *Physiologic Role* section). It has been estimated based on studies of ATP turnover during cycling and electrical stimulation of the quadriceps muscle that creatine phosphate stores may be depleted within 10 s. During recovery, creatine phosphate is regenerated from the increased free creatine stores that accumulate during exercise. Results of several studies demonstrate that complete resynthesis of creatine phosphate during recovery takes at least 5 min (Balsom et al., 1994). Creatine supplementation is thought to aid exercise performance by facilitating generation of intramuscular creatine phosphate and subsequent ATP formation, thus prolonging the duration of high-intensity physical activity (Williams and Branch, 1998). This effect is sometimes referred to as "energy buffering." By accepting a hydrogen ion (H^+) when donating a phosphate group to ADP to form ATP, creatine may buffer the H^+ produced during anaerobic glycolysis, thus helping to maintain normal muscle pH necessary for optimal performance (Demant and Rhodes, 1999; Balsom et al., 1994). Creatine supplementation also increases the rate of creatine phosphate resynthesis during recovery. Creatine phosphate is thought to inhibit glycolysis by inhibiting phosphofructokinase (PFK), the rate-limiting enzyme of glycolysis (Demant and Rhodes, 1999). As will be discussed, evidence from human studies that creatine supplementation inhibits glycolysis is lacking.

More than 100 studies of creatine's application in sports and exercise have been published. Several high-quality, representative studies will be reviewed here. Most studies have been performed to determine the influence of creatine supplementation on repeated bouts of short-duration, maximal-intensity exercise. In the first double-blind study examining the effect of creatine monohydrate supplementation vs placebo on skeletal muscle performance (Greenhaff et al., 1993), 12 physically active (but not highly trained) volunteers ingested creatine monohydrate (5 g four times daily) plus glucose (1 g four times daily) or placebo (6 g glucose four times daily). The dose of creatine monohydrate used in this study was based on results of a study (Harris et al., 1992) in which creatine 5 g four to six times daily for 4-10 d effectively increased quadriceps creatine stores (*see Pharmacokinetics* section). Both before and after five days of supplementation, subjects performed 5 d sets of 30 knee extensions separated by 1-min recovery periods. Knee extensor torque production was measured and recorded with each contraction. Plasma ammonia and blood lactate levels were measured after each set of knee extensions. All comparisons were made using the *t*-test for paired samples.

Compared with baseline, a significant increase in total peak torque production occurred in the second ($p < 0.01$) and third ($p < 0.05$) sets in the creatine group but not in the placebo group. The increase in the fourth set in the creatine group approached statistical significance ($p = 0.056$). An increase in peak torque production was seen in these three sets in all six creatine subjects. Peak torque generated was also greater after supplementation in the last 10 contractions of set 1 ($p < 0.05$) and contractions 11–20 of set 5 ($p < 0.05$). Blood lactate concentrations were not significantly different before or after supplementation. Compared with baseline, ammonia levels were lower after the fourth ($p < 0.01$) and fifth ($p < 0.01$) sets of those subjects receiving creatine supplementation. For unknown reasons, ammonia levels were also lower ($p < 0.01$) 2 min after set 5 after placebo supplementation compared with baseline.

Creatine supplementation may provide some ergogenic benefit to competitive swimmers. In one such study (Grindstaff et al., 1997), subjects were 7 male and 11 female regionally or nationally competitive swimmers, mean age 15.3 ± 0.6 yrs. Performance time, arm ergometry, body weight, and body composition per skinfold athropometry and bioelectrical impedence were measured before and after daily supplementation with creatine monohydrate 21 g (Phosphagen) plus 4.2 g granulated maltodextrin or placebo (granulated maltodextrin 25.2 g). Subjects were paired based on similarities, including gender, body weight, event, and 100-m freestyle sprint times. One subject in each pair was randomized to creatine, and the other received placebo. The supplements were similar in taste, texture, and appearance. Compliance with the study supplement was more than 90% based on daily verbal checks and a poststudy questionnaire. After baseline data pertinent to the outcome measures were taken, subjects consumed the study supplement for 9 d. The supplement was dissolved in 500 mL of water or juice and consumed with meals, three times daily. Ergometry (three 20-s sprints separated by a 60-s rest period), body weight, body composition measurements, and swim sprints (three heats, each consisting of a 50-m and 100-m sprint) were then repeated. Statistical significance was set at p 0.05, and data were analyzed using two-way repeated measures ANOVA with the Tukey *post hoc* procedure to identify significant interactions.

Creatine-supplemented subjects swam significantly faster than placebo-supplemented subjects in heat 1 and faster than baseline significantly decreased swim time in the second 100-m sprint. There was a trend toward a decrease in total time to complete the three 100-m sprints in the creatine-supplemented subjects. Change in fat free mass was greater in the creatine group but did not reach statistical significance ($p = 0.15$). Changes in fat mass and percent body fat were lower in the creatine group but did not reach statistical significance ($p = 0.08$ and $p = 0.09$, respectively). Creatine supplementation improved total work and power output only during the first 20 s of the arm ergometry exercise. The investigators suggest that perhaps work and power output would have improved with a longer rest period between sprints to allow for regeneration of creatine phosphate stores; however, as will be discussed later, the effects of creatine supplementation may be best demonstrated under circumstances of incomplete recovery. A larger sample size may also have improved results.

Subsequently, other investigators (Theodorou et al., 1999) examined the effects of acute (2 g daily in divided doses for 4 d) and chronic (5 g creatine or placebo daily for 2 mo) supplementation on the performance of elite swimmers swimming 10×50 m ($n = 14$), 8×100 m ($n = 7$), or 15×100 m ($n = 1$), according to personal preference. Swimmers' time was first measured at baseline and then within 2 d of completing the acute loading phase. Swimmers were then randomized to ingest creatine 5 g daily or placebo for 8 wk, and swimming times were again recorded. In addition, during the chronic phase of the study, six swimmers in each of the two treatment groups were timed every 2 wk during the 8-wk study period (i.e., at weeks 2, 4, 6, and 8). At the end of the chronic phase, these 12 participants were administered a second 4-d acute creatine load.

After the first acute creatine load, there was a significant improvement in mean swimming performance ($p < 0.01$, t-test for paired samples). A Wilcoxon test for paired samples showed a significant difference from baseline after creatine supplementation for sprints 3–10 for the 50-m swimmers and sprints 6 and 7 for the 8×100-m swimmers; however, 3 of the 22 swimmers showed no improvement in performance. There was a significant increase in body mass after the acute load ($p < 0.01$, t-test for paired samples). Both the creatine and placebo groups improved significantly ($p < 0.01$, repeated-measures ANOVA) after the acute load vs baseline. There was also no significant difference between the two groups in response to the acute load and no difference between the groups before and after supplementation; therefore, the placebo and creatine groups were similar in response to the acute load. The two six-member subgroups were also shown to be similar in response to the acute load. In regard to response to chronic supplementation, there was no difference in swim time after acute load and after the maintenance phase for either group per repeated-measures ANOVA. In each group, approximately half of the swimmers improved their swimming times after the maintenance phase, and half had slower swimming times. In the subgroups, repeated-measures ANOVA revealed no significant change in swim time from after acute load to each of the four maintenance times. A paired *t*-test also showed no significant change in swim time between the end of the maintenance phase (week 8) and the end of the second acute load. There was no significant change in body mass in either subgroup.

The authors hypothesized that the initial acute load may have kept muscle creatine stores near maximum, such that maintenance supplementation and a second acute load led to no further improvement. Other studies (Lemon et al., 1995; Hultman et al., 1996) suggest that in the absence of supplementation, creatine stores return to preload values after 4–5 wk. The investigators felt that the findings of these two previous studies, which were performed in healthy active men, might not apply to highly trained athletes who train for several hours each day. They hypothesized, based on results of a previous study (Harris et al., 1992), that vigorous training during the acute load might enhance creatine storage in muscle, such that the time to return of muscle creatine to presupplementation levels might be longer in elite swimmers. Because a previous study by four of the investigators (published as an abstract) showed that placebo improved performance time by only 0.02 s, the investigators felt it unlikely that the improvement after the first acute load was a placebo effect. They also noted that a placebo effect should also have been seen after the second acute load if the response to the first acute load was owing to a placebo effect. The investigators also observed that the magnitude of improvement seen with creatine supplementation was similar to that seen in their previous study.

Previous studies (Burke et al., 1996; Mujika et al., 1996) of creatine supplementation in swimmers have shown no improvement in performance. The difference in study findings can be attributed to differences in study design. In the study by Theodorou and colleagues (1999) discussed above, swimmers performed repeated swimming sprints with only a 1–2-min rest period between sprints, resulting in incomplete recovery of creatine phosphate, whereas other studies allowed recovery times of up to 10 min. Such studies that do not deplete creatine phosphate stores and cause muscle fatigue are not appropriately designed to test the effects of creatine supplementation. Peyrebrune and colleagues (1998) compared two exercise protocols, a single-sprint effort vs multiple-sprint efforts interspersed with short recovery periods, effectively demonstrating the importance of study design. As seen in the Theodorou et al. study (1999), creatine supplementation appears to confer most benefit as the number of sprints performed increases. This information suggests that creatine supplementation may not be useful for sports competitions that require only a single-sprint effort; however, creatine supplementation may benefit athletes in training for such events because it may permit longer workout sessions (Theodorou et al., 1999).

Creatine's effect on cycle ergometer performance has also been studied. A randomized, double-blind, placebo-controlled study (Birch et al., 1994) was undertaken to document the effect of creatine monohydrate supplementation 20 g/d for 5 d on power output measured using an isokinetic cycling ergometer at a velocity of 80 rpm. Fifteen healthy males volunteered for the study. Two days before beginning the 5-d supplementation period, and on the morning of the final day of supplementation, the study subjects performed three 30-s bouts of maximal stationary cycling separated by

4-min recovery periods. This period of recovery was chosen because it had previously been shown to correspond to 80% recovery of creatine phosphate stores. Blood samples were taken before and after exercise for blood lactate and plasma ammonia assay. All statistical analyses were done using the paired t-test.

Peak power output was found to be 8% higher ($p < 0.05$) during exercise bout 1 following creatine ingestion compared with exercise bout 1 at baseline. Mean power output was 6% higher during exercise bouts 1 ($p < 0.05$) and 2 ($p < 0.05$), and total work performed was greater in bouts 1 ($p < 0.05$) and 2 ($p < 0.05$) after creatine supplementation compared with baseline. Peak plasma ammonia was lower after creatine supplementation compared with baseline ($p < 0.05$), but peak blood lactate concentrations were unchanged. The authors suggest that lack of change in lactate concentrations in their study [as well as in a previously described study (Greenhaff et al., 1993)] implies that creatine supplementation does not inhibit anaerobic glycolysis. The decrease in ammonia accumulation noted in this as well as the previous study (Greenhaff et al., 1993) was attributed to increased ATP turnover rate during muscle contraction with creatine supplementation. The authors acknowledge that the increased peak power output, mean power output, and total work seen after bout 1, as opposed to bout 3 with creatine supplementation were unexpected since creatine availability would be unlikely to be compromised at the beginning of exercise.

Dawson and colleagues (1995) compared creatine 5 g, 1 g glucose polymer (Polycose®, Ross Laboratories), and 0.2 g calcium carbonate four times daily for 5 d with placebo (6 g glucose polymer plus 0.2 g calcium carbonate) in two separate double-blind studies of creatine's effect on total work and peak power output on cycle ergometer testing. In study 1, 18 active male volunteers performed a single 10-s cycling sprint; in study 2, 22 additional male volunteers performed six 6-s sprints, with 24 s of recovery between sprints. Subjects' performance at baseline and after the 5-d treatment period was documented. At baseline, subjects performed a familiarization test, followed by two baseline tests separated by at least 2 d. After treatment, two more trials 2 d apart were performed. Blood was collected at baseline and after the post-treatment test for analysis of pH and blood lactate. Body weight was also measured before and after treatment. Paired t-tests were used to compare the two baseline trials to determine whether there was a significant difference between them. If the two were not statistically different, they were averaged, and this mean was used as the baseline value. If they were different, the better of the two was used as the baseline value.

After randomization, independent t-tests determined that there were no significant differences in the two treatment groups in baseline total work or peak power scores; nonetheless, analysis of covariance (ANCOVA) was used to adjust for minor differences between the two groups in baseline performance scores. Two-way analysis of variance and covariance with repeated measures of one variable was also performed between baseline and each postloading test to determine whether there were differences within or between groups in total work, peak power performance, pH, or blood lactate. The null hypothesis was rejected if $p < 0.05$.

In each study, and in each group, there were no significant differences between performance scores on postloading tests 1 and 2. In study 1, the creatine group increased in body mass compared with baseline ($p < 0.01$), whereas body weight decreased in the placebo group. Both groups improved their total work and peak power from baseline.

There was no significant difference between the two groups. Postsupplementation, changes in blood lactate and pH showed no significant difference from baseline or between groups. In study 2, total work ($p < 0.05$), work done in sprint 1 ($p < 0.01$), and peak power ($p < 0.01$) were higher in the creatine group compared with placebo. Blood pH was unaffected. Blood lactate levels were significantly ($p < 0.05$) higher after treatment compared with baseline for both groups. In the Greenhaff et al. (1993) and Birch et al. (1994) studies, blood lactate did not change from baseline, but in this study, lactate increased, an observation that could not be explained by the study intervention. The authors suggest that postsupplementation, muscle glycogen stores may have been increased by dietary intake, which was not controlled in the study, leading to more anaerobic glycolysis.

Creatine supplementation has also been shown to help athletes maintain cycling speed on a stationary bike during 10 6-s exercise bouts interspersed with 30-s rest periods (Balsom et al., 1993a). Although the authors noted a decrease in oxygen consumption measured after the seventh exercise bout by analysis of expired gas in Douglas bags, investigators who subsequently measured oxygen consumption using a CPX system (Medical Graphics, St. Paul, MN) found that creatine, but not placebo, increased oxygen consumption significantly ($p < 0.05$) compared with baseline in highly trained cyclists exercising at 90% maximum power output (MPO; Rico-Sanz and Marco, 2000). In this study, uric acid levels at exhaustion ($p < 0.05$) and 5 min postexercise ($p < 0.01$), as well as ammonia levels at the end of the first of two 90% MPO bouts and the third of three 30% MPO bouts ($p < 0.05$), were significantly lower than baseline in the creatine group. Creatine, but not placebo, increased time to exhaustion ($p < 0.05$).

In a crossover study, nine physically active males were supplemented in random order with 20 g/d of creatine or placebo for 3 d prior to an exercise test of maximal cycling lasting 30 s (Wingate anaerobic test; Odland et al., 1997). Although resting muscle total creatine concentration was increased, creatine phosphate concentration was not increased. The authors attributed this finding to the short duration of supplementation. There was no effect on performance as measured by peak power output on cycle ergometer. For reasons discussed previously, creatine would not be expected to benefit power output during a single 30-s bout of maximal cycle exercise. Similarly, a previous study found that creatine did not improve performance (peak power, time to peak power, total work, fatigue index) on two bouts of 15-s cycle ergometer sprints separated by a 20-min rest period (Cooke et al., 1995).

Creatine supplementation as an ergogenic aid for short running sprints has been studied. In a double-blind placebo controlled study, the effect of creatine supplementation was studied in 12 sprinters training an average of 20 h per week. All athletes performed a 150-m sprint prior to supplementation and again 2 wk later, after 3 d of supplementation with creatine monohydrate (5 g five times daily in lemon juice and water) or placebo (lemon juice in water). Blood samples were taken prior to warm-up and after each sprint. Data were analyzed using a two-way ANOVA for repeated measures. Statistical significance was accepted if $p < 0.05$.

Neither the creatine group nor the placebo group improved compared with baseline, although there was a trend toward improvement in the creatine group ($p > 0.05$). There was also no difference in performance between the placebo and creatine groups in either the first (presupplementation) or second (postsupplementation) sprints.

Plasma lactate concentrations did not differ between the placebo and creatine groups after the second sprint. At baseline, plasma creatinine levels were similar for those randomized to placebo and creatine supplementation. Plasma creatinine levels increased in the creatine group after supplementation compared with baseline ($p < 0.01$) and compared with the placebo patients immediately before ($p = 0.009$) and after ($p = 0.02$) the second sprint. The authors hypothesize that the rate-limiting factor in ATP synthesis in single, continuous, high-intensity exercise, as in this study, is not the amount of creatine phosphate available, but rather the rate of ATP regeneration by creatine kinase (Javierre et al., 1997).

Another study (Terrillion et al., 1997) found that creatine supplementation did not improve time in 12 well-trained, competitive runners performing two 700-m maximal running bouts separated by 60 min. The subjects (mean age 21 yr) had just completed a collegiate track season and/or were in training for a road race. Subjects were grouped in pairs based on similarity in time to complete a 600-m run on an outdoor track. One member of each of the six pairs was randomized to creatine monohydrate 5 g plus glucose 1 g four times daily; the other was assigned to placebo (sucrose 6 g). One week after randomization, subjects performed two baseline 700-m runs separated by a 60-min rest period. This exercise was repeated 2 wk later, after the subjects had consumed the study supplement for 5 d. In addition to performance time, blood lactate was measured after completion of each 700-m run, and subjects were weighed before the first 700-m run of each of the two trials. Statistical significance was established at p 0.05, and MANOVA was used to compare time, lactate concentrations, and weight between groups and between trials. No statistically significant differences or clear trends favoring creatine were identified. The investigators suggest that creatine supplementation may not benefit running because the rest-to-work ratio in running is very low compared with other sports (i.e., rowing, football, basketball, wrestling); thus there may not be enough time to regenerate creatine phosphate, regardless of creatine stores, because the rest period is too short. Small sample size may have contributed to the results, although it is likely that creatine supplementaion does not benefit this type of activity (i.e., high intensity, relatively long duration), as will be discussed.

Three other studies of creatine's effect on sprint velocity, one in highly trained male soccer and female field hockey athletes (Redondo et al., 1996), one in college football players (Stout et al., 1997), and one in football and track athletes (Goldberg and Bechtel, 1997), showed no improvement. The negative results of the Goldberg and Bechtel study and those of Stout and colleagues might be owing to the relatively low creatine doses used (3 g/d and 10.5 g/d, respectively), or to study design, which may not have exercised the muscles to fatigue. It is important to note that in regard to a dose-response relationship with creatine, doses as low as 7.7 g/d can improve response to resistance training, if not sprint velocity (Burke et al., 2000).

In endurance sports, athletes perform aerobic activity with intermittent spurts of anaerobic activity, such as near the finish line. In a cycle ergometer study designed to simulate an endurance sport, 12 triathletes ingested 3 g creatinine monohydrate (Creatine Pulver-Multi-power®, Haleko) twice daily for 5 d prior to testing (Engelhardt et al., 1998). Subjects performed a 30-min endurance exercise followed by 10 15-s intervals, each separated by a 45-s rest. After a 120-s rest, the 10 15-s intervals were repeated, followed by 30 min of endurance exercise. Before and after supplementation, blood lactate, glucose, creatine kinase, heart rate, oxygen consumption, body weight, creatinine and creatine excretion, serum creatine and creatinine, and number of intervals completed were measured. Blood samples for creatine, creatinine, glucose, and lactate were taken before the exercise test, at the end of the first endurance test, at the end of both interval exercises, and at the end of the second endurance test. Statistical analysis included paired t-tests to identify differences among means, and the Wilcoxon test was used to calculate the change in the number of intervals performed. Significance was accepted at $p < 0.05$.

At baseline, subjects were able to perform a mean of 4.8 ± 2.5 interval repetitions with 4.7 ± 2.3 occurring in the first set and 1 in the second set. After supplementation, this increased to 6.5 ± 2.6, with 6.3 ± 2.3 occurring in the first set and 2 in the second set. Thus, the investigators found that the number of interval repetitions performed increased significantly following supplementation ($p < 0.05$). Endurance performance, however, was not influenced by creatine supplementation. There was no significant change in heart rate, oxygen consumption, blood lactate, or creatine kinase. Blood creatine concentration increased compared with baseline pre-exercise and after both interval ($p < 0.05$) and endurance ($p < 0.01$) excercise tests. Blood creatinine increased compared with baseline pre-exercise, after intervals, and after the second endurance test ($p < 0.05$). Creatine urine elimination at rest, but not after excercise, increased compared with baseline ($p < 0.01$). Similarly, an increase from baseline in creatinine elimination at rest was also noted ($p < 0.05$), but not after exercise. Prior to creatine supplementation, pre-exercise blood glucose levels were higher compared with minute 25 of the first endurance test ($p < 0.05$) and minute 25 of the second endurance test ($p < 0.01$), but after supplementation, glucose levels did not decline with exercise. Body weight increased 0.6 kg with supplementation.

The investigators concluded that creatine monohydrate at a dose of 6 g daily may be beneficial to endurance athletes if they need to do anaerobic sprints during competition, although a double-blind, placebo-controlled trial is needed to confirm these results. This conclusion is supported by a previous study (Balsom et al., 1993b) that also found no benefit for creatine supplementation in either a 6-km run or a 3–6 min treadmill run to exhaustion, both aerobic endurance exercises. In that study, athletes randomized to creatine actually ran more slowly than placebo subjects.

A double-blind crossover study was designed not only to examine the effect of creatine supplementation on endurance capacity and intermittent sprint power in elite cyclists, but also to compare the effect of creatine loading prior to exercise with creatine supplementation during exercise in addition to preexercise loading (Vandebuerie et al., 1998). Subjects were randomized to one of three protocols separated by a washout of 5 wk. Protocol A was a creatine load consisting of 25 g creatine monohydrate (Isotar® Creatine, Isotar Sports Nutrition Foundation, Novartis Nutrition, Switzerland) daily for 4 d plus 4 doses of placebo [Isotar® Long Energy (glucose, maltodextrine, coloring, flavoring, and aspartame)] administered in 4 hourly doses beginning 1 hr prior to the exercise protocol. Protocol B was a creatine load plus 4 doses of 5 g creatine administered in 4 hourly doses beginning 1 hr prior to the exercise protocol. Protocol C was placebo. Coloring, flavoring, maltodextrine, and aspartame were added to the creatine supplement such that it was indistinguishable from placebo. The exercise protocol consisted of endurance cycling followed by intermittent cycling sprints consisting of five maximal 10-s sprints separated by 2-min recovery periods. Protocol A, but not Protocol B, consistently increased peak and mean sprint power for the five sprints by 8–9% compared with placebo ($p < 0.05$, two-way ANOVA). Time to exhaustion was not increased by either Protocol A or B. The authors concluded that creatine loading improves sprint performance, whereas creatine intake during exercise counteracts the ergogenic effect of the creatine load. In addition, creatine did not improve endurance. Adverse effects noted in this study are discussed in the Adverse Effects and Toxicity section below.

The results of these and other studies have led researchers to conclude that creatine supplementation may enhance performance in certain repetitive, high-intensity, short-term exercises, but not endurance exercise. Investigators have also concluded that creatine supplementation does not appear to benefit high intensity, prolonged exercise tasks lasting from 30 to 150 s, as in the trial of Terrillion et al. (1997) (Williams and Branch, 1998). Creatine has also not unequivocally shown benefit in studies of its effects on isometric force; a study of creatine's effect on performance on an isometric grip exercise protocol showed benefit (Kurosawa et al., 1997), but supplementation did not benefit isometric ankle extension (Lemon et al., 1995). Using ^{131}P NMR, the investigators of the latter study, which included only seven volunteers and was of crossover design, documented a carryover effect in one of the three men randomized to creatine as the first treatment.

Youthful females as well as males appear to benefit in regard to strength (Vandenberghe et al., 1997a) and body composition (Vandenberghe et al., 1997a; Mihic et al., 2000), although the increase in lean body mass is only approximately 50% of that observed in males (Mihic et al., 2000). Creatine increased peak anaerobic cycling power and maximal voluntary dorsiflexion torque in females and males equally (Tarnopolsky and MacLennan, 200). One study (Hamilton et al., 2000) that was performed exclusively in females demonstrated a benefit of creatine supplementation on work capacity during fatiguing elbow flexion, but there was no benefit on peak strength generated duing elbow flexion or internal shoulder rotation, internal shoulder rotation work to fatigue, or velocity of internal shoulder rotation. Whether these results would translate into improved performance in sports that require upper extremity anaerobic response such as volleyball, baseball, softball, or racquet sports remains to be tested.

Healthy elderly (age > 60 yr) volunteers appear to benefit little or not at all from creatine supplementation in regard to isokinetic performance (Bermon et al., 1998; Rawson et al., 1999; Rawson and Clarkson, 2000), and little or none (Rawson and Clarkson 2000) or not at all (Rawson et al., 2000; Bermon et al., 1998) in regard to body composition. Creatine also did not affect strength, activities of daily living, or disease activity in patients with rheumatoid arthritis (Willer et al., 2000).

6.8.3. Cardiovascular Effects

Because cardiac creatine levels are decreased in chronic heart failure, creatine monohydrate supplementation has been studied in this population. Patients in New York Heart Association class II ($n = 9$) and III ($n = 8$) with a left ventricular ejection fraction of 29 ± 8% who had been clinically stable for at least 3 mo on diuretics, angiotensin-converting enzyme (ACE) inhibitors, digoxin, and/or β-blockers were randomized to placebo (glucose) or creatine (5 g four times daily) plus glucose for 10 d

(Gordon et al., 1995). Prior to randomization and after supplementation, all patients' performed a unilateral knee extensor exercise, wherein 60 contractions of the quadriceps femoris were performed per minute, with work load increased by 5 W each min. Work capacity (the highest load endured) was recorded. Patients also performed cycle ergometry, with an increase of 10 W/min. Heart rate and blood pressure were measured, and again, work capacity was measured was defined as the highest load achieved. Patients' muscle strength (peak torque) on bilateral knee extension was measured twice, at 14-d intervals, during 100 maximal contractions. The mean for the two legs was used in the statistical analysis. Angiography was performed at rest and during exercise, and muscle samples were taken from the quadriceps femoris for analysis of creatine, phosphocreatine, and total creatine. Intragroup differences were calculated using two-way ANOVA and paired t-tests. Intergroup differences were calculated using two-way ANOVA. Significance was accepted at $p < 0.05$.

Ejection fraction at rest and during exercise did not differ between the two groups. In the creatine group, total creatine in skeletal muscle increased compared with baseline ($p < 0.01$) and compared with the placebo group ($p < 0.01$). Phosphocreatine also increased in this group compared with baseline ($p < 0.01$) and placebo ($p < 0.05$). Free creatine increased in the creatine group compared with the placebo group ($p < 0.05$). Performance on the cycle ergometer increased with creatine supplementation compared with both baseline ($p < 0.01$) and placebo ($p < 0.05$). Performance on the unilateral extensor exercise and the bilateral extensor exercise increased in the creatine group compared with baseline ($p < 0.05$) and with the placebo group ($p < 0.05$). The authors concluded that although creatine supplementation did not improve ejection fraction, it did increase muscle strength and endurance.

Creatine may have other effects on cardiovascular health via reduction in plasma total cholesterol (TC), triglycerides (TAGs), and very low-density lipoprotein (VLDL) cholesterol. In this 12-wk study (Earnest et al., 1996b) sponsored by the product manufacturer, 34 male and female volunteers with moderate hypercholesterolemia (TC > 200mg/dL) who were not taking any cholesterol-lowering medications were randomized to receive creatine monohydrate (Phosphagen, Experimental and Applied Sciences, Golden, CO) 5 g plus glucose 1 g four times daily for 9 d, followed by 10 g for 51 d. Placebo was glucose 6 g. Study subjects maintained their usual activity 4 d/wk throughout the study. Blood lipids were measured at baseline and at weeks 4, 8, and 12. TC decreased compared with baseline ($p < 0.01$) at weeks 4 and 8, and differed from the placebo group at week 8 ($p < 0.05$, two-way ANOVA). Although at baseline females in the placebo group had a significantly lower TAG level than the creatine group ($p < 0.05$), at week 12 the creatine group had a lower TAG than the placebo group ($p < 0.05$). Compared with baseline, TAG decreased in the creatine group at weeks 4, 8, and 12 ($p < 0.01$). VLDL cholesterol, a calculated value (TAG ÷ 5), paralleled the findings for TAG. High-density lipoprotein (HDL) cholesterol, TC/HDL cholesterol ratio, and low-density lipoprotein (LDL) cholesterol did not differ from baseline or between the groups at any time. Results were consistent when analyzed by gender. Although the absolute magnitude of decrease for TC was unimpressive, TAG decreased 26% compared with baseline at week 12. Whether creatine monohydrate is an option in the treatment of hypertriglyceridemia requires more study, as does the mechanism behind creatine's effect on lipid metabolism.

Kreider and associates (1998) also found that supplementation with creatine monohydrate 15.75 g/d in combination with resistance training and sprint/agility exercises for 4 wk increased HDL 13% and decreased VLDL by 13% in 11 NCAA division IA football players.

A subsequent study examined the effect of a combination of heavy resistance training plus creatine monohydrate on blood lipids (Volek et al., 2000). Nineteen resistance-trained male subjects who had never used creatine or anabolic steroids participated. Subjects were matched in pairs according to physical characteristics and strength at baseline testing. One subject from each pair was randomly assigned in double-blind fashion to creatine monohydrate (Muscular Development Creatine®, Twin Laboratories, Hauppauge, NY), and the matched subject was assigned to the placebo (powdered cellulose) group. For the first 7 d of the study, creatine 5 g was taken five times daily. Thereafter, the supplement was taken once daily. A supervised resistance training program was started the same day as supplementation and lasted for 12 wk. Subjects completed a food diary daily. Body mass, body density using hydrodensitometry, and body fat calculated from body density were determined at baseline, at the end of week 1, and at the end of the study. Blood lipids were assessed at baseline, at the end of the loading period, and at the end of the study. Data analysis was performed using two-way ANOVA for repeated measures, and Fischer's LSD test was used to identify pairwise differences between means. Pearson's product-moment correlation coefficient was calculated to identify any relationship between body composition and serum lipids. Statistical significance was accepted if p 0.05. Compliance with the study protocol was 100%, based on pill counts. One patient in the placebo group did not complete the study for reasons unrelated to the study.

Body mass increased in the creatine subjects over the 12-wk study period. Fat-free mass was significantly higher than baseline in the creatine group at weeks 1 and 12. Change in fat-free mass from baseline to week 1 and from baseline to week 12 was significantly greater in the creatine group compared with the placebo group. In the placebo group, fat-free mass was slightly lower at wk 1 compared to baseline and had significantly increased by the end of the study. In placebo subjects, body mass decreased from baseline to week 1 and had increased significantly by 12 wk. Creatine had no effect on lipids. Unlike the Earnest et al. study (1996b), which showed a beneficial effect of creatine on serum lipids, the subjects in this study had normal blood lipid concentrations and were younger (mean age 25.6 yr) than the middle-aged subjects in the Earnest study. In addition, the creatine dose was lower in this study than in both the Earnest et al. study (1996b) and the study by Kreider et al. (1998).

The use of creatine phosphate, which is given as an injection, for intermittent claudication (Panchenko et al., 1994) and myocardial ischemia (Sharov et al., 1986) has also been studied.

6.9. PHARMACOKINETICS

Endogenous creatine is synthesized from glycine, arginine, and S-adenosylmethionine (Halkerston, 1998) in the pancreas, kidney, and liver (Balsom et al., 1994; Greenhaff, 1997; Feldman, 1999), with the liver being the main site of synthesis (Greenhaff, 1997). Most of the creatine is then transported via the bloodstream to skeletal muscle, where approximately 95% of the creatine in the body is stored (Feldman, 1999). Type I muscle fibers in the resting state have a lower concentration of creatine phosphate than type II fibers (Balsom et al., 1994). Most of the remaining 5% is found in the heart, brain, and testes (Balsom et al., 1994; Demant and Rhodes, 1999). The daily requirement of creatine needed to replace the amount broken down during normal body catabolism in a 70-kg individual is 2 g (Balsom et al., 1994; Williams et al., 1998).

The intramuscular total creatine concentration is approximately 118 mmol/kg dry muscle in healthy subjects (Jacobs, 1999). Sixty to 70% of total muscle creatine is stored in the phosphorylated form (creatine phosphate), with the remainder in the form of free creatine (Demant and Rhodes, 1999; Jacobs, 1999; Feldman, 1999). Females may have a higher total creatine level in relation to tissue weight than males, although only one study supports this (Forsberg et al., 1991). Lower levels of resting creatine phosphate have been found in the elderly in comparison with younger individuals, but no differences in total creatine levels were found. This may be a result of inactivity, rather than advancing age *per se* (Jacobs, 1999). Normal mean plasma concentrations of creatine determined in one study were 40.8 μmol/L (men) and 50.2 μmol/L (women), but in vegetarians mean levels of 25.1 μmol/L (men) and 32.4 μmol/L (women) were noted (Delanghe et al., 1989).

The first study of creatine supplementation in humans was done by Harris and colleagues (1992). In the "dose-finding" portion of this study, the investigators' goal was to identify a creatine monohydrate dose that would produce a peak plasma creatine concentration of at least 500 μmol/L. They demonstrated that creatine monohydrate solution 5 g (approximately equivalent to the creatine content of 1.1 kg fresh uncooked steak) administered orally to three volunteers weighing 76–87 kg produced a mean peak plasma level 1 h post dose of 795 μmol/L (SD ± 104 μmol/L), with a return almost to baseline after 5 h. Repeated dosing of 5 g every 2 h resulted in a plasma concentration of 1000 μmol/L for most of the dosing interval. Plasma creatinine was unchanged from baseline.

After this preliminary dose-finding study, the investigators administered creatine monohydrate to five volunteers at a dose of 5 g four times daily for 4.5 d (*n* = 2), 7 d (*n* = 2), and 10 d (*n* = 1). Seven additional subjects received 5 g six times daily for 7 d (*n* = 3), and every other day for 21 d (*n* = 4). Mean baseline total creatine muscle content was 126.8 mmol/kg dry muscle (DM). With the exception of two volunteers with relatively high (>140 mmol/kg DM) baseline total muscle creatine, supplementation increased total creatine content of the vastus lateralis. After supplementation, creatine content rose to 140–160 mmol/kg DM in all subjects. The increase was greatest in individuals with the lowest baseline muscle creatine content, with an increase of up to 50%. In three subjects it was demonstrated that uptake of creatine into the muscle was greatest (32% of the administered dose) during the first 2 d of supplementation, whereas renal excretion of the administered dose increased from 40% on day 1 to 61% on day 2, and to 68% on day 3. At least 20% of the creatine taken up into the muscle was converted to creatine phosphate. Despite an increase in phosphocreatine content, the percentage of total creatine that was phosphocreatine decreased slightly post supplementation (i.e., there was a greater increase in free creatine than in phosphocreatine).

Based on the results of this study, the authors hypothesized that a physiologic ceiling for total muscle creatine of approx 155 mmol/kg dry muscle weight might exist, at least at the doses used in this study. Based on animal data, this "ceiling" might be caused by the presence of a saturable transporter for creatine, although there is evidence that some skeletal muscles do not have this saturable transporter (Greenhaff, 1997). Harris and colleagues (1992) also tested the effect of exercise on creatine muscle uptake by administering creatine phosphate 5 g four times daily for 3.5 d ($n = 1$), six times daily for 4 d ($n = 3$), and six times daily for 7 d ($n = 1$) with daily measurement of performance on a cycle ergometer using one leg. Creatine content of the two legs was compared, and exercise was found to increase creatine uptake into muscle ($p < 0.05$). The Harris study was the first to demonstrate that oral creatine supplementation can increase both creatine and phosphocreatine stores in muscle, prompting additional clinical investigations (*see Clinical Studies* section).

Although creatine supplementation increases muscle creatine stores, continued dosing is required to maintain benefit. After supplementation with 20 g/d for 6 d followed by 2 g/d for 28 d, total muscle creatine increased approx 20% but returned to presupplementation levels after 30 d (Hultman et al., 1996). This information is important in evaluating studies in which participants receive creatine and placebo in a crossover fashion because it suggests an appropriate washout period between treatments.

Serum creatine concentrations and peak times increase linearly with creatine ingestion. Following a 20-g creatine supplementation, a peak serum creatine concentration of 2170 ± 660 mmol/L was observed approx 2 1/2 h after ingestion (Schedel et al., 1999). These investigators also found that creatinine concentrations rose by 13%, perhaps owing to conversion of creatine to creatinine in the gut. As creatine dose was increased, serum creatine concentrations and time to peak concentration increased linearly. Unpublished observations suggest that creatine in solution increases blood creatine levels more than creatine tablets (Greenhaff, 1997). There is also speculation that creatine bioavailability might be lower when it is taken as a combination product rather than as pure creatine monohydrate (Jacobs, 1999). There are no published studies comparing the bioavailability of different creatine monohydrate products or dosage forms.

Compared with placebo, muscle uptake of creatine 5 g dissolved in 250 mL of hot, sugar-free orange juice was increased by ingestion of 92.5 g carbohydrate (glucose and simple sugars) in the form of 500 mL Lucozade® (SmithKline Beecham, Coleford, UK) 30 min post dose. Ingestion of carbohydrate resulted in a 60% greater increase in total muscle creatine compared with creatine alone. This effect was attributed to a 17-fold increase in insulin secretion stimulated by the glucose load. In patients receiving carbohydrate, the increase in muscle creatine did not depend on baseline creatine muscle content, and a "ceiling effect," as documented by Harris and colleagues (1992) was not observed (Green et al., 1996). Triiodothyronine (T_3) also appears to enhance creatine uptake in vitro (Odoom et al., 1993).

A constant percentage of creatine phosphate spontaneously cyclizes to form creatinine (Halkerston, 1988). Excess creatine and its metabolite creatinine are excreted via the kidney (Demant and Rhodes, 1999; Feldman, 1999).

6.10. ADVERSE EFFECTS AND TOXICITY

A 25-yr-old man with an 8-yr history of focal segmental glomerulosclerosis frequently required treatment with corticosteroids for nephrotic syndrome. Beginning 3 yr after presentation, cyclosporine was prescribed in an effort to decrease the number of episodes. His cyclosporine levels during this time ranged from 75–125 ng/mL. Renal function remained normal, with serum creatinine values of 1.1–1.2 mg/dL, creatinine clearance of 91–141 mL/min, and an isotopic glomerular filtration rate (GFR) of 122 mL/min (July 1993). In June 1997, his serum creatinine was 1.2 mg/dL, and creatinine clearance was 93 mL/min. Twelve weeks later, his serum creatinine was 1.8 mg/dL, and creatinine clearance had dropped to 61 mL/min. By October, renal function had declined even further, with a serum creatinine of 2 mg/dL and a creatinine clearance of 54 mL/min. He had no proteinuria, his blood pressure was normal, and his cyclosporine level was therapeutic. He admitted that since August, he had been taking creatine to enhance his soccer performance. He began with a loading dose of 5 g three times daily for 1 wk, followed by a maintenance dose of 2 g/d. He was advised to discontinue this product. Isotopic GFR measured 3 d later was 67 mL/min. One mo later, his serum creatinine was 1.4 µmol/L, and creatinine clearance was 115 mL/min.

Because the time-course of renal function deterioration coincided with creatine use, the authors of this case report suggested that the decline in creatinine clearance might have been caused by tubular damage secondary to myoglobinuria, or increased creatinine production (Pritchard and Kaira 1998). Other possible mechanisms of creatine-induced renal impairment include renal hyperfiltration, vasodilation, and inhibition of tubular protein reabsorption secondary to excess dietary protein and amino acid loading (Poortmans and Francaux, 1999). Cyclosporine, a known nephrotoxin, may also have played a role in this case.

An additional case report implicated creatine monohydrate (Pro Performance Pure Creatine Monohydrate) as a cause of interstitial nephritis in an otherwise healthy 20-yr-old man (Koshy et al., 1999). The young man presented with a 4-d history of nausea, vomiting, and bilateral flank pain that began 4 wk after beginning a regimen of creatine monohydrate 5 g four times daily. He stopped taking the supplement with symptom onset and had not taken any other medications or supplements. Physical exam revealed dehydration and diffuse abdominal tenderness, with a blood pressure (BP) of 140/90 mmHg. Serum creatinine (SCr) was 1.4 mg/dL, and complete blood count, antistreptolysin O, antinuclear antibody, and plasma complement C3 and C4 were normal. Spiral computed tomographic (CT) scan was unremarkable, but urinalysis revealed 4[+] protein and 1[+] blood, with dysmorphic red cells and white cell casts. The patient was admitted to the hospital, where he received fluid replacement and analgesics. His BP peaked at 160/100 mmHg, and SCr increased to 2.3 mg/dL. Protein excretion was 472 mg/d. Renal biopsy was diagnostic for acute focal interstitial nephritis with focal tubular injury. Effacement of the glomerular foot processes and focal thickening of the basement membrane were noted on electron microscopy. BP, SCr, and urinalysis eventually returned to normal.

Despite these case reports, small studies of short duration suggest that creatine has no effect on renal function in individuals without underlying renal disease. In one such study (Poortmans et al., 1997), five healthy male volunteers ingested creatine monohydrate (Ultimate Nutrition Products, Plainville, NJ) 5 g mixed with Gatorade® powder (containing sucrose and dextrose) in warm water four times daily for 5 d. At the end of the 5-d treatment, a 24-h urine collection was performed in the laboratory, and arterial blood was drawn for creatine and creatinine analysis. Creatinine clearance, and urine creatine, creatinine, total protein, and albumin levels were determined. After a 2-wk washout, the same protocol was repeated using placebo (Gatorade powder). Differences between the creatine supplementation and placebo were determined using the Wilcoxon signed-rank test for paired samples, with statistical significance accepted at $p < 0.05$ (two-tailed). Creatine supplementation increased arterial blood creatine concentrations 3.7-fold, urine creatine excretion increased 90-fold, and creatine clearance increased 27-fold ($p < 0.05$). Creatinine clearance, urine creatinine excretion, arterial blood creatinine concentration, and protein excretion were unchanged. The short duration of this study limits the utility of the results.

Hepatorenal effects of creatine supplementation were examined in a longer term study. Creatine monohydrate (Phosphagen) 20 g daily for 5 d followed by 10 g daily for 51 d had no effect on serum creatinine, bilirubin, or total protein in 20 healthy volunteers; however, BUN was significantly increased at week 8 compared with baseline and week 4 ($p < 0.04$) in the 11 females in the study, perhaps owing to an increase in dietary protein intake which was not controlled (Earnest et al., 1996a).

In a subsequent placebo-controlled study, 20 men took creatine monohydrate (supplied by Flamma SpA, Italy) 21 g daily for 5 d, followed by 3 g daily for 58 additional d, or placebo (sucrose) in at the same dose as creatine. Blood samples and a 24-h urine sample for determination of creatinine clearance, urea clearance, and albumin excretion rate were collected at baseline and at days 5, 20, 51, and 63. Using nonparametric tests, no statistically significant difference was found between groups at any time. The investigators did suggest, however, that periodic measurement of albumin excretion would be prudent in creatine users (Poortmans and Francaux, 1998).

In a cohort study by these same investigators (Poortmans and Francaux, 1999), eight males and one female who competed in track and field and volleyball on the national and international level, and who used creatine monohydrate supplements on a regular basis, were compared with 85 male physical education and physical therapy students who did not consume creatine supplements. In the creatine group, creatine consumption varied, with athletes consuming 2–30 g daily 6–7 days per week for 0.8–5 yr (mean 2.7 yr). A fasting blood sample and a 24-h urine collection were taken from all study subjects for determination of plasma and urine creatine, creatinine, and albumin; urinary clearance of creatine, creatinine, urea, and albumin; urine creatine/creatinine ratio; and urine output as well as amount of creatine, creatinine, urea, and albumin excreted in 24 hr. The Mann-Whitney two-sample rank sum test was used to compare differences between the creatine group and the control group. Statistical significance was set at $p < 0.05$.

Urine creatine, creatine/creatinine ratio, and creatine clearance were significantly higher in the creatine users than in the control group ($p < 0.001$). Markers of renal function [creatinine clearance (a marker for GFR), urea clearance (tubular reabsorption), and albumin clearance (glomerular permeability)] were normal in both groups. Plasma creatine, creatinine, urea, and albumin did not differ between groups, and urine excretion of creatinine, urea, and albumin were within the normal range and did not differ between groups. The investigators concluded that creatine does not have detrimental renal effects in persons without underlying renal disease, although they caution that its use should be avoided in patients with known or suspected renal dysfunction.

Patients consuming creatine may have urecognized renal disease at baseline and therefore may unknowingly be at risk for adverse renal effects. For example, between 1 in 500 and 1 in 1000 persons have polycystic kidney disease, symptoms of which may not present until an individual is in his/her 20s, 30s, or 40s. Because of this public health concern, a study of creatine's effects in an animal model of this autosomal dominant disease was undertaken (Edmunds et al., 2001). In this study, Han:SpPRD-cy rats consumed creatine 0.3 g/kg/d for 7 d, followed by creatine 0.03–0.05 g/kg/d for 35 d. This dose reflects the regimen used by athletes. Kidney weight, cyst score, and kidney fluid content increased, whereas creatinine clearance decreased in the creatine-supplemented animals. The investigators hypothesized that creatine may act as an osmotic agent in renal cysts, causing fluid secretion into cysts. Because there is some evidence that creatine downregulates endogenous creatine production, arginine (used in the endogenous production of creatine) may accumulate and lead to an increase of polyamine growth factors, which cause proliferation of tubular epithelial cells, a finding in polycystic kidney disease. Even if creatine is safe in individuals with normal renal function, it may not be safe for persons with subclinical polycystic kidney disease.

In a study designed to evaluate the effects of creatine on serum lipids (Volek et al., 2000), subjects consumed creatine 5 g five times daily for 7 d, followed by creatine 5 g/d for the remainder of the 12-wk study period. Ten subjects were randomized to creatine and nine to placebo. Compared with baseline, serum creatinine was higher in the creatine group after the loading period and at week 12; however, serum creatinine remained within the normal range. In another study of creatine's effects on lipids (Earnest et al., 1996b), there was an increase in BUN in women taking creatine at week 8 compared with baseline ($p < 0.05$); BUN returned to baseline after 4 wk. The increase may have been owing to a direct effect of creatine, dietary protein intake, or timing of blood sampling relative to the menstrual cycle.

In the study described above (Volek et al., 2000), adverse effects were evaluated at the end of the 7-d loading period (25 g/d) and at the end of the remainder of the 12-wk placebo-controlled study. A questionnaire was used to assess change in thirst, appetite, skin changes, muscle soreness, muscle cramping, stomach distress, diarrhea, flatulence, headache, libido, drowsiness, nervousness, and aggression. Adverse effects reported at a higher rate than in the placebo group at the end of the loading period were decreased appetite, decreased thirst, muscle soreness, nervousness, and aggression in 10% of the creatine subjects, and stomach distress in 20%. At week 12, 50% of the creatine subjects reported increased appetite, and 10% reported increased aggression.

Liver function tests were monitored in a study utilizing Phosphagen HP™ (Experimental and Applied Sciences) (Kreider et al., 1998). Eleven study subjects (NCAA division IA football players) ingested 12 tablespoonfuls of product daily, supplying 99 g glucose, 3 g taurine, 1.1 g disodium phosphate, 1.2 g potassium phosphate, and 15.75 g creatine monohydrate. Fourteen subjects ingested placebo, which, except for the absence of creatine monohydrate, was identical to Phosphagen HP. Compared with baseline, small elevations in creatine kinase (CK) ($p < 0.05$), lactate dehydrogenase (LDH) ($p < 0.05$), and alanine aminotrasferase (ALT) ($p < 0.05$) were noted in the Phosphagen HP group. Compared with baseline, there was no increase in aspartate aminotransferase (AST) or γ-glutamyltransferase (GGT), a more specific test of liver function. CK also increased in the placebo group. The investigators attributed the increase in these enzymes, which are present in the liver and muscle, to increased training intensity. Blood creatinine concentration increased in the Phosphagen HP group compared with baseline ($p < 0.05$) but remained within normal limits for persons training intensely.

The deaths of three college wrestlers were initially suspected to be associated with their use of creatine supplements (Poortmans and Francaux, 1999); however, the wrestlers' deaths were subsequently associated with hyperthermia and dehydration caused by practices designed to achieve rapid weight loss, including wearing vapor-impermeable suits under cotton warm-up suits, vigorous exercise in a hot environment, and restricted food and water intake (CDC, 1998). In a related placebo-controlled study (Oöpik et al., 1998), six male martial arts athletes simulated the rapid weight loss program followed by wrestlers to "make weight." Subjects were asked to lose 5% of their body weight over a 5-d period using any technique desired except pharmacologic intervention. Subjects were randomized to receive creatine 20 g or placebo daily during the 5-d weight-loss period. Weight loss was greater with placebo than with creatinine ($p = 0.03$). This finding might be caused by fluid retention within the muscle, despite a decrease in plasma volume ranging from 2–4.6%. Further study is needed to ascertain whether such a decrease in plasma volume may interfere with sweating and thermoregulation.

In a survey of 52 collegiate baseball and football players using creatine, diarrhea ($n = 16$), muscle cramps ($n = 13$), weight gain perceived negatively by athlete ($n = 7$), dehydration ($n = 7$), and muscle sprain or tear ($n = 2$) were reported (Juhn et al., 1999). Reports of seizures, atrial fibrillation, ventricular fibrillation, nose bleeds, intracerebral hemorrhage, myopathies, muscle cramps, rhabdomyolysis, dyspnea, fatigue, nausea, vomiting, pituitary tumor, diarrhea, stomach cramps, stomach pain, burning sensation in the throat and stomach, severe chest pain, back pain, leg numbness, hyperuricemia, change in urine color, facial and laryngeal edema, rash, ruptured aneurysm, nervousness and anxiety, violent and aggressive behavior, migraine headache, speech impairment with loss of muscle control and foaming at the mouth, deep vein thrombosis (DVT), and death in people taking creatine have been filed with the Food and Drug Administration (FDA), but no causality has been established (FDA, 2000), and adverse effects rarely have been reported in controlled trials. Although in a study in NCAA division IA football players, creatine kinase (CK) increased significantly compared with baseline in both the placebo and creatine supplement groups, muscle cramps were not reported (Kreider et al., 1998). Because athletes typically use doses higher than those used in clinical studies (e.g., doses > 5g/d), clinical study results might not represent the real-life adverse effect profile of creatine. For example, gastrointestinal side effects such as diarrhea may result from the excessive osmotic load placed on the intestine by high doses, and creatine-associated water retention in muscle may cause weight gain or muscle cramps (Juhn et al., 1999).

Concerns have been raised that adolescents taking creatine could become predisposed to tendon and apophyseal avulsions and disruptions of bone growth plates caused by a rapid increase in strength (Pepping, 1999). No such adverse effects were noted in a study of 18 teenage (mean age 15.3 yr) competitive swimmers (Grindstaff et al., 1997).

A recent case report (Vahedi et al., 2000) describes a 33-yr-old male who presented with Wernicke's aphasia and mild right-sided face and arm weakness 6 wk after beginning a regime of "energy pills" supplying ephedra alkaloids (contains ephedrine) 40–60 mg, caffeine 400–600 mg, L-carnitine 200–300 mg, chromium 400–600 µg, creatine monohydrate 6000 mg, taurine 1000 mg, inosine 100 mg, and coenzyme Q10 5 mg daily. Babinski sign was present on the right. Serum creatinine was slightly increased but was within normal limits. CT of the brain showed an extensive left middle cerebral artery infarct. Blood pressure was 140/60, and pulse was 54 beats per min. An electrocardiogram (ECG) was normal, and transesophageal echocardiography revealed a patent foramen ovale. Because the patient had recently returned from a transatlantic flight (he had purchased the "energy pills" in Miami), a paradoxical embolism through the patent foramen ovale was suspected; however, d-dimers were normal, and DVT was ruled out. The authors felt that other potential causes of stroke, in whole or in part, in this patient included ephedra, caffeine, and creatine, although no evidence associating creatine with adverse cardiovascular events was proffered.

In the study of elite cyclists described previously (Vandbuerie et al., 1998), one subject dropped out because of severe diarrhea experienced during creatine loading (25 g creatine daily plus colored and flavored maltodextrine and aspartame). In addition, 4 of the 12 subjects experienced "distress" and syncope following exercise, during which they had received 4 hourly doses of creatine beginning 1 hr prior to exercise. These adverse effects were not reported with placebo (glucose, colored and flavored maltodextrine, and aspartame). The authors attributed these adverse effects to hypoglycemia caused by an additive effect of increased peripheral insulin sensitivity caused by exercise in conjunction with hyperinsulinemia caused by creatine intake. The authors cite animal studies to support the latter hypothesis.

6.11. INTERACTIONS

Sarcolemmic uptake of creatine is dependent on the concentration gradient for sodium between the extracellular space and the sarcolemma. Although in theory, caffeine, an adrenergic agent, should enhance creatine uptake into muscles by stimulating activity of the sodium-potassium-ATPase pump, caffeine has been found to counteract the ergogenic effects of creatine supplementation (Vandenberghe et al., 1996). In a double-blind, placebo-controlled crossover study, the effects of placebo, creatine (0.5 g/kg/d administered for 6 d), and creatine with caffeine (5 mg/kg/d administered on the final 3 d of creatine supplementation) on muscle creatine phosphate content and peak knee extension torque were documented. Compared with placebo, both treatment groups increased muscle creatine phosphate levels ($p < 0.05$, two-tailed paired t-test), with an increase of 4% in the creatine group and 6% in the creatine plus caffeine group (NS). Compared with placebo, neither treatment group improved static isometric torque production by the knee extensor muscles. Creatine supplementation improved dynamic knee extension torque compared with placebo ($p < 0.05$), but performance in the creatine plus caffeine group was similar to that with placebo. Since caffeine was ingested 20 h prior to exercise testing (caffeine $t_{1/2}$ 3–5 h), the results were not owing to an acute effect. The exact mechanism of caffeine's effect is unknown, but it might involve creatine phosphate resynthesis, not creatine uptake and storage (Vandenberghe et al., 1996).

A subsequently published study (Vandenberghe et al., 1997b) compared creatine (25 g/d for 5 d), creatine plus caffeine (5 mg/kg/d), and placebo in regard to effect on muscle phosphocreatine concentration and effect on isokinetic contractions of the quadriceps. ^{131}P NMR spectroscopy revealed that although resting muscle phosphocreatine increased 8–15% compared with baseline ($p < 0.05$) in both the creatine and creatine/caffeine groups, caffeine decreased phosphocreatine synthesis during recovery compared with placebo ($p < 0.05$). In addition, dynamic torque production increased with creatine supplementation ($p < 0.05$), whereas the combination of creatine and caffeine did not.

It has been suggested that patients taking medications with nephrotoxic potential, such as, cyclosporin, ACE inhibitors, and nonsteroidal antiinflammatory drugs, should avoid creatine supplementation owing to the possibility of increased adverse renal effects (Pepping, 1999). Likewise, drugs that inhibit the active tubular secretion of creatinine, such as cimetidine, trimethoprim, or probenecid, could theoretically increase creatine levels and thus the adverse effects of creatine. These possible interactions, however, are based on theory and not studies or documented cases.

Manufacturers of creatine monohydrate supplements often recommend mixing the product with juices or sports drinks. Athletes routinely dilute the powder in hot water with glucose or sucrose added (Poortmans and Francaux, 1999). The stability of creatine once mixed with juice has been debated by consumers on bulletin-board type postings on the Internet (NutritionalSupplements.com., 2000), with some users advising that it is unstable in orange juice and should only be mixed with apple or grape juice, others claiming it causes grape juice to ferment into wine, and still others claiming it is unstable in any juice. Other consumers advise that it is stable for only 10 min in water, whereas others claim it is stable for 8–10 h when mixed with liquids. There are no published stability studies of creatine monohydrate in juice, but dissolution of creatine in warm-to-hot water results in no detectable formation of creatinine (Harris et al., 1992). In other studies, subjects were advised to dissolve the creatine powder in warm or hot tea, coffee (Birch et al., 1994; Dawson et al., 1995), sports drinks (Poortmans et al., 1997), orange drink (Birch et al., 1994), orange juice (Green et al., 1996), or fruit juice (Oöpik et al., 1998; Rico-Sanz and Marco, 2000) before consumption.

6.12. REPRODUCTION

There is no information available on the safety of creatine supplementation during pregnancy or lactation or its excretion in breast milk.

6.13. CHEMICAL AND BIOFLUID ANALYSIS

Some analytical methods for creatine determination have drawbacks that should be kept in mind when comparing study results. Although the Jaffe reaction was commonly used in the past to estimate creatine content of tissues, it suffers from lack of specificity and other problems (Kammermeir, 1973), resulting in several published modifications (e.g., Slot, 1965). An enzymatic method described by German researchers was more specific and reproducible but took more time and cost more. To address these problems, a highly specific and sensitive paper or thin-layer chromatographic separation combined with a specific fluorescence reaction was developed (Kammermeir, 1973). The original enzymatic method has subsequently been modified (Harris et al., 1974). Blood creatine levels in one recent pharmacokinetic study were measured using an enzymatic method of SRL Inc. of Japan (Schedel et al., 1999).

For the purpose of facilitating separation of creatine from other endogenous compounds and thus permitting more accurate determinations, Scott and associates (1992) reported an HPLC method whereby creatine and phosphocreatine can be measured in plasma with a total run time of less than 15 min (following a modest sample prep). Blood is collected into preweighed, chilled syringes containing 4 mM 8-azaguanine (internal standard) and 4 mM EDTA. The blood is then centrifuged at 1000g for 15 min (4°C). A 500-µL aliquot of the plasma is then placed in a Centricon 10 microconcentrator and centrifuged at 5000g for 3 h (4°C). Fifty microliters of the ultrafiltrate is then directly injected onto the HPLC system. An Ultrasphere XL ODS (70 × 4.6 mm i.d.) column is used for component separation. Mobile phase A consists of 0.1 M anhydrous dipotassium hydrogen phosphate and 0.01 mM tetrabutylammonium phosphate. Mobile phase B consists of 0.1 M anhydrous dipotassium hydrogen phosphate and 0.01 mM tetrabutylammonium phosphate-methanol (60:40, v/v). Using a flow rate of 1 mL/min, a linear gradient of 0–50% B over 3 min is performed, followed by maintenance of these conditions for 4 min and then a return to 100% A for 4 min (again, in a linear fashion). Finally, the column is allowed to re-equilibrate in 100% A for four minutes prior to the next injection. Creatine (and phosphocreatine) concentrations are monitored using ultraviolet detection at a 214-nm wavelength. The method gives linear calibration curves from 10 nM to 1 mM creatine concentrations. Furthermore, this method allows separation of creatine and phosphocreatine from other endogenous compounds such as inosine, AMP, ADP and ATP, showing specificity of the method.

The use of reverse-phase ion-pairing HPLC to measure equine muscle content of phosphocreatine, creatine, and creatinine has been described (Dunnett et al., 1991). This method has also been used to measure muscle creatine, phosphocreatine, and creatinine content, as well as plasma creatine and creatinine in dogs (Lowe et al., 1998). These authors hypothesize that hydrolysis of phosphocreatine may occur during sample collection and preparation, making determinations of phosphocreatine, creatine, and creatinine muscle content, as opposed to total creatine (the sum of phosphocreatine, creatine, and creatinine), inaccurate (Lowe et al., 1998). Although creatine levels are unaffected by the freezing process, the biopsy procedure itself activates cellular energy utilization, resulting in a decrease in creatine phosphate. The sample should thus be allowed to equilibrate in room air for 1–2 min after collection before freezing so that the creatine phosphate concentration better approximates that in resting muscle. It should be noted that such a delay in freezing will lead to increased muscle lactate concentrations (Soderlund and Hultman, 1986).

Other HPLC methods have also been developed for the measurement of creatine in serum. Werner and colleagues (1990) describe a method to measure creatine (as well as creatinine and uric acid) in serum using HPLC with direct serum injection and multi-wavelength detection. This method is somewhat more complicated than that listed above in that a "column-switching" technique is required for separation of the analytes. Murakita (1988) also described an HPLC method for determining creatine and creatinine in serum, but this method requires a much more extensive sample clean-up and is less sensitive in its concentration determinations. Use of capillary electrophoresis to determine creatine concentrations in human urine has been described (Burke et al., 1999) and the findings confirmed by HPLC analysis. Magnetic resonance spectroscopy is a noninvasive method of continuously measuring relative concentrations of creatine phosphate in muscle during exercise. This method has been reviewed elsewhere (McCully et al., 1988).

6.14. REGULATORY STATUS

Creatine monohydrate is regulated as a dietary supplement in the United States. It does not appear on the International Olympic Committee banned substance list and is not banned by the National Collegiate Athletic Association or any other national competitive sport regulatory authorities (Anonymous, 1998). It is classified as a food in the United Kingdom (Pritchard and Kaira, 1998). It is banned in France because of concerns that it causes cancer (Ursell, 2001); however, a literature search did not reveal any studies regarding creatine monohydrate's ability to cause cancer.

6.15. SUMMARY

- Creatine is an endogenous substance important in production of ATP for muscle contraction.
- Creatine is used most commonly as a supplement by athletes and fitness enthusiasts to enhance strength and sprint activities, but studies also suggest efficacy in diseases involving inborn errors of metabolism and neuromuscular diseases.
- Despite two case reports of creatine-associated interstitial nephritis and worsening focal segmental glomerulosclerosis, studies designed specifically to examine creatine's effect on renal function have not shown detrimental effects in subjects with normal baseline renal function.
- Although creatine has been well tolerated in clinical trials, various adverse effects have been reported to the FDA, none of which have yet been definitively linked to creatine use.

REFERENCES

Anonymous. Creatine and androstenedione—two "dietary supplements." Med Lett Drugs Ther 1998;40:105–6.
Balsom PD, Ekblom B Soderland K, Sjodin B, Hultman E. Creatine supplementation and dynamic high-intensity intermittent exercise Scand J Med Sci Sports 1993a;3:143–9.
Balsom PD, Harridge SDR, Soderland K, Ekblom B. Creatine supplementation per se does not enhance endurance exercise performance. Acta Physiol Scand 1993b;149:521–3.
Balsom PD, Soderlund K, Ekblom B. Creatine in humans with special reference to creatine supplementation. Sports Med 1994;18:268–80.
Bermon S, Venembre C, Sachet S, Valour S, Dolisi C. Effects of creatine monohydrate ingestion in sedentary and weight-trained older adults. Acta Physiol Scand 1998;164:147–55.
Bessman SP, Geiger PJ. Transport of energy in muscle: the phosphorylcreatine shuttle. Science 1981;211:448–52.
Bianchi MC, Tosetti M, Fornai F, et al. Reversible brain creatine deficiency in two sisters with normal blood creatine level. Ann Neurol 2000;47:511–3.

Birch R, Noble D, Greenhaff PL. The influence of dietary creatine supplementation on performance during repeated bouts of maximal isokinetic cycling in man. Eur J Appl Physiol 1994;69:268–70.

Burke DG, MacLean PG, Walker RA, Dewar PJ, Smith-Palmer T. Analysis of creatine and creatinine in urine by capillary electrophoresis. J Chromatogr B Biomed Sci Appl 1999;732:479–85.

Burke DG, Silver S, Holt LE, et al. The effect of continuous low dose creatine supplementation on force, power, and total work. Int J Sport Nutr Exerc Metab 2000;10:235–44.

Burke LM, Payne DB, Telford RD. Effect of oral creatine supplementation on single-effort sprint performance in elite swimmers. Int J Sport Nutr 1996;6:222–33.

CDC. Hyperthermia and dehydration-related deaths associated with intentional rapid weight loss in three collegiate wrestlers—North Carolina, Wisconsin, and Michigan, November–December 1997. MMWR 1998;47:105–8.

Clark JF. Creatine: a review of its nutritional applications in sport. Nutrition 1998;14:322–4.

ConsumerLab.com. News. Consumberlab.com finds that not all creatine supplements meet label claims. Popular sports supplement test results released online. Available from: http://www.consumerlabs.com/news/news_80700.html. Accessed September 26, 2000.

Cooke WH, Grandjean PW, Barnes WS. Effect of oral creatine supplementation on power output and fatigue during bicycle ergometry. J Appl Physiol 1995;78:670–3.

Dawson B, Cutler M, Moody A, et al. Effects of oral creatine loading on single and repeated maximal short sprints. Aust J Sci Med Sport 1995; 27:56–61.

Delanghe J, De Slypere JP, De Buyzere M, et al. Normal reference values for creatine, creatinine and carnitine are lower in vegetarians. Clin Chem 1989;35:1802–3.

Demant KM, Rhodes EC. Effects of creatine supplementation on exercise performance. Sports Med 1999;28:49–60.

Dunnett M, Harris RC, Orme CE, Reverse-phase ion-pairing high-performance liquid chromatography of phosphocreatine, creatine, and creatinine in equine muscle. J Clin Lab Invest 1991;51:137–41.

Earnest C, Almada A, Mitchell T. Influence of chronic creatine supplementation on hepatorenal function [abstract]. FASEB J 1996a;10:A790.

Earnest CP, Almada AL, Mitchell TL. High-performance capillary electrophoresis—pure creatine monohydrate reduces blood lipids in men and women. Clin Sci 1996b;91:113–8.

Edmunds JW, Jayapalan S, DiMarco NM, Saboorian MH, Aukema HM. Creatine supplementation increases renal disease progression in Han:SPRD-cy rats. Am J Kidney Dis 2001;37:73–8.

Engelhardt M, Neumann G, Berbalk A, Reuter I. Creatine supplementation in endurance sports. Med Sci Sports Exerc1998;30:1123–9.

FDA (Food and Drug Administration). The SN/AEMS web report search results for creatine. Available at: URL: http://vm.cfsan.fda.gov/cgi?QUERY=creatine&STYPE=Exact. Accessed Sept 1, 2000.

Feldman EB. Creatine: a dietary supplement and ergogenic aid. Nutr Rev 1999;57:45–50.

Forsberg AM, Nilsson E, Werneman J, Bergstrom J, Hultman E. Muscle composition in relation to age and sex Clin Sci 1991;81:249–56.

Gordon A, Hultman E, Kaijser L, Kristjansson S, Rolf CJ, Nyquist O, Sylven C. Creatine supplementation in chronic heart failure increases skeletal muscle creatine phosphate and muscle performance. Cardiovasc Res 1995;30:413–8.

Goldberg PG, Bechtel PJ. Effects of low dose creatine supplementation on strength, speed, and power events by male athletes [abstract]. Med Sci Sports Exerc 1997;29:S251.

Green Al, Hultman E, MacDonald IA, Sewell DA, Greenhaff PL. Carbohydrate feeding augments skeletal muscle creatine accumulation during creatine supplementation in humans. Am J Physiol 1996;271:E821–6.

Greenhaff PL. The nutritional biochemistry of creatine. J Nutr Biochem 1997;11:610–8.

Greenhaff PL, Casey A, Short AH, et al. Influence of oral creatine supplementation of muscle torque during repeated bouts of maximal voluntary exercise in man. Clin Sci 1993;84:565–71.

Grindstaff PD, Kreider R, Bishop R, et al. Effects of creatine supplementation on repetitive sprint performance and body compostition in competitive swimmers. Int J Sport Nutr 1997;7:330–46.

Halkerston IDK. Biochemistry, 2nd ed. New York: John Wiley & Sons; 1988.

Hamilton KL, Meyers MC, Skelly WA, Marley RJ. Oral creatine supplementation and upper extremity anaerobic response in females. Int J Sport Nutr Metab 2000;10:227–89.

Harris RC, Hultman E, Nordesjo L-O. Glycogen, glycolytic intermediates and high-energy phosphates determined in biopsy samples of musculus quadriceps femoris of man at rest: methods and variance of values. Scand J Clin lab Invest 1974;33:109–20.

Harris RC, Soderlund K, Hultman E. Elevation of creatine in resting and exercised muscle of normal subjects by creatine supplementation. Clin Sci 1992;83:367–74.

Horn M, Frantz S, Remkes H, et al. Effects of chronic dietary creatine feeding on cardiac energy metabolism and on creatine content in heart, skeletal muscle, brain, liver and kidney. J Mol Cell Cardiol 1998;30:277–84.

Hultman E, Soderlund K, Timmons JA, Cederblad G, Greenhaff PL. Muscle creatine loading in men. J Appl Physiol 1996;81:232–7.

Jacobs I. Dietary creatine monohydrate supplementation. Can J Appl Physiol 1999;24:503–14.

Javierre C, Lizarraga MA, Ventura JL, Garrido E, Segura R. Creatine supplementation does not improve physical performance in a 150 m race. J Physiol Biochem 1997;53:343–48.

Jellen J, ed. Natural Medicines Comprehensive Database. Stockton, NY: Therapeutic Research Faculty; 1999.

Juhn MS, O Kane JW, Vinci DM. Oral creatine supplementation in male collegiate athletes: a survey of dosing habits and side effects. J Am Diet Assoc 1999;99:593–5.

Kammermeir H. Microassay of free and total creatine from tissue extracts by combination of chromatographic and fluorimetric methods. Anal Biochem 1973;56:341–5.

Khanna NK, Madan BR. Studies on the antiinflammatory activity of creatine. Arch Int Pharmacodyn Ther 1978;231:340–50.

Klivenyi P, Ferrante RJ, Matthews RT, et al. Neuroprotective effects of creatine in a transgenic animal model of amyotrophic lateral sclerosis. Nat Med 1999;5:347–50.

Koshy KM, Griswold E, Schneeberger EE. Interstitial nephritis in a patient taking creatine. N Engl J Med 1999;340:814–5.

Kreider RB, Ferreira M, Wilson M, et al. Effects of creatine supplementation on body composition, strength, and sprint performance. Med Sci Sports Exerc 1998;30:73–82.

Kurosawa Y, Iwane H, Hamaoka T, et al. Effects of oral creatine supplemetation on high- and low-intensity grip exercise performance [abstract]. Med Sci Sports Exerc 1997;29:S251.

Lemon P, Boska M, Bredle D, et al. Effect of oral creatine supplementation on energetics during repeated maximal muscle contraction [abstract]. Med Sci Sports Exerc 1995;27:S204.

Lowe JA, Murphy M, Nash V. Changes in plasma and muscle creatine concentration after increases in supplementary dietary creatine in dogs. J Nutr 1998;128(suppl):2691S–3S.

Matthews RTL, Yang L, Jenkins BG, et al. Neuroprotective effects of creatine and cyclocreatine in animal models of Huntington's disease. J Neurosci 1998;18:156–63.

McCully KK, Kent JA, Chanve B. Application of ^{131}P magnetic resonance spectroscopy to the study of athletic performance. Sports Med 1988;5:312–21.

Mihic S, MacDonald JR, McKenzie S, Tarnopolsky MA. Acute creatine loading increases fat-free mass, but does not affect blood pressure, plasma creatinine, or CK activity in men and women. Med Sci Sports Exerc 2000;32:291–6.

Mujika I, Chatard J, Lacoste L, Barale F, Geyssant A. Creatine supplementation does not improve sprint performance in competitive swimmers. Med Sci Sports Exerc 1996;28:1435–41.

Mujika I, Padilla S. Creatine supplementation as an ergogenic aid for sports performance in highly trained athletes: a critical review. Int J Sports Med 1997;18:491–6.

Murakita H. Simultaneous determination of creatine and creatinine in serum by high-performance liquid chromatography. J Chromatogr 1988;431:471–473.

NutritionalSupplements.com. Consumer review: when I mixed creatine with grape juice, it fermented and turned into wine. Responses 1–7. Available at URL: http:// www.nutritional supplements.com/creatineR34.html. Accessed Aug. 4, 2000.

Odland LM, MacDougall JD, Tarnopolsky MA, Elorriaga A, Borgmann A. Effect of oral creatine supplementation on muscle [PCr] and short-term maximum power output. Med Sci Sports Exerc 1997;29:216–9.

Odoom JE, Kemp GJ, Radda GK. Control of intracellular creatine concentration in a mouse myoblast cell line [abstract]. Biochem Soc Trans 1993;21:441S.

Oöpik V, Paasuke M, Timpmann S, et al. Effect of creatine supplementation during rapid body mass reduction on metabolism and isokinetic performance capacity. Eur J Appl Physiol 1998;78:83–92.

Pacific Nutrition. Prolab Nutrition creatine monohydrate. Available at: URL: http:// www.pacific-nutrition.com/creatine-prolab.htm. Accessed July 30, 2000.

Panchenko E, Dobrovolsky A, Rogoza A, et al. The effect of exogenous phosphocreatine on maximal walking distance, blood rheology, platelet aggregation, and fibrinolysis in patients with intermittent claudication. Int Angiol 1994;13:59–64.

Pepping J. Creatine. Am J Health Syst Pharm 1999 Aug 15;56:1608–10.

Peyrebrune MC, Nevill ME, Donaldson FJ, Cosford DJ. The effects of oral creatine supplementation on performance in single and repeated sprint swimming. J Sports Sci 1998;16:271–9.

Poortmans JR, Auquier H, Renaut V, et al. Effect of short-term creatine supplementation on renal responses in men. Eur J Appl Physiol 1997;76:566–7.

Poortmans JR, Francaux M. Reply to: renal dysfunction accompanying oral creatine supplements [letter]. Lancet 1998;352:234.

Poortmans JR, Francaux M. Long-term oral creatine supplementation does not impair renal function in healthy athletes. Med Sci Sports Exerc 1999;31:1108–10.

Pritchard NR, Kaira PA. Renal dysfunction accompanying oral creatine supplementation. Lancet 1998;351:1252–1253.

Rawson ES, Clarkson PM. Acute creatine supplementation in older men. In J Sports Med 2000;21:71–5.

Rawson ES, Wehnert ML, Clarkson PM. Effects of 30 days of creatine ingestion in older men. Eur J Appl Physiol 1999;80:139–44.

Redondo D, Dowling EA, Graham BL, Almada AL, Williams MH. The effect of oral creatine monohydrate supplementation on running velocity. Int J Sports Nutr 1996;6:213–21.

Rico-Sanz J, Marco MTM. Creatine enhances oxygen uptake and performance during alternating intensity exercise. Med Sci Sports Exerc 2000;32:379–85.

Schedel JM, Tanaka H, Kiyonaga A, Shindo M, Schutz Y. Acute creatine ingestion in humans: consequences on serum creatine and creatinine concentrations. Life Sci 1999;65:2463–70.

Scott MD, Baudendistel LJ, Dahms TE. Rapid separation of creatine, phosphocreatine and adenosine metabolites by ion-pair reversed-phase high-performance liquid chromatography in plasma and cardiac tissue. J Chromatogr 1992;576:149–154.

Seraydarian MW, Artaza L, Abbott BC. Creatine and the control of energy metabolism in cardiac and skeletal muscle cells in culture. J Mol Cell Cardiol 1974;6:405–13.

Seraydarian MW, Artaza L, Abbott BC. The effect of adenosine on cardiac cells in culture. J Mol Cell Cardiol 1972;4:477–84.

Seraydarian MW, Sato E, Savageau M, Harary I. In vitro studies of beating heart cells in culture. XII. The utilization of ATP and phosphocreatine in oligomycin and 2-deoxyglucose inhibited cells. Biochim Biophys Acta 1969;180:264–70.

Sharov VG, Afonskaya NI, Ruda MY, et al. Protection of ischemic myocardium by exogenous phosphocreatine (Neoton): pharmacokinetics of phosphocreatine, reduction of infarct size, stabilization of sarcolemma of ischemic cardiomyocytes, and antithrombotic action. Biochem Med Metab Biol 1986;35:101–14.

Sheppard HL, Raichada SM, Kouri KM, Stenson-Bar-Maor L, Branch JD. Use of creatine and other supplements by members of civilian and military health clubs: a cross-sectional survey. Int J Sport Nutr Exerc Metab 2000;10:245–9.

Sipila I, Rapola J, Simell O, Vannas A. Supplementary creatine as a treatment for gyrate atrophy of the choroids and retina. N Engl J Med 1981;304;867–70.

Slot C. Plasma creatinine determination. A new and specific Jaffe reaction method. Scand J Clin Lab Invest 1965;17:381–387.

Smith JC, Stephens DP, Hall EL, Jackson AW, Earnest CP. Effect of oral creatine ingestion on parameters of the work rate-time relationship and time to exhaustion in high-intensity cycling. Eur J Appl Physiol 1998a;77:360–65.

Smith SA, Montain SJ, Matott RP, et al. Creatine supplementation and age influence muscle metabolism during exercise. J Appl Physiol 1998 Oct;85:1349–56.

Soderlund K, Hultman E. Effects of delayed freezing on content of phosphagens in human skeletal muscle biopsy samples. J Appl Physiol 1986;61:832–5.

Spande JI, Schottelius BA. Chemical basis of fatigue in isolated mouse soleus muscle. Am J Physiol 1970;219:1490–5.

Stockler S, Hanefeld F, Frahm J. Creatine replacement therapy in guanidinoacetate methyltransferase deficiency, a novel inborn error of metabolism. Lancet 1996;348:789–90.

Stockler S, Marescau B, De Deyn PP, Trijbels JM, Hanefelf F. Guanidino compounds in guanidinoacetate methytransferase deficiency, a new inborn error of creatine synthesis. Metabolism 1997;46:1189–93.

Stout JR, Echerson J, Noonan D, Moore G, Cullen D. The effects of a supplement designed to augment creatine uptake on exercise performance and fat free muscle in football players [abstract]. Med Sci Sports Exerc 1997;29:S251.

Sullivan PG, Geiger JD, Mattson MP, Scheff SW. Dietary supplement creatine protects against traumatic brain injuty. Ann Neurol 2000;48:723–9.

Tarnopolsky MA, MacLennan DP. Creatine monohydrate supplementation enhances high-intensity exercise performance in males and females. Int J Sport Nutr Exerc Metab 2000;10:452–63.

Tarnopolsky MA, Roy BD, MacDonald JR. A randomized, controlled trial of creatine monohydrate in patients with mitochondrial cytopathies. Muscle Nerve 1997;20:1502–9.

Terrillion KA, Kolkhorst FW, Dolgener FA, Joslyn SJ. The effect of creatine supplementation on two 700m maximal running bouts. Int J Sport Nutr 1997;7:138–43.

Theodorou AS, Cooke CB, King RFGJ, et al. The effects of longer-term creatine supplementation on elite swimming performance after an acute creatine loading. J Sports Sci 1999;17:853–9.

Ursell, A. Is the 'safe steroid' safe? The Daily Telegraph (London) 2001 August 15, p. 16.

Vahedi K, Domigo V, Amarenco P, Bousser M-G. Ischaemic stroke in a sportsman who consumed MaHuang extract and creatine monohydrate for body building [letter]. J Neurol Neurosurg Psychiatry 2000;68:112–3.

Vandebuerie F, Vanden Eynde B, Vandenberghe K, Hespel P. Effect of creatine loading on endurance capacity and power cyclists. In J Sports Med 1998;19:490–5.

Vandenberghe K, Gillis N, Van Leemputte M, et al. Caffeine counteracts the ergogenic action of muscle creatine loading. J Appl Physiol 1996;80:452–7.

Vandenberghe K, Goris M, Van Hecke P, et al. Long-term creatine intake is beneficial to muscle performance during resistance training. J Appl Physiol 1997a;83:2055–63.

Vandenberghe K, Van Hecke P, Van Leemputte M, Vanstapel F, Hespel P. Inhibition of muscle phosphocreatine resynthesis by caffeine after creatine loading [abstract]. Med Sci Sports Exerc 1997b;29:S249.

van der Knaap MS, Verhoeven NM, Maaswinkel-Mooij P, et al. Mental retardation and behavioral problems as presenting signs of a creatine synthesis defect. Ann Neurol 2000;47:540–3.

Vannas-Sulonen K, Sipila I, Vannas A, Simell O, Rapola J. Gyrate atrophy of the choroid retina. A follow-up of creatine supplementation. Opthalmology 1985;92:1719–27.

Volek JS, Duncan ND, Mazzetti SA, et al. No effect of heavy resistance training on creatine supplementation on blood lipids. Int J Sport Nutr Exerc Metab 2000;10:144–56.

Vorgerd M, Grehl T, Jager M, et al. Creatine therapy in myophosphorylase deficiency (McArdle disease): a placebo-controlled crossover trial. Arch Neurol 2000;57:956–63.

Wallack RM. Creatine: the magic bullet? Available from: URL: http://www.more.com/dept_info/index.html?skuld=400156. Accessed July 27, 2000.

Werner G, Schneider V, Emmert J. Simultaneous determination of creatine, uric acid and creatinine by high-performance liquid chromatography with direct serum injection and multiwavelength detection. J Chromatogr 1990;525:265–275.

Willer B, Stucki G, Hoppeler H, Bruhlmann P, Krahenbuhl S. Effects of creatine supplementation on muscle weakness in patients with rheumatoid arthritis. Rheumatology 2000;39:293–8.

Williams MH, Branch JD. Creatine supplementation and exercise performance: an update. J Am Coll Nutr 1998;14:322–4.

Chapter 7

Dehydroepiandrosterone (DHEA) (Prasterone)

John Edward Pope, Melanie Johns Cupp,
and Timothy S. Tracy

7.1. HISTORY

Dehydroepiandrosterone (DHEA) is an endogenous steroid that is produced by the zona reticularis of the adrenal cortex (Gurnell and Chatterjee, 2001). It was first isolated in 1934 from urine by Butenandt and Dannenbaum. In 1944, dehydroepiandrosterone sulfate (DHEA-S), DHEA's sulfated metabolite, was isolated from the urine. In 1954, DHEA was isolated from the blood, and in 1959 the chemist E.E. Baulieu discovered that DHEA-S was the most abundant form of the hormone found in human plasma. In 1965, De Neve and Vermeulen reported an association between DHEA-S levels and aging; it was found that as people age, DHEA-S levels decline in a linear fashion (Lieberman, 1995; Yen, 2001). This discovery led to numerous studies that focused on the link between DHEA and DHEA-S levels and the aging process.

In the early 1980s, DHEA was described as a miracle drug with antiaging, antiobesity, and anticancer properties. DHEA was available by prescription as a weight loss product in the United States until 1985 when the Food and Drug Administration (FDA) banned its marketing. It reappeared as an over-the-counter supplement after the passage of the Dietary Supplement Health and Education Act (DSHEA) of 1994 (Corrigan, 1999).

7.2. CHEMICAL STRUCTURE

The chemical structure of DHEA is shown in Fig. 7-1.

From: *Forensic Science: Dietary Supplements: Toxicology and Clinical Pharmacology*
Edited by: M. J. Cupp and T. S. Tracy © Humana Press Inc., Totowa, New Jersey

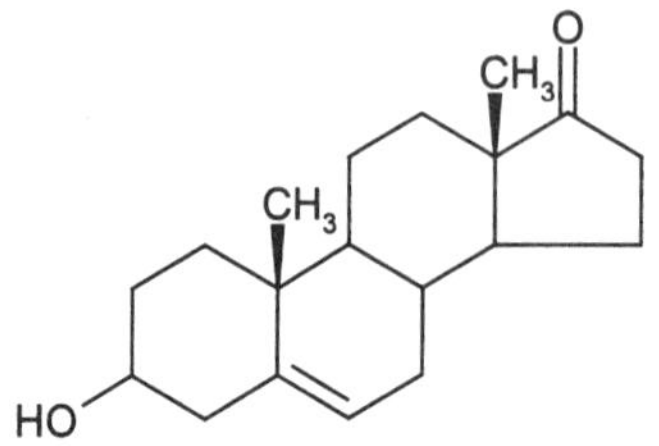

Fig. 1. Chemical structure of dehydroepiandrosterone.

7.3. CURRENT PROMOTED USES

DHEA is promoted as a hormone replacement for individuals older than 40 yr of age. Claims that have not yet been clinically substantiated include reversing the aging process, slowing Parkinson's disease and Alzheimer's disease progression, improving body composition and cognitive function, preventing cancer and heart disease, and improving sexual function. DHEA has been touted as the "mother hormone," a "fountain of youth," a "miracle pill," and an "antidote for aging," among other monikers (Baulieu et al., 2000).

The use of over-the-counter steroids by athletes has surged since baseball star Mark McGwire admitted to his use of androstenedione as a dietary supplement (Birchard, 1999). Athletes use DHEA for two major reasons. One rationale for use is DHEA's role as a precursor for the anabolic steroid testosterone. The other reason that athletes use DHEA is its effect as an anticatabolic agent; DHEA is an antiglucocorticoid that is said to accelerate recovery after sporting events or heavy training sessions (Corrigan, 1999).

7.4. SOURCES AND CHEMICAL COMPOSITION

In 1935, various articles were published on how DHEA acetate could be formed by the debromination of cholesteryl acetate dibromide with chromic acid in acetic acid. In 1949, Merck developed a synthetic pathway using bile acids to form cortisone as the precursor to DHEA. Roussel Uclaf, a French pharmaceutical company, obtained the license to make DHEA through the method developed by Merck. By 1960, Roussel Uclaf produced over one-third of the world's corticosteroids. Today, DHEA is readily prepared from cholesterol (Petrow, 1996). Commercially available DHEA supplements manufactured by Experimental and Applied Sciences (EAS) are derived from wild yams (Brown et al., 1999).

7.5. PRODUCTS AVAILABLE

Many companies distribute DHEA as a nutritional supplement. Popular branded products include Natures Blend DHEA®, DHEA Max®, Natrol DHEA®, GNC A-Z DHEA®, and EAS DEA. The latter product has been found to be 98–99% pure by two independent laboratories using high-performance liquid chromatography (HPLC) (Brown et al., 1999). There is great variation in DHEA content compared with label claims both within and between DHEA products. In a study performed to assess the DHEA content of DHEA products available at health food stores in the United States, only 7 of 16 products tested contained 90–110% of the labeled DHEA content. One product contained no DHEA, and two products with no labeled strength contained less than 1 mg. One product contained an average of 150% of the labeled amount of DHEA per dosage unit, with a coefficient of variation of 32% (Parasrampuria et al., 1998).

The typical dose of DHEA seen in many of the over-the-counter supplements is 25–50 mg. Many DHEA product distributors recommend a cyclic regimen of 1 wk off DHEA after each 2-wk supplementation period to minimize side effects such as gynecomastia and adverse effects on the lipid profile (Brown et al., 1999).

7.6. PHYSIOLOGIC EFFECTS

The human adrenals secrete large amounts of DHEA and its sulfated metabolite DHEA-S. These hormones are converted to biologically active estrogens and androgens in peripheral tissues. Over 30% of the total androgens in males and more than 90% of the total estrogens in postmenopausal women are produced by peripheral conversion of DHEA (Yen, 2001).

During the development of the fetus, the fetal adrenal gland produces high amounts of DHEA and DHEA-S, which provide essential estrogen to the placenta. After birth, the production of DHEA from the child's adrenals is minimal. Once the child reaches adrenarche, which occurs between the ages of 6 and 8 yr, there is an increase in the synthesis of DHEA. This surge of DHEA leads to an increase in testosterone in males and estrogen in females, which result in the development of pubic and axillary hair. DHEA production continues to increase from the time of adrenarche until the third decade of life, when DHEA is at its highest level. Once this peak is reached, DHEA concentrations decline approximately 2% each year. By the time an individual reaches 80 yr of age, DHEA levels are only 10–20% of the levels seen during the third decade of life (Gurnell and Chatterjee, 2001).

Because of the age-associated decrease in DHEA levels, many studies have focused on the effects of low levels of DHEA on the health of the elderly. Some of these findings include an inverse relationship between DHEA-S levels and cardiovascular disease in elderly males; an association with breast cancer risk in premenopausal women; a positive correlation between DHEA-S levels and bone mineral densities of the spine, hip, and radius in women between the ages of 45 and 69; a positive correlation between depression and DHEA-S levels in women; an inverse correlation between DHEA-S levels and insulin resistance; and a correlation between a higher cortisol/DHEA ratio and cognitive decline in both men and women (Gurnell and Chatterjee, 2001).

DHEA appears to have a role in immune function. In vitro data suggest that local DHEA concentrations influence which type of T-lymphocytes (helper type 1 cells vs helper type 2 cells) dominate in various tissues. Other observations underscoring DHEA's relationship to immune function include relatively low DHEA and DHEA-S levels in patients with lupus (van Vollenhoven, 2000) and the correlation between low DHEA levels (less than approx 2.0 µg/L) and progression to AIDS in HIV-infected patients (Centurelli and Abate, 1997).

7.7. In Vitro Effects and Animal Data

Animal studies suggest that DHEA may be beneficial in improving memory and helping to prevent the development of atherosclerosis, cancer, obesity, and diabetes (Pepping, 2000). DHEA has also been shown to ameliorate autoimmune nephritis in a murine model of lupus (van Vollenhoven et al., 1995). Other effects on the murine immune system, reported by Ray Daynes and associates in the early 1990s, include increased production of interleukin-2 (IL-2) and interferon-γ by activated T-lymphocytes and decreased production of IL-4, IL-5, and IL-6 (van Vollenhoven et al., 1998; van Vollenhoven et al., 2000). Suzuki and colleagues also demonstrated that DHEA increases IL-2 production by activated human T-lymphocytes (van Vollenhoven, 2000). Feeding mice DHEA-S 100 µg/mL in drinking water from weaning until death did not affect survival, incidence of lethal illness, or cellular or humoral immunity compared with controls (Miller and Chrisp, 1999). There was also no beneficial effect on lifespan or cancer incidence in a study in which middle-aged mice were fed DHEA-S 25 µg/mL in drinking water (Pugh et al., 1999).

7.8. Clinical Studies

7.8.1. Exercise Performance

Forty male subjects, aged 40–60 yr (mean age 48.1 yr) with weight training experience were randomized to androstenedione 50 mg twice daily, DHEA 50 mg twice daily, or placebo for 3 mo. At baseline and at weeks 6 and 12, body composition, hormone profile, prostate-specific antigen (PSA), glucose, insulin, lipids, alanine aminotransferase (ALT), well-being, libido, strength, and aerobic capacity were measured. Patients were instructed to maintain their normal diet. Two-way ANOVA was used to analyze the data, along with the Scheffe test for identification of specific pairwise differences. Baseline vs postsupplementation data were analyzed using t-tests. Pearson product moment correlation analysis was performed to identify significant correlations between variables. Statistical significance was accepted at the $p < 0.05$ level. DHEA had no effect on any variable studied (Wallace et al., 1999).

A study published that same year examined the effects of DHEA (Experimental and Applied Sciences, Golden, CO) on serum hormone levels and resistance training in 30 men aged 19–29 yr (Brown et al., 1999). Study subjects denied previous resistance training or use of any supplement. Twenty subjects were randomly assigned to receive DHEA 150 mg or placebo during weeks 1 and 2, 4 and 5, and 7 and 8 of an 8-wk training program. Body composition was assessed at baseline and at the end of weeks 4 and 8. Serum free and total testosterone, androstenedione, estrone, estriol, estradiol, luteinizing hormone (LH), and follicle-stimulating hormone (FSH) were measured at baseline and at the end of weeks 2, 5, and 8. A glucose tolerance test was also performed at baseline, and within 3 d of the end of supplementation. Insulin levels as well as glucose levels were measured as part of the glucose tolerance test. Muscle biopsies were obtained before and after the 8-wk training period. Compliance was measured using a patient diary and a pill count at the end of the study. Subjects were instructed with regard to a diet supplying 150 g/d carbohydrate but were otherwise advised to maintain their normal diet. Subjects kept a diet history for 3 d prior to the baseline glucose tolerance test and were instructed to ingest the same diet prior to the second glucose tolerance test.

In a second part of study, the effects of a single dose of DHEA 50 mg on serum androstenedione, free testosterone, estradiol, LH, and FSH were evaluated in 10 of the subjects prior to administration and every 30 min. for 6 h. Subjects received DHEA or placebo in a double-blind, randomized fashion, with washout of at least 1 wk between treatments. Data were analyzed using two-way repeated measured ANOVA with the Newman-Keuls test for multiple comparisons. The DHEA and placebo groups were similar in age, fitness, and exercise experience. One subject in the resistance training group withdrew from the study.

After single-dose administration of DHEA 50 mg, androstenedione levels increased within 30 min, peaked 30 min later, and remained elevated for 6 h ($p <$ 0.05). No other hormone levels were altered compared with placebo. In the resistance training phase of the study, the DHEA group did not differ from the placebo group in number of sets, repetitions, intensity of exercise, body composition, or muscle strength. To exemplify the small effect of DHEA in increasing upper body muscle strength, the investigators calculated that 475 patients would have to be treated with DHEA to produce a statistically significant difference from placebo if statistical significance was accepted at the $p = 0.05$ level with a 20% chance of type II error. Compared with placebo, DHEA did not affect lipids, liver function tests, hemoglobin, hematocrit, total iron, glucose tolerance, or insulin senstivity.

Because of a power failure resulting in loss of frozen samples, muscle samples from only nine patients were usable for analysis. There was no significant difference between the placebo and DHEA groups in percentage of type I fibers, mean cross-sectional area of type I fibers, or mean cross-sectional area of type II fibers in these nine subjects. DHEA and DHEA-S levels could not be measured owing to thawing of samples. There were no significant changes in LH, FSH, total testosterone, free testosterone, or estrogen levels. Compared with baseline, androstenedione levels were higher in the DHEA group at weeks 2 and 5, but not at week 8. The cause of the decrease in mean androstenedione level in the DHEA group at week 8 was postulated to involve inhibition by DHEA of 3-β-hydroxysteroid dehydrogenase (the enzyme responsible for androstenedione production), increased clearance, or decreased DHEA entry into the systemic circulation. An initial increase in androstenedione levels followed by a return to baseline was also observed in a previous study (Mortola and Yen, 1990) described below in the Replacement in Aging Section. As in the previous study (Mortola and Yen, 1990), Brown and colleagues (1999) found no effect of DHEA on FSH or LH, suggesting that DHEA does not interact with the hypothalamic-pituitary axis. Despite the initial increase in androstenedione levels, estrogen levels did not increase. This finding was unexpected by the investigators because androstenedione administration had led to increased estrogen levels in a previous study (King et al., 1999).

7.8.2. Systemic Lupus Erythematosus

A double-blind, placebo-controlled study of DHEA (Diosynth, Chicago, IL) 200 mg/d in mild-to-moderate lupus was undertaken based on human and animal data suggesting a link between sex hormones and the disease (van Vollenhoven et al., 1995).

Thirty women diagnosed with lupus per the American College of Rheumatology criteria were included in the study. None of the patients had kidney involvement requiring high-dose glucocorticoids or cyclosporine. Patients were treated throughout the study per the professional judgment of their physicians; no medications were prohibited. Outcome measures included the previously validated systemic lupus erythematosus (SLE) Disease Activity Index (SLEDAI) score, patient and physician assessment of disease activity on a 100-point visual analog scale (VAS), number of disease flares, prednisone use, erythrocyte sedimentation rate (ESR), anti-DNA antibodies, complement, platelets, and hematocrit. Lipids and fasting glucose were also measured as a part of side effect monitoring. Chi-squared analysis was used to compare the number of disease flares. Other data were analyzed using t-tests for determination of differences between groups, followed by ANCOVA with baseline disease activity index score and glucocorticoid use as covariates with treatment group. One patient in each treatment group was lost to follow-up.

At baseline, prednisone dose was higher in the DHEA group. At the end of the 3-mo study, the only significant differences in changes from baseline between the placebo and treatment groups were a decrease in patient's assessment of disease activity in the DHEA group ($p = 0.022$, ANCOVA) and an increase in platelet count compared with baseline in the placebo group ($p < 0.003$, t-test). Patient's assessment of disease activity was significantly higher in the placebo group ($p < 0.05$). Although the DHEA group showed improvement only in a subjective outcome measure, trends in improvement in other outcomes suggest that significant differences might have been seen if the study had included more subjects. Also, variations in medical treatment among patients may have confounded the results. Because the appearance of acne in the DHEA group could have unblinded the study, data were analyzed separately for patients with acne vs patients who did not develop acne. Separate analysis of the data, however, did not change the results. When asked, 10 patients in the DHEA group guessed that they had received DHEA, whereas 9 patients in the placebo group guessed that they had received DHEA, further suggesting that blinding was not compromised. After the 3-mo study, open-label use of DHEA 50–200 mg/d was studied for up to 6 mo. Similar results were reported in placebo patients switched to DHEA as in the double-blind portion of the study. Patients who continued DHEA showed further improvement, suggesting that a study of longer duration is needed.

In another randomized, placebo-controlled study of DHEA treatment of lupus erythematosus, patients with severe disease were randomized to capsules containing placebo or DHEA (Diosynth) 200 mg/d for 6 mo (van Vollenhoven et al., 1999). All patients had been diagnosed as having severe disease using American College of Rheumatology criteria. Because a previous study (van Volllenhoven et al., 1995) had demonstrated only modest benefit from DHEA, DHEA monotherapy was not attempted. At study enrollment all patients were receiving high-dose glucocorticoids with or without additional immunosuppressives. The mean baseline prednisone dose was 49.4 mg/d in the DHEA group and 52.6 mg/d in the placebo group (NS). During the course of the study, patients' drug therapy regimen was adjusted per their physician's clinical judgment. The primary outcome measure was response to therapy defined as disease stabilization. Very specific criteria for disease stabilization were delineated for each major manifestation of lupus: nephritis, hematologic lupus, and serositis. Other outcomes included Systemic Lupus Activity Measure (SLAM) and SLEDAI scores, physician and patient global assessment, prednisone dose, ESR, and bone mineral density (BMD). Patients were assessed monthly, and BMD was measured at baseline and at 6 mo. Chi-squared analysis was used to compare the number of responders in each group. Paired or unpaired t-tests, as appropriate, were used to assess other data. Of the 21 patients initially enrolled, 1 was lost to follow-up and 1 died. Two patients dropped out owing to perceived lack of efficacy, but data continued to be collected from these patients and were included in the intention-to-treat analysis.

Placebo-treated patients, but not patients in the DHEA group, experienced a significant decrease in spinal BMD compared with baseline ($p < 0.05$) attributed to the continued need for high-dose prednisone. There were nonsignificant trends in improvement in SLEDAI and SLAM scores favoring DHEA. Sixteen study subjects opted to continue DHEA 200 mg/d in open-label fashion for an additional 6 mo. No significant changes in outcome measures occurred during the open-label portion of the study. The minimal benefit of DHEA in this study may be attributed to severity of disease, small sample size, potential for differences between the two groups in disease treatment, and a significantly greater baseline disease severity per physician global assessment in the DHEA group ($p = 0.04$).

A double-blind phase III study involving patients with steroid-dependent disease was published as an abstract (Petri et al., 1997). All patients were receiving prednisone 10–30 mg/d. One hundred ninety-one women were randomized to DHEA (Genelabs, Redwood City, CA) 100 mg/d, DHEA 200 mg/d, or placebo for 7–9 mo. Prednisone dose was reduced monthly to maintain stable or decreased disease activity per the SLEDAI activity index. The ability to decrease the corticosteroid dose to the physiologic range (7.5 mg/d) for at least 2 mo, including the month 7 visit, was defined as the primary outcome measure. Among patients with active disease at baseline, significantly more patients in the DHEA 200 mg/d group could be titrated to a physiologic corticosteroid dose than in the placebo group ($p = 0.03$).

In an open-label study of DHEA use in patients with lupus (van Vollenhoven et al., 1994), DHEA (Sigma, St. Louis, MO) 200 mg/d was administered for 3–6 mo to nine premenopausal women and one postmenopausal woman with mild or moderate lupus. Disease activity was measured using the SLEDAI measurement of lupus activity as well as patient and physician overall assessment of disease activity using a VAS. Physician's overall assessment improved from baseline to month 3 ($p = 0.040$, paired t-test). By month 6, patient's global assessment and the SLEDAI had improved compared with baseline ($p < 0.05$ using both paired t-tests and Wilcoxon's signed rank test). Of the six patients who completed 6 mo of the study and who were taking corticosteroids at study entry, the mean daily corticosteroid dose decreased compared with baseline ($p = 0.042$).

These 10 patients plus 40 other women with mild-to-moderate lupus (absence of severe nephritis or central nervous system involvement) subsequently participated in an open-label study of DHEA (Diosynth) 200 mg/d (van Vollenhoven et al., 1998). Thirty-seven patients were premenopausal, and 9 of the 13 postmenopausal patients were taking estrogen replacement therapy. DHEA dose was decreased to 50 or 100 mg/d if necessary because of development of side effects. Doses of corticosteroids and other lupus treatments were adjusted at the discretion of the attending physician. Complete blood cell count, ESR, and lipids were measured at each visit. SLEDAI, patient and physician assessment of overall disease activity using a VAS, and corticosteroid dose were assessed each month for up to 12 mo. Statistical analysis of changes in these outcome measures was performed using paired t-tests. Results pertaining to androgen levels in this study are presented in the *Pharmacokinetics* section.

Twenty-one patients were able to continue DHEA treatment for 12 mo. When all patients were assessed regardless of treatment duration, prednisone dose was significantly lower at months 3, 6, 9, and 12 ($p < 0.05$) compared with baseline. SLEDAI was also significantly lower than baseline at all time points ($p < 0.01$, paired t-test). Patient assessment of disease activity was lower at months 3, 6 ($p < 0.01$, paired t-test), and 12 ($p < 0.05$), whereas physician assessment was significantly lower than baseline only at 12 mo ($p < 0.05$). When analyzing only those patients able to complete 12 mo of treatment, prednisone dose was significantly lower than baseline at months 6, 9, and 12 ($p < 0.05$). In this group of patients, SLEDAI was significantly lower than baseline at months 3, 9, and 12 ($p < 0.05$). Physician assessment of disease activity was significantly lower at months 3 ($p < 0.01$) and 12 ($p < 0.05$), whereas patient assessment of disease activity was lower at all assessment periods ($p < 0.01$). There were no differences in response between pre- and postmenopausal women or between postmenopausal women taking estrogen and those not taking estrogen. DHEA did not affect any laboratory values.

7.8.3. Replacement in Aging

Because DHEA and DHEA-S are in part responsible for the circulating androgens and estrogens in postmenopausal women, DHEA may be useful as an addition to estrogen replacement therapy in this population (Buster et al., 1992) (see Pharmacokinetics section below for further discussion of this study). Mortola and Yen (1990) examined the effects of DHEA (Sigma) in a small ($n = 6$), short-term, double-blind, placebo-controlled crossover study in six obese postmenopausal women. The women ranged in age from 46 to 61 yr, were 30–50% above their ideal body weight, had not taken hormone replacement therapy or any other prescription medication within 1 yr, and were free of disease. Women were randomized to two DHEA 200 mg doses or two placebo capsules four times daily for 28 d. Subjects were crossed over to the alternate treatment after a 2-wk washout. A 75-g glucose tolerance test was performed at baseline, with serum glucose and insulin measured 0, 30, 60, 120, and 180 min after administration. This test was repeated at the end of each 28-d treatment period. Serum DHEA, DHEA-S, androstenedione, testosterone, dihydrotestosterone, estrone, estradiol, and sex hormone-binding globulin were measured at baseline and at 30, 60, 120, 180, and 240 min after the first dose of DHEA. These tests were repeated weekly, along with serum glucose, lipids, thyroid function tests, liver function tests, renal function tests, electrolytes, complete blood counts, and urinalysis. Weight, percent body fat, FSH, and LH were measured at baseline and after each 28-d treatment phase. Twenty-four h diet recall was performed randomly throughout the study, and body fat was determined at baseline and at the end of each treatment phase. Differences in hormone, steroid-binding globulin, glucose, and insulin levels were compared with baseline using two-way ANOVA and the Newman-Keuls test for multiple comparisons. Changes in lipids as a percent of baseline values were analyzed using two-way

ANOVA with the Duncan test. Differences in body weight, percent body fat, thyroid function tests, FSH, and LH were analyzed using ANOVA.

Compared with baseline, DHEA, DHEA-S, androstenedione, testosterone, and dihydrotestosterone levels were significantly higher 120, 180, and 240 min after the first 400-mg dose of DHEA ($p < 0.05$). Levels of these hormones were also significantly higher than baseline at weeks 1, 2, 3, and 4 ($p < 0.05$); however, levels peaked at week 2 and then declined. There was no change from baseline in estrogen or sex hormone-binding globulin levels after the single dose of DHEA. Although sex hormone-binding globulin did not change with chronic therapy, the area under the curve of sex hormone-binding globulin was lower during DHEA treatment compared with placebo treatment ($p < 0.05$, t-test). Estrone, but not estradiol, levels were higher compared with baseline at weeks 3 and 4 of DHEA administration. Percent change from baseline in estrone and estradiol levels was significantly higher at weeks 1, 2, 3, and 4 ($p < 0.05$) than observed with placebo treatment. FSH and LH levels remained unchanged, suggesting that the decrease in androgens noted after week 2 was not caused by alteration of gonadotropin release from the pituitary. Within the first week of DHEA administration, the percent change in total cholesterol and HDL compared with baseline was less in the DHEA group compared with placebo treatment ($p < 0.05$). In subjects receiving DHEA, insulin levels were significantly higher 60, 120, and 180 min. after the second glucose tolerance test compared with the baseline test ($p < 0.05$), and the area under the curve for insulin was higher after the second test ($p < 0.05$, t-test). Dietary intake, body weight, and percent body fat were not altered by DHEA therapy. A decrease in total T4, an increase in T3 resin uptake, and a decrease in thyroid-binding globulin were seen with DHEA administration but not with placebo ($p < 0.05$ compared with baseline).

Aging is associated with a decrease in protein synthesis, a decrease in lean body mass and bone mass, and an increase in body fat. A randomized, double-blind, placebo-controlled, crossover study was conducted to determine the effects DHEA on body composition, psychological and physical health, sexual function, urologic function, blood chemistry and hematology, and endocrinology in 39 males with an age range of 60–84 yr (Flynn et al., 1999). The patients received either micronized DHEA 100 mg in a wax vegetable oil matrix (Belmar Pharmacy, Lakewood, CO) or placebo for 3 mo. After 3 mo, the patients were crossed over to the other therapy. The 6-mo supplementation period was followed by a 3-mo washout. Blood and urine collection, dietary analysis, body composition determination, assessment of activities of daily living, and assessment of sexual function were performed at baseline, after each 3-mo supplementation period, and after the washout period. T-tests and Chi-squared analysis were used to compare placebo and DHEA responses.

During the periods when subjects ingested DHEA, significant decreases in mean blood values for blood urea nitrogen (BUN)/creatinine ratio ($p < 0.003$), uric acid concentration ($p < 0.003$), ALT ($p < 0.006$), total cholesterol ($p < 0.009$), and high-density lipoprotein (HDL) cholesterol ($p < 0.02$) were noted. Significant increases in hemoglobin concentration ($p < 0.03$), serum potassium ($p < 0.04$), DHEA concentration, DHEA-S concentration, estradiol concentration ($p < 0.0005$), and free testosterone concentration ($p < 0.0013$) were also observed. Little change was noted in voiding, sexual function, food intake, activities of daily living, lean body mass, percent body fat, body composition, and total weight. All the statistically significant changes noted in the study returned to baseline after the 3-mo washout period (Flynn et al., 1999). It is important to note that the DHEA preparation used in this study was a special micronized lipophilic preparation designed to enhance DHEA bioavailability and prepared by a compounding pharmacy; thus, the results of this study may not be applicable to most common DHEA supplements available without a prescription (see *Pharmacokinetics* section for further discussion of this particular preparation).

A subsequent study examined long-term DHEA replacement in both elderly men and women (Baulieu et al., 2000). Two-hundred eighty subjects 60–79 yr of age participated. Subjects were recruited from a geriatric clinic and had presented with age-related complaints including asthenia, memory difficulties, anxiety, or pain. Subjects were free of depression, dementia, history of hormone-dependent cancer, elevated PSA, and abnormal prostate findings on digital exam. Subjects were randomized to receive DHEA (Diosynth-France, St. Denis, France) 50 mg/d or placebo. Compliance was confirmed every 3 mo by pill counts and DHEA-S levels. Quality of life, mood, cognitive function, sexual function (assessed by questionnaire), hand grip, and epidermal thickness were measured. In addition, the following were assessed: insulin-like growth factor, lipids, ALT, glucose, homocysteine levels, DHEA-S, testosterone, 5α-androstanediol glucuronide (a DHEA metabolite), estradiol, estrone, estrone sulfate, 5α-dihydrotestosterone, creatinine, and serum markers of bone turnover. The above parameters were measured at baseline and at months 6 and 12 following initiation of therapy. Body composition, bone density, sebum production, skin hydration, skin pigmentation, vascular structure and function, and blood pressure were measured at baseline and at the end of the study. The Wilcoxon rank sum test and Chi-squared analysis were used to compare effects in the DHEA and placebo groups. Two-way ANOVA was also used to determine whether DHEA had any effect on vascular parameters. Data for subjects younger than 70 yr were analyzed separately from data for subjects 70 and older.

By mo 6, DHEA-S levels had increased in male subjects in both age groups to levels similar to those of young adult men, and in female subjects, levels had exceeded those of young adult women. At 12 mo, DHEA-S levels were decreased significantly in all subjects younger than 70 yr compared with 6-mo levels ($p < 0.05$ for men, $p < 0.01$ for women). DHEA-S levels also were decreased in women 70 yr and older ($p < 0.01$) but not in men of this same age group. In male subjects, 12-mo estradiol levels were elevated compared with baseline regardless of age ($p < 0.05$). Estradiol levels increased in women ($p < 0.001$) but did not reach those typically observed during the early follicular phase of menstruating women. At 6 mo, testosterone levels were increased in women of both age groups and in 14 subjects exceeded those of premenopausal women. Conversely, by month 12, testosterone levels were subsequently decreased in women regardless of age group ($p < 0.001$ and $p < 0.05$, younger and older groups, respectively), with four subjects (21%) exhibiting levels above the normal range for premenopausal women.

Six-month 5α-androstanediol glucuronide levels were similar in men and women, and were higher than those typically observed in premenopausal women. By month 12, 5α-androstanediol glucuronide levels had decreased in women younger than 70 yr

($p < 0.05$) but remained above premenopausal levels. The increase in 5α-androstanediol glucuronide seen in men in the absence of an increase in testosterone levels suggests that DHEA is metabolized preferentially to 5α-androstanediol glucuronide as opposed to testosterone. Reflecting the findings of Mortola and Yen (1990) and Brown and colleagues (1999), the decrease in 5α-androstanediol glucuronide in men and women from month 6 to month 12 and the decrease in testosterone in women from month 6 to month 12 suggest that some adaptation or negative feedback occurs with long-term DHEA use in regard to androgen production, particularly in subjects younger than 70 yr. There was no similar evidence of an adaptive response in regard to estradiol production.

DHEA did not cause a statistically significant change in PSA, lipids, glucose, ALT, LH, FSH, triiodothyronine, or thyroid-stimulating hormone. The lack of effect of DHEA administration on FSH or LH, also noted in previous studies (Mortola and Yen, 1990; Brown et al., 1999), absence of effect on thyroid function, and lack of evidence of downregulation of estrogen production with long-term use suggests that DHEA administration does not affect the hypothalamic-pituitary axis. In contrast to the findings of previous studies (Morales et al., 1994; Goldberg, 1998), DHEA did not increase insulin-like growth factor levels in this study. In women older than 70 yr, a decrease in serum phosphate was documented, suggesting decreased osteoclastic activity. Radial bone density also increased significantly in this group. Hip BMD increased in women younger than 70 yr. Levels of type I collagen telopeptide, a marker of bone resorption, decreased significantly in women 70 and over. Sexual function improved in women, but not in men. Skin hydration ($p < 0.003$) and sebum production were higher, and skin color was less yellow ($p < 0.03$) at the end of the study compared with baseline. Epidermal thickness was increased at 6 months and remained stable at 12 mo ($p < 0.05$). Neither arterial wall thickness, distensibility, stiffness, nor diameter was affected by DHEA.

These authors concluded that DHEA is well tolerated and produces beneficial effects on bone density and libido in women and on skin in both genders. However, this study used otherwise healthy volunteers, and the safety and efficacy of DHEA replacement in elderly patients with serious medical or psychiatric illness is unknown. Additional study is needed in patients with lower DHEA-S levels, in patients 80 yr and older, and in patients with specific age-related problems (Baulieu et al., 2000).

A systematic review of all pertinent randomized controlled trials of either DHEA or DHEA-S supplementation concluded that the available data do not support use of these products for improving cognitive function or slowing the rate of cognitive function decline either in normal elderly individuals or in those with dementia, perhaps because studies to date have included small numbers of patients or have been of short duration. A study of DHEA supplementation in Alzheimer's disease has been completed, but the results are not yet available (Huppert and Van Niekerk, 2001).

7.8.4. Depression

Several open-label or single-blind studies have been conducted investigating the use of DHEA as an antidepressant. Morales and colleagues (1994) noted that a higher percentage of both men and women receiving DHEA 50 mg/d reported improved well-being after 12 wk of treatment ($p < 0.005$, paired *t*-test) compared with patients treated with placebo. Wolkowitz and colleagues (1999) conducted a double-blind, placebo-controlled trial to test the antidepressant efficacy of DHEA. Twelve men and 10 women, with unipolar or bipolar type II clinical depression, were enrolled in the study. All of the patients had Hamilton Depression Rating Scale (HAM-D) scores of 16 or greater and were medication-free or had been receiving stable doses of an antidepressant for 2 or more mo. For the first week, all subjects received placebo capsules to eliminate placebo responders. One subject was deemed a placebo responder and was eliminated from the study. The remaining 22 patients received either DHEA 30 mg or a placebo daily for the first 2 wk, then DHEA 30 mg or placebo two times daily for 2 wk, and finally DHEA 30 mg or a placebo three times daily for 2 wk. Upon completion of the 6-wk treatment period, patients were reevaluated using the same depression scale. Of the 11 patients receiving DHEA, 5 patients were treatment responders, defined as a 50% or greater decrease in depressive symptoms and a HAM-D score of 10 or less. There were no treatment responders in the placebo group. A mean decrease of 30.5% ($p < 0.04$, repeated measures ANOVA) in the HAM-D score was observed in patients receiving DHEA. This study, along with other studies conducted evaluating the use of DHEA as an antidepressant, suggests that DHEA may be useful in the treatment of depression.

7.8.5. HIV/AIDS

An uncontrolled study presented at the International Conference on AIDS in 1996 reported reductions in viral load in AIDS patients (Anonymous, 1996). In another uncontrolled study of 12 patients with AIDS receiving an average DHEA dose of 75 mg/d, increases in CD4+ cell counts were reported, but because controls were not employed, it is unclear whether the effect was caused by the DHEA or concurrent administration of antiviral drugs (Hasheeve et al., 1994). In a study of tolerability of DHEA (250, 500, or 750 mg given three times daily) in HIV patients, Dyner et al. (1993) observed a reduction in the decline of CD4+ counts in patients receiving 750 mg three times daily compared with 250 mg dosing. Mild adverse effects were noted in all patients, but no serious toxicities were observed. A dose of 50 mg/d was shown to improve quality of life in HIV-positive subjects but did not affect CD4+ cell counts (Piketty et al., 2001).

7.8.6. Other Clinical Studies

DHEA has also been investigated clinically as a hormone replacement therapy in patients with low DHEA levels caused corticosteroid therapy, Addison's disease, or hypopituitarism (Gurnell and Chatterjee, 2001); and to help increase the rate of reepithelialization in burn patients undergoing autologous skin grafting (Pepping, 2000). Subjective improvements in strength, stamina, and well-being have been noted in uncontrolled studies in multiple sclerosis patients (Anonymous, 1996).

7.9. PHARMACOKINETICS

After parenteral injection, DHEA's pharmacokinetics can be described by a two-compartment model, whereas DHEA-S is most accurately depicted by a one-compartment model. The half-lives of DHEA and DHEA-S differ owing to differences in protein binding; DHEA-S has stronger serum albumin binding affinity compared with DHEA and thus a longer half-life (Longcope,1996).

The mean bioavailability of exogenously administered DHEA is 50% (Corrigan, 1999). Oral DHEA is subject to first-pass metabolism to androsterone and etiocholanolone. It is also rapidly converted to DHEA-S (Callies et al., 2000). DHEA-S, the sulfated metabolite of DHEA, is found in higher quantities in the plasma than is DHEA (Kroboth, 1999). Most circulating DHEA-S, 77.8 ± 17.3%, is converted to DHEA in males; and 60.5 ± 8.2% is converted to DHEA in females (Longcope, 1996). Once DHEA-S is converted to DHEA by peripheral and adrenal sulfohydrolases, it is difficult to reverse the process (Kroboth et al., 1999). The percentage of DHEA that is converted back to DHEA-S is only 5.2 ± 0.7% in males and 6.25 ± 0.54% in females (Longcope, 1996). DHEA-S can be metabolized to androstenedione by 3β-hydroxysteroid dehydrogenase (Brown et al., 1999) and to testosterone. The percentage of DHEA that forms androstenedione and testosterone is 4.7 ± 0.3% and 0.62 ± 0.06% in males and 7.1 ± 1.7% and 0.87 ± 0.02% in females, respectively (Longcope, 1996). Androstenedione can be aromatized to estrone and estradiol and can also be converted to estriol. Testosterone is also aromatized to estradiol (King et al., 1999); thus, DHEA is an important source of estrogens in postmenopausal women. Urinary metabolites of DHEA include androstenediol sulfate, androsterone, etiocholanolone, isoandrosterone, 5β-etiocholanolone (Longcope, 1996), and 5α-androstanediol glucuronide (Baulieu et al., 2000).

One small study demonstrated that exogenous DHEA can increase testosterone levels in normal women (Mahesh and Greenblatt, 1962). DHEA 100 mg was administered to two women subjects. Blood samples for determination of plasma testosterone levels were drawn before DHEA administration, and 30, 60, and 90 min after dose. There was a three- to fourfold increase in plasma testosterone in both women. Peak plasma testosterone levels were reached in 60 min in one subject, and in 90 min in the other. In addition, there was an increase in DHEA-S levels after DHEA administration. Androsterone sulfate levels also increased after DHEA administration, but only after DHEA-S levels had peaked. These results suggest that rapid sulfation of DHEA is followed by metabolism of DHEA-S to androsterone sulfate. Although this study demonstrates that DHEA administration can elevate testosterone levels in women, similar results have not been demonstrated in men. In men, exogenous DHEA appears to be preferentially metabolized to 5α-androstanediol glucuronide (Baulieu et al., 2000).

Tummala and Svec (1999) examined 18 published articles to study the correlation between the administration of DHEA and serum levels of DHEA and DHEA-S in humans. In most of the reviewed articles, the typical daily dose of DHEA administered was 300 mg or less. Only seven studies utilized daily doses greater than 300 mg. The researchers concluded that the serum DHEA and DHEA-S levels increased in a logarithmic fashion as the dose of DHEA was increased. The dose of DHEA that produced the greatest effect on DHEA and DHEA-S serum levels was 300 mg/d. Any dose above 300 mg/d showed no additional beneficial effect, as a plateau is reached. Theoretically, above this point there is a higher risk of experiencing side effects without a significant increase in the effective level of DHEA.

In a study described earlier (van Vollenhoven et al., 1998), 50 premenopausal women were administered DHEA 50–200 mg/d, and DHEA, DHEA-S, and testosterone levels were measured at baseline and every 3 mo. Androgen levels increased and reached a plateau after 3 mo of treatment. DHEA and DHEA-S levels were in the high normal or supraphysiologic range; testosterone levels remained in the normal range. There was substantial interindividual variation in androgen levels among patients receiving the same DHEA dose. The DHEA product used in this study was obtained from Diosynth and prepared as capsules by the hospital pharmacy.

In the study by Mortola and Yen (1990) described in the Clinical Studies section, androgenic effects such as insulin resistance, decreased sex hormone-binding globulin, and increases in serum testosterone and dihydrotestosterone within hours of the first dose reflect the pharmacokinetics of orally administered plain, milled, crystalline DHEA, the form used in this and most studies. This DHEA formulation undergoes first-pass metabolism in the liver to androgens before reaching the systemic circulation. Based on a study demonstrating that the first-pass metabolism of orally administered progesterone could be reduced (i.e., its bioavailability could be increased) by administering it in a cholesterol fatty acid ester preparation, the bioavailability of a preparation of micronized DHEA (Sigma) 150 mg in a wax vegetable oil matrix tablet prepared by Belmar Pharmacy (Lakewood, CO) was investigated (Buster et al., 1992). Theoretically, not only would this fatty preparation be absorbed primarily through the lymphatic rather than the portal circulation, the micronized particles would enter the portal circulation rapidly so as to overwhelm the capacity of first-pass metabolism, leading to enhanced DHEA bioavailability with lower androgen levels.

In a study using this formulation, eight postmenopausal women who had not taken estrogen replacement therapy for at least 2 wk were randomized to receive a single dose of DHEA 150 mg, DHEA 300 mg, and placebo in a randomized, crossover design. There was a washout period of at least 1 wk between treatments. Blood samples were drawn 20 min and 5 min prior to the dose, at the time of dose administration, and at various times up to 720 min after dosing. Plasma concentrations of estradiol, DHEA, DHEA-S, and testosterone were measured. Data were analyzed using repeated measures ANOVA with the Newman-Keuls test for multiple comparisons.

As opposed to standard crystalline preparations, androgen levels increased in a linear fashion with this preparation. Mean peak DHEA-S and testosterone levels were significantly higher than the peaks occurring with placebo ($p < 0.05$), and the peaks occurring with the 300-mg dose [1688 µg/dL (DHEA-S) and 311 ng/dL (testosterone)] were higher than after the 150-mg dose [1185 µg/dL (DHEA-S) and 183 ng/dL (testosterone)] ($p < 0.05$). It should be noted that the direct ^{125}I radioimmunoassay used to measure testosterone in this study was determined to overestimate testostereone levels by approximately 300%. After taking this difference into account, the testosterone levels seen in this study up to 12 hr after the 150-mg dose were similar to those seen in premenopausal women. Like peak DHEA-S levels, peak DHEA levels were also superphysiologic and were higher than with placebo after either dose amount [1617 µg/dL (150 mg dose) and 2639 µg/dL (300 mg dose)] ($p < 0.05$), but there was no significant difference in peak DHEA levels between the two doses. Single-dose administration of this DHEA preparation did not increase estradiol levels, as opposed to increases in estrone and estradiol seen with chronic administration in the study by Mortola and Yen (1990). DHEA levels were higher (suggesting better bioavailability), and DHEA-S and testosterone levels were comparable to those achieved with 1600 mg/d in the earlier study. The investigators suggest that a dose of 50–75 mg of this micronized, lipophilic DHEA preparation would supply androgen levels similar to those seen in premenopausal women.

Callies and colleagues (2000) examined the effects of oral DHEA on urinary steroid metabolite levels in males and females. Fourteen healthy elderly men and nine healthy young women were included in the study. The researchers obtained a baseline 24-h urine sample from each volunteer. Urine DHEA, androsterone, etiocholanolone, and 16-α DHEA levels were determined at baseline. Androsterone, etiocholanolone, and 16-α DHEA are major metabolites of DHEA that are excreted primarily in the urine. The nine women were treated with dexamethasone 4 d prior to the administration of the DHEA to simulate DHEA suppression due to aging. After pretreatment with dexamethasone, the women were administered a placebo, DHEA 50 mg, or DHEA 100 mg. The administration of DHEA 50 mg led to steroid metabolite urinary excretion amounts comparable to those at baseline prior to the administration of dexamethasone. The administration of DHEA 100 mg increased urinary metabolite excretion approximately fourfold over the baseline level. The elderly, male volunteers were given either DHEA 50 mg or DHEA 100 mg after establishing a baseline urinary excretion amount. Their results were compared with that of a control group made up of young, healthy men. DHEA 50 mg increased the urinary metabolite excretion of the elderly men slightly above the levels of the control group, but administration of DHEA 100 mg led to urinary excretion amounts approximately six to seven times higher than observed in the control group. This led the researchers to conclude that DHEA 50 mg is a suitable replacement dose for the elderly and other patients with DHEA deficiency.

As previously discussed, an inverse correlation between endogenous concentrations of DHEA and DHEA-S and the age of patients has been observed. Furthermore, endogenous DHEA-S concentrations in women are approximately 50–70% less than levels seen in men at any point throughout their lifetimes. A single-blind, placebo-controlled study was conducted to identify sex differences in the pharmacokinetics of DHEA after single and multiple dosing in older adults (Frye et al., 2000b). Previous studies had examined only single-dose pharmacokinetics. Six men and seven women aged 65–79 yr were enrolled in the study, which lasted for 29 d. On days 1–7, all subjects received a placebo. On days 8–22, they received DHEA 200 mg/d. Days 23–29 represented a washout period. Blood samples for determination of plasma DHEA and DHEA-S were drawn on days 1, 8, 15, 22, and 29 of the study just prior to the administration of the daily dose of DHEA or placebo and then 1, 2.5, 3.5, 4, 5, 6, 7, 9, 11, 14, and 23.5 h after the dose. Data were analyzed using repeated-measures ANOVA.

Baseline DHEA concentrations were similar in women and men in this study, whereas other investigators have found higher DHEA concentrations in women. The DHEA area under the curve (AUC) and maximum DHEA concentrations (C_{max}) in women were higher than those observed in men after doses 1, 8, and 15. In women, the AUC was lower after doses 8 and 15 than after the first dose, whereas in men, the AUC remained the same with multiple dosing. The mean half-life of DHEA steadily decreased in women during the administration of DHEA 200 mg from 11.7 to 6.9 h, whereas the half-life in men stayed relatively constant at 8 h.

The largest difference seen between men and women in the studies was the DHEA-S level. The endogenous DHEA-S level in men was 3.7 times greater than the level in women at the beginning of the study. The observation that endogenous DHEA-S levels are higher in men is consistent with findings of previous studies. During the administration of DHEA 200 mg, the DHEA-S levels between men and women showed no significant differences; thus, the net change in DHEA-S concentrations was greater in women. After the washout period, the DHEA-S levels returned to normal in both groups. The results from the study showed that DHEA and DHEA-S pharmacokinetics differ between men and women.

It should be noted that the half-life observed by Frye and colleagues (2000b) was shorter than that observed in another study of older subjects (67.8 ± 4.3 yr) in which DHEA was found to have a half-life of approx 20 h after administration of 25- or 50-mg tablets (Legrain et al., 2000). However, in the study by Legrain et al. (2000), the dose of DHEA was much smaller (50 mg) and thus produced DHEA concentrations just slightly higher than baseline endogenous concentrations. This resulted in these endogenous concentrations providing a larger percentage of the DHEA concentration measured and thus "artificially" elevating the concentrations measured at later time points, contributing to estimation of a longer half-life in the study by Legrain and coworkers (2000).

7.10. ADVERSE EFFECTS AND TOXICITY

Anabolic steroids are known to affect mood and can cause depression, euphoria, psychosis, and mania. A case report described a 51-yr-old man who required hospitalization for delusions of grandeur, irritable and expansive mood, and agitation approximately 5 mo after beginning self-medication with DHEA 50 mg/d to increase his energy level (Kline and Jaggers, 1999). He was also taking multivitamins and a beef liver extract tablet. He noted an increase in energy within days of beginning DHEA supplementation, and his wife noted that within 2 wk of beginning DHEA, he exhibited progressively worsening insomnia, irritability, grandiosity, hyperactivity, and irrational behavior. Because of her concerns, he decreased the dose to 25 mg/d the week prior to admission. In the hospital, he was treated with haloperidol 10 mg/d and divalproex 1500 mg/d (serum level 81.3 ng/mL). His condition improved over the course of several weeks, and haloperidol was tapered and discontinued without symptom recurrence. He remained well at 4-mo follow-up on divalproex. Although this patient had no personal history of psychiatric illness or substance abuse, his baseline mood was described as "mildly hypomanic, with a high level of energy." DHEA is present in relatively large concentrations in the limbic system and may function as an excitatory neurotransmitter (Kline and Jaggers, 1999) by acting as an antagonist at the γ-aminobutyric acid receptor or as an agonist at the N-methyl-D-aspartate receptor (Gurnell and Chatterjee, 2001). Thus, DHEA may be capable of precipitating a manic episode, particularly in predisposed patients.

In another published case report, a 55-yr-old man developed heart palpitations within 2 wk of beginning supplementation with DHEA 50 mg/d (Sahelian and Borken, 1998). His only other medication was the anorexiant dexfenfluramine (Redux), which he had discontinued 2 wk prior to beginning DHEA. Premature atrial contractions and premature ventricular contractions were documented in the emergency room. Thyroid function, potassium and other blood chemistries, echocardiogram, and a stress test were all normal. Propranolol 10 mg three times daily was prescribed, and DHEA was continued without further palpitations. The patient discontinued DHEA but restarted the supplement 4 mo later, with return of premature atrial contractions and premature ventricular contractions within 36 h. The palpitations were controlled with atenolol 25 mg twice daily. Although the temporal association between cardiac arrhythmias and DHEA use and their rapid reappearance with rechallenge suggest a cause–effect relationship between use of the supplement and the patient's symptoms, the DHEA product was not analyzed; therefore, a supplement ingredient other than DHEA may have been responsible for this adverse effect.

In an uncontrolled pilot study of DHEA 200 mg/d in 10 women, 3 developed mild acne responsive to topical therapy. One patient developed moderate acne and chose to withdraw from the study. Two patients receiving prednisone 10–20 mg/d reported hirsutism after 5–6 mo of DHEA treatment, and some noted a decrease in menstrual flow (van Vollenhoven et al., 1994).

Adverse effects reported in 14 women with lupus receiving DHEA 100 mg/d in a double-blind study included acne ($n = 8$), hirsutism ($n = 2$), weight gain ($n = 2$), emotional changes ($n = 1$) and abnormal menses ($n = 1$) (van Vollenhoven et al., 1995). In a study that included 19 women with lupus receiving DHEA 200mg/d for 6 mo, adverse effects deemed possibly or probably related to DHEA and occurring in more DHEA than placebo-treated patients during the double-blind portion of the trial included acne ($n = 6$), menstrual irregularities ($n = 8$), and hirsutism ($n = 4$) (van Vollenhoen et al., 1999).

In a study in which DHEA 50–200 mg/d was administered to 50 women with lupus (van Vollenhoven et al., 1998), mild acne responsive to topical treatment occurred in 62% of the premenopausal women and 31% of the postmenopausal women. In this 12-mo study, acne was worse during the first 4 mo of therapy. Mild hirsutism occurred in 22% of the premenopausal women, whereas oily skin, hair loss, breast tenderness, and vertigo were reported by 15–23% of the postmenopausal subjects. There were no differences in adverse effects between postmenopausal women taking estrogen and those not taking estrogen. One subject in this study with a history of asthma experienced increased bronchospasm after 3 d of treatment, which improved with DHEA discontinuation.

Genelabs (Redwood City, CA) which is pursuing FDA approval of DHEA for the treatment of lupus, reports that among the 600 patients who have received their DHEA product at a dose of 100–200 mg/d during clinical trials, mild-to-moderate acne and hirsutism were the most frequently reported adverse effects and were generally reversible with product discontinuation (Genelabs, 2001). The study by Petri and colleagues (1997), described in the Clinical Studies: Systemic Lupus Erythematosus section was in fact part of the Genelabs data described previously. In this study, acne occurred in almost half of the patients receiving DHEA, and hirsutism occurred in approximately 10% (Petri et al., 1997).

Voice deepening has also purportedly occurred in women. It is warned that hirsutism and voice changes may not be reversible (Anonymous, 1996).

Mild headache and insomnia, which resolved with DHEA discontinuation and reappeared upon rechallenge, were the only adverse effects reported in a dose-ranging study in which HIV-infected patients received DHEA 250–750 mg three times daily

(Centurelli and Abate, 1997). DHEA 50 mg/d was well tolerated in a quality of life study in HIV-positive patients (Piketty et al., 2001).

Insulin resistance has been reported in women receiving DHEA (Mortola and Yen, 1990). This observation is in contrast to reports of an inverse relationship between DHEA-S levels and type 2 diabetes (Gurnell and Chatterjee, 2001) and increased DHEA-S levels with insulin-sensitizing drugs such as metformin (Kroboth et al., 1999; Gurnell and Chaterjee, 2001). DHEA 150 mg/d did not affect glucose tolerance or insulin levels in young men, although in this study, the subjects were undergoing resistance training, which may have offset any adverse effect of DHEA or its metabolite, androstenedione, on insulin sensitivity (Brown et al., 1999).

Because DHEA is metabolized to testosterone and androstenedione, which can be aromatized to estradiol and estrone, estrogenic adverse effects may be problematic in men (Birchard, 1999; Kroboth et al., 1999; Leder et al., 2000). Increased estrogen levels in men are associated with gynecomastia and an increase in the risk of developing cardiovascular disease (King et al., 1999). In addition, one of the adverse effects documented in males using DHEA is a decrease in HDL cholesterol, which is a risk factor associated with the development of cardiovascular disease (Flynn et al., 1999; King et al., 1999). Conversely, as previously discussed, an inverse relationship between DHEA-S levels and cardiovascular disease has been documented. In a study of healthy young men, DHEA 300 mg three times daily for 2 wk inhibited arachidonate-stimulated platelet aggregation completely in one of five subjects, and slowed the rate of platelet aggregation in three others (Jesse et al., 1995). Platelet aggregation was not affected in the placebo group. Adverse effects were not reported. Inhibition of platelet aggregation may explain DHEA's reputed beneficial effect on cardiovascular disease. At this time, concerns that DHEA may increase the risk of cardiovascular disease or cause increased bleeding or bruising remain theoretical.

Reversible toxic hepatitis has also been documented (Buster et al., 1992). In this study, as described under Pharmacokinetics, an increase in liver function tests was noted at study completion in one subject, who developed symptoms of liver dysfunction 2 wk later. This patient had preexisting antinuclear antibodies; thus, the etiology of the hepatitis may have been autoimmune in nature.

Despite evidence from animal studies that DHEA may inhibit growth of certain experimental cancers, patients who have a personal or family history of breast, ovarian, endometrial, or prostate cancer should use DHEA with caution, and probably only under medical supervision, because it is not yet clear how it may affect these hormone-dependent cancers. For example, prosate cancer has been associated with high levels of endogenous insulin-like growth factor, which are increased by administration of DHEA to middle-aged and elderly men (Morales et al., 1994; Goldberg, 1998). Although increased PSA has not been documented in studies of DHEA supplementation in men (Goldberg, 1998; Wallace et al., 1999; Baulieu et al., 2000), it has been recommended that PSA, insulin-like growth factor levels, and DHEA levels should be monitored in men taking DHEA supplements (Goldberg, 1998). It has also been suggested that DHEA be used with caution in men suffering from benign prostatic hypertrophy (Pepping, 2000). In a rat model of hormone-dependent prostate cancer, DHEA prevented prostate cancer induction even when administered after pre-cancerous lesions were present (McCormick and Rao, 1999); however, these results cannot be extrapolated to humans without further study because of interspecies differences in metabolism, differences in the endogenous hormone milieu between experimental animals and men at risk for prostate cancer, and dosage considerations.

Although DHEA has been shown to protect against development of nitrosourea-induced mammary cancer in rats (Lubet et al., 1998), DHEA's protective effect is estrogen-dependent; in the absence of estrogens, DHEA stimulates breast cancer growth (Gatto et al., 1998). DHEA's protective effect has been demonstrated to involve stimulation of androgen receptors by DHEA (Gatto et al. 1998); however, in an estrogen-deficient state, such as would be seen in postmenopausal women, DHEA's predominant effect may be estrogenic (Stoll, 1999). DHEA at physiologic concentrations has estrogen-like effects in both hormome-dependent and non-hormone-dependent breast cancer cell lines, perhaps by conversion of DHEA to estrogens by aromatase or to other estrogen receptor agonists by other enzymes (LeBail et al., 1998). In mature female rodents with functioning ovaries, DHEA had uterotrophic effects at a dose of 2000 mg/kg of food (but not at lower doses) for 28 d (Nephew et al., 2000).

In the studies of DHEA in women with lupus conducted by Genelabs, use of mammography, uterine ultrasound, and endometrial biopsy were added to the study protocol beginning in January 1999. Among 600 women, almost half of whom had been exposed to DHEA for over 1 yr, an increased risk of breast cancer was not observed, nor was endometrial hyperplasia noted (Genelabs, 2001). Menstrual irregularities occurred in similar numbers of placebo and DHEA-treated patients (Petri, 1997). Longer follow-up is needed to rule out an increased risk of breast cancer with DHEA supplementation.

Although high estrogen levels have been associated with development of pancreatic cancer in men (King et al., 1999), pretreatment with dietary DHEA 0.6% inhibited the growth of pancreatic cancer xenografts in male nude, athymic mice (Muscarella et al., 1998).

7.11. INTERACTIONS

Certain medications can increase serum levels of endogenous DHEA and/or DHEA-S. Alprazolam and diltiazem increase DHEA levels, whereas amlodipine, danazol, diltiazem, and metformin increase DHEA-S levels. Danazol is thought to increase DHEA-S levels by inhibiting its conversion to DHEA because it also decreases DHEA levels. Insulin is a regulator of DHEA metabolism; increased insulin levels increase DHEA and DHEA-S clearance, thus decreasing their concentrations. Insulin levels are decreased by diltiazem, amlodipine, and metformin (Kroboth et al., 1999). This suggests that decreased circulating insulin is the mechanism behind the effects of these medications on DHEA and DHEA-S levels. Zidovudine increases DHEA levels in HIV-infected patients with low baseline DHEA levels (Centurelli and Abate, 1997). Theoretically, the use of DHEA supplements in patients taking medications that increase endogenous DHEA and/or DHEA-S levels might lead to an increase in the risk of developing adverse effects.

Aminoglutethamide decreases DHEA-S levels by decreasing the conversion of cholesterol to pregnenolone, DHEA's precursor. Carbamazepine also decreases DHEA-S levels, possibly by enzyme induction, but it has not been demonstrated to affect

DHEA levels. Dexamethasone decreases both DHEA and DHEA-S levels, perhaps owing to inhibition of anterior pituitary release of adrenocorticotrophin (ACTH), which stimulates release of DHEA and DHEA-S from the adrenal cortex. Morphine administration has been shown to decrease DHEA levels in mice (Kroboth et al., 1999). DHEA does not appear to alter prednisone metabolism (Genelabs, 2001).

In a study of the effects of DHEA administration on CYP3A-mediated metabolism of triazolam, 13 elderly men and women, ages 65–79 yr, were administered placebo for 1 wk, followed by DHEA 200 mg/d for 2 wk (Frye et al., 2000a). Triazolam 0.25 mg was administered on days 1–22. DHEA decreased triazolam clearance to a variable extent (0.6–42.2% decrease). This variability might reflect the interindividual variability in CYP3A concentrations among individuals. Inhibition of CYP3A was probably owing to DHEA-S, rather than DHEA, based on data using human liver microsomes. The results of this study suggest that there may be other potential drug interactions with DHEA because CYP3A is involved in the metabolism of many common drugs used therapeutically. CYP3A4 substrates include calcium channel blockers; alprazolam, midazolam, atorvastatin, lovastatin; carbamazepine, indinavir, ritonavir, saquinavir, clarithromycin, erythromycin, donepezil, fentanyl, methadone, ethinyl estradiol; cyclosporine, tacrolimus, sirolimus, itraconazole, ketoconazole, nefazodone, sertraline, quinine, quinidine, finasteride, tamoxifen, doxorubicin, etoposide, vincristine, and vinblastine (Lingtak-Neander and Horn, 1999).

7.12. REPRODUCTION

Embryotoxicity and fetotoxicity were reported in pregnant rats administered DHEA at a dose of 15 mg/kg/d while pregnant. At least six women taking DHEA 100–200 mg/d have become pregnant. Three pregnancies were terminated, and three resulted in normal offspring with no evidence of teratogenicity (Genelabs, 2001). Product labeling on all DHEA supplements recommends that women not use DHEA if they are pregnant, nursing, capable of bearing children, or taking any other prescription medications, especially hormone products.

7.13. CHEMICAL AND BIOFLUID ANALYSIS

Drug testing for anabolic steroids is based on the ratio of testosterone (T) to epitestosterone (E; an inactive testosterone isomer produced in the testes). Normally, the T/E ratio is 1:1, but it is increased with use of anabolic steroids. The International Olympic Committee (IOC) considers a T/E ratio of greater than one positive for anabolic steroid use. Because DHEA is metabolized to testosterone, it increases both testosterone and epitestosterone, and the ratio usually remains below the cutoff, although with higher doses athletes may test positive. In Australia, a soccer player tested positive with a T/E ratio of 14.5 although he was allegedly consuming only DHEA 50 mg/d (Corrigan, 1999).

DHEA and DHEA-S can be measured by a number of commercial kits from a variety of manufacturers; of a saliva sample is required. These kits generally involve the use of radioimmunoassay (RIA) techniques for quantitation and are rapid and sensitive. Either kits can be purchased for testing by clinical labs or samples can be sent to a variety of commercial labs for sample quantitation. Additionally, an enzyme-linked immunosorbent assay (ELISA) methodology has been developed for the quantitation of DHEA-S (Lewis et al., 1996). However, with both the RIA and ELISA kits, crossreactivity with other steroids can be problematic (Chasalow et al., 1989), and thus the specificity of the assay should be monitored. A number of researchers have developed techniques using gas chromatography with mass spectrometric or electron capture detection for the purpose of measuring DHEA or DHEA-S, reducing the chances of cross-reactivity (Johnson et al., 1980; Gaskell et al., 1980; Finlay et al., 1982; Chabraoui et al., 1991; Wudy et al., 1992, 1993). However, each of these assays requires separate analysis for DHEA and DHEA-S.

Recently, Zemaitis and Kroboth (1998) published a method for measuring both DHEA and its sulfate conjugate in human serum in one analytical run. Briefly, to 0.5 mL of spiked serum, 10 μL of 5-androsten-3β-ol-16-one methyl ester (internal standard) in methanol (50 ng/μL) and 0.5 mL of 0.01 M phosphate buffer (pH = 7) are added. The samples are then mixed and sonicated for 5 min. Solid phase extraction columns (1 mL) are preconditioned with 1 mL of methanol followed by 1 mL of water. The sample is then loaded onto the column and drawn through under vacuum at a rate of 1 mL/min. The cartridge is washed with 1 mL of 5% methanol in water and allowed to dry for 20 min under vacuum. The analytes are then eluted with two 0.6-mL portions of acetonitrile with the eluent subsequently evaporated to dryness. The dried residue is then reconstituted in methanol for injection (3 μL) into the gas chromatograph. Separation of the analytes (DHEA, DHEA-S, and internal standard) is achieved with a DB-5MS capillary column (30 m × 0.25 mm i.d., 0.25-μm film thickness). Helium, flowing at 40 cm/s, is used as the carrier gas. The injector temperature is set to 270°C, the transfer line temperature to 280°C, and the ion source temperature to 175°C. The oven temperature is programmed as follows: the temperature is started at 130°C, held for 1 min, and then increased at a rate of 15°C/min up to a temperature of 280°C, at which it is held for 3 min. Injections are made in splitless mode with a dwell time of 0.7 min before the purge valve is turned on. Parent masses of m/z 288 (DHEA) and 302 (internal standard) are monitored along with daughter ion spectra being recorded from m/z 195 to m/z 320. DHEA-S "desulfated" isomers are monitored at an m/z of 270. This monitoring of daughter ion spectra allows positive confirmation of the analyte and gives high specificity to the analysis.

7.14. REGULATORY STATUS

DHEA is available in the United States without a prescription. It is currently regulated as a dietary supplement, despite its absence from usual human foods (Parasrampuria et al., 1998). In 2001, Genelabs submitted a New Drug Application to the FDA for their DHEA formulation, Aslera®, for treatment of lupus (Genelabs, 2001). The effect of future FDA approval of Aslera as a prescription medication on over-the-counter availability of DHEA remains to be seen.

DHEA is banned in Canada, the United Kingdom (Dupee, 2002), and Australia, but because of Internet sales, DHEA may be available to residents of countries in which it is banned (Corrigan, 1999). In 1997, the IOC added DHEA to its list of banned substances (Corrigan, 1999). Use of DHEA is also banned by the National Collegiate Athletic Association (NCAA, 2001).

7.15. SUMMARY

- DHEA and its sulfate form DHEA-S are androgenic hormones that are converted in the body to androstenedione, testosterone, and estrogens.
- Levels of DHEA appear to decrease with age, suggesting that supplementation with exogenously administered DHEA might reverse the aging process. These claims have not been substantiated in clinical trials.
- DHEA administration does not appear to produce substantial improvement in exercise performance but does appear to exert positive effects in patients suffering from systemic lupus erythematosus.
- Adverse effects associated with androstenedione use are generally androgenic in females (e.g., hirsutism, acne, menstrual irregularities) and largely estrogenic in males (e.g., gynecomastia).
- DHEA is regulated and sold as a dietary supplement in the United States. However, its use is banned by several amateur and professional sports organizations and sale is banned in several foreign countries.

REFERENCES

Anonymous. Dehydroepiandrosterone (DHEA). Med Lett Drugs Ther 1996;38:91-2.

Ballantyne CS, Phillips SM, MacDonald JR, Tarnopolsky MA, MacDougall JD. The acute effects of androstenedione supplementation in healthy young males. Can J Appl Physiol 2000;25:68–78.

Baulieu E, Thomas G, Legrain S, et al. Dehdroepiandrosterone (DHEA), DHEA sulfate, and aging: contribution of the DHEAge study to a sociomedical issue. Proc Natl Acad Sci USA 2000;97:4279–84.

Birchard K. Body-building supplement fails to strengthen muscle and may harm health. Lancet 1999;353:1943.

Brown GA, Vukovich MD, Sharp RL, et al. Effect of oral DHEA on serum testosterone and adaptations to resistance training in young men. J Appl Physiol 1999;87:2274–83.

Buster JE, Casson PR, Straughn AB, et al. Postmenopausal steroid replacement with micronized dehydroepiandrosterone: preliminary oral bioavailability and dose proportionality studies. Am J Obstet Gynecol 1992;166:1163–70.

Callies F, Arlt W, Siekmann L, et al. Influence of oral dehyroepiandrosterone (DHEA) on urinary steroid metabolites in males and females. Steroids 2000;65:98–102.

Centurelli MA, Abate MA. The role of dehydroepiandrosterone in AIDS. Ann Pharmacother 1997;31:639–2.

Chabraoui L, Mathian B, Patricot MC, Revol A. Specific assay for unconjugated dehydroepiandrosterone in human plasma by capillary gas chromatography with electron-capture detection. J Chromatogr 1991;567:299–307.

Chasalow FI, Blethen SL, Duckett D, Zeitlin S, Greenfield J. Serum levels of dehydroepiandrosterone sulfate as determined by commercial kits and reagents. Steroids 1989;54:373–83.

Corrigan AB. Dehydroepiandrosterone and sport. MJA 1999;171:206–8.

Dupee R. Can we prevent aging? Available from: http://www.msnbc.com/news/691799.asp?pre=msnandcp1=1. Accessed January 24, 2002.

Dyner TS, Lang W, Geaga J, et al. An open-label dose escalation trial or oral dehydroepiandrosterone tolerance and pharmacokinetics in patients with HIV disease. J Acquir Immune Defic Synd 1993;6:459–65.

Finlay EM, Morton MS, Gaskell SJ. Identification and quantification of dehydroepiandrosterone sulphate in saliva. Steroids 1982;39:63–71.

Flynn MA, Weaver-Osterholtz D, Sharpe-Timms KL, Allen S, Krause G. Dehydro-epiandrosterone replacement in aging humans. J Clin Endocrinol Metab 1999;84:1527–33.

Frye RF, Kroboth PD, Folan RN, et al. Effect of DHEA on CYP3A-mediated metabolism of triazolam [abstract]. Clin Pharmacol Ther 2000a;67:109.

Frye RF, Kroboth PD, Kroboth FJ, et al. Sex differences in the pharmacokinetics of dehydroepiandrosterone (DHEA) after single- and multiple-dose administration in healthy older adults. J Clin Pharmacol 2000b;40:596–605.

Gaskell SJ, Pike AW, Griffiths K. Analysis of testosterone and dehydroepiandrosterone in saliva by gas chromatography-mass spectrometry. Steroids 1980;36:219–28.

Gatto V, Aragno M, Gallo M, et al. Dehdroepiandrosterone inhibits the growth of DMBA-induced rat mammary carcinoma via the androgen receptor. Oncol Rep 1998;5:241–3.

Genelabs. GL701(DEA, prasterone) for the treatment of systemic lupus erythematosus (SLE) in women. Briefing document. FDA Arthritis Advisory Committee, April 19, 2001. Available from: www.fda.gov/ohrms/dockets/ac/01/briefing/Briefing%20 information/3740b1_01_gendlabs.htm. Accessed December 29, 2001

Goldberg M. Dehydroepiandrosterone, insulin-like growth factor-I, and prostate cancer [letter]. Ann Intern Med 1998;129:587–8.

Gurnell EM, Chatterjee VKK. Dehydroepiandrosterone replacement therapy. Eur J Endocrinol 2001;145:103–6.

Hasheeve D, Salvato P, Thompson C. DHEA: a potential treatment for HIV disease [abstract]. International Conference on AIDS, Institute, TX. 1994;10:223.

Huppert FA, Van Niekerk JK. Dehydroepiandrosterone (DHEA) supplementation for cognitive function (Cochrane Review). In: The Cochrane Library, issue 4. Oxford: Update Software, 2001.

Jesse RL, Loesser K, Eich DM, et al. Dehydroepiandrosterone inhibits human platelet aggregation in vitro and in vivo. Ann NY Acad Sci 1995;774:281–90.

Johnson DW, Phillipou G, James SK, Seaborn CJ, Ralph MM. Specific quantitation of plasma dehydroepiandrosterone-sulphate by GC-MS: comparison with a direct RIA. Clin Chim Acta 1980;106:99–101.

King DS, Sharp RL, Vukovich MD, et al. Effect of oral androstenedione on serum testosterone and adaptations to resistance training in young men: a randomized controlled trial. JAMA 1999;281;2020–8.

Kline MD, Jaggers ED. Mania onset while using dehydroepiandrosterone. Am J Psychiatry 1999;156:971.

Kroboth PD, Salek FS, Pittenger AL, Fabian TJ, Frye RF. DHEA and DHEA-S: a review. J Clin Pharmacol 1999;39:327–48.

LeBail JC, Allen K, Nicolas JC, Habrioux G. Dehydroepiandrosterone sulfate estrogenic action at its physiological plasma concentration in human breast cancer cell lines. Anticancer Res 1998;18:1683–8.

Leder BZ, Longcope C, Catlin DH, Ahrens B, Schoenfeld DA, Finkelstein, JS. Oral androstenedione administration and serum testosterone concentrations in young men. JAMA 2000;283:779–82.

Legrain S, Massien C, Lahlou N, et al. Dehydroepiandrosterone replacement administration: pharmacokinetic and pharmacodynamic studies in healthy elderly subjects. J Clin Endocrinol Metab 2000;85:3208–17.

Lewis JG, Bason LM, Elder PA. Production and characterization of monoclonal antibodies to dehydroepiandrosterone sulfate: application to direct enzyme-linked immunosorbent assays of dehydroepiandrosterone sulfate and androsterone/epiandrosterone sulfates in plasma. Steroids 1996;61:682–7.

Lieberman S. An abbreviated account of some aspects of the biochemistry of DHEA, 1934–1995. Ann NY Acad Sci 1995;774:1–15.

Lingtak-Neander C, Horn J. Management of metabolic drug interactions, in: Carter BL, ed. Pharmacotherapy Self-Assessment Program, module 8, 3rd ed. Kansas City, MO: American College of Clinical Pharmacy, 1999.

Longcope C. Dehydroepiandrosterone metabolism. J Endocrinol 1996;150:S125–7.

Lubet RA, Gordon GB, Prough RA, et al. Modulation of methylnitrosourea-induced breast cancer in Sprague-Dawley rats by dehydroepiandrosterone: dose-dependent inhibition, effects of limited exposure, effects on peroxisomal enzymes, and lack of effects on levels of Ha-Ras mutations. Cancer Res 1998;58:921–36.

Mahesh VB, Greenblatt RB. The in vivo conversion of dehydroepiandrosterone and androstenedione to testosterone in the human. Acta Endocrinol 1962;41:400–6.

McCormick DL, Rao KV. Chemoprevention of hormone-dependent prostate cancer in the Wistar-Unilever rat. Eur Urol 1999;35:464–7.

Miller RA, Chrisp C. Lifelong treatment with oral DHEA sulfate does not preserve immune function, prevent disease, or improve survival in genetically heterogenous mice. JAGS 1999;47:960–6.

Morales AJ, Nolan JJ, Nelson JC, Yen SC. Effects of replacement dose of dehydroepiandrosterone in men and women of advancing age. J Clin Endocrinol Metab 1994;78:1360–8.

Mortola JF, Yen SS. The effects of oral dehydroepiandrosterone on endocrine-metabolic parameters in postmenopausal women. J Clin Endocrinol Metab 1990;71:696–704.

Muscarella P, Boros LG, Fisher WE, Rink C, Melvin WS. Oral dehydroepiandrosterone inhibits the growth of human pancreatic cancer in nude mice. J Surg Res 1998;72:154–7.

NCAA. 2002–2003 NCAA Banned Drug Classes. Avaialbe from: URL: http://www.ncaa.org. Accessed Sept. 4, 2002.

Nephew KP, Osborne E, Lubet RA, Grubbs CJ, Khan SA. Effects of oral administration of tamoxifen, toremifene, dehydroepiandrosterone, and vorozole on uterine histomorphology in the rat. Proc Soc Exp Bio Med 2000;223:288–94.

Parasrampuria J, Schwartz K, Petesch R. Quality control of dehydroepiandrosterone dietary supplement products [letter]. JAMA 1998;280:1565.

Pepping J. DHEA: dehyroepiandrosterone. Am J Health Syst Pharm 2000;57:2048–56.

Petri M, Lahita R, McGuire J, et al. Results of the GL701 (DHEA) multicenter steroid-sparing SLE study. Arthritis Rheum 1997;40(suppl):S327.

Petrow V. A history of steroid chemistry: some contributions from European industry. Steroids 1996;61:473–5.

Piketty C, Jayle D, Leplege A, et al. Double-blind placebo-controlled trial of oral dehydroepiandrosterone in patients with advanced HIV disease. Clin Endocrinol 2001;55:325–30.

Pugh TD, Oberly TD, Weindruch R. Dietary intervention at middle age: caloric restriction but not dehydroepiandrosterone sulfate increases lifespan and lifetime cancer incidence in mice. Cancer Res 1999;59:1642–8.

Sahelian R, Borken S. Dehydroepiandrosterone and cardiac arrhythmia [letter]. Ann Intern Med 1998;129:588.

Stoll BA. Dietary supplements of dehydroepiandrosterone in relation to breast cancer risk. Eur J Clin Nutr 1999;53:771–5.

Tummala S, Svec F. Correlation between the administered dose of DHEA and serum levels of DHEA and DHEA-S in human volunteers: analysis of published data. Clin Biochem 1999; 32: 355–61.

van Vollenhoven RF. Dehydroepiandrosterone in systemic lupus erythematosus. Rheum Dis Clin North Am 2000;26:349–62.

van Vollenhoven RF, Engleman EG, McGuire JL. An open study of dehydroepiandrosterone in systemic lupus erythematosus. Arthritis Rheum 1994;37:1305–10.

van Vollenhoven RF, Engleman EG, McGuire JL. Dehydroepiandrosterone in systemic lupus erythematosus: results of a double-blind, placebo-controlled, randomized clinical trial. Arthritis Rheum1995;38:1826–31.

van Vollenhoven RF, Morabito LM, Engleman EG, McGuire JL. Treatment of systemic lupus erythematosus with dehydroepiandrosterone: 50 patients treated up to 12 months. J Rheumatol 1998;25:285–9.

Van Vollenhoven RF, Park JL, Genovese MC, West JP, McGuire JL. A double-blind, placebo-controlled, clinical trial of dehydroepiandrosterone in severe systemic lupus erythematosus. Lupus 1999;8:181–7.

Wallace MB, Lim J, Cutler A, Bucci L. Effects of dehyroepiandrosterone vs androstenedione supplementation in men. Med Sci Sports Exerc 1999;31:1788–92.

Wellman M, Shane-McWhorter L, Orlando PL, Jennings JP. The role of dehydroepiandrosterone in diabetes mellitus. Pharmacotherapy 1999;19:582-91

Wolkowitz OM, Reus VI, Keebler A, et al. Double-blind treatment of major depression with dihydroepiandrosterone. Am J Psychiatry 1999;156:646–9.

Wudy SA, Wachter UA, Homoki J, Teller WM, Shackleton CHL. Androgen metabolism assessment by routine gas chromatography mass spectrometry profiling of plasma steroids: part 1, unconjugated steroids. Steroids 1992;57:319–24.

Wudy SA, Wachter UA, Homoki J, Teller WM. Determination of dehydroepiandrosterone sulfate in human plasma by gas chromatography/mass spectrometry using a deuterated internal standard: a method suitable for routine clinical use. Horm Res 1993;39:235–40.

Yen S. Dehydroepiandrosterone sulfate and longevity: new clues for an old friend. Proc Natl Acad Sci USA 2001;98:8167–9.

Zemaitis MA, Kroboth PD. Simplified procedure for measurement of serum dehydroepiandrosterone and its sulfate with gas chromatography-ion trap mass spectrometry and selected reaction monitoring. J Chromatogr B Biomed Sci Appl 1998;716:19–26.

Chapter 8

Dimethylglycine (N,N-Dimethylglycine)

Melanie Johns Cupp and Timothy S. Tracy

8.1. HISTORY

Dimethylglycine was discovered in 1943 (Tonda and Hart, 1992). It is found in some but not all formulations of pangamic acid (vitamin B15). Pangamic acid is not an identifiable substance because of the variety of products that have been marketed as such. One pangamic acid formulation that contains dimethylglycine is the "Russian formula," which was patented in 1975 and contains 61.5% calcium gluconate and 38.5% dimethylglycine (Gray and Titlow, 1982a). This is not the same as the pangamic acid isolated by Krebs and associates in 1951, which was studied in the treatment of cardiovascular disease in the 1950s and is structurally distinct from dimethylglycine (Kemp, 1959). Pangamic acid has been sold as a dietary supplement in the United States at least since the late 1970s, when the lay press celebrated its benefits (Colman et al., 1980). Although pangamic acid is also known as vitamin B15, it is not actually a vitamin because no deficiency state has been identified, and it has no known nutritional value (Colman et al., 1980; Gray and Titlow, 1982a). FoodScience Laboratories was the original distributor of vitamin B15 in the United States, and the Food and Drug Administration (FDA) challenged the company in court in the early 1980s in an attempt to remove the product from the market (Gray and Titlow, 1982a). As a result of this litigation, dimethylglycine continued to be marketed, but the use of the terms "vitamin B15" and "pangamic acid" fell out of favor (Hoorn, 1989). Currently, however, products labeled as vitamin B15, pangamic acid, and diemthylglycine are available. Some Internet sites incorrectly use the terms pangamic acid and vitamin B15 as synonyms for dimethylglycine.

8.2. CHEMICAL STRUCTURE

See Fig. 8-1 for the chemical structure of *N,N*-dimethylglycine.

From: *Forensic Science: Dietary Supplements: Toxicology and Clinical Pharmacology*
Edited by: M. J. Cupp and T. S. Tracy © Humana Press Inc., Totowa, New Jersey

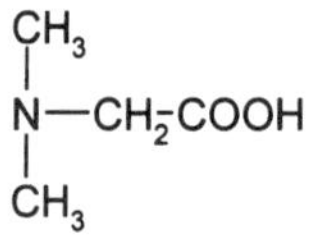

$$CH_3$$
$$|$$
$$N\text{---}CH_2\text{---}COOH$$
$$|$$
$$CH_3$$

Fig. 1. Chemical structure of N,N-Dimethylglycine

8.3. CURRENT PROMOTED USES

Dimethylglycine is promoted as an athletic performance enhancer and as a supplement for patients with autism or pervasive developmental disorder (Kern et al., 2001).

8.4. SOURCES AND CHEMICAL COMPOSITION

Dimethylglycine is a tertiary amine with the empiric formula $C_4H_9NO_2$ (Porter et al., 1985; Anonymous, 1996). It is an analog of glycine in which the amine hydrogens of glycine have been replaced with two methyl groups (Roach and Carlin, 1982). Dimethylglycine is formed in the liver mitochondria by the action of β-homocysteine methyltransferase during the metabolism of homocysteine to methionine (Porter et al., 1985; Roach and Carlin, 1982). Betaine, which is formed from choline, is the methyl donor in this reaction, and dimethylglycine is formed by the removal of one methyl group from betaine (Freed, 1984). Dimethylglycine is sold commercially as the hydrochloride salt, but it is present in meat as dimethylglycine; this difference may have implications for carcinogenicity (*see Adverse Effects and Toxicity* section; Colman et al., 1980).

8.5. PRODUCTS AVAILABLE

Dimethylglycine is generally sold as the hydrochloride salt in tablets, capsules, or (less commonly) lozenges. Most products are purported to contain 50, 125, or 135 mg of dimethylglycine per dosage unit. Dimethylglycine is also available in bulk for veterinary (equine) use. It is more readily available via the Internet than in retail outlets and health food stores.

8.6. ANIMAL DATA

8.6.1. Anticonvulsant Activity

In response to a case report that dimethylglycine may be effective in the treatment of epilepsy (Roach and Carlin, 1982), Freed (1984) administered saline or various doses of dimethylglycine intraperitoneally to mice, followed 10 min later by intraperitoneal pentylenetetrazol 60 mg/kg to induce seizures. Dimethylglycine caused a dose-dependent decrease in the incidence of seizures ($p < 0.001$, Fischer's exact test) as well as a significant increase in the time to the first seizure ($p = 0.0012$, Kruskal-Wallis test).

Ward and colleagues (1985) fed 36 female Sprague-Dawley rats dimethylglycine in water (0.026 mg/mL) *ad libitum* for 2 wk. Water consumption was 120–240 mL/d. Thirty-six rats were used as controls. Each group was divided into six groups, and each was administered penicillin G intraperitoneally at doses of 2200–4200 mg. Survival was measured 12 h after injection. All rats demonstrated lethargy, myoclonus, ataxia, and posturing at penicillin doses greater than 2200 mg. Only one rat treated with dimethylglycine died vs 18 in the control group ($p < 0.001$, Chi-squared). The mechanism of action of dimethylglycine in preventing seizure activity is unknown. Glycine is an inhibitory neurotransmitter, and dimethylglycine, being methylated, is more lipid-soluble than glycine and might more easily cross the blood-brain barrier. The investigators hypothesized that once inside the central nervous system, dimethylglycine might act directly as an inhibitory neurotransmitter, or indirectly by conversion to glycine.

8.6.2. Exercise Performance

Dimethylglycine's effect on exercise performance in horses has been studied. Levine and associates (1982) utilized Spur-15®, a product containing dimethylglycine 400 mg, calcium gluconate 600 mg, vitamin A 25,000 IU, vitamin E 500 IU, vitamin D3 250 IU, iron 5 mg, copper 1.5 mg, and manganese 5 mg per packet. Twenty racing standardbreds were randomly assigned to 11/2 packets of Spur-15 or placebo twice daily in their usual grain ration. Horses were raced and trained normally throughout the study. Blood levels for determination of complete blood cell count, creatinine phosphokinase, lactic acid (the primary outcome measure), calcium, cholesterol, glucose, blood urea nitrogen, uric acid, creatinine, total bilirubin, alkaline phosphatase, lactate dehydrogenase, and aspartate aminotransferase were drawn prior to supplementation, following training on day 2, on day 34, and after training on day 35. Statistical analysis was not described. Lactic acid levels after training were lower on days 2 and 35 (posttraining levels) in the treatment group than in the placebo group. The statistical significance of these differences is unclear.

8.6.3. Immunomodulating Effects

In vitro testing of dimethylglycine's effects on blast transformation was performed using lymphocytes from 30 normal volunteers, 15 patients with sickle cell disease, and 30 patients with insulin-dependent diabetes (Graber et al., 1981). A number of lymphocytes were incubated with dimethylglycine 1 mg/mL, and other lymphocytes served as a control. Phytohemagglutinin, concanavalin A, and pokeweed mitogen were used to stimulate lymphocyte proliferation. Cell proliferation, as determined by thymidine uptake, doubled or tripled in the dimethylglycine-exposed cells from sickle cell patients and diabetic patients and almost doubled in cells from healthy subjects.

A rabbit model was used to investigate further dimethylglycine's immunomodulating activity, with specific attention to possible mechanisms of action and whether its action depends on the character of the antigenic stimuli (Reap and Lawson, 1990). Rabbits were randomized to two test groups and two control groups, each consisting of six rabbits. The 12 rabbits in the test group were force-fed dimethylglycine (DaVinci Laboratories, Essex Junction, VT) 20 mg/kg/d in distilled water using a syringe. Control rabbits were force-fed distilled water. Typhoid vaccine (Wyeth Laboratories, Atlanta, GA) was administered intradermally on day 14 and intramuscularly on day 23 to six rabbits in each group, and formalin-treated influenza

A was administered intramuscularly on days 14 and 23 to the remaining six rabbits in each group. Blood samples were taken on days 14, 23, and 44 for determination of antibody titers. Blood was also collected on day 30 for T-cell proliferation testing. Data were analyzed using two-tailed Student's *t*-test.

None of the animals initially had an appreciable influenza or typhoid antibody titer. Rabbits in the dimethylglycine group achieved a higher mean influenza antibody titer than the control group ($p = 0.0006$). After the booster vaccination, mean titer was fourfold higher in the dimethylglycine group, but this difference was not statistically significant ($p = 0.1$). Mean antibody titer to typhoid O antigen (somatic antigen) was higher in the dimethylglycine group than in the control group after the first injection ($p = 0.0302$), as well as after the booster ($p = 0.0047$). Dimethylglycine-treated animals had a higher mean antibody titer to typhoid H antigen (flagellar antigen) after both the first and second injections, but these differences were not statistically significant. T-cells from dimethylglycine-treated rabbits exhibited a greater in vitro response to antigenic stimuli than those of control animals, both in the animals injected with influenza antigen ($p = 0.0024$) and in those injected with typhoid vaccine ($p = 0.018$).

In their discussion, the authors describe an unpublished study in which guinea pigs fed dimethylglycine did not develop an enhanced antibody response to an anthrax vaccine; however, the dimethylglycine-treated animals were more likely to survive anthrax infection than the control animals, implying enhanced cellular immune response. Although the investigators did not elucidate the mechanism of dimethylglycine's immunostimulatory action, they proposed the hypothesis of potentiation of T-cell expression of the OKT4 antigen or inhibition of T-suppressor cells, thereby enhancing cell-mediated immunity.

8.7. CLINICAL STUDIES

8.7.1. Enhanced Athletic Performance

Girandola and colleagues (1980a) studied the effect of dimethylglycine on oxygen consumption, blood lactate levels, and heart rate in eight moderately fit volunteers (seven men and one woman) performing maximal cycle ergometry. Subjects took two 400-mg tablets of "pangamic acid" three times each day for 2 wk. The tablets contained an equimolar mixture of calcium gluconate and dimethylglycine (Gluconic 15®, Da Vinci Laboratories). Cycle ergometry was performed before and after supplementation. Outcome measures were assessed during exercise and after recovery. Supplementation had no statistically significant effect on any of the measured parameters. This study was also published as an abstract (Girondola et al., 1980b).

Black and Sucec (1981) administered calcium pangamate, an equimolar mixture of calcium pangamate and dimethylglycine, to 18 active males in a crossover study. Maximum oxygen consumption (VO_2 max), anaerobic threshold, and running performance were measured at baseline, after 2 wk of supplementation with calcium pangamate 100 mg three times daily with meals, and after 2 wk of placebo. Calcium pangamate had no effect on any of the outcome measures.

Gray and Titlow (1982b) studied the effects of "pangamic acid" containing 61.5% calcium gluconate and 38.5% dimethylglycine on blood glucose, blood lactate levels, and performance on the Bruce Multistage Treadmill Test in 16 athletes engaged in daily cross-country workouts. All study subjects were male and ranged in age from 18 to 22 yr. Subjects were paired based on running performance, and members of each matched pair were randomized to either placebo or pangamic acid. Baseline and post-workout blood samples were drawn for determination of blood lactate and blood glucose levels. Other measures of exercise performance were maximum heart rate, treadmill time, and recovery heart rate 1 and 3 min post exercise. Subjects then began supplementation with pangamic acid (DaVinci Laboratories) 300 mg/d or identical placebo for 21 d. Blood and treadmill testing was repeated. Data were analyzed using multivariate ANOVA.

Baseline data were similar between the two groups, except for maximum heart rate and heart rate 3 min post exercise, which were lower in the pangamic acid group ($p < 0.05$). These values were also lower in the dimethylglycine group than in the placebo group post treatment when subjects were examined individually ($p < 0.05$). This probably does not reflect a treatment effect of pangamic acid, but rather baseline differences between the two groups, particularly since no statistically significant difference was found when all dependent variables were analyzed simultaneously.

Bishop and associates (1987) studied the effects of acute dimethylglycine supplementation on running performance. Sixteen members of a United States National Collegiate Athletic Association Division I varsity track team (13 men and 3 women) participated. Subjects were administered 1 mL dimethylglycine (Nutritional Logic, Seacliffs, NJ) or placebo in water flavored with mouthwash 5 min and 2 min prior to exercise. One minute prior to exercise, 0.5 mL of the solution was administered. Subjects were instructed to hold the solution sublingually and then swallow. The total dimethylglycine dose administered was 135 mg. After supplement or placebo administration, treadmill exercise was performed, and ventilation, oxygen consumption, heart rate, respiratory quotient, and perceived exertion were measured. Repeated measures ANOVA was used to analyze data. Dimethylglycine did not affect any of the outcome measures.

Dimethylglycine did not appear to have any effect on metabolic or circulatory responses to exercise in any of these studies, perhaps owing to the small sample size; however, Gray and Titlow (1982b) described a Soviet study of "pangamic acid" that demonstrated better maintenance of blood sugar and a reduction of blood lactate during exercise, particularly as exercise intensity increased. This study was not blinded or placebo-controlled. In another study with positive results (Pipes, 1980), 12 male track athletes aged 18–21 yr ingested "pangamic acid" 5 mg/d or placebo for 7 d. Exercise treadmill performance was measured before and after supplementation. The treatment group showed a 23.6% increase in time to exhaustion compared with baseline vs a 0.9% increase in placebo-treated subjects. Maximum oxygen consumption increased 27.5% in the treatment group, whereas the placebo group showed only a 3.3% increase.

8.7.2. Anticonvulsant Activity

Roach and Carlin (1982) presented a case report of a 22-yr-old mentally retarded man with mixed complex, partial, and grand mal seizures who demonstrated a decrease in seizure activity within 1 wk of taking dimethylglycine 90 mg twice daily. Dimethylglycine was initiated by the patient's mother when a health food store employee suggested that it might improve the patient's stamina. The patient had failed to respond to phenytoin, acetazolamide, and diazepam, and despite therapeutic levels of carbamazepine and phenobarbital, the patient's electroencephalogram (EEG) had routinely showed right temporal lobe spikes and he had previously suffered 16–18 generalized seizures per week. The number of seizures decreased to three per week with dimethylglycine. Two attempts to withdraw dimethylglycine resulted in an increase in seizure frequency. It was hypothesized that dimethylglycine's antiepileptic activity may be owing to conversion in the CNS to the inhibitory neurotransmitter glycine; action as an agonist at the glycine receptor; modification of the balance of inhibitory and excitatory amino acids in the central nervous system by competing for transport mechanisms into the central nervous system; or inhibition of inactivation of glycine in the synapse.

Following this report, Roach and Gibson (1983) designed a double-blind, placebo-controlled pilot study of dimethylglycine in five patients aged 5–19 yr with refractory seizures. Three patients had complex partial seizures, one had grand mal seizures, and one had akinetic seizures. Study subjects (three males and two females) received dimethylglycine 270 mg or placebo for 30 d. They were then crossed over to the opposite treatment arm. Seizure frequency was reported by family members and teachers for at least 1 mo. No statistically significant improvement in seizure frequency was reported in any of the test subjects. It was suggested that the original case report patient may have had a metabolism defect that was corrected by the administration of dimethylglycine.

Haidukewych and Rodin (1984), as part of a research program for new anticonvulsants, submitted dimethylglycine to the Epilepsy Branch of the National Institute of Neurological and Communicative Disorders and Stroke for screening as an anticonvulsant. Dimethylglycine showed no anticonvulsant activity in mice at any dose tested. These investigators suggested that the patient in the case report published by Roach and Carlin (1982) had a unique, previously undescribed requirement for dimethylglycine, or that the results were due to a placebo effect.

In a double-blind study in patients with epilepsy, Gascon and colleagues (1989) randomized 19 residents of a school for the mentally retarded to dimethylglycine or placebo. Study subjects were taking at least two antiepileptic drugs. The experimental group received dimethylglycne 100 mg three times daily for 2 wk, followed by 200 mg three times daily for for 2 wk. Antiepileptic drug trough plasma levels were drawn within 2 wk of starting supplementation. Once supplementation was started, antiepileptic plasma levels were measured on days 2, 5, 8,15, and 30. Levels were also drawn 1 and 2 wk after the study ended. A seizure log and record of medication administration were maintained by institution staff, as was their usual practice. Mean seizure frequency was analyzed for each subject before the study, during the first 2 wk of supplementation, during the second 2 wk of supplementation, and post supplementation using a multivariate version of Student's *t*-test called Hotelling's r^2.

Seizure frequency decreased approx 30% in both groups, suggesting no therapeutic effect of dimethylglycine. Levels of all antipiletic drugs except valproic acid were within the therapeutic range in all patients at baseline and during supplementation. Baseline valproic acid levels were subtherapeutic (< 50 mg/dL) in 4 of 9 dimethylglycine patients and in 4 of 10 placebo patients at baseline. In two of the dimethylglycine patients, serum levels increased into the therapeutic range during supplementation. Valproic acid levels increased in two of the placebo-treated patients, but levels did not reach the therapeutic range. The investigators noted that these changes in valproic acid levels were not unexpected because valproic acid levels tend to fluctuate in patients on multiple antiepileptic drugs.

8.7.3. Immunomodulating Effects

Based on a 1972 study published in a Russian veterinary journal showing that "calcium pangamate" (composition not described) restored immune response in irradiated rabbits and guinea pigs, Graber and associates (1981) conducted a double-blind study designed to examine the effects of dimethylglycine on cell-mediated and humoral immune response. Twenty healthy volunteers were recruited from the Medical University of South Carolina faculty and their families. Eleven men and nine women, aged 18–64 yr, participated. Age pairing of individuals within families was done such that dietary habits were similar between the two groups. Test subjects received 120 mg of dimethylglycine and 180 mg of calcium gluconate each day for 10 wk. The control group recived calcium gluconate 300 mg. Pneumovax® (14-valent *Streptococus pneumoniae* vaccine) 0.5 mL was administered to all subjects intramuscularly on study day 14. Blood was obtained from the subjects on days 0,14, 35, and 56 and was tested for anti-pneumococcal antibodies. Response was analyzed using repeated measures ANOVA.

Treatment subjects exhibited a fourfold increase in antibody response to pneumococcal vaccine compared with the control group ($p < 0.01$). To test the effect of dimethylglycine on cell-mediated immune response, monocytes isolated from all subjects were cultured in the presence of concanavalin A, streptokinase-streptodornase, and Pneumovax. Production of leukocyte inhibition factor (LIF) was measured by incubating the supernatants with granulocytes from a single donor. Granulocyte migration was then measured to determine the LIF index. The two-tailed Student's *t*-test was used to compare migration indexes between the two groups. When streptokinase-streptodornase and Pneumovax were used as stimulants, the LIF index was lower ($p < 0.001$) in the dimethylglycine group than in the control group, indicating increased lymphocyte responsiveness. These results support earlier animal studies reporting that dimethylglycine enhances both humoral and cell-mediated immune responses. The investigators suggest that dimethylglycine may make a useful vaccine adjunct.

8.7.4. Autism

Based on anecdotal reports of the efficacy of dimethylglycine in autism and a theoretical basis for its mechanism of action, Bolman and Richmond (1999) undertook a placebo-controlled study of dimethylglycine in eight autistic patients. Subjects were selected from a local autism organization in Hawaii. The diagnosis of autism was made by the investigators using the DSM-III-R criteria. Ten males, ages 4–30 yr, were included. After a 2-wk baseline period, subjects received placebo or dimethylglycine in a double-blind fashion. Dimethylglycine was dosed based on weight. Subjects weighing less than 70 kg received 125 mg/d, subjects weighing 70–120 kg received 250 mg, and the single subject weighing 120 kg received 375 mg. After a 2-

wk washout, subjects were crossed over to the other therapy. The second supplementation period was followed by 2 wk of observation without supplementation. Subjects were evaluated weekly using the Autism Rating Scale from the Children's Psychiatric Rating Scale measuring social relatedness, speech characterisitics, activity, affect, and abnormal movements; a newly developed rating scale evaluating changes in speech, eye contact, cooperation, understanding, attention, sleep, bizarre behavior, anger/tantrums, activity level, and overall behavior; and a scale tailored to the symptoms of each individual subject, designed with the help of each child's parents, rating attention, social relationships, sensory-motor behaviors, language/communication, self-help skills, and any unique symptoms. Eight subjects completed the study.

Dimethylglycine did not produce any statistically significant beneficial effects, and there were several trends suggesting a negative effect for dimethylglycine. Possible reasons for the negative results included low dosage of dimethylglycine, small sample size, and insensitive outcome measures given the variability in autistic symptomatology. Subgroup analysis of data from those patients who appeared to benefit from dimethylglycine may be necessary to show benefit.

In a second double-blind study (Kern et al., 2001), a higher dose of dimethylglycine was used. Thirty-nine children aged 3–11 yr meeting the DSM-IV criteria for autism or pervasive developmental disorder were randomized to placebo or dimethylglycine (FoodScience Laboratories). The dose of dimethylglycine was 125 mg for subjects weighing less than 40 lbs, 250 mg for subjects weighing 41–70 lbs, 375 mg for subjects weighing 71–100 lbs, 500 mg for subjects weighing 101–130 lbs, and 625 mg for subjects weighing more than 131 lbs. Behavior was assessed using the Vineland Maladaptive Behavior Domain of the Vineland Adaptive Scales Survey Form (a parent interview tool) and the Abberrant Behavior Checklist, Subscales I–V. The latter was completed with parent input and by observing the subjects' behavior in a child-friendly room with toys and activity centers. The Vineland Maladaptive Behavior Domain measures eye contact; eating and sleeping problems; attention; concentration; aggressiveness; peculiar preoccupations, mannerisms, or habits; self-injurious behavior; awareness of surroundings; bizarre speech; and rocking. The Abberrant Behavior Checklist is a tool used to evaluate the effects of psychotropic medications on inappropriate or maladaptive behavior and contains items pertinent to patients with autism or pervasive developmental disorder, including self-injurious behavior; isolation; presence of fixed facial expression; lack of emotional responsiveness; and repetitive speech, hand, body, or head movements. The 58 individual items on the checklist are grouped into five subcales. Subjects were assessed at baseline and at week 4 by the same investigator. A pediatric neurologist examined 33 of the subjects, including assessment of alertness, eye contact, ability to follow commands, gait, strength, muscle tone, deep tendon reflexes, and fine motor skills.

Statistical analysis using ANOVA and t-tests showed no improvement in behavior scores for the treatment group compared with the placebo group. Dimethylglycine did not affect the overall neurologic exam ($p < 0.57$, Chi-squared), but three children in the dimethylglycine group exhibited improvement in gross motor function, including improved muscle tone and coordination, and less posturing and toe walking. No improvements in neurologic parameters were noted in the placebo group. Fifty-eight percent of the children in the dimethylglycine group were said to respond positively to the treatment according to parental report, whereas 53% of the children in the placebo group were said to respond positively.

8.8. PHARMACOKINETICS

Dimethylglycine is a small water-soluble molecule (Anonymous, 1996), and absorption is likely to be rapid and complete. Dimethylglycine is oxidized in the liver to sarcosine (monomethylglycine) by dimethylglycine dehydrogenase (Porter et al., 1985; Kern et al., 2001). Dimethylglycine may be sufficiently lipophilic to cross the blood-brain barrier (Ward et al., 1985).

8.9. ADVERSE EFFECTS AND TOXICITY

Based on prior evidence that dimethylglycine could be nitrosated to nitrososarcosine, which is a weak carcinogen, and also to dimethylnitrosamine, which is a potent carcinogen, Colman and colleagues (1980) tested the mutagenicity of dimethylglycine HCl using the Ames assay with and without exposure to sodium nitrite. After incubation of dimethylglycine with sodium nitrite at 37°C for 45 min, ascorbate and oxygen were added to consume any residual nitrites that could induce mutagenesis. Controls included nitrite alone, nitrosated dimethylglycine not exposed to ascorbate and oxygen, and nitrite that had been exposed to ascorbate and oxygen. Commercially purchased dimethylnitrosamine was used as a positive control. Of the five *Salmonella typhimurium* strains used in the test, mutagenicity caused by nitrosated dimethylglycine was observed only in the TA100 and TA1535 strains. When the test solutions containing dimethylglycine were incubated with rat liver microsomal enzymes (S9 supernatant), evidence of mutagenicity was "unequivocal"; however, dimethylglycine alone was only weakly mutagenic. Similarly, dimethylnitros- amine was mutagenic only when incubated with the S9 supernatant. Although nitrite alone was strongly mutagenic for both organisms with and without exposure to the S9 supernatant, treatment with ascorbate and oxygen abolished this effect, suggesting that the mutagenicity of nitrosated dimethylglycine was not caused by unconsumed nitrites. The investigators concluded that dimethylglycine is nitrosatable and that the mutagenic nitrosated moiety is not dimethylnitrosamine, but rather nitrososarcosine or another nitrosated product. The concentration of dimethlyglycine used in this study was less than would be predicted after ingestion of 50 mg of dimethylglycine.

Because nitrites are present in human saliva and the pH conditions of the study were comparable to those to which dimethylglycine would be exposed after ingestion, this in vitro study has potential clinical implications. It has been argued that because the nitrite concentrations used in this study are far in excess of those present in human saliva, the results cannot be extrapolated to ingestion of dimethylglycine as a dietary supplement (Kendall, 1994). It is important to note that the hydrochloride salt of dimethylglycine was used in the Colman study and is the form of dimethylglycine used in commercial products. Whether these results would apply to dimethylglycine present in meat, which is not the hydrochloride salt and is present intracellularly in low concentrations, is unknown.

Based on a subsequent unpublished study that failed to reproduce the results of Colman and colleagues (1980) under the same experimental conditions, Hoorn (1989) examined dimethylglycine's mutagenicity in *Salmonella typhimurium* strains TA 100 and TA 135 using the Ames assay as described above. Mutagenicity was assessed both with and without exposure of dimethylglycine HCl to sodium nitrite. Dimethylglycine did not increase the number of revertants, with or without metabolic activation, compared with the control solution. The mutagenicity profile of sodium nitrite alone was similar to the profiles of the nitrosated product and the control mixture. Hoorn concluded that the mutagenicity observed in the Colman et al. study (1980) was owing to unconsumed nitrite, not dimethylglycine or its nitrosated product.

In one study of dimethylglycine in children with autism (Kern et al., 2001), one child was withdrawn owing to possible adverse behavioral changes; however, only 16% of the children were reported to have negative behavioral effects, compared with 32% of the children in the placebo group. These negative effects included hyperactivity, difficulty sleeping, and aggressiveness.

No adverse reactions or effects on body temperature or blood pressure were noted in a 10-wk study of healthy adult volunteers (Graber et al., 1981). Dimethylglycine was not associated with any adverse effects or toxicity in a 30-d rabbit study (Reap and Lawson, 1990).

8.10. INTERACTIONS

No dimethylglycine-drug interactions have been reported.

8.11. REPRODUCTION

No information on the effects of dimethylglycine on reproduction exist.

8.12. CHEMICAL AND BIOFLUID ANALYSIS

Assays for *N,N*-dimethylglycine have involved a variety of techniques such as enzymatic assay (Porter et al., 1985), gas chromatography-mass spectrometry (GC-MS) (Allen et al., 1993), and liquid chromatography-ultraviolet (LC-UV) detection (Laryea et al., 1994). Recently, Laryea and colleagues (1998) developed a straightforward and sensitive method for detecting *N,N*-dimethylglycine concentrations in both blood and urine. First, a derivatizing reagent solution is prepared by dissolving in 100 mL of acetonitrile 66 mg of 18-crown-6 and 1390 mg of 4-bromophenacyl bromide. Urine samples are then diluted 10-fold; plasma samples are used undiluted. Fifty microliters of KH_2PO_4 (100 mM) is added to 50 μL of sample and vortexed; then 900 μL of derivatizing reagent is added with continued mixing. Samples are then capped and heated at 80°C for 60 min. After cooling, the samples are mixed again and centrifuged at 1000g. Fifteen microliters of the resulting supernate is then injected directly onto the high-performance liquid chromatography (HPLC) device. An LC-SCX (5 μm, 250 × 4.6 mm i.d.) column is used for chromatographic separation. An isocratic elution profile is used with a total run time of 20 min. The mobile phase consists of 22 mM choline in a 90:10 mixture of acetonitrile/water. A flow rate of 1.5 mL/min is used for sample elution, and the eluate is monitored with an ultraviolet detector set to 254 nm.

The retention time for the phenylacyl bromide ester derivative of *N,N*-dimethylglycine is approximately 13 min. The limit of detection for the assay is 2 μM, although this could potentially be improved by injecting a larger volume of sample into the chromatographic system. Recovery of *N,N*-dimethylglycine at various concentrations is greater than 98% in both plasma and urine. Although a derivatizing step is required, the method is relatively simple, with limited sample cleanup required and good assay sensitivity achieved.

Other methods, as mentioned above, exist for the analysis of *N,N*-dimethylglycine. Although functional, they suffer from limitations. The enzymatic method of Porter and associates (1985) can suffer from interferences from endogenous compounds, and thus care must be taken to include appropriate controls. The mass spectrometric method of Allen and colleagues (1993) is both sensitive and specific but requires extensive sample cleanup and preparation as well as expensive equipment. Finally, the LC-UV method originally published by Laryea and colleagues (1994) suffers from a lack of sensitivity, which may become problematic under certain circumstances.

8.13. REGULATORY STATUS

Products labeled as vitamin B15, pangamic acid, and dimethylglycine are regulated as dietary supplements.

8.14. SUMMARY

- Dimethylglycine is the methylated analog of the amino acid and inhibitory neurotransmitter glycine. It is formed during the conversion of homocysteine to methionine.
- Dimethylglycine is one component of some formulations of pangamic acid (vitamin B15). Pangamic acid (vitamin B15) is sometimes erroneously used as a synonym for dimethylglycine.
- Dimethylglycine has been studied as an exercise performance enhancer in humans and horses, as an anticonvulsant, and as treatment for autism; however, findings have been inconsistent. It may be useful as an immunostimulant, particularly as a vaccine adjuvant.
- Dimethylglycine is a small, water-soluble molecule that is probably well absorbed after oral administration. It may be sufficiently lipid-soluble to cross the blood-brain barrier. It is metabolized in the liver.
- Dimethylglycine has been well tolerated in clinical studies. It is does not appear to be mutagenic.

REFERENCES

Allen RH, Stabler SP, Lindenbaum J. Serum betaine, N,N-dimethylglycine and N-methylglycine levels in patients with cobalamin and folate deficiency and related inborn errors of metabolism. Metabolism 1993;42:1448–60.

Anonymous. N-N-dimethylglycine, in: Budavari, ed. The Merck Index, 12th ed. Whitehouse Station, NJ: Merck Research Laboratories, 1996.

Bishop PA, Smith JF, Young B. Effects of N,N-dimethylglycine on physiological response and performance in trained runners. J Sports Med 1987;27:53–6.

Black DG, Sucec AA. Effects of calcium pangamate on aerobic endurance parameters, a double blind study [abstract]. Med Sci Sports Exerc 1981;13:93.

Bolman WM, Richmond JA. A double-blind, placebo-controlled, crossover pilot trial of low dose dimethylglycine in patients with autistic disorder. J Autism Dev Disord 1999; 29:191–4.

Colman N, Herbert V, Gardner A, Gelernt M. Mutagenicity of dimethylglycine when mixed with nitrite: possible significance in human use of pangamates. Proc Soc Exp Biol Med 1980;164:9–12.

Freed WJ. N,N-Dimethylglycine, betaine, and seizures [letter]. Arch Neurol 1984;41:1129–30.

Gascon G, Patterson B, Yearwood K, Slotnick H. N,N dimethylglycine and epilepsy. Epilepsia 1989;30:90–3.

Girandola RN, Wiswell RA, Bulbulian R. Effects of pangamic acid (B-15) ingestion on metabolic response to exercise. Biochem Med 1980a;24:218–22.

Girandola RN, Wiswell RA, Bulbulian R. Effects of pangamic acid (B-15) ingestion on metabolic response to exercise [abstract]. Med Sci Sports Exerc 1980b;12:98.

Graber CD, Goust JM, Glassman AD, Kendall R, Loadholt CB. Immunomodulating properties of dimethylglycine in humans. J Infect Dis1981;143:101–5.

Gray and Titlow. B15: Myth or miracle? Physician Sportsmed 1982a;10:107–12.

Gray ME, Titlow LW. The effect of pangamic acid on maximal treadmill performance. Med Sci Sports Exerc 1982b;14:424–7.

Haidukewych D, Rodin EA. N,N-dimethylglycine shows no anticonvulsant potential [letter]. Ann Neurol 1984;15:405.

Hariganesh K, Prathiba J. Effect of dimethylglycine on gastric ulcers in rats. J Pharm Pharmacol 2000;52:1519–22.

Hoorn AJW. Dimethylglycine and chemically related amines tested for mutagenicity under potential nitrosation conditions. Mutat Res 1989; 222:343–50.

Kemp GL. A clinical study and evaluation on pangamic acid. JAOA 1959; 58: 714-5.

Kendall RV. Comment: N,N-dimethylglycine and L-carnitine as performance enhancers in athletes [letter]. Ann Pharmacother 1994;28:973.

Kern JK, Miller VS, Cauller L, et al. Effectiveness of N,N-dimethylglycine in autism and pervasive developmental disorder. J Child Neurol 2001;16:169–73.

Laryea MD, Steinhagen F, Pawliczek S, Wendel U. Simple method for the routine determination of betaine and N,N-dimethylglycine in blood and urine. Clin Chem 1998;44:1937–41.

Laryea MD, Zass R, Ritgen J, Wendel U. Simultaneous determination of betaine and N,N-dimethylglycine in urine. Clin Chim Acta 1994;230:169–75.

Levine SB, Myhre GD, Smith GL, Burns JG. Effect of nutritional supplement containing N,N-dimethylglycine (DMG) on the racing standardbred. Equine Pract 1982;4:17–20.

Pipes TV. The effects of pangamic acid on performance in trained athletes [abstract]. Med Sci Sports Exerc 1980;12:98.

Porter DH, Lin M, Wagner C. Measurement of dimethylglycine in biological fluids. Anal Biochem 1985;151:299–303.

Reap EA, Lawson JW. Stimulation of the immune response by dimethylglycine, a nontoxic metabolite. J Lab Clin Med 1990;115:481–6.

Roach ES, Carlin L. N,N-dimethylglycine for epilepsy [letter]. N Engl J Med 1982;307:1081–2.

Roach ES, Gibson P. Failure of N,N-dimethylglycine in epilepsy [letter]. Ann Neurol 1983;14:347.

Tonda ME, Hart LL. N,N dimethylglycine and L-carnitine as performance enhancers in athletes. Ann Pharmacother 1992;26:935–7.

Ward TN, Smith EB, Reeves AG. Dimethylglycine and reduction of mortality in penicillin-induced seizures [letter]. Ann Neurol 1985;17:213.

Chapter 9

Fish Oil

Laura Martin, Melanie Johns Cupp, and Timothy S. Tracy

9.1. HISTORY

In the 1950s, fish oil was found to have hypolipidemic effects similar to those of linoleic acid, a polyunsaturated n-6 fatty acid found in vegetable oil. This observation was not pursued further until the 1970s, when it was noted that Greenland Eskimos had a lower incidence of mortality from heart disease than Danish people. The diet of the latter group was high in saturated fat compared with the Eskimo diet, which was rich in fish oil. Since then, fish oil has been studied for its cardiovascular, antiinflammatory, and central nervous system effects (Connor and Connor, 1997). Fish oil has been a health food store staple for over a decade.

9.2. CHEMICAL STRUCTURES

Refer to Fig. 9-1 for chemical structures of the n-3 polyunsaturated fatty acids eicosapentaenoic acid (EPA) and docosahexaenoic acid (DHA).

9.3. CURRENT PROMOTED USES

Fish oil is promoted to support cardiovascular, neurologic, and joint health.

9.4. SOURCES AND CHEMICAL COMPOSITION

The n-3 polyunsaturated fatty acids eicosapentaenoic acid (EPA) and docosahexaenoic acid (DHA) are the active components of fish oil. They are synthesized in oceans, lakes, and rivers by phytoplankton, which are then ingested by fish (Connor and Connor, 1997). In n-3 fatty acids, the first double bond in the molecule occurs three carbon atoms away from the terminal end of the carbon chain (Stone, 1996). EPA and DHA contain 20 and 22 carbon atoms, respectively (Pawlosky, 2001).

From: *Forensic Science: Dietary Supplements: Toxicology and Clinical Pharmacology*
Edited by: M. J. Cupp and T. S. Tracy © Humana Press Inc., Totowa, New Jersey

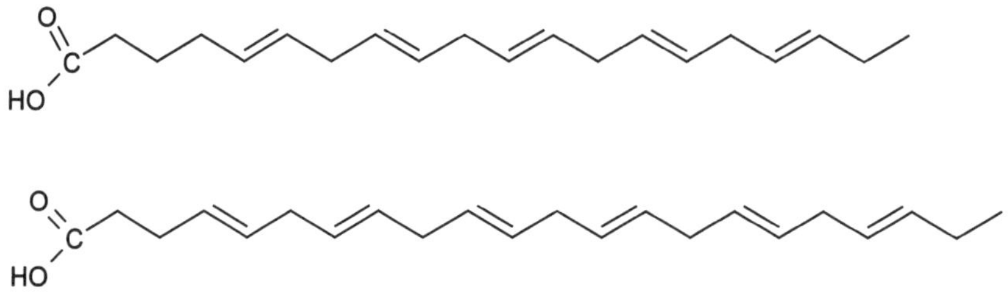

Fig. 1. Chemical structure of (top) 5, 8, 11, 14, 17-eicosapentaenoic Acid (EPA) and (bottom) 4, 7, 10, 13, 16, 19-docohexaenoic Acid (DHA).

Herring, sardines, and anchovies have high concentrations of EPA and DHA, salmon has medium concentrations, and sole, halibut, cod, and shellfish have low concentrations (Uauy-Dagach et al., 1996).

9.5. PRODUCTS AVAILABLE

Fish oil is typically available as clear gelcaps. Popular products include MaxEPA™ (R.P. Scherer, Clearwater, FL), Mega Twin EPA (Twin Laboratories, Inc., Hauppauge, NY), and GNC's products. K85® (Pronova, Oslo, Norway) contains 85% EPA and DHA. This is approximately threefold higher than the EPA/DHA content of MaxEPA. K85 also contains vitamin E 4 IU/g (Goodfellow et al., 2000). Small amounts of vitamin E are added to some products as an antioxidant to prevent spoilage (Stone, 1996).

Fish oil preparations that are produced in room air at ambient temperatures can oxidize, resulting in the capsule having a fishy odor and taste. Concentrated and purified fish oil prepared by vacuum distillation at low temperatures under nitrogen can minimize the odor/taste problem by removing fishy smelling impurities and minimizing oxygen exposure (Stoll et al., 2000). Contaminants are also removed during this process (Stoll et al., 2000). The use of purified products is preferred in clinical studies, in which blinding can be problematic owing to the taste or odor associated with lower quality products (Stoll et al., 2000).

The independent laboratory ConsumerLab.com has tested the potency and purity of 20 brands of fish oil products commonly available through catalogs, retail stores, multilevel marketing companies, and the Internet. Six of the products tested failed to meet ConsumerLab.com's standards because they contained only 50–80% of the labeled amount of DHA, and two of the six contained only 33% and 82% of the labeled content of EPA. None of the products contained detectable levels of mercury, and none showed evidence of decomposition (ConsumerLab.com, 2002). A list of products that passed testing and details about the testing methodology are available at the web site www.consumerlabs.com.

Fish oil products differ in their content of DHA, EPA, other fatty acids, cholesterol, and other substances. DHA and EPA may be present in the form of triglycerides, free fatty acids, methyl esters, or ethyl esters (Nordøy et al., 1991). These differences may lead to difference in therapeutic effect.

9.6. IN VITRO EFFECTS AND ANIMAL DATA

In vitro data suggest that fish oil's beneficial cardiovascular effects may involve increased incorporation of EPA and DHA into endothelial cell membranes, leading to improved membrane fluidity and production of the vasodilator nitic oxide (NO). Fish oil's ability to decrease oxygen-derived free radical production in neutrophils and monocytes suggests that the increased endothelial NO release may be secondary to a decrease in endothelial oxygen-derived free radical production (Goodfellow et al., 2000). In addition, unlike most prostaglandins derived from arachidonic acid, those derived from EPA are not proarrhythmic. Incorporation of EPA into cell membranes may therefore cause a beneficial shift in the balance of prostaglandins (Leaf, 2002). Indeed, there is clinical evidence to suggest that fish oil has an antiarrhythmic effect (Marchioli et al., 2002).

Fish oil has several proposed psychiatric indications, including depression, bipolar disorder, and schizophrenia. Cell membranes and their fatty acids play an integral role in neurotransmission because they are the matrix in which receptors are embedded, and they help the receptors hold their shape. Biochemical studies show that omega-3 fatty acids can be incorporated into cell membranes where they can affect neurotransmission, in part by suppressing phophatidylinositol second messenger activity. Red blood cell membrane fatty acid composition is thought to mirror that of neuronal cell membranes and can be measured conveniently and noninvasively. Evidence supporting a role of omega-3 fatty acids in the treatment of depression includes the inverse correlation between red blood cell membrane omega-3 fatty acid content and depression and the progressive decrease in maternal plasma and red blood cell DHA content during pregnancy, which may culminate in postpartum depression. A paucity of red blood cell membrane DHA has also been noted in schizophrenic patients, which may lead to oxidative damage to the membrane phospholipids, resulting in altered information processing. Evidence supporting a role for fish oil in bipolar disorder includes the dampening effect of ingestion of large amounts of omega-3 fatty acids on signal transduction (Cott, 1999).

Fish oil decreases proteinuria and improves mortality in the murine model of lupus nephritis, perhaps via antithrombotic and/or antiinflammatory effects (Clark and Parbtani, 1994). Fish oil's utility in inflammatory conditions probably stems from its ability to competitively inhibit the formation of proinflammatory prostaglandins and leukotrienes, such as leukotriene B4; it may also serve as a substrate for the synthesis of eicosanoids with lesser inflammatory activity, as well as antithrombotic prostaglandins (Kremer et al., 1987).

9.7. CLINICAL STUDIES

Most studies of fish oil have focused on its beneficial effects on cardiovascular outcomes; such studies have utilized dietary modification or have been epidemiologic in nature, as opposed to studies of commercially available fish oil capsules. This section will review representative clinical studies in which fish oil capsules, as opposed to dietary interventions or other sources of omega-3 fatty acids, were studied. Because of variations in the DHA and EPA content of various fish oil products, it may not be possible to extrapolate data from one study to another that used a different product. In addition, fish contain nutrients other than fish oil that may be beneficial; therefore, data from studies involving dietary changes may not apply to fish oil capsules. Compliance with the large number of capsules used in some studies may be problematic and may limit the actual effectiveness of fish oil in clinical practice.

9.7.1. Cardiovascular Indications

A recent systematic review concluded that modification of fat intake, such as increasing dietary omega-3 fatty acids and decreasing total fat, has only a small benefit in regard to cardiovascular morbidity and mortality (Hooper et al., 2001). Studies in which modification of omega-3 fatty acid intake was the only dietary intervention were excluded from the analysis.

One study included in the analysis was a randomized controlled trial (DART) with factorial design by Burr and colleagues (1989). In this landmark study, 2033 men younger than 70 yr were followed for 2 yr after a diagnosis of acute myocardial infarction to determine whether dietary intervention would prevent a second myocardial infarction. Patients were excluded if they were diabetic, awaiting cardiac surgery, or intended to follow one of the intervention diets independently of the study. The men were randomly assigned to receive or not receive instruction on three dietary interventions. One intervention was advice on how to reduce fat intake to less than 30% of total caloric intake. The second intervention was advice to eat at least two weekly portions (200–400 g) of fatty fish. If individuals receiving this advice could not tolerate fish, they were instructed to take MaxEPA 0.5 g three times daily. Finally, the third intervention was advice to increase cereal fiber intake to 18 g/d. The major endpoints of the study were total mortality and ischemic heart disease events. The latter included ischemic heart disease death and nonfatal myocardial infarction.

A 6 mo, 14% of the patients who had received fish advice were taking MaxEPA as a partial or total substitute for fish. At 2 yr, 22% of these patients were taking MaxEPA. Subjects who received fat intake advice did not show a decrease in mortality compared with subjects who did not receive this advice. Those who received education regarding fiber had a higher, although not significant, incidence of mortality compared with subjects who did not receive this advice. Subjects advised to eat fatty fish, however, showed a 29% decrease in the incidence of overall mortality ($p < 0.05$, log rank test), attributable to a decrease in ischemic deaths in this group ($p < 0.01$, log rank test). The incidence of reinfarction plus death from ischemic heart disease was not significantly affected by any of the regimens. The investigators believed that fish oil could exert its beneficial effects by inhibiting clotting mechanisms and platelets as well as preventing ventricular fibrillation during acute myocardial ischemia.

A prospective, placebo-controlled, randomized, double-blind, parallel-group study was conducted by Goodfellow and colleagues (2000) to ascertain whether fish oil supplementation could improve large artery endothelial function in hypercholesterolemic patients. Thirty subjects with hypercholesterolemia despite adhering to a low-fat diet for 3 mo were enrolled. Patients were excluded if they had smoked within the previous 2 yr; if they had had diabetes or hypertension; or if they had a history of coronary, cerebral, or peripheral vascular disease. Individuals receiving hormone supplements, vasoactive medications, vitamins, antioxidants, or fish oils were excluded as well. Subjects were assessed at baseline and again after 4 mo. Endothelial function was assessed using ultrasonic measurement of flow-mediated dilation in the brachial artery. The study group received K85 2 g twice daily, and the placebo group received 2 corn oil capsules daily. Two patients in the fish oil group did not complete the study for unknown reasons. There was a 95% compliance rate for both the fish oil and placebo groups.

There were no significant differences between the groups at baseline. The blood flow in the brachial artery after wrist cuff release was similar in both groups before and after treatment; however, flow-mediated dilation increased significantly after fish oil treatment compared with placebo ($p < 0.05$, unpaired t-test). Fish oil did not affect cholesterol, or very low-density, low-density, or high-density lipoproteins (VLDLs, LDLs, or HDLs) but did significantly reduce triglycerides ($p < 0.05$, unpaired t-test). Placebo did not have any significant effect on lipid profiles. The investigators concluded that fish oil improves large artery endothelium-dependent dilation in subjects with hypercholesterolemia without affecting endothelium-independent dilation caused by sublingual administration of glyceryl trinitrate. The investigators suggest that this benefit may be caused by an increase in NO.

In an open-label study (Marchioli et al., 2002), 11,323 subjects who had suffered a heart attack within 3 mo of study enrollment were randomized to fish oil 1 g/d (850–882 mg EPA/DHA ethyl esters), vitamin E 300 mg/d, a combination of the two, or no treatment. All patients received standard medical treatment and advice on lifestyle modifications. Patients randomized to fish oil achieved a survival benefit after only 3 mo of treatment (RR 0.59; 95% CI 0.36–0.97, $p = 0.037$), which persisted throughout the 3.5 yr study (RR 0.79; 95% CI 0.66–0.93, $p = 0.006$). This mortality benefit was attributed to a decrease in sudden death, suggesting an antiarrhythmic effect of fish oil. Subject demographics, social history, and medical history revealed that the population studied had a relatively low-risk cardiac profile. This may limit the ability to extrapolate the study results to the general population of myocardial infarction survivors.

Although fish oil may cause some reduction in blood pressure, this benefit has not been demonstrated in all studies (Toft et al., 1995). Fish oil has been shown to control blood pressure in heart transplant patients (Holm et al., 2001); however, a randomized, double-blind, placebo-controlled trial in 21 men with uncontrolled hypertension does not support the use of fish oil as anadjuvant to conventional antihypertensives (Gray et al., 1996). The antihypertensive effects of fish oil appear to be conferred principally by the DHA component (Mori et al., 1999). Differences in study results may be a function of dose, DHA vs EPA concentration, or study population. In contrast to its variable effects on blood pressure, the ability of fish oil to decrease triglyceride concentrations has been fairly consistent across various populations. Fish oil 3 g/d did not provide additional benefit in preventing restenosis after angioplasty when added to standard treatment with aspirin and a calcium channel blocker.

9.7.2. Diabetes

Farmer and colleagues (2001) systematically reviewed 18 randomized, placebo-controlled trials of fish oil supplementation in patients with type 2 diabetes to examine the effects of fish oil on lipids, glucose levels, and cardiovascular events. Fish oil was administered in capsule form in 17 of the studies, and in liquid form in one. EPA doses ranged from 1.08 to 5.2 g, and DHA doses ranged from 0.3 to 4.8 g. The reviewers concluded that fish oil decreases triglycerides, increases LDL, and has no effect on glucose control. Similarly, glucose control was not affected in a large study in which approximately 15% of the study participants had diabetes (Marchioli et al., 2002).

9.7.3. Psychiatric Indications

Fish oil 9.6 g/d was compared with olive oil placebo in a double-blind study of 30 patients meeting the DSM-IV criteria for bipolar disorder (Stoll et al., 1999). Other medications were allowed if doses were stable, and patients continued to be managed routinely by their usual clinician throughout the 4-mo study, although no change in medications or medication dosages was allowed. The primary outcome measure was time to mood destabilization, which was longer in the fish oil group ($p = 0.002$, Mantel-Cox). Three of 14 patients in the fish oil group suffered a change in mood vs 10 of the 16 patients in the placebo group. Interestingly, the patients in the fish oil group who relapsed exhibited mood elevation, whereas 9 of 10 placebo patients who relapsed experienced depressive symptoms. This suggests that fish oil may be better at preventing depression than mania (Su and Shen, 2000). More study of fish oil in bipolar disorder is needed and has been funded (Cott, 1999).

Although there have been several studies and case reports supporting the efficacy of EPA or DHA as single-entity agents in schizophrenia and depression, no randomized, placebo-controlled studies of fish oil *per se* in schizophrenia or depression have been published to date. Administration of MaxEPA 10 g/d for 6 wk to 20 patients with schizophrenia increased red blood cell omega-3 fatty acid composition and improved negative symptoms using the Positive and Negative Syndrome Scale (PANSS; Laugharne et al., 1996). As with bipolar disorder, additional studies of fish oil in schizophrenia and depression are forthcoming (Cott, 1999).

9.7.4. Other Uses

A double-blind crossover study supports the use of fish oil (EPA 1080 mg and DHA 720 mg/d) in dysmenorrhea (Harel et al., 1996). Randomized, double-blind studies also support the use of fish oil to decrease the need for nonsteroidal anti-inflammatory drugs (NSAIDs), improve symptoms, and stabilize disease progression in rheumatoid arthritis (Kremer et al., 1987; Lau et al., 1993), and as adjunctive therapy in inflammatory bowel disease (Stenson et al., 1992; Kim, 1996). More study is needed in these disorders. Fish oil has been shown to slow progression of IgA nephropathy, prevent thrombosis in polytetrafluorethylene dialysis grafts, and minimize cyclosporine-associated nephrotoxicity. It may also decrease calciuria in patients predisposed to kidney stones (Donadio et al., 2001).

Other proposed uses have less supporting data. A phase I dose-ranging study of fish oil capsules for cancer cachexia has been published (Burns et al., 1999), but placebo-contolled efficacy studies in humans have not yet been published. Although fish oil benefited children with asthma in a hospital setting in which allergen exposure and diet were carefully controlled (Nagakura et al., 2000), there are few additional data to support the use of fish oil in asthma (Woods et al., 2001). Despite benefical effects in animal models, a double-blind crossover study failed to demonstrate benefit of MaxEPA 15 g/d in lupus nephritis. More study is needed because of the potential for crossover effects or therapeutic effects from olive oil, which was used as a placebo (Clark and Parbtani, 1994).

9.8. PHARMACOKINETICS

Conflicting data exist on whether the bioavailability of DHA and EPA differ depending on whether they are administered as free fatty acids, triglycerides (e.g., MaxEPA), or ethyl esters (e.g., K85; von Schacky and Weber, 1985; Nordøy et al., 1991) Some reports have suggested that EPA incorporation into triglycerides was reduced and delayed when it was formulated as the ethyl ester compared with the triglyceride (von Schacky and Weber, 1985). However, others have found no difference in either EPA or DHA incorporation, regardless of the formulation (Nordøy et al., 1991). Thus, the individual formulation rather than the type of fatty acid delivery vehicle (e.g., ethyl ester or triglyceride) may be the limiting factor.

With the triglyceride formulations, EPA and DHA plasma concentrations are similar and are gender-independent. Plasma concentrations of EPA achieved were highly dose-dependent, whereas plasma concentrations of DHA achieved were only marginally dose-dependent. With these formulations, a dose of 12 g/d provides plasma concentrations of DHA that are only marginally higher than those produced with a dose of 6 g/d. Doses higher than 6 g/d may therefore not be clinically warranted (Marsen et al., 1992) with respect to producing increased DHA concentrations in the body.

9.9. ADVERSE EFFECTS AND TOXICITY

Fish oil preparations, particularly cod liver oil, may contain considerable amounts of vitamin A; however, with consumption of recommended dosages, toxicity is not a concern. Hypervitaminosis A was diagnosed in a patient who consumed fish oil 30–50 capsules/d for 1 yr. In addition to taking several different brands of fish oil capsules, he also took an unknown number of cod liver oil capsules. Symptoms, which included myalgias, anorexia, nausea, vomiting, fatigue, pruritis, dry skin, and angular chelitis resolved within 1 wk of discontinuation of fish oil supplementation (Grubb, 1990).

A 35-yr-old woman with a history of depression began taking a product containing DHA 330 mg and EPA 220 mg per capsule, two capsule three times daily, at the advice of a friend, who suggested it would improve her mood. She had not taken antidepressants for 8 mo, and had never experienced a manic episode. Five d later, she became hyperactive and grandiose and behaved inappropriately toward men. Two d after discontinuing the product, the patient's mood and behavior normalized (Kinrys, 2000).

A diet providing EPA 2–3 g prolongs bleeding time by 42%, an effect that is at least additive with the antiplatelet effects of therapeutic doses of aspirin (Thorngren and Gustafson, 1981). Individuals taking fish oil should be therefore be monitored for unusual bleeding or bruising.

A study of MaxEPA 750 mg administered five times weekly for 6 mo to diabetic rats demonstrated acceleration of progression of diabetic retinopathy compared with untreated animals (Hammes et al., 1996). The potential benefit of fish oil in persons with diabetes in regard to cardiovascular risk should be weighed against the theoretical risk of worsening retinopathy.

Fish oil is generally fairly well tolerated, with diarrhea being the most common side effect in patients receiving up to 21 1-g fish oil capsules/d providing DHA and EPA 13.1 g/d (Burns et al., 1999). Other adverse effects include fishy breath, nausea (Stoll et al., 2000), and elevated LDL (Grubb, 1990; Gray et al., 1996; Farmer et al., 2001), the risk of which increases as triglyceride levels and fish oil doses increase (Farmer et al., 2001). Five patients with excessive drowsiness ($n = 2$), urticarial rash, and abdominal pain and distention were reported by a dermatologist treating 100 patients with MaxEPA. These symptoms resolved within 1 d of product discontinuation and reappeared with rechallenge (Mehta, 1992).

There is a theoretical risk of exposure to pollutants such as mercury, dioxins, furans, or PCBs in unpurified fish oil products because these toxins accumulate in fish. Another theoretical concern is methanol toxicity from the use of products that deliver EPA and DHA as methyl esters (Nordøy et al., 1991). Weight gain and pancreatitis could potentially occur with high doses. There is evidence that fish oil may cause central venous pooling in the lung, leading to a drop in hematocrit (Nordøy et al., 1991) or, hypothetically, respiratory distress in patients with heart failure or chronic lung disease.

In an open study using fish oil capsules providing DHA 2.2 g and EPA 0.6 g/d for prevention of colorectal cancer in patients with familial adenomatous polyposis ($n = 3$) and multiple colorectal polyps ($n = 2$), three patients developed endometrial cancer after 1 yr of therapy, colon cancer after 2 yr of therapy, and lung cancer after 1 yr of therapy. The fish oil product used in this study had a higher concentration of DHA than EPA, whereas most previous studies used products higher in EPA. In addition, the duration of this study was longer than that of most previous studies. These differences may account for the investigators' findings. More study is needed (Akedo et al., 1998).

Interestingly, MaxEPA increased the risk of azaserine-induced precancerous pancreatic nodules in rats, perhaps by altering relative levels of various eicosanoids (Appel and Woutersen, 1996).

9.10. INTERACTIONS

Because of its antiplatelet effects and documented additive effects with aspirin (Thorngren and Gustafson, 1981), fish oil should be used cautiously with drugs that have antiplatelet effects such as aspirin, NSAIDs, and clopidogrel. In a placebo-controlled 4-wk study, anticoagulation clinic patients with stable international normalized ratios (INRs) were randomized to fish oil 3 g/d, fish oil 6 g/d, or placebo. Fish oil did not appear to affect INR in this small ($n = 16$) study. One patient experienced bruising. The lack of effect on INR does not rule out increased risk of bleeding caused by additive anticoagulant and antiplatelet effects (Bender et al., 1998).

9.11. REPRODUCTION

Randomized, placebo-controlled studies have failed to demonstrate a benefit of fish oil for preventing pregnancy-induced hypertension and proteinuria or intrauterine growth retardation in high-risk women (Onwude et al., 1995; Olsen et al., 2000); however, it may decrease the risk of preterm labor in women with a history of preterm labor (Olsen et al., 2000). Only high-quality products known to be free of mercury should be used during pregnancy.

9.12. CHEMICAL AND BIOFLUID ANALYSIS

Analysis of fatty acids in serum is typically accomplished using gas chromatography (GC) with various types of detection, although liquid chromatography (LC) methods do exist (Wang and Peter, 1983; Baty et al., 1986; Liebich et al., 1991). Baty and colleagues (Baty et al., 1986) developed both GC and LC methods for analysis of ester-derivatized fatty acids and found the methods to be comparable. One of the more recent methods, developed specifically for analyzing polyunsaturated fatty acids in patients receiving fish oil, was developed by Liebich and colleagues (1991). This method utilizes GC with flame ionization detection. The fatty acids, specifically 5,8,11,14,17-eicosapentaenoic acid (EPA) and 4,7,10,13,16,19-docosahexaenoic acid (DHA), are converted into their methyl esters through a derivatization reaction. Briefly, 2 mL of methanol-toluene (4:1, v/v) in which 40 µg of 13,16,19-docosatrienoic acid (internal standard) has been dissolved and 200 µL of acetyl chloride are added to 100 µL of serum. This mixture is then reacted for 60 minutes at 100°C, followed by neutralization with 5 mL of 6% potassium carbonate. Following centrifugation at 1800g for 10 min, the toluene phase is separated and directly injected onto the GC column.

Chromatographic separation is achieved on a fused silica column coated with 25 µm free fatty acid phase, polyethylene glycol 2-nitroterephthalate (FFAP; column, 25 m × 0.25 mm i.d.). Nitrogen is used as the carrier gas with a split ratio of 1:25. Two microliters of sample are injected onto the column. A temperature program is used for analysis in which the temperature is ramped from 80 to 160°C at a rate of 6°C/min (i.e., over 13.3 min) and then ramped to 200°C at a rate of 0.5°C/min (i.e., over another 20 min) and held at that temperature. Retention times for each of the analytes are as follows: EPA 79.6 min; internal standard 98.4 min; and DHA 108.2 min. This lengthy run time is necessary to achieve chromatographic separation of EPA and DHA from the numerous other fatty acids present in serum. The assay listed above can also be used to detect and quantitate concentrations of caprylic acid, capric acid, myristic acid, palmitic acid, palmitoleic acid, stearic acid, oleic acid, cis-vaccenic acid, linoleic acid, 6,9,12,15-octadecatetraenoic acid, 11-eicosenoic acid and 7,10,13,16,19-docosapentaenoic acid. Limits of sensitivity for the assay are less than 2 ng/mL for EPA and less than 5 ng/mL for DHA. This method has the advantage that it has proven utility in patients receiving fish oil supplementation in that it is sensitive enough to detect concentrations of these fatty acids (EPA and DHA) prior to fish oil administration as well as during treatment.

9.13. REGULATORY STATUS

Fish oil products are regulated as dietary supplements by the Food and Drug Administration.

9.14. SUMMARY

- Fish oil has potential therapeutic utility as an adjunct to standard therapy in heart disease, rheumatoid arthritis, hypertriglyceridemia, and inflammatory bowel disease. It is considered a standard therapy for IgA nephropathy.
- Fish oil is generally well tolerated. Diarrhea and other gastrointestinal complaints are the most common adverse effects. Cases of hypervitaminosis A have been reported, as well as mood elevation.
- Fish oil may potentially increase the risk of bleeding or bruising when taken with antiplatelet drugs or anticoagulants.

REFERENCES

Akedo I, Ishikawa H, Nakamura T, et al. Three cases with familial adenomatous polyposis diagnosed as having malignant lesions in the course of a long-term trial using docosahexanoic acid (DHA)-concentrated fish oil capsules. Jpn J Clin Oncol 1998;28:762–5.

Appel MJ, Woutersen A. Dietary fish oil (MaxEPA) enhances pancreatic carcinogenesis in azaserine-treated rats. Br J Cancer 1996;73:36–43.

Baty JD, Willis RG, Tavendale R. A comparison of methods for the high-performance liquid chromatographic and capillary gas-liquid chromatographic analysis of fatty acid esters. J Chromatogr 1986;353:319–28.

Bender NK, Kraynak MA,Chiquette E, et al. Effects of marine fish oils on the anticoagulation status of patients receiving chronic warfarin therapy. J Thromb Thrombolysis 1998;5:257–61.

Burns CP, Halabi S, Clamon GH, et al. Phase I clinical study of fish oil fatty acid capsules for patients with cancer cachexia: cancer and leukemia group B study 9473. Clin Cancer Res 1999;5:3942–7.

Burr ML, Gilbert JF, Holliday RM, et al. Effects of changes in fat, fish, and fibre intakes on death and myocardial reinfarction: diet and reinfarction trial (DART). Lancet 1989;2:757–61.

Clark WF, Parbtani A. Omega-3 fatty acid supplementation in clinical and experimental lupus nephritis. Am J Kidney Dis 1994;23:644–7.

Connor SL, Connor WE. Are fish oils beneficial in the prevention and treatment of coronary artery disease? Am J Clin Nutr 1997;66(suppl):1020S–31S.

ConsumerLab.com. News. Consumberlab.com finds fish oil supplements free of mercury, but 30% lacking in key ingredient—meet label claims—test results of omega-3 fatty acid (EPA and DHA) products released today. Available from: http://www.consumerlabs.com/news/news_112001.asp. Accessed January 25, 2002.

Cott J. Omega-3 fatty acids and psychiatric disorders. Alt Ther Women Health 1999;1:97–101.

Donadio JV. N-3 Fatty acids and their role in nephrologic practice. Curr Opin Nephrol Hypertens 2001;10:639–42.

Farmer A, Montori V, Dinneen S, Clar C. Fish oil in people with type 2 diabetes mellitus (Cochrane Review). In: The Cochrane Library, Issue 4. Oxford: Update Software, 2001.

Goodfellow J, Bellamy MF, Ramsey MW, Jones CJH, Lewis M. Dietary supplementation with marine omega-3 fatty acids improve systemic large artery endothelial function in subjects with hypercholeterolemia. J Am Coll Cardiol 2000;35:265–70.

Gray DR, Gozzip CG, Eastham JH, Kashyap ML. Fish oil as an adjuvant in the treatment of hypertension. Pharmacotherapy 1996;16:295–300.

Grubb BP. Hypervitaminosis A following long-term use of high-dose fish oil supplements. Chest 1990;97:1260.

Hammes HP, Weiss A, Fuhrer D, Kramer HJ, Papavassilis C, rimminger F. Acceleration of experimental diabetic retinopathy in the rat by omega-3 fatty acids. Diabetalogia 1996;39:251–5.

Harel Z, Biro FM, Kottenhahn RK, Rosenthal SL. Supplementation with omega-3 polyunsaturated fatty acids in the management of dysmenorrhea in adolescents. Am J Obstet Gynecol 1996;174:1335–8.

Holm T, Andreassen AK, Aukrust P, et al. Omega-3 fatty acids improve blood pressure control and preserve renal function in hypertensive heart transplant recipients. Eur Heart J 2001;22:428–36.

Hooper L, Summerbell CD, Higgins JP, et al. Reduced or modified dietary fat for preventing cardiovascular disease (Cochrane Review). In: The Cochrane Library, Issue 3. Oxford: Update Software, 2001.

Kim YI. Can fish oil maintain Crohn's disease in remission? Nutr Rev 1996;54:248–52.

Kinrys G. Hypomania associated with ω3 fatty acids [letter]. Arch Gen Psychiatry 2000;57:715–6.

Kaul U, Sanghvi S, Bahl VK, Dev V, Wasir HS. Fish oil supplements for prevention of restenosis after coronary angioplasty. Int J Cardiol 1992;35:87–93.

Knapp HR, FitzGerald GA. The antihypertensive effects of fish oil. A controlled study of polyunsaturated fatty acid supplements in essential hypertension. N Engtl J Med 1989;320:1037–43.

Kremer JM, Jubiz W, Michalek A, et al. Fish-oil fatty acid supplementation in active rheumatoid arthritis. Ann Intern Med 1987;106:497–503.

Lau CS, Morley KD, Belch JJ. Effects of fish oil supplementation on non-steroidal anti-inflammatory drug requirement in patients with mild rheumatoid arthritis—a double-blind placebo controlled study. Br J Rheumatol 1993;32:982–9.

Laugharne JD, Mellor JE, Peet M. Fatty acids and schizophrenia. Lipids 1996;31(suppl):S163–5.

Leaf A. On the reanalysis of the GISSI-Prevenzione [editorial]. Circulation 2002;105:1874–5.

Liebich HM, Wirth C, Jakober B. Analysis of polyunsaturated fatty acids in blood serum after fish oil administration. J Chromatogr 1991;572:1–9.

Marchioli R, Barzi F, Bomba E, et al. Early protection against sudden death by n-3 polyunsaturated fatty acids after myocardial infarction. Time-course analysis of the results of the Gruppo Italiano per lo Studio della Sopravvivenza nell Infarcto Miocardico (GISSI)-Prevenzione. Circulation 2002;105:1897–1903.

Marsen TA, Pollok M, Oette K, Baldamus CA. Pharmacokietics of omega-3 fatty acids during ingestion of fish oil preparations. Prostaglandins Leukot Essent Fatty Acids 1992;46:191–6.

Mehta VR. Side effects of eicosapentaenoic acid and docosahexaenoic acid (MaxEPA). J Assoc Physicians India 1992;40:486.

Mori TA, Bao DQ, Burke V, Puddey IB, Beilin LJ. Docosahexaenoic acid but not eicosapentaenoic acid lowers ambulatory blood pressure and heart rate in humans. Hypertension 1999;34:253–60.

Nagakura T, Matsuda S, Shichijyok K, Sugimoto H, Hata K. Dietary supplementation with fish oil rich in omega-3 polyunsaturated fatty acids in children with bronchial asthma. Eur Respir J 2000;16:861–5.

Nordøy A, Barstad L, Connor WE, Hatcher L. Absorption of the n-3 eicosapentaenoic and docosahexaenoic acid as ethyl esters and triglycerides by humans. Am J Clin Nutr 1991;53:1185–90.

Olsen SF, Secher NJ, Tabor A, et al. Randomized clinical trials of fish oil supplementation in high risk pregnancies. Fish Oil Trails in Pregnancy (FOTIP) team. Br J Obstet Gynecol 2000;107:382–95.

Onwude JL, Lilford RJ, Hjartardottir H, Staines A, Tuffnell D. A randomized double blind placebo controlled trial of fish oil in high risk pregnancy. R J Obstet Gynaecol 1995;102:95–100.

Pawlosky, RJ. Physiological compartmental analysis of alpha-linolenic acid metabolism in adult humans. J Lipid Res 2001;42:1257–65.

Reis GJ, Sipperly ME, McCabe CH, et al. Randomized trial of fish oil for prevention of restenosis after coronary angioplasty. Lancet 1989;2:177–81.

Stenson WF, Cort D, Rodgers J, et al. Dietary supplementation with fish oil in ulcerative colitits. Ann Intern Med 1992;15:609–14.

Stoll AL, Damico KE, Marangell LB, Severus WE. In reply. Arch Gen Psychiatry 2000;57:716–7.

Stoll AL, Severus WE, Freeman MP, et al. Omega 3 fatty acids in bipolar disorder: a preliminary double-blind, placebo-controlled trial. Arch Gen Psychiatry 1999;56:407–12.

Stone NJ. Fish consumption, fish oil, lipids, and coronary heart disease. Circulation 1996;94:2337–40.

Su K, Shen WW. Are ω 3 fatty acids beneficial in depression but not mania [letter]? Arch Gen Psychiatry 2000;57:716.

Thorngren M, Gustafson A. Effect of 11-week increases in dietary eicosapentaenoic acid on bleeding time, lipids, and platelet aggregation. Lancet 1981;2:1190–3.

Toft I, Bønaa KH, Ingebretsen OC, Nordøy A, Jenssen T. Effects of polyunsaturated fatty acids on glucose homeostasis and blood pressure in essential hypertension. A randomized, controlled trial. Ann Intern Med 1995;123:911–8.

Uauy-Dagach R, Valenzuela A. Marine oils: the health benefits of n-3 fatty acids. Nutr Rev 1996;54:S102-8.

Von Schhacky C, Weber PC. Metabolism and effects on platelet function of the purified eicosapentaenoic and docosahexaenoic acids in humans. J Clin Invest 1985;76:2446-50.

Wang ST, Peter F. Gas-liquid chromatographic determination of fatty acid composition of cholesteryl esters in human serum using silica Sep-Pak cartridges. J Chromatogr 1983;276:249–256.

Woods RK, Thien FCK, Abramson MJ. Dietary marine fatty acids (fish oil) for asthma (Cochrane Review). In: The Cochrane Library, Issue 4. Oxford: Update Software, 2001.

Chapter 10

γ–Hydroxybutyric Acid (GHB), γ-Butyrolactone (GBL), and 1,4-Butanediol (BD)

Betsy Meredith, Melanie Johns Cupp, and Timothy S. Tracy

10.1. History

γ-hydroxybutyric acid (GHB) was synthesized in 1960 by the French physician Henry Labroit (Ropero-Miller and Goldberger, 1998). Because of its then reported low toxicity and lack of side effects, the use of GHB in anesthesia and psychiatry was initially endorsed (Labroit, 1964), but it soon fell out of favor as an anesthetic owing to its unpredictable actions and adverse effects (Ropero-Miller and Goldberger, 1998). GHB has also been studied as a treatment for opioid and ethanol withdrawal; as a treatment for narcolepsy; and in the management of shock. In the 1980s, GHB was promoted in the United States as a growth hormone stimulator (Chin et al., 1998). After the Food and Drug Administration (FDA) banned the over-the-counter sales of L-tryptophan in 1989, GHB was promoted as a replacement sleep aid (Ropero-Miller and Goldberger, 1998). Beginning in 1990, the FDA began an investigation into several reports of GHB-associated vomiting, dizziness, tremors, and seizures resulting in hospitalization and death (FDA, 1997). GHB gained public notoriety with the death of actor River Phoenix, which was purportedly associated with GHB use. At that time, GHB was popular in Los Angeles nightspots, where it was commonly found in powder form. GHB then began appearing on college campuses, first in Florida and Georgia (Minai, 2001). The FDA and the Department of Justice took action against several manufacturers, distributors, and promoters of GHB. Through these actions and the use of embargos and public education campaigns, the distribution and abuse of GHB began to decrease. There was then a resurgence in the use of GHB and accompanying reports of GHB-associated adverse effects and deaths with the creation of clandestine labs (FDA, 1997). Subsequently, the GHB precursors γ-butyrolactone (GBL) and 1,4-butanediol (BD) began to be marketed as natural, nontoxic dietary supplements (FDA 1999a, b).

From: *Forensic Science: Dietary Supplements: Toxicology and Clinical Pharmacology*
Edited by: M. J. Cupp and T. S. Tracy © Humana Press Inc., Totowa, New Jersey

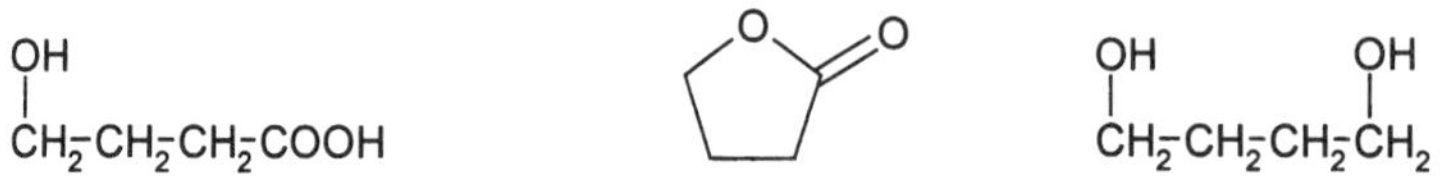

OH
|
CH₂-CH₂-CH₂-COOH

OH   OH
| |
CH₂-CH₂-CH₂-CH₂

Fig. 1. Chemical structures of (left) γ-hydroxybutyric acid, (center) γ-butyrolactone, and (right) 1,4-butanediol.

10.2. CHEMICAL STRUCTURES

See Fig. 10-1 for chemical structures of γ-hydroxybutyric acid, γ-butyrolactone and 1,4-butanediol.

10.3. CURRENT PROMOTED USES

GHB has enjoyed recent popularity as an illicit drug for its purported use as a euphoriant, a sexual enhancer, and a steroid alternative for body builders (Chin et al., 1998). In addition, GHB has been characterized as a "date rape drug" (CDC, 1997).

GBL is claimed to build muscles, improve physical performance, enhance sex, reduce stress, induce sleep (FDA, 1999b), stimulate growth hormone release, and relieve addictions (Hardy et al., 1999).

10.4. SOURCES AND CHEMICAL COMPOSITION

GHB is an endogenous four-carbon, water-soluble molecule (Li et al., 1998a). GHB is found in the central nervous system with binding sites present in the cortex, hippocampus, midbrain, basal ganglia, and substantia nigra. Nonneuronal tisses such as the kidney also contain GHB. In fact, the kidney contains more than 10 times the concentration of GHB that is found in the brain, whereas the amounts found in the heart and muscle are fivefold greater than those in the brain (Cash, 1994).

GHB is produced by adding sodium hydroxide to GBL (Ropero-Miller and Goldberger, 1998), the cyclic ester of GHB (Fessenden and Fessenden, 1986; Zvosec et al., 2001). The consequent ester hydrolysis of GBL yields a clear solution that is approximately 70% GHB by weight (Ropero-Miller and Goldberger, 1998).

GBL is also known by the names 2[(³H)]-furanone dihydro, dihydro-2(³H)-furanone, 4-butanolide, butyrolactone, 4-butyrolactone, tetrahydro-2-furanone, and butyrolactone-γ (FDA, 1999b).

BD is a substituted furanone (Higgins and Borron, 19966) that is rapidly converted to GHB upon ingestion. It is also commonly referred to as tetramethylene glycol and butylene glycol (Zvosec et al., 2001).

10.5. PRODUCTS AVAILABLE

GHB is known by a variety of names including sodium oxybate, sodium oxybutyrate (CDC, 1990), 4-hydroxybutyrate (Helrich et al., 1964), liquid ecstasy, liquid x, cherry meth, soap, growth hormone booster (Li et al., 1998b), Georgia home boy, grievous bodily harm, G, GMB, easy lay, great hormones at bedtime, GH beers

(Zvosec et al., 2001), everclear, poor man's heroin, goops, nature's quaalude, salt water, water, wolfies, scoop, and zonked (Ropero-Miller and Goldberger, 1998). GHB products illegally imported from Europe include Alcover, Gamma-OH, Somatomax-PM, Anectamine, Somsanit, and Natural Sleep 500 (Zvosec et al., 2001).

GHB is distributed as a sodium salt in tablet or powder form, which is commonly dissolved in water (CDC, 1990), fruit juice, a carbonated beverage, or alcohol. It is also available as a putty, gel, and liquid (Zvosec et al., 2001). Undiluted GHB liquid is clear, oily, and slightly more viscous than water, with a salty or "solvent" taste (hence the street name "salt water"). Cinnamon or a food dye may be added to make it more palatable (Ropero-Miller and Goldberger, 1998).

GBL is an acrylate polymer (e.g., Super Glue®) solvent (CDC, 1999) used in the textile industy and found in household wood cleaners and paint removers (Ropero-Miller and Goldberger, 1998). It is promoted as a "nontoxic" or "organic" cleaner. Products include Verve, Verve 5.0, and Miracle Cleaning Products. Ingredients may or may not be listed (Zvosec et al., 2001).

GBL products promoted for human consumption are commonly liquids and may be labeled as furanone, lactone, or furanone dihydro. Products include Beta-Tech, Blue Nitro, Blue Nitro Vitality, Eclipse 4.0, Firewater, Furomax, Furan, Furanone, Gamma G, Gamma Ram, G3®, GenX, GH Gold, GH Revitlizer, Insom-X, Invigorate, Jolt, Nu-Life, ReActive, Regenerize, Remforce, Renewsolvent, Rest-Eze, Revivarant G, Thunder, V3, Verve, and Verve 5.0. RenewTrient™ is available in capsule as well as liquid form (Zvosec et al., 2001). Revivarant, a liquid GBL product in a 32-ounce bottle, and Revivarant G, which contained 200 mg in powder form in a pill bottle, were recalled by the Trimfast Group in response to a voluntary recall requested by the FDA (1999b).

BD products are usually clear oily liquids with a citrus or ketone odor (Higgins and Borron, 1996; Dyer et al., 1997). Products containing BD include Cherry fX Bombs, Lemmon fX Drops, Orange fX Drops, Revitalize Plus, Serenity, Enliven, GHRE, NRG3 (FDA, 1999a), Thunder Nectar, Thunder (there is also a GBL product by this name), SomatoPro (liquid and capsules), X-12, Rest-Q, Biocopia PM, Dormir, Amino Flex, RejuvNite, Ultradiol, N-Force, Liquid Gold, Soma Solutions, Blue Raine, InnerG, and Zen (Zvosec et al., 2001). BD has also been sold as "pine needle oil" in 3-ounce opaque white spray bottles (Dyer et al., 1997).

Like GBL, BD is also marketed as a "nontoxic" or "organic" liquid cleaning solvent or acrylate polymer solvent and is found in some paint removers (Higgins and Barron, 1996; Zvosec et al., 2001). BD-containing cleaning products include Blue Raine, Thunder, Serenity II, Mystik, Midnight, Miracle Cleaning Products, Weight Belt Cleaner (Zvosec et al., 2001) and Bullet" (Higgins and Borron, 1996). The ingredients may not be listed (Zvosec et al., 2001).

The BD content of some of these products has been determined using gas chromatography-mass spectroscopy (GC-MS). Thunder Nectar contains 10% BD. NRG3 is labeled as 18% BD but has been found to contain only 5% using GC-MS. InnerG is labeled to contain 5% BD but has been found to contain 7% using GC-MS. Zen is labeled to contain 14% BD but has been found to contain 16% using GC-MS. Serenity is labeled to contain 7% but contains 6% per GC-MS (Zvosec et al., 2001).

10.6. IN VITRO EFFECTS AND ANIMAL DATA

GHB may act as a neurotransmitter (Vayer et al., 1987). Unlike other neurotransmitters, GHB is able to cross the blood-brain barrier after peripheral administration. When administered peripherally at high doses, it induces responses such as sedation and eventually anesthesia, which may be accompanied by an electroencephalographic (EEG) response in some animal species similar to that seen in human absence seizures (Cash, 1994). GHB thus can be used to produce an animal model of absence seizures for study (Dyer, 1991). Convulsions have been produced in the cat following tactile stimuli after GHB administration (Winters and Spooner, 1965).

Endogenous GHB may be involved in the modulation of dopaminergic activity (Snead, 1977). Dopamine levels in the brain doubled in rats 1 h after iv injection of 20 mmol GHB (Gessa et al., 1966). In an additional study, significant increases in dopamine levels were observed 1 h after GHB administration (50 and 100 mg/kg) in male rats. However, there were no significant changes in serotonin metabolism. It was concluded that low doses of GHB selectively affect dopaminergic activity (Miguez et al., 1988). Subanaesthetic doses of intravenous GHB (50–400 mg/kg) have resulted in dose-related stimulation of the firing of nigral dopaminergic neurons in unanesthetized rats whereas high doses (1000 and 1500 mg/kg) inhibited the firing almost completely (Diana et al., 1991). It has also been proposed that GHB acts as a major endogenous inhibitor of energy metabolism and may take on a protective role on both neuronal and peripheral tissues when energy supplies are limited (Mamelak, 1989). For example, animal studies suggest that GHB may protect against anoxic brain injury and induced arrhythmias (Vickers, 1969).

A sustained hypertensive effect was achieved upon the intraperitoneal or intravenous injection of GHB in rats at a dose of 1 g/kg. Cerebral blood flow did not change significantly in the GHB treated rats vs controls (Johansson and Hardebo, 1982).

10.7. CLINICAL STUDIES

Depite claims, there are no studies demonstrating GHB's ability to improve physical or sexual performance. Several published studies have shown GHB to be effective in the treatment of narcolepsy. At one sleep disorders clinic, nightly use of GHB in over 120 patients with narcolepsy over a 15-yr period has provided over 750 patient-yr of experience with GHB in this disorder (Scharf et al., 1998).

GHB has been studied as a general anesthetic in humans since the 1960s. Vickers (1969) and Dyer (1991) reviewed the findings of several of these studies. Early investigators discovered that doses of 40–50 mg/kg administered orally or intravenously produce somnolence within 15 min. Patients may then fall asleep but can be aroused. Smaller doses occasionally cause agitation or hypomania. Higher doses, corresponding to a blood level of 2.5 µmol/L, result in a coma within 30–40 min from which the patient cannot be aroused for 1–2 h (Helrich et al., 1964; Vickers, 1969; Dyer, 1991).

During GHB-induced light coma, rapid-eye-movement (REM) sleep occurs periodically. The patient can protect his or her airway in this state and may even fight attempts to obstruct it on purpose. Nevertheless, it should be assumed that the patient's airway is compromised under GHB anesthesia, because with deeper coma, the EEG resembles that produced by barbiturate anesthesia, and pharyngeal and laryngeal reflexes are impaired (Vickers, 1969). Myoclonic movements may occur during induction or emergence (Borgen et al., 2002). GHB's effects are relatively specific to the cerbral cortex, thus sparing the brainstem. Without input from the cerebral cortex, respirations become slow and deep (Vickers, 1969). Because tidal volume increases, minute ventilation remains normal despite slowed respirations. Cheynes-Stokes respirations may occur with an incidence of 9.5–28% (Vickers, 1969; Dyer, 1991). As with normal sleep, pCO_2 decreases by approx 2 mmHg. Blood pressure may remain stable, drop approx 10 mmHg, or even increase slightly with light coma (Vickers, 1969). During deep coma, pupils are constricted and unresponsive (Dyer, 1991). Because GHB is not an analgesic, surgical stimuli cause vasoconstriction, reflex movements, vocalization, sweating, and increased heart rate, blood pressure, and cardiac output (Vickers, 1969; Dyer, 1991).

Growth hormone and cortisol levels increase with GHB administration (Vickers, 1969; Dyer, 1991). Hopes that use of GHB during induction could produce an anabolic state post surgery were never realized, although there is evidence that it can produce a positive nitrogen balance when administered with parenteral nutrition over several days (Vickers, 1969). Long-term GHB administration did not have an anabolic effect in alcoholic patients (Addolorato et al., 1999).

Since 1990, 14 studies of GHB's use as a general anesthetic or sedative have been published, mostly in non-English journals. Most studies were performed in Germany and Russia. The results of these studies highlight the potential clinical utility of GHB in cardiac bypass surgery owing to its lack of effect on hemodynamics (Kleinschmidt et al., 1997, Kleinschmidt et al., 1998). Supplementary analgesia with narcotics is typically used (Kleinschmidt et al., 1997; Kleinschmidt et al., 1998). GHB has also shown promise as a sedative for use as an adjunct to spinal anesthesia. In this setting, GHB has shown no important effects on hemodynamics or respiratory depression (Kleinschmidt et al., 1999). Other desirable properties of GHB demonstrated in recent studies include preservation of cerebral blood flow and the cerebral vascular response to carbon dioxide (Detsch et al., 1999).

10.8. Pharmacokinetics

In a study in which ^{14}C-labeled GHB was administered orally to rats, the area under the radioactivity vs time curve was 65% that after intravenous administration. The amount of radioactivity recovered in the feces was very small, suggesting that first-pass metabolism is responsible for GHB's low bioavailability. It is possible that the radioactive GHB was metabolized by gut flora to volatile products that escaped detection; however, it was demonstrated that little loss of radioactivity occurred with sample storage. There was large interanimal variability in absorption (Lettieri and Fung, 1976).

In humans, GHB absorption is prompt, and onset of effect correlates with attainment of peak concentrations. Because absorption is saturable, peak levels are delayed, and peak concentration (C_{max}) increases less than expected with increasing dose. Peak concentrations occur 25, 30, and 45 min after oral doses of 12.5, 25, and 50 mg/kg, respectively (Palatini et al., 1993).

GHB is not bound to plasma proteins. The time course of GHB in plasma follows a two-compartment model (Palatini et al., 1993). Using data collected by Helrich and associates (1964) after intravenous administration, Dyer (1991) calculated a volume of distribution for GHB of 0.4 L/kg in the first compartment and 0.58 L/kg in the second compartment. Mean volume of distribution was calculated to be 0.307 L/kg in a study in which GHB was administered orally (Scharf et al., 1998).

A semi-log plot of plasma concentration vs time reveals an initial rapid decline in plasma concentrations representing tissue distribution. This is followed by a curve that becomes increasingly convex with increasing dose, representing nonlinear elimination. GHB's nonlinear absorption and elimination are thought to be the result of saturable active transport (Palatini et al., 1993).

GHB is metabolized to a limited extent to γ-aminobutyric acid (GABA). GABA formation may be greater at higher GHB concentrations (Zvosec et al., 2001). GHB is also catabolized to succinic semialdehyde in the brain and peripheral organs, eventually entering the Krebs cycle and exiting the body as water and carbon dioxide in expired air (Li et al., 1998b; Zvosec et al., 2001). Only 2–5% of a given dose is excreted unchanged in the urine, where it begins to appear within 4 h of ingestion (Helrich et al., 1964; Ropero-Miller and Goldberger, 1998). This value is consistent with a study in rats in which a mean of only 5.45% of the administered radioactivity (^{14}C-labeled GHB) was recovered unchanged in the urine (Lettieri and Fung, 1976). GHB's rapid metabolism renders urinary recovery essentially complete within 8 h of a 25 mg/kg dose. At this dose, plasma elimination is virtually complete 2–4 h post dose (Ferrara et al., 1992). After a dose of 100 mg/kg, GHB is undetectable in the urine 12 h post dose and undetectable in blood 8 h post dose (Dyer, 1991).

The mean half-life of GHB is 20 min after a single 12.5-mg/kg dose and 23 min after a single 50-mg/kg dose in healthy volunteers. Elimination is saturable, and clearance decreases by approximately 50% when the dose is increased from 12.5 to 50 mg/kg. Although half-life increased slightly, it did not increase as much as would be expected given the decrease in clearance. This is because half-life was calculated from the terminal portion of the plasma concentration vs time curve: lower GHB concentrations were not sufficient to saturate active cellular transport mechanisms (Palatini et al., 1993). In a study of 10 alcoholic patients administered GHB 25 mg/kg every 12 h for 1 wk, only 5 patients (4 with biochemical evidence of liver function abnormalities) exhibited saturable elimination. Administration of a dose of 50 mg/kg to the patients who exhibited linear elimination kinietics at a dose of 25 mg/kg resulted in a disproportionate rise in the area under the plasma concentration vs time curve (AUC), confirming capacity-limited elimination of GHB. A mean half-life of 27 min was reported (Ferrara et al., 1992). In a study of six patients with narcolepsy administered two doses of GHB 4 h apart, at doses ranging from approximately 25–50 mg/kg, mean half-life was 53 min, with a range of 26.9–71.4 min (Scharf et al., 1998). Note that the GHB half-life reported by these investigators differs substantially from that published by Palatini and associates (1993) and Ferrara and colleagues (1992). This is probably because Scharf and colleagues (1998) used a less senstitve assay, limiting their ability to measure the low GHB levels that exist during the true terminal (β) elimination phase. The half-life reported by Scharf and colleagues therefore appears mainly to reflect the half-life of the distributive phase ($t1/2\alpha$) rather than the terminal elimination half-life ($t1/2\beta$).

GHB blood concentrations caused by endogenous GHB production range from 20 to 52 mg/L; blood concentrations in six fatalities reported at the California Association of Toxicologists Annual Meeting in 1997 ranged from 98 to 596 mg/L (Ropero-Miller and Goldberger, 1998).

GBL is metabolized to GHB in the body by lactonases in the bloodstream (LoVecchio et al., 1998; CDC, 1999; Zvosec et al., 2001) and appears to be better absorbed than GHB (CDC, 1999). This observation may be explained by conversion of GHB to GBL by cyclic esterification in the presence of stomach acid (Gorton, 1998; Fessenden and Fessenden, 1986). Animal data suggest that GHB can also be converted to GBL in the liver and that GBL is the active moiety. GHB brain concentrations are actually at maximum levels when animals awaken from GHB-induced anesthesia, suggesting that some metabolic product is the hypnotic agent. Further evidence that GBL is the active form is the observation that after intravenous administration of GHB in humans, maximum clinical effect lags behind time of peak plasma concentration (T_{max}) by approximately 15 min (Helrich et al., 1964).

BD is metabolized to γ-hydroxybutyraldehyde in the brain and liver by alcohol dehydrogenase. This intermediate is then converted to GHB by aldehyde dehydrogenase (Zvosec et al., 2001). When it is administered intravenously to rats, the half-life is less than 1 min, owing to rapid hydrolysis in the bloodstream to GHB, which is excreted as CO_2 (Anonymous, 1999).

10.9. ADVERSE EFFECTS AND TOXICITY

10.9.1. GHB

In studies of GHB use as a general anesthetic, emergence reactions occurred in 7–8% of patients. Hypothermia was seen in 25% of pediatric patients in one report but could be prevented by use of blankets (Dyer, 1991). Excessive salivation (and vomiting in more than 50% of patients) can occur, particularly with movement during the first h of anesthesia, or during recovery (Vickers, 1969; Dyer, 1991). It has been suggested that vomiting is more frequent with oral administration; however, it is thought that GHB-associated vomiting is centrally mediated. Vomiting can be prevented with traditional antiemetics. Moderate bradycardia occurs under unopposed influence of the vagus nerve. This may compromise cardiac output, but both heart rate and cardiac output will increase with atropine administration (Vickers, 1969). Often accompanying the onset of coma are clonic or extrapyramidal movements of the arms or face, which can be prevented with concomitant use of small doses of barbiturates, phenothiazines, or anticonvulsants (Vickers, 1969; Dyer, 1991). Movements resembling tonic-clonic seizures have been reported (Dyer, 1991). Although these movements are often described as seizures, they are said to be more appropriately characterized as myoclonus (Borgen et al., 2002). Hypomania and agitation have been domumented with small doses (Vickers, 1969). Initial reports warned that GHB causes an intracellular potassium shift, resulting in hypokalemia, and concomitant potassium supplementation was once routinely used; however, subsequent study revealed that decreases were small, if they occurred at all. Use of preoperative diuretics, which cause urinary potassium loss, and administration of GHB in an insulin and glucose infusion, which can cause an intracellular potassium shift, may have contributed to early reports of GHB-induced hypokalemia. Other metabolic effects include hypernatremia owing to its sodium content, metabolic alkalosis, and hyperglycemia (Vickers, 1969).

In a study of healthy volunteers, a dose of 12.5 mg/kg caused slight dizziness in three of eight healthy volunteers. Onset of dizziness correlated with time of peak plasma concentration (25 min post dose) and lasted approximately 15 min. At doses of 25 and 50 mg/kg, all subjects complained of mild dizziness and/or drowsiness, which resolved within 1 hr. One subject complained of nausea lasting 60–90 min after the 50 mg/kg dose (Palatini et al., 1993). Higher doses result in coma (Vickers, 1969).

Animal experiments have shown that the median lethal dose (LD_{50}) is 1.7 g/kg, 5–15 times the coma-inducing dose. Death may be caused by sodium overload or respiratory depression (Vickers, 1969; Dyer, 1991).

GHB toxicity may include manifestations of coma, seizure-like movements, respiratory depression, vomiting, amnesia, and hypotonia (associated with doses of 10 mg/kg body weight), a normal sequence of REM and non-REM sleep (doses of 20–30 mg/kg body weight), and anesthesia (doses of approximately 50 mg/kg body weight). Severe respiratory depression, seizure-like activity, coma, and decreased cardiac output may occur with doses of more than 50 mg/kg body weight. Concomitant use of alcohol may also potentiate coma and respiratory depression (CDC, 1997). Other adverse effects include myoclonus, bradycardia, hypotension, transient metabolic acidosis, and mild hypothermia. Treatment for GHB overdose is restricted to supportive care because no specific antidote exists. As with other acute intoxications, establishing intravenous access and cardiovascular, respiratory, and neurologic monitoring are recommended. After 6 h of observation, patients who have recovered can be discharged or admitted if still clinically intoxicated (Li et al., 1998a). Resolution of symptoms can be expected within 2–96 h with supportive care.

The first published case of GHB intoxication presented on June 4, 1990 (Dyer, 1991). The patient was a 23-yr-old man who took 1 teaspoonful of GHB dissolved in orange juice. Two and a half hours later, he was unconscious and vomiting. In the emergency room, he responded only to deep pain, moving all extremities. Pupils were sluggish and 6 mm. Blood pressure was 159/90 mmHg, heart rate was 60 beats per min, and respirations were 20 breaths per min. Four h later, the patient awoke while being intubated. His only complaint was dizziness. Electrolytes were normal. Urine pH was 5, and urine glucose was 100 mg/dL. Toxicology testing of urine and blood were negative.

Several important features of GHB intoxication were identified in a review of cases at a New Orleans hospital during the period between September and November 1995. These seven cases were characterized by acute delirium and respiratory depression with intermittent violent outbursts, especially during intubation attempts. The behavior was described by one physician as "a drowning swimmer flailing for air." After supportive measures, including intubation and mechanical ventilation in four cases, normal mental and respiratory function returned within 2–6 h. Patients have fully recovered even after exhibiting violent behavior during apneic spells, suggesting a neuroprotective role for GHB during hypoxic episodes. There were no reports of seizure activity in these patients. U-waves were noted on the electrocardiographs of five patients (Li et al., 1998b).

A withdrawal syndrome characterized by insomnia, tremor, and anxiety following discontinuation of GHB in chronic, high-dose users has been reported. In one case, a 24-yr-old man with attention-deficit hyperactivity disorder (ADHD) had been self-medicating with GHB liquid "to help focus" and for bodybuilding. The estimated daily dose was 70–105 g. Six h after his last dose, he presented to the emergency room with confusion, emotional lability, intermittent anxiety, tremor, nausea, and vomiting. Diazepam 10 mg to be taken as needed was prescribed, but he returned to the emergency room the next morning with agitation, tremor, and frightening hallucinations. Initially, he was oriented, but within 24 h he developed tachycardia, confusion, agitation, and combativeness requiring physical restraints and sedation with a lorazepam drip, haloperidol, and diazepam. Symptoms continued, but began to improve by hospital day 7; on day 10, the lorazepam drip was tapered. He was discharged on day 12 (Dyer et al., 2001).

In another published case (Dyer and Andrews, 1997), a 23-yr-old woman had been taking three to five capfuls of GHB liquid 721 mg/mL daily (43–144 g/d) for 1 yr to enhance her bodybuilding efforts. Three h after her last dose, she presented to her primary care physician with anxiety, insomnia, and tremor. Six wk prior, an increase in dosing frequency to one to five capfuls every 3 h was necessary to prevent anxiety. She was admitted to the hospital with paranoia, hallucinations, and agitation. Blood pressure was 138/98 mmHg, and heart rate was 110 beats per min. Propranolol was administered to control tachycardia. Physical restraint was required in addition to benzodiazepines and phenothiazine antipsychotics. She improved rapidly on day 7, and she was discharged on day 9. Urine toxicology was negative (Dyer and Andrews, 1997; Dyer et al., 2001).

Similarly, a 24-yr-old man presented to a crisis center complaining of hallucinations. He had been using GHB for 10 mo for its euphoric effects and noted that increased use was necessary to prevent hallucinations; he was consuming approximately 1 gallon every 2 wk. He was referred to drug rehabilitation. Within 2 mo, he had increased the frequency of GHB ingestion to 1.5 teaspoonful every 30 min. Twenty minutes after his last dose, he presented to a detoxification unit with a 2-mo history of nausea, vomiting, and diarrhea. More acutely, the patient also suffered from diplopia, blurred vision, dyspnea, urinary frequency, thirst, blacking out, anorexia, anxiety, tremors, mydriasis, and feeling "weak and swollen." Lorazepam was prescribed for agitation. ECG revealed left ventricular hypertrophy and possible ischemia of the inferior wall. Urine GHB concentration was 1750 mg/L, which was consistent with a previous urine concentration after GHB overdose. Tachycardia, combativeness, and hallucinations developed over the next 24 h. Physical restraint and sedation with propofol, benzodiazepines, and antipsychotics was necessary. By day 12, his symptoms were improving, and lorazepam taper began. The next day, he was delirious but arousable, and he died that evening after suffering a seizure, cardiac arrest, and bradycardia unresponsive to atropine, epinephrine, and external pacing. Autopsy revealed pulmonary edema, as well as enlarged heart, left ventricular hypertrophy, and severe focal stenosis of the left anterior descending artery, but no evidence of infarction. GHB withdrawal was ruled the cause of death. Five additional withdrawal cases were also reviewed (Dyer et al., 2001) in this same article.

In summary, the patients described in these eight cases ranged in age from 22 to 38 yr. Reasons for use included bodybuilding in two patients; as an alcohol substitute in one patient; as an alcohol substitute and for bodybuilding in one patient; and for depression and mood control in an additional patient. In four of these patients, GHB had been used every 1–2 h around the clock for 6–12 mo prior to discontinuation. Presenting withdrawal symptoms included delirium ($n = 1$), delusions ($n = 2$), confusion ($n = 2$), myoclonus or tremors ($n = 3$), thrashing ($n = 1$), hallucinations ($n = 5$), agitation ($n = 1$), hypertension ($n = 1$), incoherent speech ($n = 3$), short-term memory loss ($n = 1$), diaphoresis ($n = 5$), nausea ($n = 1$), vomiting ($n = 1$), myalgias ($n = 1$), hypertonia ($n = 1$), and mild cogwheel rigidity ($n = 1$). Treatments included benzodiazepines (lorazepam, diazepam, temazepam), antipsychotics (haloperidol, trifluoperazine), benztropine, chloral hydrate, and labetolol (for hypertension). Onset of symptoms ranged from 2 to 6 h after the last dose and lasted 5–15 d. One patient died. The necessity of increasing dosing frequency to prevent withdrawal suggests the development of pharmacologic tolerance with around-the-clock dosing. Less frequent dosing, such as that used in narcolepsy studies, does not produce tolerance. The mechanism of tolerance to GHB is unknown. The similarity between GHB withdrawal and withdrawal from other sedative hypnotics that affect GABA receptors suggests that the mechanism behind the development of tolerance and physical dependence to GHB might involve its metabolism to GABA or an effect on GABA receptors (Dyer et al., 2001).

Additional case reports of GHB intoxication/withdrawal have been reported. Most involve symptoms similar to those reported here. However, some unique symptoms have also been reported in various cases. For example, Wernicke-Korsakoff syndrome has been attributed to the abuse of GHB (Friedman et al., 1996). The patient had stopped eating for 1 wk prior to hospital admission. On presentation, the patient exhibited the classic triad of Wernicke-Korsakoff symptoms including global confusion, sixth nerve palsy, and ataxic gait. In addition, paranoid delusions and hallucinations were present. The patient was treated with supportive measures including thiamine, whereupon the symptoms resolved and the patient was completely asymptomatic after 1 mo. In another case, a 22-yr-old man presented to his personal physician complaining of progressively worsening painless hematuria that had lasted for 2 d (Wiley et al., 1998). The patient denied any kind of trauma or increase in exercise. Urinalysis and liver function tests provided little additional information other than the presence of a large amount of blood in the urine sample. The patient did report that he and a friend had been consuming home-brewed GHB, the recipe for which he had obtained form the internet, for the past 2 mo (36 mL at bedtime, four nights a week). Interestingly, the friend also reported the presence of painless dark urine. On further questioning, the individual reported that they had substituted swimming pool tablets (calcium hypochlorite) in place of the sodium hydroxide called for in the recipe. It was suggested that this change in formula probably resulted in unexpected chemical reactions that produced the hematuria. Finally, Ingels et al. (2000) reported three cases of coma and respiratory depression in patients ingesting either GHB, GBL, or BD (in each case a different compound was ingested). However, in these cases as with many cases of toxicity of GHB or its precursors, other substances of abuse were also found to be present (e.g., amphetamines, cocaine, alcohol, or benzodiazepines). This concomitant administration of various substances greatly complicates diagnosis and treatment of these situations.

When the FDA prohibited the commercial sale of GHB, mail order kits and instructions for making GHB from GBL began to appear on the Internet. These instructions call for sodium hydroxide to be added to GBL to open the lactone ring, forming GHB. If the unreacted sodium hydroxide is not neutralized with acid, alkali burns can result from use of the product. This is illustrated by the case of a 19-yr-old woman who presented to the emergency room with severe dysphagia and burning pain of the mouth, tongue, and esophagus after drinking a liquid purported to be GHB. Physical exam revealed uvular edema and erythema of the posterior pharynx. She exhibited no signs or symptoms of GHB toxicity, and urine drug testing was negative for GHB. On endoscopy, the esophagus was noted to be red, diffusely ulcerated in a circumferential pattern, and edematous from the epiglottis to the gastric fundus. The patient developed a midesophageal stricture that required repeated dilations (Dyer and Reed, 1997).

10.9.2. GBL

GBL produces a clinical picture similar to that of GHB intoxication. Between April 1998 and April 1999, the FDA received 119 reports of adverse events associated with GBL. The median age of patients was 27 yr (range 11–71 yr). Sixty-three percent were male. Symptoms included central nervous system depression, repiratory depression (requiring intubation in 19 patients), bradycardia, myoclonus, vomiting, confusion, combativeness, and addiction or withdrawal (9 patients; Hardy et al., 1999). Seizures and death have also been reported (FDA, 1999b). These reports prompted the FDA to issue a public warning and request a voluntary recall of GBL-containing products (Hardy et al., 1999).

The features of GBL intoxication are illustrated in the following case report (LoVecchio et al., 1998). A 36-yr-old man was stopped by police for irregular driving. The police noted that he was lethargic, diaphoretic, and vomiting. At the hospital, he appeared to be intoxicated, and physical exam was noncontributory. Within 1 hr, his mental status returned to normal, and he was able to explain that approximately 30 min prior to being picked up by police, he had ingested 2 ounces (60 mL) of a product called RenewTrient, which contains GBL. At the time, this product was available in health food stores. He denied ingestion of alcohol or other substances. Blood alcohol content, urine toxicology screen with enzyme-multiplied immunoassay, thin-layer chromatography, and GC-MS were negative. Using GC with flame ionization detection, butyrolactone was identified in the patient's urine. The label for RenewTrient cautioned against seeking help should intoxication occur because this might result in "uninformed" medical personnel using unnecessary or dangerous treatments. The label also advised users to inform others that normal use of the product would result in unarousable sleep and that high doses could result in sweating, muscle spasms, vomiting, bedwetting, and diarrhea. The manufacturer's recommended dose for sleep is 1 ounce, which purportedly will induce stage 3 and 4 sleep within 30 min lasting 3–6 h. In a response to the case report by LoVecchio and colleagues (1998), the manufacturer maintained that the only treatment necessary is to "sleep it off," although they also claim its effects can be reversed using physostigmine 2 mg (Gorton, 1998).

Seven case reports of GBL toxicity were reported in Minnesota, 14 in Mexico, and 20 in Texas in 1998 and 1999 (CDC, 1999). In one report, a 24-yr-old man vomited and had seizures after consuming 3–4 ounces of Revivarant. He exhibited unusual behavior, with periods of agitation punctuated by episodes of profound calm. Emergency medical assistance was required. He was found to be diaphoretic and bradycardic (heart rate 45), and his skin was warm and flushed. Pulse oximetry revealed oxygen saturation of 96%. Systolic blood pressure was 110 mmHg, and blood glucose was 90 mg/dL. He was transported to the hospital. In route, he exhibited 30–60 s periods of combativeness followed by a comatose state for 1–3 min. He was unconscious upon arrival at the hospital but would spontaneously open his eyes. He withdrew to painful stimuli but did not speak. Glasgow Coma Scale was 7. Rectal temperature was 94.8°F. Urine drug screen and blood alcohol content were negative. A diagnosis of toxic encephalopathy was made, and he was intubated and transferred to the intensive care unit. He recovered over the next 7 h, with an increase in heart rate to 116 beats per min and an improvement in mental status. He was able to recall that he had ingested Revivarant but could not recall subsequent events (CDC, 1999).

A 46-yr-old woman who ingested 2.7 ounce of Revivarant plus alcohol subsequently had a seizure and lost consciousness. Emergency medical personnel found her unconscious and bradycardic (heart rate 54 beats per min) with respiratory depression requiring oxygen by facemask and later mechanical ventilation. Temperature was 96.1°F, and pupils were miotic. Blood alcohol content was 0.11%. She recovered quickly and was discharged the next morning. She could not recall the events surrounding the incident (CDC, 1999).

A third patient reported to the CDC by an emergency department in Minnesota was a 31-yr-old man who lost consciousness and fell after drinking 1 ounce of Revivarant, four beers, and a "large sip" of wine. Upon regaining consciousness, he was ambulatory but exhibited muscle twitching, confusion, anxiety, agitation, and amnesia. Pulse was 64 beats per min, and oral temperature was 95.2°F. Alcohol breath level was 0.08%. He denied illicit drug use, including previous GBL use. He recovered and was discharged (CDC, 1999).

Two additional cases of GBL toxicity occurred in 24- and a 26-yr-old men who ingested 10–13 ounces of Revivarant in a bar in conjunction with alcohol. They lost consciousness upon exiting the bar and were transported to the hospital. At the hospital, mental status alternated between somnolence and confusion, with neither patient being able to follow commands. Vitals were normal in both patients, but one man had loss of bowel control. Breath alcohol levels were 0.09 and 0.15%. Both recovered within 2 h and denied use of illicit substances. They were unable to recall most of the events of evening (CDC, 1999).

Two women, aged 19 and 22 yr, experienced vomiting and reduced consciousness after ingesting Revivarant. The 19-yr-old ingested 2 ounces of the product plus one beer, and the other patient ingested an unknown amount of Revivarant and no alcohol. The former patient exhibited lethargy and disorientation, and the other required pharmacologic and physical restraint for agitation alternating with moments of quiet. Physical exam revealed normal vitals except for respiratory depression. Both patients quickly recovered and were discharged from the emergency department 4 h later (CDC, 1999).

Fourteen cases of GBL toxicity were reported to the New Mexico Poison Center in an approximately 4-mo period from late 1998 to early 1999. Twenty cases were reported to Texas poison control centers during this same period. Nine of the New

Mexico patients were male, and ages ranged from 14 to 36 yr. The ages of the Texas patients ranged from 11 to 41 yr, and 13 were male. Ten of the Texas patients and five of the New Mexico patients had also used alcohol and/or other drugs. Most patients were discharged from the emergency department within 13 h, but three were hospitalized. The mean amount of GBL ingested was 3 ounces (range 1–10 ounces). Signs and symptoms included nausea and vomiting ($n = 16$), obtundation ($n = 22$), bradycardia ($n = 7$), tachycardia ($n = 3$), prolonged unconsiousness ($n = 15$), seizures ($n = 4$), confusion ($n = 10$), combativeness ($n = 7$), repiratory depression ($n = 12$), anxiety or nervousness ($n = 7$), tremors/twitching ($n = 4$), amnesia ($n = 2$), euphoria ($n = 2$), cardiac arrest ($n = 1$), and respiratory arrest ($n = 2$). One motor vehicle accident occurred as a result GBL use. No deaths were reported.

As with GHB, a GBL withdrawal syndrome has been described. A 36-yr-old woman presented to the emergency room with acute psychosis characterized by thought blocking, tangential thinking, delusions, and hallucinations. No autonomic symptoms were evident. She had been taking 10–15 ml/d of a product called Invigorate (3.5 g GBL/oz) but had discontinued the product 2 d prior to presentation. She denied the use of other drugs, and toxicology testing was negative. Computed tomography (CT), ECG, and routine labs were normal. White blood cell count (WBC) was elevated at 13,400/mm^3. Lorazepam 1 mg and haloperidol improved her mental status, and she recovered within 48 h (Greene et al., 1999).

10.9.3. BD

Use of the BD-containing products Cherry fX Bombs, Lemmon fX Drops, and Orange fX Drops were tied to illness reported in 100 attendees of a 1996 New Year's Eve party in Los Angeles. The products were traced to a California chiropractor, who was fined $2000 and imprisoned in February 1998 (FDA, 1999a).

Although BD intoxication typically occurs as a result of intentional abuse and misuse of the product, the first published U.S. case report of BD ingestion involved ingestion of approximately 1 ounce of the BD product Bullet® by a 2-yr-old boy (Higgins and Borron, 1996). The patient arrived at the emergency room approx 40 min after ingestion. Vitals were blood pressure 87/52 mmHg, heart rate 56 beats per min, respirations 3 breaths per min, and rectal temperature 36.3° C. Glasgow Coma Score was 3. Pupils were 2–3 mm, equal, and sluggish. Rhonchi were noted throughout the lungs, and a chest X-ray revealed a small left lower lobe infiltrate consistent with aspiration pneumonitis. Gag reflex was poor. The patient was flaccid and unresponsive and required intubation. Some vocal cord edema was noted. Blood gas on 100% oxygen revealed metabolic acidosis. Serum calcium, total protein, albumin, and phoshorus were low. The child was extubated approximately 6 h after admission, and was discharged the following day. The authors of this case report found only one previously published case series of BD intoxication, which occurred in Denmark.

Other early U.S. case reports of BD intoxication involved a product referred to by the patients as "pine needle oil." In one case, a 20-yr-old man experienced nausea and vomiting after ingesting four times the usual dose of the product. Two and a half hours later, he became comatose and required intubation. Vitals included blood pressure 136/60 mmHg, heart rate 30 beats per min, and respirations 12 breaths per min. Glucose was 153 mg/dL. Blood alcohol content was 0 mg/dL, and a urine drug screen was positive for tetrahydrocannabinol, a marijuana metabolite. He did not respond to naloxone but awoke spontaneously 50 min after presentation and was extubated. In the second case, a 44-yr-old man was arrested for public intoxication and taken to the emergency room after becoming agitated, losing consciousness, and vomiting. In the emergency room, he was comatose and exhibited myoclonus. Vitals included heart rate 40 beats per min and respiration 8 breaths per min. Blood alcohol content was 0 mg/dL. The patient awakened within 3 h and reported having taken nine yohimbine tablets and a few sprays of "pine needle oil" prior to presentation. The "pine needle oil" was analyzed and identified as BD (Dyer et al., 1997).

Zvosec and colleagues (2001) described nine episodes of BD intoxication in eight patients. Six of these cases presented between June and December 1999 to the investigators' emergency departments. Three additional cases were identified through public health officials. Two patients, a husband and wife ages 32 and 29 yr, respectively, ingested the BD-containing product Thunder Nectar, which a friend had given them. Their friend had purchased the product at a health food store, and he assured them that it was nontoxic. The bottle was unlabeled, and he provided no dosage instructions. The husband ingested 200 mL (20 g BD; 300 mg/kg) of the product to increase libido, and his wife ingested 110–140 mL (11–14 g BD). The wife recalled that approx 15 min after ingesting the product, she felt lightheaded and sat down in a chair. Her next memory was awakening 7 h later on the floor and finding her husband dead beside her and covered with vomitus. He had also lost bowel control. Blood GHB concentration was 432 mg/L, urine GHB concentration was 5430 mg/L, and urine BD concentration was 845 mg/L measured using GC-MS. Toxicologic testing was also positive for marijuana. Other toxicologic testing was negative. Toxicologic testing was not performed on the decedent's wife.

A third patient, a 42-yr-old woman, ingested 30–60 mL (5.4–10.8 g BD; 95–189 mg/kg) of NRG3 for insomnia. She was also taking sertraline for depression. Three h after ingesting NRG3, her boyfriend reported that she was talking to him and that 1 h later, when he left, she was sleeping. He returned 8 h later and found her dead. Blood GHB level was 837 mg/L, blood BD level was 220 mg/L, urine GHB was 1161 mg/L, and urine BD was 1756 mg/L measured by GC-MS. The stomach contained 201 mg/kg GHB and 579 mg/kg BD. Additional toxicologic testing of the urine and blood was negative (Zvosec et al., 2001).

Another patient, a 26-yr-old man, ingested an unknown quantitiy of NRG3 prior to speaking with his brother on the phone. The patient's brother noticed that his speech was slurred, and he heard him fall to the floor. Paramedics found him unconscious. Food was burning on the stove, and there was smoke in the house. He was transported to the emergency room, where his heart rate was 110 beats per min, and his blood pressure was 180/90 mmHg. Naloxone and dextrose were administered. He required mechanical ventilation for 3 h, but recovered rapidly. Toxicologic screening and routine laboratory tests were negative. The patient had a 2-yr history of increasing use of BD and GBL, escalating to around-the-clock use for bodybuilding and prevention of BD/GBL withdrawal symptoms. According to the patient, these symptoms included auditory hallucinations, insomnia, vomiting, tachycardia, sweating, tremor, depression, anxiety, and agitation (Zvosec et al., 2001).

As with GHB and GBL, seizure-like activity has been associated with BD ingestion. A 39-yr-old man purchased a 1-L container of BD from a chemical supply company after learning from an Internet chat room that it might help his occasional insomnia. He began taking 10 mL of the solution each night. On the seventh night of BD ingestion, he experienced a 3-min tonic seizure, mental status changes, and fecal incontinence. He was taken to the emergency room, where neurologic evaluation, including EEG, was normal. Electrolytes were normal, and toxicologic testing was negative. The seizure was attributed to BD, or its metabolite GHB (Cisek et al., 1999); however, the patient had a history of depression and was also taking bupropion 200 mg twice daily, which can lower the seizure threshold.

In a case that illustrates well the addiction and physical dependence that may be associated with use of BD and other GHB precursors, a 37-yr-old woman had a 1-yr history of use of eight different brands of BD and GBL for treatment of insomnia and depression. Over the previous 6 mo, she had presented to the emergency room twice with BD intoxication and once with GBL intoxication, the latter after being picked up by police for driving erratically. The patient related that around-the-clock dosing was necessary to prevent withdrawal symptoms, which included anxiety, chest tightness, palpitations, and tremor beginning 4–6 h after the last dose. During one withdrawal episode, she experienced auditory, visual, and tactile hallucinations, paranoid delusions, insomnia, agitation, and tremor for 5 d after product discontinuation, necessitating hospitalization. Three and a half months after this hospitalization, she ingested 90 ml of InnerG. Although she had been taking InnerG 30 mL every 4 h for the previous 4 wk, she increased the dose to 90 mL (4.5 g BD) to "increase energy." Ninety minutes later, she was found shouting and thrashing on the ground, confused and incontinent of urine. In the hospital, her behavior alternated between episodes of screaming and thrashing and periods of quiet. She was oriented to person only, was easily startled, and could follow commands only briefly. Her behavior necessitated sedation with droperidol and physical restraints. On recovery, she exhibited withdrawal symptoms, including hypervigilance and insomnia. Urine GHB was 716 mg/L, urine BD was undetectable, and serum GHB was 317 mg/L measured using GC-MS. Additional toxicologic screening was negative, and she denied use of alcohol or other drugs.

She was discharged after refusing treatment for withdrawal and 2 mo later was brought to the emergency department after paramedics found her moaning and banging her head on the floor of her residence after ingesting an unknown amount of Zen, a BD-containing product. She was admitted to the hospital. Mechanical ventilation was necessary for 3 d, with sedation using propofol, diazepam, and lorazepam for the first 2 d. Urine GHB was 5140 mg/L, and urine BD was undetectable measured by GC-MS. Upon recovery, she enrolled in a substance abuse program and was discharged on day 8. She withdrew from the program after 2 wk and was brought to the emergency room twice more in the subsequent 2 1/2 mo for treatment of BD intoxication. She finally completed an inpatient substance abuse treatment program with subsequent outpatient treatment (Zvosec et al., 2001).

Intoxication after use of the product InnnerG was described in an additional case. This 51-yr-old man ingested 60 mL (3 g BD) of InnerG before exercise, and 1 h later was found unconscious at a traffic light. He could be aroused only with great effort.

He recovered within 2 h, and reported that he had been using a GBL supplement (Revivarant) for 4 mo to increase athletic and sexual performance prior to switching to InnerG (Zvosec et al., 20001).

Another patient in this case series was a 22-yr-old man who was found unconscious by friends 1 h after ingesting 90–120 mL (6.3–8.4 g BD) of the product Serenity to increase energy. When paramedics arrived, he was vomiting and was unresponsive to painful stimuli. Naloxone was administered. He was bradycardic (heart rate 50 beats per min), hypotensive (systolic blood pressure 100 mmHg), and incontinent of urine. Respiratory rate was 10, and oxygen saturation was 92%. Intubation and mechanical ventilation were required. Urine GHB was 415 mg/L, and urine BD was undetectable using GC-MS. Additional toxicologic screening was negative. Within 4 h, he had fully recovered and was discharged (Zvosec et al., 2001).

Although these reports of BD intoxication involved products promoted as dietary supplements, the next case illustrates that BD users may also purchase concentrated industrial BD from chemical supply companies as a cheaper alternative. Neighbors reported seeing this 29-yr-old patient wandering partially naked and disoriented. Physical exam initially revealed shallow and slow respiration (12 breaths per min), sweating, twitching of the arms and legs, and central nervous system depression, which was followed 30 min later by agitation requiring lorazepam. Naloxone was also administered. He recovered within 5 h and related that he had been using 5–7.5 mL of his own dilution of concentrated industrial BD every four h for the past 6 mo for treatment of alcohol addiction. He had read on Internet web sites that BD and GHB could be used for this purpose (Zvosec et al., 2001)

10.9.4. Carcinogenicity/Mutagenicity

BD does not appear to be carcinogenic or mutagenic, although the available human data are insufficient to make a definitive determination. A case control study found that two cases with non-Hodgkin's lymphoma and three controls had had occupational exposure to BD as pesticide production workers or sprayers (odds ratio 3; 95% CI 0.5–18). Oral, subcutaneous, and topical application of BD to mice and oral and subcutaneous administration to rats failed to produce carcinogenic effects. There was no evidence of mutagenicity in bacteria, yeast, fruit flies, rat liver cells, mouse bone marrow, or cultured human cells; however, an increase in sister chromatid exchanges and chomosmal aberrations was noted in Chinese hamster ovary cells in the presence of BD and a metabolic activation system (Anonymous, 1999).

10.9.5. Pharmacologic Treatment

Treatment for GHB overdose has to date been restricted to supportive care because no specific antidote exists. Two case reports of reversal of GHB-induced coma by physostigmine have been noted (Viera and Yates, 1999). A clinical study also has reported that physostigmine can reverse GHB-induced sedation in patients undergoing elective anesthesia (Henderson et al., 1976). Naloxone has been reported to inhibit the actions of GHB in rodents (Snead and Bearden, 1980) but no effect on GHB symptoms has been observed in humans (Ross, 1995; Thomas et al., 1997; Ingels et al., 2000). With respect to the treatment of GHB (or GBL) withdrawal, high doses of benzodiazepines (up to 507 mg of lorazepam and 120 mg of diazepam given over 90 h) have been used in some cases (Craig et al., 2000) but Sivilotti and colleagues (2001) report the use of pentobarbital to be more effective in relieving the withdrawal symptoms.

10.10. INTERACTIONS

GHB, BD, or GBL would be expected to potentiate the central nervous system and respiratory depressant effects of drugs such as alcohol, narcotic analgesics, benzodiazepines, and other drugs with sedative effects. Indeed, various animal studies and human case reports have demonstrated an additive effect of sedative agents, including ethanol and thiopental, when taken together with GHB (Dyer, 1991; Li et al., 1998b).

The actions of GHB may be potentiated by HIV protease inhibitors, according to a case report (Harrington et al., 1999). A 29-yr-old man became unresponsive and exhibited clonus of both legs and then the left side of his body 20 min after ingesting approx 1/2 teaspoonful of GHB. The patient had been diagnosed with AIDS and had a history of *Pneumocystis carinii* pneumonia, Kaposi's sarcoma, thrush, and neutropenia. Medications included ritonavir 400 mg three times daily, saquinivir 400 mg twice daily, granulocyte-colony stimulating factor 300 µg thrice weekly, azithromycin 1200 mg once daily, acyclovir 400 mg thrice daily as needed, multivitamins daily, and aerosolized pentamidine monthly. The patient was responsive only to pain. Heart rate was 40 beats per min, and respirations were shallow. The patient was intubated by paramedics and transported to the emergency room. Heart rate increased to 117 beats per min after administration of atropine. Blood pressure was 159/120 mmHg, and body temperature was 35.3(C. Physical exam, chest X-ray, head CT, and laboratory tests were unremarkable.

Urine drug testing revealed methamphetamine, tetrahydrocannabinol, atropine, methylenedioxymethamphetamine (MDMA), and prochlorperazine. These findings were consistent with the patient's history of ingestion of two MDMA tablets approximately 29 h prior to admission, and prochlorperazine 5 mg for nausea 17 h prior to admission. The patient also admitted to smoking marijuana 3 d previously. In addition to the GHB he took just prior to losing consciousness, he had taken approx 1/2 teaspoonful 6 h prior to admission. He used GHB to offset the stimulant effects of MDMA, which he reported persisted for more than 24 h post ingestion. During this time, his friends took similar quantities of the same GHB product every 2–3 h with no ill effects. Although the patient had taken similar doses of GHB in the past on several occasions, he had never experienced any adverse effects. This was prior to being prescribed protease inhibitors, however. Ritonavir blocks the metabolism of several drugs by inhibition of cytochrome P450 isoenzymes (i.e., CYP3A4, CYP2D6, CYP2C9, and CYP2C19), and saquinavir inhibits CYP3A4. There is evidence that GHB is metabolized through first-pass metabolism, which often involves cytochrome P450 isoenzymes. The authors of the case report concluded that the patient's nearly fatal reaction to a relatively small dose of GHB was caused by inhibition of first-pass metabolism by one or both protease inhibitors, resulting in increased GHB levels.

BD is oxidized to GHB by alcohol dehydrogenase and aldehyde dehydrogenase, which are inhibited by ethanol and disulfiram (Dyer et al., 1997); however, the clinical significance of this is unknown.

10.11. REPRODUCTION

There are no data on the effects of GHB, GBL, or BD on human reproduction. BD at doses of up to 500 mg/kg/d administered to pregnant rats on days 6–15 of gestation produced no evidence of embryotoxicity on day 21 (Anonymous, 1999).

10.12. CHEMICAL AND BIOFLUID ANALYSIS

Standard gas chromatography-mass spectrometry (GC-MS) methods are readily used to detect GHB. GHB can be detected in serum, plasma, blood, and urine provided that a specific request is made to the toxicology laboratory; it will not be detected on routine urine or blood toxicology screens. Specimens may be frozen and tested elsewhere at a later date if GC-MS is not locally available (National Medical Services, Willow Grove, PA; 1-800-522-6671). Another available service for cases of sexual assault provides a combined GC-MS assay free of charge for flunitrazepam (Rohyponol®), GHB, and alcohol (Hoffman-La Roche Sexual Assault Hotline; 1-800-608-6540) (Li, 1999). It should be noted that GHB appears to be a product of the normal decomposition processes following death. Thus, GHB can be detected in blood samples from individuals post-mortem who had not ingested the substance (Fieler et al., 1998). Thus, it is recommended that urine be used as the preferred body fluid from which GHB toxicological samples are taken for post-mortem analysis since urine does not appear to be contaminated with GHB produced during the decomposition process.

A number of analytical procedures have been developed for the analysis of GHB and GBL, (Ferrara et al., 1993; McCusker et al., 1999; LeBeau et al., 2000; Couper and Logan, 2000; Frison et al., 2000), with most utilizing GC-MS. A sensitive, specific, and relatively simple procedure has been published by LeBeau and colleagues (2000) that can be used to detect GHB and GBL in either plasma or urine. The method utilizes headspace analysis via GC-MS. In this procedure, the GHB is treated with concentrated sulfuric acid to facilitate cyclization to GBL. The advantage of this procedure is that through analysis of acid-treated and untreated aliquots, it can be determined whether detected GBL was derived from GHB.

Briefly, the specimen is separated into two 1-mL aliquots, and 25 µL of the internal standard (hexadeuterated GHB and hexadeuterated GBL 100 µg/mL) are added. Concentrated sulfuric acid (150 µL) is added to one of the aliquots. The samples are then vortexed and allowed to sit for 5 min (conversion of GHB to GBL). To each tube, 5 mL of methylene chloride is added; the tubes are continuously inverted for 10 min and then centrifuged at 2000g for 5 min to facilitate separation of the layers. The aqueous layer is then removed and discarded. The methylene chloride extracts are then transferred to conical tubes and concentrated to approx 75 µL under nitrogen at 35°C. It is important not to allow the tubes to evaporate to dryness, as this will lead to additional sources of variability in the assay. The remaining volume is then transferred to a 20-mL headspace vial for analysis. Samples are heated in the autosampler at 100°C for 15 min prior to injection.

Chromatography is achieved with a DB-624 capillary column (30 m × 0.25 mm × 1.4 µm) and nitrogen as the carrier gas (34 cm/s). The injection port temperature is 150°C, initial column temperature 50°C, and initial hold time 5.8 min, followed by a temperature ramp of 20°C/min. The final column temperature is 150°C, and the final hold time is 7 min. Injections are made in split injection mode (10:1). Mass spectrometric detection is conducted in full-scan EI mode (m/z 35-200) with the electron multiplier operating at 200 eV above autotune. The retention time for GBL and its deuterated analog is approx 10.9 min. Quantitation of GBL is made using the molecular ion of the parent drug at m/z 86 and the deuterated internal standard at m/z 92. Since analysis is made from two separate aliquots, one in which all drug was converted to the butyrolactone and one not, a simple subtraction will allow determination of the GHB concentration. This method is sensitive to concentrations of 5 µg/mL in both plasma and urine. It should be noted that the hexadeuterated internal standards are commercially available.

Recently another method has been described that has a similar sensitivity (as low as 1 µg/mL in plasma and 5 µg/mL in urine) but requires a more complex sample preparation procedure (Frison et al., 2000). Again, it requires conversion of GHB to GBL with headspace analysis and GC-MS. The primary difference lies in the use of solid-phase microextraction for sample cleanup. This procedure requires a special device that transfers the analyte (in this case GBL) onto a fiber, which is then inserted into the gas chromatograph injector for direct thermal desorption. Positive ion chemical ionization is used as the mass spectrometric detection method. The method appears to be accurate and reproducible.

10.13. REGULATION

Although they are often labeled as dietary supplements, the FDA classifies GHB, GBL, and BD as unapproved new drugs (FDA, 1999a). The FDA has released reports warning physicians and consumers about GHB's toxic effects (FDA, 1997, 1999a, b). In 1999, the FDA issued press releases warning consumers about GBL (FDA, 1999a, b) and BD (FDA, 1999a). They also asked manufacturers to recall their GBL products (FDA, 1999b). The FDA has declared BD a Class I Health Hazard, meaning that its use is potentially life-threatening (FDA, 1999a). Public health officials and physicians are urged to report adverse effects of these products to the DEA at (202) 307-7183 (CDC, 1997) or the FDA MedWatch program at 1-800-332-1088 (CDC, 1999).

GHB was designated a Schedule I controlled substance at the federal level in March 2000 (DEA, 2001), and thus it is illegal to possess even for industrial use. GBL and butanediol are listed as precursor chemicals used in the illicit manufacture of GHB (i.e., List I substances), and thus it is in violation of federal law to possess these chemicals with the intent to manufacture GHB. The DEA's position on GBL and BD is that they will be treated as Schedule I substances if they are manufactured or distributed for human consumption (Sapienza, 2000). Florida law prohibits even industrial use of GBL and BD (Minai, 2001).

The FDA approved Xyrem®, a GHB product from Orphan Medical Inc., for treatment of narcolepsy-associated cataplexy (FDA, 2002). It is estimated that 180,000 patients could benefit from Xyrem, although only about 50,000 patients have been diagnosed to date. Only approx 4000 physicians nationwide currently treat narcolepsy, and Xyrem will be promoted only to those physicians. Xyrem will be a Schedule III controlled substance when prescribed for narcolepsy. A special distribution system and education program are planned to prevent diversion. Patients will be responsible for securing their Xyrem and will be required to sign a contract signifying their understanding of procedures related to Xyrem distribution and security. Physicians and patients will be informed that in the event that Xyrem is diverted, it will be treated as a Schedule I controlled substance. To minimize diversion further, Xyrem will be manufacturered by a single manufacturer, and distributed by a single pharmacy (Express Scripts). Upon receiving a prescription, the specialty pharmacy will verify the prescriber's licensure and DEA number. Xyrem will be shipped directly from the pharmacy to the patient overnight. The pharmacist will contact the patient within 24 h to confirm that the patient received the Xyrem and to counsel the patient regarding its appropriate use (Engel, 2000).

10.14. SUMMARY

- Although it was originally used as an anesthetic, GHB is now used illicitly as a euphoriant and steroid alternative. Additionally, its use has been involved in a number of "date rape" cases.
- GHB is naturally found in body tissues such as the brain, heart, and kidney.
- GBL and 1,4-butanediol are liquid cleaning solvents that are readily converted to GHB after ingestion.
- GHB ingestion can lead to drowsiness, sleep, or eventually coma, depending on the dose.
- GHB withdrawal syndrome can occur following chronic use and is characterized by insomnia, tremor, and anxiety.
- GHB has recently been designated a Schedule I drug by the Drug Enforcement Administration. Possession of GBL and BD with intent to manufacture GHB is also illegal.

REFERENCES

Addolorato G, Capristo E, Gessa GL, Caputo F, Stefanni GF, Gasbarrini G. Long-term administration of GHB does not affect muscle mass in alcoholics. Life Sci 1999;65:191–6.

Anonymous. IARC Monogr Eval Carcinog Risks Hum 1999;71:367–82.

Borgen LA, Cook HN, Hornfeldt CS, Fuller DE. Sodium oxybate (GHB) for treatment of cataphexy. Pharmacotherapy 2002;22:798–9.

Cash CD. Gammahydroxybutyrate: an overview of the pros and cons for it being a neurotransmitter and/or a useful therapeuticx agent. Neurosci Behav Rev 1994;18:291–304.

CDC. Adverse events associated with ingestion of gamma-butyrolactone—Minnesota, New Mexico, and Texas, 1998–1999. MMWR 1999;48:137–40.

CDC. Epidemiologic notes and reports multistate outbreak of poisonings associated with illicit use of gamma hydroxybutyrate. MMWR 1990;39:861–3.

CDC. Gamma hydroxy butyrate use—New York and Texas, 1995–1996. MMWR 1997;46:281–3.

Chin RL, Sporer KA, Cullison B. Clinical course of γ-hydroxybutyric acid overdose. Ann Emerg Med 1998;31:716–22.

Cisek J, Holstege C, Rose R. Seizure associated with butanediol ingestion. J Toxicol Clin Toxicol 1999;37:650.

Couper FJ, Logan BK. Determination of γ-hydroxybutyrate (GHB) in biological specimens by gas chromatography-mass spectrometry. J Anal Toxicol 2000;24:1-7.

Craig K, Gomez HF, McManus JL, Bania TC. Severe gamma-hydroxybutyrate withdrawal: a case report and literature review. J Emerg Med 2000;18:65–70.

DEA. Gamma hydroxybutyrate (GHB). Available from: URL: http://www.dea.gov/concern/ghb.htm. Accessed June 6, 20001.

Detsch O, Erkens U, Schneck H, et al. Cerebral blood flow velocity and carbon dixide vasoreactivity during γ-hydroxybutyrate/fentanyl anaesthesia in non-neurosurgical patients. Eur J Anaesthesiol 1999;16:195–200.

Diana M, Mereu G, Mura A, et al. Low doses of γ-hydroxybutyric acid stimulate the firing rate of dopaminergic neurons in unanesthetized rats. Brain Res 1991;566:208–11.

Dyer JE. γ-Hydroxybutyrate: a health-food product producing coma and seizurelike activity. Am J Emerg Med 1991;9:321–4.

Dyer JE, Andrews KM. Gamma hydroxybutyrate withdrawal. J Toxicol Clin Toxicol 1997;35:554.

Dyer JE, Galbo MJ, Andrews KM. 1,4-Butanediol, "pine needle oil": overdose mimics toxic profile of GHB. J Toxicol Clin Toxicol 1997;35:554.

Dyer JE, Reed JH. Alkali burns from illicit manufacture of GHB. J Toxicol Clin Toxicol 1997;35:533.

Dyer JE, Roth B, Hyma BA. Gamma-hydroxybutyrate withdrawal syndrome. Ann Emerg Med 2001;37:147–53.

Engel P. GHB—what are the implications for states. Presented at the National Association of State Controlled Substances Authorities (NASCSA), 16th Annual Education Conference, Louisville, KY, Nov. 1, 2000.

FDA. FDA re-issues warning on GHB. FDA talk paper T97-10. Rockville, MD: Food and Drug Administration, February 18, 1997.

FDA. FDA warns about GBL-related products. FDA talk paper T99-21. Rockville, MD: Food and Drug Administration, May 11, 1999a.

FDA. FDA warns about products containing γ butyrolactone or GBL and asks companies to issue a recall. FDA talk paper T99-5. Rockville, MD: Food and Drug Administration, January 21, 1999b.

FDA. FDA approved Xyrem for cataplexy attacks in patients with narcolepsy. FDA alk Paper T02-31. Rockville, MD: Food and Drug Administration, July 17, 2002.

Ferrara SD, Tedeschi L, Frison G, et al. Therapeutic gamma-hydroxybutyric acid monitoring in plasma and urine by gas chromatography-mass spectrometry. J Pharm Biomed Anal 1993;11:483–7.

Ferrara SD, Zotti S, Tedeschi L, et al., Pharmacokinetics of γ-hydroxybutyric acid in alcohol dependent patients after single and repreated oral doses. Br J Clin Pharmacol 1992;34:231-5.

Fessenden RJ, Fessenden JS. Organic Chemistry, 3rd ed. Monterey, CA: Brooks/Cole Publishing Company; 1986.

Fieler EL, Coleman DE, Baselt RC. γ-Hydroxybutyrate concentrations in pre-and postmortem blood and urine. Clin Chem 1998;44:692-3.

Friedman J, Westlake R, Furman M. Grievous bodily harm: γ-hydroxybutyrate abuse leading to a Wernicke-Korsakoff syndromes. Neurology 1996;46:469-71.

Frison G, Tedeschi L, Maietti S, Ferrara SD. Determination of γ-hydroxybutyric acid (GHB) in plasma and urine by headspace solid-phase microextraction and gas chromatography/positive ion chemical ionization mass spectrometry. Rapid Commun Mass Spectrom 2000;14:2401–7.

Gessa GL, Vargiu L, Crabai F, et al. Selective increase of brain dopamine induced by γ-hydroxybutyrate. Life Sci 1966;5:1921–30.

Gorton C. Reply to: butyrolactone-induced central nervous system depression after ingestion of RenewTrient, a "dietary supplement" [letter]. N Engl J Med 1998;339:848.

Greene T, Dougherty T, Rodi A. γ-Butyrolactone (GBL) withdrawal presenting as acute psychosis. J Toxicol Clin Toxicol 1999;37:651.

Harrington RD, Woodward JA, Hooton TM, Horn JR. Life-threatening interactions between HIV-1 protease inhibitors ad the illicit drugs MDMA and γ-hydroxybutyrate. Arch Intern Med 1999;159:2221–4.

Hardy LJ, Slifman NR, Klontz KC, et al. Adverse events reported with the use of gamma butyrolactone products marketed as dietary supplements. J Toxicol Clin Toxicol 1999;37:649–50.

Helrich M, McAslan TC, Skolnik S, Bessman SP. Correlation of blood levels of 4-hydroxybutyrate with state of consciousness. Anesthesiology 1964;25:771–5.

Higgins TF, Borron SW. Coma and respiratory arrest after exposure to butyrolactone. J Emerg Med 1996;14:435–7.

Ingels M, Rangan C, Bellezzo J, Clark RF. Coma and respiratory depression following the ingestion of GHB and its precursors: three cases. J Emerg Med 2000;19:47–50.

Johansson B, Hardebo J. Cerebrovascular permeability and cerebral blood flow in hypertension induced by γ hydroxybutyric acid: an experimental study in the rat. Acta Neurol Scand 1982;65:448–57.

Kleinschmidt S, Grundmann U, Janneck U, et al. Total intravenous anaesthesia using propofol, gamma-hydroxybutyrate or midazolam in combination with sufentanil for patients undergoing coronary artery bypass surgery. Eur J Anaesthesiol 1997;14:590–9.

Kleinschmidt S, Grundmann U, Knocke T, et al. Total intravenous anaesthesia with gamma-hydroxybutyrate (GHB) and sufentanil in patients undergoing coronary artery bypass graft surgery: a comparison in patients with unimpaired and impaired left ventricular function. Eur J Anaesthesiol 1998;15:559–64.

Kleinschmidt S, Schellhase C, Mertzlufft F. Continuous sedation during spinal anaesthesia: gamma-hydroxybutyrate vs. propofol. Eur J Anaesthesiol 1999;16:23–30.

LeBeau MA, Montgomery MA, Miller ML, Burmeister SG. Analysis of biofluids for gamma-hydroxybutyrate (GHB) and gamma-butyrolactone (GBL) by headspace GC-FID and GC-MS. J Anal Toxicol 2000;24:421–8.

Labroit H. Sodium 4-hydroxybutyrate. Int J Neuropharmacol 1964;3:433–52.

Lettieri J, Fung H. Absorption and first-pass metabolism of ^{14}C-gamma-hydroxybutyric acid. Res Commun Chem Pathol Pharmacol 1976;13:425–37.

Li J. γ-Hydroxybutyrate intoxication and overdose [reply]. Ann Emerg Med 1999;33:475–6.

Li J, Stokes SA, Woeckener A. A Tale of novel intoxication: a review of the effects of γ-hydroxybutyric acid with recommendations for management. Ann Emerg Med 1998a;31:729–36.

Li J, Stokes SA, Woeckener A. A tale of novel intoxication: seven cases of γ-hydroxybutyric acid overdose. Ann Emerg Med 1998b;31:723–8.

LoVecchio F, Curry SC, Bagnasco T. Butyrolactone-induced central nervous system depression after ingestion of RenewTrient, a "dietary supplement." N Engl J Med 1998;339:847–8.

Mamelak M. Gammahydroxybutyrate: an endogenous regulator of energy metabolism. Neurosci Biobehav 1989;13:187–98.

McCusker RR, Paget-Wilkes H, Chronister CW, Goldberger BA. Analysis of gamma-hydroxybutyrate (GHB) in urine by gas chromatography-mass spectrometry. J Anal Toxicol 1999;23:301–305.

Minai L. GHB's 'stupor effect' has made it popular. Los Angeles Times, January 29, 2001.

Miguez I, Aldegunde M, Duran R, et al. Effects of low doses of gammahydroxybutyrate on serotonin, noradrenaline, and dopamine concentrations in rat brain areas. Neurochem Res 1988; 13: 531–3.

Palatini P, Tedeschi L, Frison G, et al. Dose-dependent absorption and elimination of gamma-hydroxybutyric acid in healthy volunteers. Eur J Clin Pharmacol 1993;45:353–6.

Ropero-Miller J, Goldberger BA. Recreational drugs. Current trends in the 90s. Clin Lab Med 1998;18:727–46.

Ross TM. Gamma hydroxybutyrate overdose: Two cases illustrate the unique aspects of this dangerous drug. J Emerg Nurs 1995;21:274–6.

Sapienza, F. Presentation at National Assicoation of State Controlled Substances Authorities (NASCSA) 16th Annual Education Conference, Louisville, KY, Nov. 1, 2000.

Scharf MB, Lai AA, Branigan B, Stover R, Berkowitz DB. Pharmacokinetics of gammahydroxybutyrate (GHB) in narcolepsy patients. Sleep 1998;21:507–14.

Sivilotti ML, Burns MJ, Aaron CK, Greenberg MJ. Pentobarbital for severe gamma-butyrolactone withdrawal. Ann Emerg Med 2001;38:660–5.

Snead OC. Gammahydroxybutyrate. Life Sci 1977;126:1935–44.

Thomas G, Bonner S, Gascoigne A. Coma induced by abuse of gamma-hydroxybutyrate (GHB or liquid ecstasy). BMJ 1997;314:35–6.

Wiley J, Dick R, Arnold T. Hematuria from home-manufactured GHB. J Toxicol Clin Toxicol 1998;36:502–3.

Vayer P, Mandel P, Maitre M. Gammahydroxybutyrate, a possible neurotransmitter. Life Sci 1987;1547–57.

Vickers MD. Gammahydroxybutyric acid. Int Anesth Clin 1969;7:75–89.

Winters WD, Spooner CE. Various seizure activities following gamma-hydroxybutyrate. Int J Neuropharmacol 1965;4:197–200.

Zvosec DL, Smith SW, McCutcheon JR, et al. Adverse events, including death, associated with the use of 1,4-butanediol. N Engl J Med 2001;344:87–94.

Chapter 11

Germanium

Thomas A. Chase, Melanie Johns Cupp, and Timothy S. Tracy

11.1. History and Traditional Uses

Germanium, an element with both metallic and nonmetallic properties, was discovered in 1886. Germanium supplements became popular in the 1970s in Japan to prevent and treat disease, and their use had spread to Britain and other countries by the mid-1980s (Tao and Bolger, 1997).

11.2. Chemical Structure

Refer to Fig. 11-1 for the chemical structure of germanium sesquioxide.

11.3. Current Promoted Uses

Germanium is promoted for treatment of rheumatoid arthritis, osteoarthritis, depression, cirrhosis, food allergies, candidiasis, chronic viral infections including hepatitis and HIV, heavy metal poisoning, cataracts, glaucoma, heart disease, high cholesterol, high blood pressure, cancer, low energy, osteoporosis, and pain relief.

11.4. Sources and Chemical Composition

Germanium has an atomic number of 32 and a weight of 72.6. Although some medicinal plants, (including ginseng, aloe, and garlic) purportedly have relatively high germanium concentrations, they actually contain concentrations only on the order of parts per billion. The earth's crust contains germanium at a concentration of 7 ppm, freshwater contains 0.6 mg/L, and soil contains 0.6–1.3 mg/kg. Accordingly, germanium is present in nearly all food in trace amounts and is the main source of germanium for humans (Tao and Bolger, 1997).

From: *Forensic Science: Dietary Supplements: Toxicology and Clinical Pharmacology*
Edited by: M. J. Cupp and T. S. Tracy © Humana Press Inc., Totowa, New Jersey

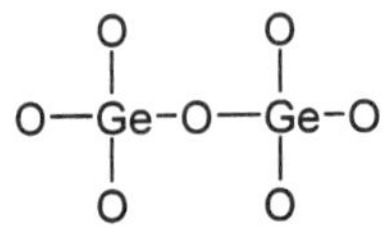

$$O-\underset{\underset{O}{|}}{\overset{\overset{O}{\|}}{Ge}}-O-\underset{\underset{O}{|}}{\overset{\overset{O}{\|}}{Ge}}-O$$

Fig. 1. Chemical structure of germanium sesquioxide.

Two of the most toxic germanium compounds are germanium dioxide (GeO_2) and germanium sesquioxide $(GeCH_2 CH_2CO_2H)_2O_3$ (Tao and Bolger, 1997). The latter is arranged three-dimensionally as two cubic triangles with a shared base consisting of three oxygen atoms (Goodman, 1988).

11.5. PRODUCTS AVAILABLE

The most commonly advertised organic germanium compound on the Internet is germanium sesquioxide, also known as bis-betacarboxyethylgermanium sesquioxide (Mainwaring et al., 2000), carboxyethyl germanium sesquioxide (Schauss, 1991), carboxyethylgermanium sesquioxide (Shinohara et al., 1999), carboxyethylgermanium (Gerber and Leonard, 1997; Mainwaring et al., 2000), propagermanium, SK-818 (Tao and Bolger, 1997), and 3-oxygermylpropionic acid polymer (Ishiwata et al., 1998). Germanium-132 and Ge-132 were purportedly once brand names for germanium sesquioxide from Global Marketing (San Francisco, CA) (Schauss, 1991). These terms are commonly used by commercial web sites as well as medical authors as generic synonyms for germanium sesquioxide. Germanium-132 will be the focus of this chapter owing to its popularity in the United States among germanium compounds. Germanium-132 preparations generally come in powder, capsule, or liquid form.

Another organic germanium product used by consumers, particularly in Europe, is germanium lactate citrate (Hess et al., 1993), also known as lactate-citrate germanium and brand-named Sanumgerman® by the German company Sanum-Kehlbeck (Schauss, 1991).

Spirogermanium (Unimed) is a germanium compound with a heterocyclic ring structure that was formerly studied as an antineoplastic (Schauss, 1991). This product is not typically promoted to consumers and is not discussed in any detail in this chapter.

Inorganic germanium compounds such as germanium dioxide are sold as nutritional supplements in some countries (Schauss, 1991) but not typically in the United States. Germanium dioxide is used in the production of germanium-132 and may be found as a contaminant in some germanium-132 products (Tao and Bolger, 1997). For this reason, and because, like germanium-132, germanium dioxide has been associated with nephrotoxicity, its toxicities will be covered in some detail under the Adverse Effects and Toxicity section.

11.6. IN VITRO EFFECTS

Spirogermanium was shown to have synergistic activity against human colorectal cancer and transitional cell carcinoma of the bladder in vitro when combined with cisplatin or 5-fluorouracil, but not when combined with doxorubicin, methotrexate, vinblastine, vincristine, or radiation (Hill et al., 1984). Spirogermanium also showed cytotoxic activity in a wide range of cancer using NIL 8 hamster cells (Goodman, 1988).

11.7. CLINICAL STUDIES

Despite the promising results of in vitro studies using several tumor cell lines, investigation of spirogermanium and germanium-132 as antineoplastics was abandoned owing to toxicity and lack of efficacy in phase I and II clinical trials in advanced lung, breast, renal, and prostate cancer (Mainwaring et al., 2000).

An anecdotal report describes a 47-yr-old woman diagnosed with pulmonary spindle cell carcinoma who failed conventional therapy with one cycle of etoposide/ifosfamide, one cycle of paclitaxel/cisplatin, radiation therapy, and two cycles of mesna, ifosfamide, doxorubicin, and dacarbazine (Mainwaring et al., 2000). Six weeks after discontinuing treatment because of worsening symptoms and tumor progression, the patient began self-medicating with a tapering regimen of germanium sesquioxide with a starting dose of 7.2 g. The regimen was recommended by an acquaintance who claimed this regimen had cured him of oat cell carcinoma 15 yr before. The patient noted symptomatic improvement within a few days, and 3 mo later, a chest X-ray showed a 60% decrease in tumor size, with almost complete resolution by computed tomography (CT) 5 and 7 mo after beginning the germanium compound. Four years later, the patient was tumor-free and still taking germanium sesquioxide without any reported side effects. The authors did not discuss assessment of renal function. The authors concluded that spontaneous remission is unlikely but cannot be ruled out.

11.8. PHARMACOKINETICS

Radiolabeled germanium dioxide administered to rabbits and dogs was found to be almost completely eliminated in the urine and feces within 72 hr of administration, with only small amounts remaining in the kidneys (Schauss, 1991). In rats, germanium was detected in the serum 15 min after administration of germanium dioxide, and peak serum concentrations occurred in 2 h. Its distribution can be described using a two-compartment model. The volume of distribution of the central compartment is 3.1 ± 0.3 L, and the volume of distribution of the tissue compartment was 8.5 ± 2.9 L. Tissue concentrations were highest in the sciatic nerve and the kidney, reflecting the toxicities reported with germanium dioxide in rat studies. Its distibution and elimination follow first-order kinetics. The elimination rate constant is 0.3 h^{-1}, and the elimination half-life is 2.3 h (Lin et al., 1999).

The pharmacokinetics of germanium-132 are similar in rats and humans. Approximately 30% of a given germanium-132 dose is absorbed orally. Peak plasma levels occur in 2 h. Germanium is not protein bound and is widely distributed throughout the body. Eighty-five percent of a given dose is eliminated renally (Goodman, 1988).

11.9. ADVERSE EFFECTS AND TOXICITY

The oral median lethal dose (LD_{50}) of germanium dioxide is 3.7 g/kg for male rats and 6.3 g/kg for male mice (Schauss, 1991; Tao and Bolger, 1997). The LD_{50} for intraperitoneal germanium dioxide is 2.025 mg/kg for female mice and 1.62 mg/kg for female rats (Schauss, 1991). Toxicities of germanium dioxide reported in mice and rats include tremors, sedation, cyanosis, vasodilation, ptosis, hypothermia, reduced spontaneous activity, and respiratory failure resulting in death (Schauss 1991).

For germanium-132, the LD_{50} is 11.7 g/kg and 11 g/kg for male and female rats, respectively, and 6.3–12.5 g/kg for male and 11.4 g/kg for female mice (Tao and Bolger, 1997).

In vitro spirogermanium cytotoxicity studies using Chinese hamster cells and Hela cells demonstrated a significant inhibition of protein, RNA, and DNA synthesis at micromolar concentrations (Goodman, 1988). Low-dose sodium germanate administered for life was not tumorigenic in mice (Tao and Bolger 1997).

In a phase I study of germanium-132 performed by theAsai Germanium Research Institute, the maximum tolerated dose was 50–100 mg/kg. Soft stool was reported by some subjects. No hematologic or biochemical abnormalities were noted (Goodman, 1988).

Case reports of renal toxicity associated with the use of germanium supplements began in the early 1980s (Tao and Bolger, 1997). These reports first surfaced in Japan and then were seen Europe, reflecting the geographic spread of germanium's popularity. Although the actual germanium compound consumed in most cases is unknown (Tao and Bolger, 1997), germanium-132 and germanium dioxide appear to be the principal germanium compounds associated with nephrotoxicity (Schauss, 1991; Shinohara et al., 1999). Germanium lactate citrate has also been implicated.

At least 31 cases of germanium-associated nephrotoxicity, including nine fatalities, have been reported, and the most common signs and symptoms have been reviewed by Tao and Bolger (1997). Anorexia, weight loss, fatigue, nausea, vomiting, anemia, and muscle weakness accompanied renal failure. All patients had degeneration of the tubular epithelial cells with vacuolization and electron-dense mitochondrial inclusions. Despite these pathologic changes, urinalysis was normal. In addition to kidney involvement, other organ toxicities included hypoplastic bone marrow; peripheral and central neuropathy with severe axonal degeneration, sensory impairment; truncal and cerebellar ataxia; swollen skeletal and cardiac myocytes; mitochondria with electron-dense deposits; and hepatosteatosis. One patient had paresthesias and vomiting for 2 mo after product discontinuation. The mechanism of toxicity in these case reports is thought to involve disruption of mitochondrial function or cytotoxicity because neither immunoglobulin nor complement involvement appears to be important. Vomiting may be caused by impairment of gastrointestinal motor activity, as evidenced by a delay in intestinal transit time in one patient with frequent vomiting. Details of select individual case reports follow. The specific germanium compound used by each patient is listed if known.

A 55-yr-old ill-appearing woman presented to the hospital with several complaints after having taken 47 g of elemental germanium in elixir form over the preceding 19 mo (Takeuchi et al., 1992). The earliest symptom to appear was anorexia, which first occurred 15 mo after beginning to take the product, followed by malaise after 18 mo of therapy. Other complaints included weakness, weight loss, and paresthesia and hypesthesia of the proximal upper and lower extremities and the tongue. One month earlier, she had been diagnosed with anemia and renal failure at another hospital. Pertinent physical findings on the latter admission included pale conjunctiva, hypoactive deep tendon reflexes, and decreased muscle tone in the extremities.

Hemoglobin and hematocrit were 9.1 g/dL and 25%, respectively. Urinalysis was normal. BUN was 44 mg/dL, and serum creatinine was 21.3 mL/min with fractional excretion of sodium 0.56. Serum protein and albumin were only slightly depressed. Uric acid was 15 mg/dL. Alanine aminotransferase and aspartate aminotransferase were 48 U/L and 133 U/L, respectively. Lactate dehydrogenase (LDH) was 642 U/L, creatine kinase (CK) was 2658 U/L, and serum myoglobin was 1500 ng/ml. Muscle biopsy revealed necrosis and muscle fiber regeneration, but no inflammatory infiltrate. Although nerve conduction was normal shortly after admission, a repeat electromyogram during hospital week 11 showed delayed conduction.

Despite improvement in CK and myoglobin, and initiation of prednisone at week 5 for treatment of polymyositis, weakness and sensory defects progressed to the point that 6 weeks after admission, the patient had difficulty standing, swallowing, and moving. Hand and perioral tremors akin to those seen in parkinsonism were noted. The patient died from undertermined causes during week 12 of hospital admission.

Both biopsy and autopsy renal findings included periodic acid-Schiff (PAS)-positive yellow/brown granules in the thick ascending limb of the loop of Henle and in the distal tubular epithelium, which were identified as lipofuscin using Schmorl's stain. The basement membrane in these areas was thickened, and the epithelial cells were flattened and had undergone vacuolar degeneration and desquamation. Myoglobin was found in intact proximal tubular epithelial cells and in the tubular lumen. Grossly, the kidney was relatively intact, and glomerular vascular lesions were minimal, with no inflammatory infiltrate. In the biopsy specimens, which were the only specimens so examined, there was weak immunofluorescent staining of the glomerular capillary walls. Nonrenal autopsy findings included degeneration of cardiac and skeletal muscle, vacuolization and fatty degeneration of the hepatocytes, hypoplastic bone marrow, and a decrease in cerebellar Purkinje cells. Compared with a cohort of patients with renal failure, this patient had higher serum, urine, spleen, kidney, adrenal gland, and myocardial germanium levels. Germanium was not detected in the brain or skeletal muscle. The autopsy did not provide a definitive cause of death, although death was attributed to some effect associated with germanium.

A similar case was subsequently published (Kim et al., 1998). A 53-yr-old ill-appearing man presented to the hospital with several symptoms, including weakness and a 16-kg weight loss over 3 mo. He had a taken a total of 400 g of lysine germanium oxide powder over 17 mo. Anorexia first occurred 14 mo after beginning the supplement. BUN and serum creatinine were 60 and 2.6 mg/dL, respectively, at that time. One month later, the patient noted tingling of the palms and soles and asthenia of the lower extremities. Upon admission, the patient had no deep tendon reflexes. BUN and serum creatinine on admission were 62 and 3 mg/dL, respectively, with a creatinine clearance of 39 mL/min. Serum uric acid was 18.8 mg/dL. The patient was anemic, with a hemoglobin of 10.5 g/dL. Urinalysis was essentially normal, but urine β_2-microglobulin was elevated. Serum LDH was 519 U/L, CK was 2005 U/L, and myoglobin was greater than 300 U/L. Serum protein and albumin were 6.6 and 3.8 g/dL, respectively. Ionized calcium was low, at 0.79 mmol/L, and parathyroid hormone was depressed, which could reflect nephritis or a direct effect of germanium on the parathyroid gland. Liver function tests were essentially normal. Serum sodium, potassium, chloride, and bicarbonate were low. Phosphorus was slightly elevated at 6.1 mg/dL. Blood and urine germanium concentrations were elevated, at 62.7 and 2190 µg/L, respectively. Renal ultrasound showed no structural abnormalities. Electromyography was consistent with polyneuropathy affecting mainly the sensory nerves. On renal biopsy, the glomeruli were essentially normal, although they were slightly enlarged, with a segmentally increased matrix. The tubular epithelial cells were severely necrotic and contained PAS-positive granules. The interstitium was mildly fibrotic. There was no evidence of antibody deposits using immunofluorescence microscopy. No electron-dense mitochondrial inclusions were noted in the tubular epithelium. Two months after product discontinuation, BUN and serum creatinine remained elevated at 48 and 3.6 mg/dL, respectively, although weakness had improved slightly.

Okada and others (1989) reported three cases of renal failure associated with germanium. The first case involved a 24-yr-old woman nurse who presented to her physician with malaise and fatigue. She was pale and cachectic, with anemic-appearing conjunctiva. She was hospitalized and diagnosed with hepatitis B. Upon the advice of a friend, she began self-medicating with germanium 90 mg/d. Approximately 18 mo later, she was found to have a creatinine clearance of 19 ml/min and had metabolic acidosis.

Another patient in this same series, a 37-yr-old housewife, presented with anorexia, malaise, fatigue, and lower extremity mylagia after taking the same germanium product at the same dose as the first patient for approximately 1 1/2 yr for self-treatment of hepatitis B. Creatinine clearance was 34.3 mL/min. She was mildly anemic and had an elevated erythrocyte sedimentation rate. The third case reported by these clinicians involved a 36-yr-old man taking the same germanium preparation at a dose of 90 mg/d for 6 mo for treatment of hepatitis. Creatinine clearance was 16.5 mL/min. He was mildly anemic, and complained of general malaise.

Urinalysis was essentially normal in the two patients in which urinalysis was performed; however, a renal biopsy from the first patient revealed extensive tubular atrophy with epithelial degeneration and interstitial fibrosis as well as an inflammatory infiltrate of lymphocytes and plasma cells. Using immunofluoroscopy, IgG was identified on the glomerular capillary wall and the tubular basement membrane. Electron microscopy revealed many cytoplasmic vacuoles in the glomerular epithelial cells and in the proximal and distal tubular epithelial cells, as well as electron-dense material in the mitochrondria of cells in the distal nephron. Many epithelial cells were degenerated and had pycnotic nuclei. All three patients had very high concentrations of germanium in their hair, fingernails, and toenails. The first patient had germanium 56.4, 15.7 and 14.6 µg/g dry weight of hair, fingernails, and toenails, respectively. The second patient had germanium 173.7, 5.4, and 15.8 µg/g dry weight of hair, fingernails, and toenails, respectively. The third patient had 88 µg per gram dry weight of hair and 35 µg per gram dry weight of finger- plus toenails. Germanium was not detected in the hair or nails of control subjects not consuming germanium supplements. The germanium product consumed by all three patients was analyzed and was found to contain germanium 1500 µg/mL. No carbon was detected in the product, suggesting that inorganic germanium was the main ingredient.

Hess and colleagues (1993) reported two cases of renal failure associated with germanium use by HIV-positive patients. A 25-yr-old woman ingested a product labeled "organic germanium" containing 18% germanium lactate citrate to stimulate her immune system. Forty-seven grams of germanium (260 g of the compound) were ingested over a 9-mo period. She was taking no other medications. On presentation, she complained of fatigue, severe abdominal pain, nausea, and diarrhea. Serum creatinine was 4.6 mg/dL, and hemoglobin was 9.1 g/dL. Within 19 d, her creatinine reached 9.1 g/dl, protein excretion was 280 mg/24 h, and her creatinine clearance had fallen to 7 mL/min/1.73 m², necessitating hemodialysis. Ultrasound revealed an enlarged liver (15 cm). Alkaline phosphatase, γ-glutamyltransferase, alanine aminotransferase, and aspartate aminotransferase were elevated at 189, 159, 75, and 102 U/L, respectively. Plasma lactate was elevated at 7.3 mEq/L, arterial pH was 7.337, and bicarbonate was 4.4 mEq/L, reflecting metabolic acidosis. Liver failure and lactic acidosis resolved within 5 mo. Dialysis was discontinued after approximately 3 mo, and 10 mo after presentation, creatinine clearance had risen to 13 mL/min/1.73 m², but serum eythropoietin was only 7.8 mU/mL (normal 15–30 mU/mL), necessitating replacement. Twenty months after discontinuing the germanium product, creatinine clearance was 11 mL/min/1.73 m², and protein excretion was 1.01 g/d. Hyperkalemia also persisted, with values ranging from 4.9 to 5.9 mEq/L. Two years after presentation, creatinine clearance was 14 mL/min/1.73 m², and protein excretion was 0.84 g/d.

The second case reported by these authors was the 26-yr-old male housemate of the first patient. He was taking the same germanium regimen as she, although reportedly on a more irregular schedule. He presented for examination after his friend developed an adverse reaction to the product. Serum creatinine was found to be 2.9 mg/dL, with a creatinine clearance of 43 mL/min/1.73 m². Protein excretion was 0.36 g/d. Nine months after product discontinuation, creatinine clearance was unchanged. Renal biopsies, obtained immediately after product discontinuation, revealed cell degeneration with vacuolization, particularly in the distal tubule, with electron-dense mitochndrial deposits. PAS-positive intracellular deposits were present in the distal tubular cells. A focal interstitial inflammatory infiltrate of plasma cells was also noted.

A second renal biopsy was performed on the first patient 20 mo after product discontinuation. The second biopsy showed striking focal atrophy of tubular cells with minor interstitial fibrosis, a small number of granular intracellular inclusions, and interstitial infiltration with plasma cells. There was slight mesangial proliferation. The electron-dense deposits noted in the first biopsy were absent in the second. The woman patient also underwent a liver biopsy, which demonstrated severe steatosis. Spherical electron-dense inclusions, similar to those seen in the kidney, were noted. Kidney and liver germanium concentrations were elevated. Kidney concentrations of germanium were still elevated.

Use of spirogeranium has not been associated with nephrotoxicity, but it has been associated with transient dizziness, vertigo, ataxia, and paresthesia; thus, its side effect profile suggests neurotoxicity rather than nephrotoxicity (Schauss, 1991).

Tao and Bolger (1997) reviewed animal studies that reproduce the germanium-associated toxicities reported in humans. Rats fed germanium dioxide 150 mg/kg/d for 13 wk exhibited decreased body weight, increased BUN and serum creatinine, and decreased creatinine clearance. The renal tubular cells were degenerated, and the mitochondria were swollen and contained electron-dense inclusions. Glomeruli were normal, and there was no evidence of immune involvement. In the liver, centrilobular vacuolization was noted, and liver enzymes were elevated. The myocardium was also affected; vacuoles and a waxy cytoplasm were seen. Biochemical and histologic evidence of kidney dysfunction were present in rats treated for only 4 wk. Five weeks after germanium discontinuation, these abnormalities persisted, suggesting long-term injury.

In a study using only 75 mg/kg for 24 wk, liver function returned to normal 14–16 wk after germanium discontinuation, but tubulointerstitial fibrosis remained, and treated rats had lower hematocrits and higher germanium tissue levels than controls. Germanium-associated growth retardation, anemia, and nephrotoxicity are dose- and duration-dependent. Treatment with germanium dioxide 13 mg/kg for 6 mo resulted in kidney dysfunction and skeletal muscle myopathy, with distal tubule degeneration and electron-dense inclusions in swollen mitochondria evident after 9–10 mo. As is typical of germanium-associated nephrotoxicity, the glomeruli appeared normal. Both skeletal and cardiac muscle cells showed focal atrophy and mitochondrial swelling. At a higher dose of 69 mg/kg, rats with unilateral nephrectomies exhibited elevated BUN and serum creatinine after only 6 wk, with dramatic increases after 10 wk. Histologic changes were similar to those seen with the lower dose. Mortality was 40%.

Several additional rat studies demonstrated myopathy, evidenced by reduced skeletal muscle weight, enlarged mitochondria with electron-dense inclusions and numerous cristae, abundant ragged red fibers, cytochrome c oxidase deficiency, and muscle cell degeneration and phagocytosis, as well as accumulation of fat droplets in muscle cells. These changes were evident after 4 mo of treatment with a diet containing 0.2% germanium dioxide (100–150 mg/kg) and after 23 wk of treatment with a diet comprised of germanium dioxide 0.15%. Peripheral neuropathy was also seen in young rats fed a diet comprised of 0.15% germanium dioxide for 6–8 mo; thus, germanium-associated myopathy precedes other toxicities. Histologically, the first neurologic changes were noted in the cytoplasm of Schwann cells. Subsequently, nerves demonstrated edema as well as segmented demyelination and remyelination. Rats fed sodium germanate 5 ppm in their water throughout their lifetimes exhibited elevated tissue germanium levels as well as nephro- and hepatotoxicity. No effect on body weight was noted. Unlike germanium dioxide, rat studies using germanium-132 do not consistently demonstrate kidney damage, even when administered at doses providing equivalent amounts of germanium. In one study, germanium-132 accumulated in the kidney to a lesser extent than germanium dioxide; however, in another study in which rats were fed either compound at a dose of 50 ppm of diet for 6 wk, urinary germanium levels were higher in the germanium-132 group than in the germanium dioxide group. Kidney germanium concentrations were low with both compounds, but renal pathology was evident. In another study, male but not female rats exhibited renal tubular casts and swelling of tubular cells when administered germanium-132 at a dose of 714 mg/kg/d for 6 mo. Germanium accumulated in the spleen and liver as well as the kidney.

11.10. INTERACTIONS

A 63-yr-old man with membranous glomerulosclerosis began taking Uncle Hsu's® Korean ginseng, a ginseng and germanium-containing product, 10–12 tablets/d (Becker et al., 1996). He was receiving furosemide and cyclosporine for treatment of his kidney disease. Ten days after beginning the supplement, he required hopitalization because of edema and hypertension. Although his usual weight was 74.5 kg, he weighed 87.3 kg on admission. Blood pressure was 186/100 mmHg, and serum creatinine was 1.3 mg/dL. Furosemide 240 mg was administered intravenously every 8 h, and the supplement was discontinued. Renal ultrasound was unremarkable. He was discharged with a blood pressure of 138/84 mmHg and a weight of 76 kg. He was prescribed furosemide 80 mg twice daily. At home, he began taking the ginseng/germanium supplement, and his weight increased to 88 kg over the following 2 wk, despite an increase in furosemide dose to 240 mg twice daily. His cysclosporine level ranged from 167 to 231 mg/L. Serum creatinine was 1.4 mg/dL. He was admitted to the hospital and was once again treated with furosemide 240 mg every 8 h, and the supplement was discontinued. His weight decreased to 73.6 kg, and his blood pressure decreased to 128/78 mmHg over 2 d. Because pathologic changes in the kidney with chronic germanium ingestion have been noted in the asceding limb of the loop of Henle where furosemide acts, the clinicians attributed the patient's diuretic resistance to germanium.

A concern with germanium lactate citrate is its citrate content. Citrate chelates and enhances the absorption of aluminum, which could be particularly detrimental to dialysis patients, who are at risk of aluminum toxicity (Hess et al., 1993).

11.11. REPRODUCTION

Germanium-132 administered intraperitoneally to rats and intravenously to rabbits at doses of 1000 and 500 mg/kg, respectively, demonstrated no teratogenicity. A dose of 4000 mg/kg was said to show teratogenicity compared with control rats, but specific effects were not described (Tao and Bolger, 1997). A study performed with rats according to the advice of the World Health Organization and the Canadian Ministry of Health found that an older formulation of Sanumgerman® caused fetal anomalies, resulting in skeletal malformations and defects of the bones. The influence on the pregnant female rats was minimal, and no damaging effects to the mothers were seen (Goodman, 1988). Dimethyl germanium oxide has been shown to produce anophthalmia, umbilical hernias, and limb abnormalities in chick embryos. Germanium trioxide 40 and 100 mg/kg administered intravenously to hamsters on gestation day 8 caused an increased embryonic resorption rate but did not cause any apparent malformations (Gerber and Leonard, 1997).

11.12. CHEMICAL AND BIOFLUID ANALYSIS

Different techniques are used to measure germanium. Inductively coupled plasma-mass spectrometry (ICP-MS) is a new technique used specifically for trace element analysis. Normally ICP-MS is used to measure air and water in our natural surroundings. This test has now found a new niche in analyzing biologic specimens such as serum, liver, and kidney (Lin et al., 1999). Other methods used to indentify germanium in urine, hair, nails, and plasma are graphite furnace atomic absorption spectrometry (GFAAS) and microwave-induced plasma mass spectrometry (MIP-MS) (Shinohara et al., 1999). Schauss suggests that hair analysis may be used as an early indicator of germanium toxicity (1991).

The most common method for measuring germanium concentrations is graphite furnace atomic absorption spectrophotometry. Shinohara and colleagues (1999) report the use of this methodology to measure germanium concentrations in human nails, hair, blood, urine, and organ specimens. For this method, hair and nail samples are washed with deionized water and then air-dried before weighing. One milliliter of urine, 10–100 mg of hair or nail, or 200–400 μL of plasma are required for the analysis. The glass tubes used should be demetalolyzed prior to use to avoid background. Two milliliters of HNO_3 and 0.2 mL $HClO_4$ are added, and the samples are heated at 120–140°C. The samples are then diluted with 0.5% HNO_3 prior to analysis. To increase assay sensitivity, 10 μL of Ni (100 μg/mL) are injected with 10 μL of sample into the furnace. A hollow cathode Ge tube is used as the resonance source, with a lamp current of 12.5 mA. The analytical wavelength is 265.2 nm, with polarized-Zeeman background correction and a slit width of 0.4 nm. Samples are subjected to a furnace heating program whereby they are dried for 30 s at 80–120°C and a gas flow of 200 mL/min (argon), charred for 30 s at 700°C and gas flow of 200 mL/min argon, and atomized for 10 s at 2700°C with no gas flow; finally, the chamber is cleaned for 4 s at 2900°C, again at an argon gas flow of 200 mL/min. The detection limit for germanium under these conditions is 3 ng/mL (or 0.03 ng/10 μL).

These same investigators also report a novel MIP-MS method for measuring germanium concentrations (Shinohara et al., 1999). This method is approximately 60 times more sensitive than atomic absorption spectrophotometry. For patients who have ingested germanium, the atomic absorption spectrophotometry method appears to be adequate; however, to measure germanium concentrations in patients who have not been exposed to germanium (i.e., control subjects), the mass spectrometry method will be required since background plasma, urine, and hair levels are generally less than 3 ng/mL (detection limit), although nail concentrations may be detectable.

11.13. REGULATORY STATUS

The Food and Drug Administration has banned importation of germanium because of its nephrotoxicity and "unapproved new drug" status when labeled for use in the prevention or cure of disease (FDA, 2000). The Attorney General of the State of Minnesota has taken action against an Internet vendor of Vitalium Plus®, a product containing germanium-132 and feverfew, for allegedly advertising the product in a misleading and unbalanced fashion (Consumer Fraud Alert Network, 2000). Germanium compounds, particularly germanium-132, are marketed as dietary supplements in the United States. In Canada, germanium is banned as a dietary supplement or drug (Buche, 2000).

11.14. SUMMARY

- Germanium is a metalloid found in several organic and inorganic compounds that have been used as supplements or investigational drugs in humans. Germanium-132 is the most common germanium compound sold as a dietary supplement in humans.
- Germanium is eliminated renally.
- Germanium compounds have been associated with nephrotoxicity, myopathy, weight loss, anemia, central and peripheral neurotoxicity, hepatotoxicty, and bone marrow suppression.
- Hallmarks of germanium-associated nephrotoxicity include renal tubular damage with electron-dense mitrochondrial inclusions, normal-appearing glomeruli, little or no immunofluorescence, and normal urinalysis.

- Germanium may cause diuretic resistance, and germanium lactate citrate may enhance aluminum toxicity in dialysis patients.
- Germanium is banned in Canada, but is available as a dietary supplement in the United States.

REFERENCES

Becker BN, Greene J, Evanson J, Chidsey G, Stone WJ. Ginseng-induced diuretic resistance [letter]. JAMA 1996;276:606–7.

Buche J. How to take germanium. Available from: URL: http://seasilver.threadnet.com/Preventorium/germados.htm. Accessed July 17, 2000.

Consumer Fraud Alert Network. Vitalium Plus health scam. Available from: URL: http://www.microsmarts.com/fraudalert/mcccom.htm. Accessed July 17, 2000.

FDA. Import alert IA5407. Revised 9/13/95. Available from: URL:http://www.fda.gov/ora/fiars/ora_import_ia5407.html. Accessed July 26, 2000.

Gerber GB, Leonard A. Mutgenicity, carcinogenicity, and teratogenicity of germanium compounds. Mutat Res 1997;387:141–6.

Goodman S. Therapeutic effects of organic germanium. Med Hypotheses 1988;26:207–15.

Hess B, Raisin J, Zimmermann A, et al. Tubulointerstitial nephropathy persisting 20 months after discontinuation of chronic intake of germanium lactate citrate. Am J Kidney Dis 1993;21:548–52.

Hill BT, Bellamy AS, Metcalfe S, et al. Identification of synergistic combinations of spirogermanium with 5-fluorouracil or cisplatin using a range of human tumour cell lines in vitro. Invest New Drugs 1984;2:29–33.

Ishiwata Y, Yokochi S, Hashimoto H, Ninomiya F, Suzuki T. Protection against concanavalin A-induced murine liver injury by the organic germanium compound, propagergermanium. Scand J Immunol 1988;48:605–14.

Kim KM, Lim CS, Kim S, et al. Nephropathy and neuropathy induced by a germanium-containing compound. Nephrol Dial Transplant 1998;13:3218–9.

Lin C, Chen T, Hsieh Y, Jiang S, Chen S. Kinetics of germanium dioxide in rats. Toxicology 1999;132:147–53.

Mainwaring MG, Poor C, Zander DS, Harman E. Complete remission of pulmonary spindle cell carcinoma after treatment with oral germanium sesquioxide. Chest 2000;117:591–3.

Okada K, Okagawa K, Kawakami K, et al. Renal failure caused by long-term use of a germanium preparation as an elixir. Clin Nephrol 1989;31:219–24.

Schauss AG. Nephrotoxicity and neurotoxicity in humans from organogermanium compounds and germanium dioxide. Biol Trace Element Res 1991;29:267–80.

Shinohara A, Chiba M, Inaba Y. Determination of germanium in human specimens: comparative study of atomic absorption spectrometry and microwave-induced plasma mass spectrometry. J Anal Toxicol 1999;23:625–31.

Takeuchi A, Yoshizawa N, Oshima S, et al. Nephrotoxicity of germanium compounds. Nephron 1992;60:436–42.

Tao S, Bolger M. Hazard assessment of germanium supplements. Regul Toxicol Pharmacol 1997;25:211–9.

Chapter 12

Glucosamine and Chondroitin

Melanie Johns Cupp and Timothy S. Tracy

12.1. HISTORY

In the 1950s, in vitro studies of glucosamine demonstrated its potential to increase fibroblast production of collagen and mucopolysaccharides. These findings led to studies of glucosamine for the treatment of osteoarthritis (OA) in humans, first with an injectable product, and then with oral supplementation (McCarty, 1994). Public interest in the use of glucosamine for OA increased in the late 1990s, in some measure owing to the publication of two books for laypersons on the subject, *The Arthritis Cure* and *Maximizing the Arthritis Cure* (Thie et al., 2001).

12.2. CHEMICAL STRUCTURES

See Fig. 12-1 for the chemical structures of glucosamine and chondroitin.

12.3. CURRENT PROMOTED USES

Although glucosamine/chondroitin products cannot be promoted for the treatment of OA in the United States, they are generally advertised as nutrients that decrease joint pain, improve joint strength and function, and rebuild and maintain connective tissue by stimulating the synthesis of new cartilage and inhibiting cartilage breakdown. Most advertising is geared toward older persons, although some products are promoted to athletes, bodybuilders, and fitness enthusiasts.

12.4. SOURCES AND CHEMICAL COMPOSITION

Glucosamine and chondroitin are cartilage constituents. Glucosamine, an aminomonosaccharide synthesized from glucose (Reichelt et al., 1994), is a small (mol wt 179.17) organic base with a pKa of 6.91 at 37°C. It is highly soluble in water and in hydrophilic organic solvents such as methanol (Setnikar et al., 1986). In vivo, fruc-

From: *Forensic Science: Dietary Supplements: Toxicology and Clinical Pharmacology*
Edited by: M. J. Cupp and T. S. Tracy © Humana Press Inc., Totowa, New Jersey

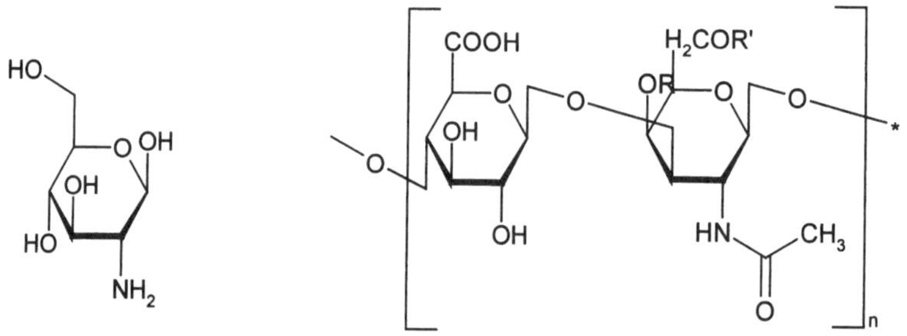

Fig. 1. Chemical structures of (left) glucosamine and (right) chondroitin sulfate. R = H or SO_3H; R' = H or SO_3H.

tose-6-phosphate, formed during glycolysis, is aminated in a reaction using glutamine as an amine donor to yield glucosamine-6-phosphate. Exogenously administered glucosamine is thought to be converted directly to glucosamine-6-phosphate. Glucosamine-6-phosphate is then acetylated and conjugated with uridine diphosphate (UDP). This product is then incorporated into cartilage (McCarty, 1994).

The glycosaminoglycans (GAGs) known as chondroitin sulfates are polysaccharide chains of disaccharide units. Each disaccharide unit is composed of sulfated residues of β-D-glucuronic acid (uronic acid) and α-D-*N*-acetyl-galactosamine. There are three positions in the disaccharide structure that may be sulfated, resulting in disaccharides with different physicochemical properties. Examples include chondroitin sulfate A, or chondroitin-4-sulfate, and chondroitin sulfate C, or chondroitin-6-sulfate. The heterogeneity of the disaccharides and polysaccharide chains results in glycosaminoglycans with different biologic and pharmacologic activity (Conte et al., 1995). Thus, results of a study using a particular chondroitin sulfate may not apply to other products of a different structure.

Glucosamine is ubiquitous in meat, fish, and poultry (McCarty, 1994). Manufacturers of glucosamine-containing products obtain glucosamine from the hydrolysis of chitin, a polysaccharide that is a major component of crustacean shells (Horstman and Wood, 1998; Bodewes, 2000; Nutrasense™ Company, 2000; Rexall Sundown, 2000a; Reginster et al., 2001); the chondroitin used in dietary supplements is derived from bovine trachea cartilage (Horstman and Wood, 1998; Bodewes, 2000; Conte et al., 1995) or shark cartilage (Conn et al., 1999; Donohoe, 2000).

12.5. PRODUCTS AVAILABLE

Glucosamine and chondroitin, usually found together in combination products, accounted for over $500 million in retail sales from July 1998 to May 1999 (American Nutraceutical Association, 2000). Most products are capsules, although tablets are also fairly common. Other formulations include softgels, liquids, and chewables. According to the labels, products generally contain 100, 250, 350, 500, 750, or 1500 mg of glucosamine sulfate, glucosamine HCl, or *N*-acetyl glucosamine per tablet or capsule. Chondroitin sulfate content also varies, with each tablet or capsule said to contain 16.7, 20, 200, 250, 400, 500, or 600 mg. Some products also contain manganese, vitamin D, calcium, methylsulfonyl methane (MSM), collagen, B vitamins, vitamin C, niacin, L-arginine zinc, molybdenum, selenium, boron, and/or herbs such as willow bark extract. Manufacturers' dosage recommendations vary widely, but most fall in the range of three to six capsules daily. Some manufacturers recommend decreasing the dose after the first 60 d of therapy.

Osteo Bi-flex® by Rexall Sundown is the industry leader in glucosamine/chondroitin combination product sales (Anonymous, 1999). Regular strength Osteo Bi-flex caplets and softgels contain glucosamine HCl 1500 mg and chondroitin sulfate 1200 mg per six-caplet/softgel serving; this same amount is provided by three of the double strength softgels. Other popular products include Cosamin® DS by Nutramax Laboratories, which contains glucosamine HCl 500 mg, chondroiton sulfate 400 mg, and manganese ascorbate 76 mg (Nutramax Laboratories, 2000d); Schiff's Move Free™ Joint Care Formula, which contains glucosamine HCl and *N*-acetyl D-glucosamine sulfate 500 mg, and chondroitin sulfate 400 mg; and McNeil Consumer Healthcare's Aflexa™, which contains glucosamine 340 mg per 500 mg glucosamine sulfate and glucosamine HCl tablet. Glucosamine and chondroitin products are available in retail stores, pharmacies, and mail order catalogs and via the Internet. Cosamin DS is an exception in that it is available only from pharmacists, physicians, and other health care professionals, although a prescription is not required (Nutramax Laboratories, 2000d).

Nutramax Laboratories also makes Cosequin® DS for large dogs. This product contains the same ingredients as Cosamin DS for humans. Cosequin®, which is half as potent as Cosequin® DS, is available for cats and small dogs (Nutramax Laboratories, 2000a). A Cosamin powder containing glucosamine 1800 mg, chondroitin sulfate 600 mg, and manganese ascorbate 120 mg per scoop is available for horses. Veterinarians are also purportedly using these Cosaquin products for birds and exotic animal species (Nutramax Laboratories, 2000c). Dona™, a glucosamine sulfate powder for oral solution, is approved in several countries as a prescription treatment for OA, and was used in several glucosamine studies. It has been marketed abroad as Dona™, Viartril-S™, and Xicil™. Dona™ is now available in the United States without a prescription from Rotta Pharmaceuticals, Inc.

Glucosamine sulfate contains glucosamine, sulfate, chloride, and sodium in a stoichiometric ratio of 2:1:2:2 (Reginster et al., 2001). Glucosamine hydrochloride is the predominant glucosamine salt found in U.S. products. Because of to the difference in molecular weight between glucosamine sulfate and glucosamine hydrochloride, glucosamine hydrochloride contains approximately one-third more glucosamine per unit weight than glucosamine sulfate.

A study done at the University of Maryland School of Pharmacy and published in the Spring 2000 issue of the *Journal of the American Nutraceutical Association* showed that of 32 chondroitin products tested, only 5 products contained more than 90% of the chondroitin content claimed on the label, and 17 products contained less than 40%. Contents ranged from 0 to 110% of the label claim (American Nutraceutical Association, 2000), as measured by high-performance liqiud chromatography (HPLC). Variability among chondroitin capsules from the same manufacturer was significant, reflecting quality control problems. Fourteen glucosamine or glucosamine/chondroitin products were also analyzed using HPLC (F-D-C Reports, 2000). Twelve products contained at least 90% of the labeled glucosamine content, one contained less than

40%, and one contained approx 70%. Contents ranged from 25 to over 115% of the labeled amounts (American Nutraceutical Association, 2000). The Maryland researchers noted that in general, the less expensive products showed wider variation in content compared with the label (F-D-C Reports, 2000). Based on this information, the American Nutraceutical Association CEO/executive director is calling for the U.S. Pharmacopeia (USP) to develop standards for glucosamine/chondroitin products and other supplements (American Nutraceutical Association, 2000). Subsequently, Consumer Reports found that Now Double Strength Glucosamine and Chondroitin, ArthxDS Glucosamine Chondroitin, Solgar Extra Strength Glucosamine Chondroitin Complex, and Now Chondroitin Sulfate contained less than 90% of the labeled amount of ingredients; 15 other brands were acceptable (Anonymous, 2001b).

ConsumerLab.com's study of glucosamine/chondroitin products yielded similar findings. Twenty-five glucosamine and/or chondroitin products were tested to determine whether the ingredients matched the labeled content. Overall, almost 33% of the tested products failed to meet ConsumerLab.com's standards. Six of 13 glucosamine/chondroitin products did not pass because of low chrondroitin levels (ConsumerLab, 2000). The testing details, as well as a list of products that passed, are available at www.consumerlabs.com. PhytoPharmica's glucosamine sulfate product was one of the products that passed ConsumerLab.com's independent evaluation (PhytoPharmica, 2000).

Inter- and intraproduct inconsistency among glucosamine and chondroitin products suggests that the results of clinical trials, most of which have used European products, may not predict the actual safety and efficacy of glucosamine/chondroitin products available in the United States, and that studies done with one U.S. product cannot be extrapolated to other U.S. products, even if the products appear identical based on the label contents.

12.6. IN VITRO EFFECTS AND ANIMAL DATA

Glucosamine has been shown to increase proteoglycan production in chondrocytes isolated from patients with OA (Bassleer et al., 1998). *N*-acetyl-D-glucosamine, which is found in some glucosamine products, is less active in vitro, presumably because it has less affinity for the enzyme responsible for glucosamine-6-phosphate production (McCarty, 1994). Whether these in vitro differences translate into clinical differences remains to be seen.

The first study demonstrating chondroitin sulfate's effects on cartilage biochemistry examined the synovial fluid aspirated from the knee joints of patients with OA. Eight women were randomized to receive chondroitin sulfate (Chondrosulf®) 800 mg/d for 5 d, five patients (two female) were randomized to this same treatment for 10 d, and five patients (three female) were randomized to placebo. Synovial fluid was aspirated at baseline and at days 5 and 10. An increase in hyaluronan (a cartilage component) and a decrease in the lysosomal enzyme *N*-acetylglucosaminidase compared with baseline were detected in treated but not in control patients. The molecular weight of the hyaluronan increased, suggesting a qualitative as well as a quantitative change in hyaluronan. In addition, there was a decrease in the amount of high molecular weight sulfated glycosaminoglycans in the synovial fluid, the presence of which indicates cartilage breakdown. There was also an increase in the amount of low molecular weight compounds in the synovial fluid, suggesting the presence of exogenously administered chondroitin in the synovial fluid. Leukocyte count and protein content did not change. The criteria used to diagnose OA in these patients was not specified, and the unequal gender distribution among the study groups suggest a problem with the randomization procedure, which was not described (Conte et al., 1995).

The ability of glucosamine/chondroitin to protect dogs from chemically induced synovitis of the radiocarpal joint was assessed in 32 adult mixed-breed dogs (Canapp et al., 1999). One group of dogs received glucosamine/chondroitin for 21 d, and three groups received placebo. Joints were then injected on alternate days for a total of three injections. After induction of synovitis, one group continued to receive placebo, and two were given glucosamine/chondroitin. Lameness was evaluated daily, and nuclear scintigraphy was performed at baseline and on days 13, 20, 27, 34, 41, and 48. Dogs given oral glucosamine/chondroitin prior to chymopapain injection had less joint inflammation by nuclear scintigraphy in days 41 and 48 after joint injection and lower lameness scores in days 12, 19, 23, and 24 after injection compared with the other groups.

The rationale for use of glucosamine and chondroitin in combination stems from glucosamine's ability to stimulate GAG production and chondrointin sulfate's ability to inhibit GAG breakdown, which would theoretically result in a synergistic effect if they were used together. In vitro and animal data presented at the American College of Rheumatology's Annual Scientific Meeting in 1999 support such a synergistic effect.

The reasoning behind inclusion of manganese in some glucosamine/chondroitin products stems from its function as a cofactor for enzymes responsible for GAG synthesis, as well as its function as a cofactor for superoxide dismutase, an enzyme that inactivates oxygen free radicals, thus inhibiting oxidative tissue damage. Unrecognized manganese deficiency may be involved in the pathogenesis of OA (Das and Hammad, 2000).

12.7. CLINICAL STUDIES

Interest in glucosamine and chondroitin has focused on their potential as treatments for OA. OA is primarily a disorder of the hyaline cartilage, which coats the bony surface of synovial joints. Hyaline cartilage is a matrix of collagen, proteoglycans, and chondrocytes, which produce the matrix, and water (March, 1997). Proteoglycans (PGs) have a protein core and many negatively charged GAG chains, which allow it to retain water. Under pressure from load bearing, the hydrated PG gel releases water, thus serving as a "shock absorber." In OA, there is a decrease in cartilage PG accompanied by a decrease in compressibility, exposing the underlying bone to stresses that stimulate hypertrophic repair with resulting bone remodeling and limitation of joint motion. The pathogenesis of OA involves mechanical stress with an accompanying imbalance between cartilage degeneration and normal repair. In osteoarthritis, levels of chondrocyte-derived metalloproteinases such as stromelysin and collagenase, which are responsible for removal of both normal and abnormal cartilage, increase more rapidly than endogenous inhibitors, resulting in a net loss of PGs. Interleukin-1 (IL-1), IL-6, and tumor necrosis factor-α (TNF-α) may be involved in suppression of normal chrondrocyte function, leading to deceased synthesis of collagen and proteoglycans, increased production of degradative enzymes, and inhibition of chondrocyte proliferation (Pinals, 1996). Glucosamine and chondroitin sulfate are substrates for GAG synthesis; they also stimulate GAG synthesis and inhibit its degradation (Morreale et al., 1996; Talent and Garcy, 1996). Glucosamine may also have antiinflammatory activity (Talent and Garcy, 1996). There has been great interest in using these compounds in the treatment of OA, and hence these studies will be described in some detail.

Studies of OA have been noted to have deficiencies that hinder one's ability to make reliable interpretations of the literature. OA studies may lack both a standardized diagnosis and a standardized outcome assessment. For example, several studies do not present specific diagnostic criteria, but instead make the ambiguous statement that the patient suffers from OA. In addition, although common variables measured include pain and range of motion, the methods used to measure these variables differ. Even though standardized, validated instruments exist to measure these variables, they are not uniformly used (Towheed and Hochberg, 1997). Other basic requirements of a quality drug study include randomization, blinding, and use of controls to minimize bias. Reasons for choosing the number of subjects studied, and the inclusion as well as the exclusion criteria, should be explained. In addition, all subjects should receive the same active treatment; thus, patients taking medications that could confound the results should be excluded from participation, or analysis of covariance should be used to take into account the effects of other treatments. The investigators should have a means of measuring compliance with the prescribed regimen and confirming that patients did not take medications that could confound the study results. The investigators should clearly state the primary outcome measures, explain how they are to be measured, and discuss the appropriateness of the instruments used to measure the variables. Finally, data should be treated with the appropriate statistical tests, and dropouts should be included in the analysis (Mosdell, 1996).

The International League Against Rheumatism classifies glucosamine and chondrotin as a slow-acting drugs for osteoarthritis (SADOA). SADOAs improve pain and perhaps function after a delay (several weeks or months), and the benefits persist for at least one mo after the drug is discontinued. Studies of SADOAs, therefore, should focus on pain and function as primary outcomes. SADOAs should be distinguished from disease-modifying osteoarthritis drugs (DMOADs), which prevent, slow, or reverse the morphologic joint and cartilage changes in OA. In studies of DMOADs, primary outcome measures are radiographic changes, such as joint space narrowing (Runkel and Cupp, 1999).

Although all the studies conducted thus far have been favorable toward glucosamine and chondroitin, the conclusions that can be drawn are limited by poor study design. A recent quality assessment and metaanalysis of glucosamine and chondroitin studies (McAlindon et al., 2000) included three of the chondroitin studies reviewed here (Bourgeois et al., 1998; Busci and Poor 1998; Uebelhart et al., 1998). Six other studies were included but are not reviewed in this chapter because two utilized an intramuscular product and four were not published in English. McAlindon et al. (2000) also analyzed three of the glucosamine studies reviewed in this monograph (Pujalte et al., 1980; Noack et al., 1994; Houpt et al., 1999), plus two others not reviewed here because they employed parenteral routes of administration. Two subsequently published glucosamine studies with negative results were not included in the analysis (Hughes and Chertsey, 2000; Rindone et al., 2000). McAlindon and colleagues concluded that although these preparations are probably effective to some degree, the benefits are probably overstated due to quality issues and publication bias. An additional metaanalysis of chondroitin sulfate for OA (Leeb et al., 2000) included four of the chondroitin studies reviewed here (Morreale et al., 1996; Bourgeois et al., 1998; Busci and Poor, 1998; Uebelhardt et al., 1998) plus three others. Nine studies examined by Leeb and colleagues, including the study by Verbruggen and colleagues (1998) reviewed here, were excluded from the metaanalysis because of design flaws. The authors concluded that although chondroitin may be useful in OA, larger, long-term studies are needed to prove its efficacy. A multicenter study sponsored by the National Institutes of Health comparing glucosamine/chondroitin, glucosamine alone, and placebo in 1000 patients began enrolling patients in February 2000. Outcome measures include pain and function. Unfortunately, the study is only 16 wk in duration (Anonymous, 2000) and will not answer questions about long-term efficacy and safety.

Although intramuscular administration of both glucosamine and chondrotin, as well as intraarticular administration of glucosamine, have been studied, only studies in which these products were administered orally will be reviewed here.

12.7.1. Glucosamine vs Placebo for Osteoarthritis

Drovanti and colleagues (1980) conducted a placebo-controlled, double-blind study comparing oral glucosamine (Viartril-S®, Rotta Pharmaceuticals, Monza, Italy) 500 mg tid vs placebo for 30 d in 80 patients. Pain, tenderness, swelling, and restriction of movement were rated on a scale of 0 to 4 each wk. Using Fisher's exact test, it was determined that significantly more patients in the glucosamine group experienced complete pain relief or freedom from restricted function. In addition, treated patients experienced a 72% reduction in total symptom score from baseline compared with a 36% reduction in the placebo group. A similar pattern of improvement was seen with each symptom. Using the Wilcoxon signed-rank test, the authors determined that both groups experienced a significant reduction in symptoms compared with baseline ($p < 0.001$) and also concluded using a Student's t-test, that glucosamine produced a significantly larger decrease in a significantly shorter time ($p < 0.001$). At study completion, electron microscopy revealed that cartilage samples taken from two patients in the glucosamine group more closely resembled normal cartilage than cartilage taken from two placebo patients, but the investigators did not compare cartilage samples before and after treatment. Nausea and heartburn were reported once in the glucosamine group, and constipation was reported twice.

In a study by D'Ambrosio and colleagues (1981), 30 inpatients who had not received antiinflammatory drugs in the 2 wk prior to study enrollment were randomized to receive either 400 mg parenteral glucosamine sulfate or piperazine/chlorbutanol (an antiarthritic drug used in Italy that is visually indistinguishable from glucosamine). The active treatments were administered daily for 1 wk, followed by 14 d of oral glucosamine 500 mg tid in the glucosamine group, or 14 d of placebo in the piperazine/chlorbutanol group. Pain at rest, pain during passive and active movements, and limitation of articular function were scored on a scale of 0–3 at baseline and at days 7 and 21. The overall symptom score decreased by 58% during parenteral glucosamine therapy and by 13% more with oral therapy. Using the Mann-Whitney U-test, the authors found that this decrease was significantly larger ($p < 0.05$ at day 7 and $p < 0.01$ and day 21) than that reported in the other group, which experienced a 31% decrease in symptom score during piperazine/chlorbutanol therapy, a benefit that was lost during oral placebo treatment. Patterns of improvement were reportedly seen for each symptom measurement. No adverse effects were reported in either treatment group.

Crolle and D'Este (1980) evaluated 30 inpatients using the same study design as D'Ambrosio and colleagues described above. A trend toward greater improvement in the glucosamine group was reported at day 7, which reached statistical significance ($p < 0.01$) at day 21 per the chi-square test. Four subjects enrolled in this study had circulatory disorders, three had liver disorders, and two had diabetes. Five subjects were taking antibiotics, two were taking antidepressants, and five were taking "treatments for lung disorders." The authors noted no interaction between glucosamine and these diseases or medications, and no adverse effects were reported.

A double-blind evaluation of oral glucosamine sulfate (Viartril-S) 500 mg tid vs placebo was conducted by Pujalte and colleagues (1980) in 20 outpatients with OA of the knee. Pain, tenderness, swelling, and degree of movement restriction were rated on a scale of 0–4 by physician and self-assessment prior to treatment and every 3 d for 6–8 wk during treatment. At the end of the study, the symptom scores were averaged and treated with the Student's *t*-test and analysis of variance. A significant alleviation of pain, tenderness, and swelling was reported in the glucosamine group compared with the placebo group ($p < 0.01$). There was a trend toward greater improvement in the glucosamine group in movement restriction; the authors attributed the lack of statistical significance to patients having only mild baseline movement restriction. Patients treated with glucosamine experienced earlier alleviation of pain, tenderness, and swelling compared with the placebo group according to the Student's *t*-test ($p < 0.01$). The Fischer's exact test was used to determine that a significantly larger proportion of patients experienced decreased pain, tenderness ($p = 0.005$), and swelling ($p = 0.004$). There were no complaints of adverse effects in the glucosamine group.

The safety and efficacy of glucosamine sulfate (Dona® 200-S, Opfermann Arzneimittel, Wiehl, Germany) 500 mg three times daily were compared with that of placebo in a double-blind, randomized, multicenter study in 252 ambulatory outpatients with OA of the knee (Noack et al., 1994). Inclusion criteria were uni- or bilateral OA without signs or symptoms of inflammation. Patients had to have been symptomatic for at least 6 mo and were diagnosed using Lequesne's clinical and radiologic criteria. Radiographic grading was done using Jäger and Wirth's classification system, a modification of the Kellgren and Lawrence system that assesses progression of joint space narrowing, increase in subchondral sclerosis, and development of osteophytes and subchondral cysts. For inclusion, radiographic stage had to be I–III, with a Lequesne index of at least 4. Patients were excluded who had received intraarticular corticosteroids within 2 mo of enrollment, had used nonsteroidal anti-inflammatory drugs (NSAIDs) within 2 wk of enrollment, had had recent knee trauma, were over- or underweight, or had a clinically important hematologic, hepatic, or renal abnormality. OA treatments (including analgesics, corticosteroids, and physical therapy) were not allowed during the study.

Efficacy measures included weekly Lequesne index and the investigator's overall efficacy assessment (good, moderate, unchanged, worse) at the end of the 4-wk treatment period. The main outcome measure was the number of treatment responders in each group, defined as patients with a decrease in the Lequesne index of at least 3 points, and an overall assessment of moderate or good. Safety measures included urinalysis, blood chemistry, hematology, heart rate, blood pressure, and weight. Subjects were also asked weekly if they had experienced any adverse effects and were asked to classify any events as mild, moderate, or severe. One hundred twenty-six subjects were randomized to each treatment group. This sample size was calculated to be adequate to have 80% power to detect a statistically significant difference between groups. Success rates were compared using Fisher's exact test. Differences between mean Lequesne index scores at each clinic visit were compared using t-tests. Laboratory data were analyzed using McNemar Shift test. Adverse effects and dropout rates were assessed using Fisher's exact test. Data analysis was performed both by excluding dropouts and by intent-to-treat analysis. Demographic and baseline data were found to be comparable between the two groups using chi-square or t-tests as appropriate for the type of data being assessed.

There were more responders (55%) in the glucosamine group than in the placebo group (38%) ($p < = 0.014$), and the Lequesne index was lower at week 4 in the glucosamine group ($p < 0.05$). This latter significant finding may have been a spurious result of using multiple t-tests. Using the intent-to-treat approach, the response rate was 52% in the glucosamine group and 37% in the placebo group ($p = 0.016$). The investigators also analyzed the data after grouping patients according to baseline severity per the Lequesne index, but this maneuver did not change the outcome, perhaps due to small sample size in each group. Five patients in the glucosamine group reported gastrointestinal disturbances, two reported headache, and one reported itching.

Glucosamine HCl (Phanstiehl Laboratories) 500 mg tid was compared with placebo in 118 patients with OA of the knee (Houpt et al., 1999). Subjects were recruited through a newspaper advertisement and were included based on degree of pain, disease effect on activities of daily living, physical exam, and X-ray findings. Primary outcome measures included total scores on the Western Ontario and McMaster University Osteoarthritis Index [WOMAC; a visual analog scalde (VAS)] and its subscales for pain, stiffness, and function. The WOMAC was completed at baseline (week –2), week 0, and week 8. Secondary outcome measures were pain improvement recorded in a daily diary (–1, 0, +1), improvement on knee examination, and patients' perception at the end of the study of which product they had taken. Patients were excluded if they required a cane or other assistive device to walk, had ever taken glucosamine or corticosteroids, or had had an intra-articular injection within the past 6 mo. Acetaminophen 500 mg, supplied by the investigators, was allowed as rescue medication. Patients recorded acetaminophen use and side effects daily. Prior to the 2-wk run-in, patients were randomized to placebo or glucosamine using a computer. There were no significant differences at baseline between the two groups in regard to age, sex, weight, duration of symptoms, analgesic use prior to study, WOMAC, pain over the month prior to the trial, pain at week 0, and radiologic score. Seventeen patients dropped out during the run-in, and two placebo patients and one glucosamine patient withdrew during the study period. The investigators calculated that at least 47 patients in each treatment group would be necessary to detect a difference. Intent-to-treat analysis was used. Fisher's exact test was used to compare improvement on knee exam and the number of patients in each group who correctly guessed which treatment they were receiving. To assess number of acetaminophen tablets used, pain diary scores, and WOMAC scores, *t*-tests were used. The Mann-Whitney U test was also used to confirm the validity of the *t*-test.

Results of the pain diary and knee exam suggested improvement in the glucosamine vs placebo group. There was no significant difference between the groups in regard to acetaminophen use, total WOMAC score, or WOMAC subscale scores. The authors of a subsequent study (Das and Hammad, 2000) suggest that the VAS WOMAC might not be an appropriate assessment tool for efficacy of an slow-acting agent such as glucosamine, which provides subtle improvement over the course of several months, because there may be high intrapatient variability in rating over time, independent of disease severity, causing score variability and a resulting lack of statistically significant improvement. There was no difference between groups in the number of patients who correctly guessed which treatment they had been receiving. Adverse gastrointestinal effects (gas, cramps, bloating) occurred in approx 12% of patients in each group. The investigators point out that these symptoms may have been caused by the Krafen whey used in the placebo capsules and as a filler in the glucosamine capsules.

Hughes and Chertsey (2000) found no significant difference between glucosamine sulfate 1500 mg/d and placebo in their 6-mo study measuring global pain, pain at rest, and pain with movement using a 100-mm VAS, range of movement, the McGill Pain Questionnaire, WOMAC, and need for rescue medication. There was a large placebo response. Subgroup analysis suggested that patients with mild-to-moderate pain may benefit from glucosamine. Glucosamine was well tolerated.

Glucosamine 500 mg (Applehart Laboratories, Bedford, NH) tid was compared with placebo in a double-blind study (Rindone et al., 2000). Inclusion criteria were a history of OA of the knee and grade 1–4 arthropathy on knee radiographs evaluated by a radiologist blinded to the purpose of the study. Grading was based on criteria described by Kellgren and Lawrence: grade 0 = normal; grade 1 = doubtful narrowing of the joint space and possible osteophytic lipping; grade 2 (mild) = definite osteophytes and possible joint space narrowing; grade 3 (moderate) = moderate multiple osteophytes, definite joint space narrowing, some sclerosis, and possible deformity of bone contour; and grade 4 (severe) = large osteophytes, marked joint space narrowing, severe sclerosis, and definite deformity of bone contour (Das and Hammad, 2000). Patients who had previously taken glucosamine and/or chondroitin and those who were not ambulatory were excluded. Subjects were randomized using a computer-generated list of random numbers. Treatment was continued for 2 mo. Patients were permitted to use other analgesics during the study. Subjects were evaluated at baseline and at days 30 and 60. Pain was assessed at rest and while walking using a 10 cm VAS. Adverse effects were also assessed at each visit.

Age, baseline VAS, and duration of OA were assessed using the independent Student's *t*-test, and a z-test was used to analyze percentage of patients taking analgesics and percentage of patients with each radiographic stage. These data did not differ between the treatment groups. Changes in scores from baseline were assessed using one-way ANOVA. One hundred fourteen patients were enrolled. Five patients in each group were lost to follow-up and were not included in the data analysis. Six patients dropped out owing to adverse effects, but the investigators did not note whether their data was included in the analysis. According to the investigators' calculation, 100 patients would be required to detect an absolute difference of 1.1 on the VAS. Data were analyzed on 98 patients, 49 in each group. No significant difference was noted between the study groups in regard to resting and walking pain at either of the assessments on day 30 or day 60. There was also no difference between the groups in regard to mean change in scores from baseline. Seventeen glucosamine patients and 11 placebo patients experienced adverse effects. Most side effects were mild and self-limiting and included loose stools, nausea, heartburn, and headache. Two glucosamine patients dropped out owing to diarrhea (1 patient) and dizziness (1 patient), which resolved with product discontinuation. Four patients in the placebo group withdrew because of rash, sedation, diarrhea, and constipation.

In a 3-yr study designed to assess whether glucosamine can modify disease progression (Pavelka et al., 2000), 202 patients were randomized to glucosamine sulfate 1500 mg/d or placebo. Joint space width was measured using weight bearing, full extension, antero-posterior radiographs of the narrowest medial compartment of the tibiofemoral joint. Symptoms were assessed using the WOMAC. Joint space narrowing did not occur in the treatment group but increased by a mean of 0.2 mm in the placebo group ($p = 0.002$, ANOVA). The WOMAC score improved significantly more in the glucosamine group ($p = 0.01$).

A study designed to assess the long-term efficacy of glucosamine sulfate 1500 mg once daily on OA progression (Reginster et al., 2001) utilized the Italian product marketed as Dona, Vitartril-S, or Xilcil® (Rotta Research Group, Monza, Italy) and approved in several countries as a prescription treatment for OA. The product was administered as a powder for oral solution. Patients at least 50 yr of age with primary knee OA affecting the medial femorotibial joint (MFTJ) compartment were diagnosed using American College of Rheumatology criteria. Severity was graded using the Kellgren and Lawrence radiographic system. Exclusion criteria were history of rheumatic disease with an OA component; articular inflammation on physical exam; erythrocyte sedimentation rate more than 40 mm/h; rheumatoid factor titer more than 1:40; knee trauma; body mass index more than 30; abnormal hemtologic, hepatic, renal, or metabolic function; or corticosteroid use within the past 3 mo. Patients were randomized to glucosamine or placebo for 3 yr. Acetaminophen 500 mg, diclofenac 50 mg, piroxicam 20 mg, or proglumetacin (an NSAID available in Europe) 150 mg were allowed as rescue medications. Patients recorded use of rescue medications in a diary.

Primary outcome measures were the mean and minimum change in the joint space width in the narrowest MFTJ compartment measured using automated analysis of digitized X-rays taken at baseline at at years 1 and 3. OA symptoms were measured using the visual analog version of the WOMAC. Secondary outcome measures were use of rescue medications, withdrawal rates, adverse effects, effects on yearly routine lab tests including fasting glucose, and number of patients experiencing marked structural damage progression, defined as joint space narrowing of more than 0.5 mm. It was calculated that at least 60 patients in each group were necessary to detect a 0.5 mm difference in joint space narrowing with 80% power and statistical significance accepted at *p* 0.05. One hundred six patients were randomized to each group to allow for dropouts. Two methods of intent-to-treat analysis were used to handle data in dropouts: (1) carrying the last observation forward; and (2) as a worst-case scenario, assignment of the average change recorded in the placebo group to the dropouts. ANOVA was used to analyze change in joint space narrowing and WOMAC scores, mean number of days during which rescue medication was needed, and continuous baseline data. Chi-square was used to analyze the proportion of patients in each group with marked structural damage progression and categorical baseline characteristics. Either chi-square or Fisher's exact test, as appropriate, was used to assess adverse effects and dropout rates. The Spearman correlation test was used to determine correlation between joint space narrowing and symptoms. Two hundred twelve patients were enrolled in the study, with 36% and 33% of patients dropping out of the glucosamine and placebo groups, respectively, over the 3-yr study period ($p = 0.77$). Patients in the two groups were similar in baseline characteristics.

At the end of the study, minimum joint space narrowing ($p = 0.003$) and mean joint space narrowing ($p = 0.043$) were significantly less in the glucosamine group using the worst-case-scenario intent-to-treat analysis. The change from baseline in the WOMAC pain score ($p < 0.047$) and the WOMAC physical function score $p = 0.02$) were significantly greater in the glucosamine group. There was no correlation between symptom improvement or use of rescue medication and radiographic findings. There were no significant differences between the two groups in use of rescue medications, adverse effects, and laboratory tests. The investigators concluded that the results suggest that glucosamine may be a disease modifying treatment for OA.

12.7.2. Glucosamine vs Ibuprofen for Osteoarthritis

Vaz (1982) compared ibuprofen 400 mg tid with oral glucosamine sulfate 500 mg tid in 40 outpatients with OA of the knee in an 8-wk study. Pain was assessed using a scale of 0–3 at baseline and at weeks 1, 2, 4, and 8. Although ibuprofen had significantly decreased pain scores compared with baseline and compared with glucosamine by the end of the first week ($p < 0.001$ Student's *t*-test), glucosamine was superior to ibuprofen at week eight ($p < 0.05$). One patient taking glucosamine and two taking ibuprofen reported heartburn and epigastric pain; one patient taking glucosamine reported nausea; and a patient taking ibuprofen reported abdominal pain and headache.

Glucosamine sulfate 500 mg three times daily was compared with ibuprofen 400 mg three times daily in a 4-wk randomized, double-blind study (Müller-Faßbender et al., 1994). Inclusion criteria were mild symptoms of uni- or bilateral OA of the knee for at least 3 mo and a Lequesne index of at least 7. Patients with important hematologic abnormalities, liver or kidney disease, peptic ulcer disease, NSAID allergy, recent injury to the knee, corticosteroid injection of the knee within the preceding 2 mo, or habitual use of NSAIDs during the past 2 mo were excluded. Patients were institutionalized for physical therapy during the study. Use of medications for OA was prohibited. The investigators calculated that 180 patients would be needed in order to have an 80% chance of detecting a statistically significant difference between groups. Two hundred patients were enrolled. Almost all patients participated in physical therapy during the study.

The primary outcome measure was the Lequesne index, modified to allow assessment of pain in both knees. Other outcome measures included overall efficacy judged by the investigators as good, moderate, or poor, erythrocyte sedimentation rate, and hematology. Responders were defined as subjects with "good" overall efficacy plus a decrease in the Lequesne index of at least 2 points, or 1 point if the baseline score was 12 or less. Success rates were compared weekly using Fisher's exact test with Bonferroni's correction for repeated measures. Statistical significance was accepted when $p < 0.0125$. Differences between mean Lequesne index scores at each clinic visit were compared using t-tests. Laboratory data were analyzed using the McNemar shift test. Adverse effects were assessed using Fisher's exact test. Demographic and baseline data were found to be comparable between the two groups using chi-square or t-tests, as appropriate. One patient in the ibuprofen group was excluded after randomization, and four additional ibuprofen and six glucosamine sulfate patients were excluded owing to use of prohibited analgesics. These patients were given negative overall efficacy assessments for purposes of the intent-to-treat analysis.

Although the number of responders was higher in the ibuprofen group at week 1, suggesting quicker improvement with ibuoprofen, response did not differ significantly between groups. Lequesne index scores were also comparable between groups, with a mean decrease of 6 points by week 6. Glucosamine was better tolerated than ibuprofen, with 35% of the subjects in the ibuprofen group reporting adverse effects vs 6% in the glucosamine group ($p < 0.001$). Gastrointestinal disturbances ($n = 5$) and a dermatologic reaction ($n = 1$) were the only treatment-emergent adverse events reported in the glucosamine group. The investigators concluded that glucosamine is at least as effective as ibuprofen for symptom relief in paients with OA of the knee and is better tolerated. Hospitalization of patients and use of physical therapy limits the applicability of the results to typical outpatients.

Investigators compared glucosamine sulfate 500 mg tid (Viartril-S) with ibuprofen 400 mg tid in a 4-wk, double-blind, double-dummy study in 178 Chinese patients with OA of the knee (Qiu et al., 1998). After randomization, patients took the study treatment for 4 wk. Knee pain at rest, pain with movement, and tenderness with pressure were assessed on a scale of 0–3 before treatment, after 2 and 4 wk of treatment, and 2 wk after treatment completion. Knee swelling was also assessed on a scale of 0–3 at these same intervals. At the end of the treatment period and at 2-wk follow-up, the investigator rated improvement as "worsened, unchanged, improved, or definitely improved" and also rated the treatment's therapeutic utility (benefits vs disadvantages) as "unclear, none, moderate, or good." Adverse effects (symptoms, laboratory abnormalities), their severity, and their causality were assessed at each visit. An overall evaluation of safety was scored on a scale of 0–3. Data were treated with the Mann-Whitney U-test (ibuprofen vs glucosamine) and the Wilcoxon signed-rank test (treatment vs baseline). One patient in the glucosamine group withdrew from the study, and nine ibuprofen patients withdrew owing to adverse effects. Dropouts were not included in the analysis.

Although both treatments decreased knee pain and knee swelling compared with baseline ($p < 0.0001$), the difference between the two groups was not statistically significant. In regard to improvement, the difference between the two groups was not significant at the end of treatment, but the glucosamine patients had better improvement ratings 2 wk after study completion than the ibuprofen patients ($p = 0.01$), suggesting a continued therapeutic effect even after glucosamine discontinuation. Therapeutic utility did not differ between the two treatments ($p = 0.08$). The overall evaluation of safety was better for the glucosamine group ($p = 0.01$). Adverse effects in the glucosamine group included mild stomach discomfort (three patients), mild sleepiness (one patient), and mild nausea (one patient). Fourteen patients in the ibuprofen group experienced adverse effects.

Most of the previously described studies were limited to patients with OA of the knee. A study compared glucosamine sulfate 500 mg (Jamieson™, Windsor, Ontario, Canada) with ibuprofen 400 mg in pain reduction in patients with OA of the temporomandibular joint (Thie et al., 2001). The primary outcome measure was a 20% or greater decrease in functional joint pain on the colored analog scale (CAS; a validated and reliable modified VAS). Secondary outcome measures were pain-free and maximum jaw opening; Brief Pain Inventory (BPI) score, which measures pain intensity and effect of pain on quality of life; and masticatory muscle tenderness, measured using a pressure threshold meter. Patients were recruited from an orofacial pain clinic, through mailings to dentists, and through a newspaper advertisement. The diagnosis of OA was confirmed by X-ray. Other exclusion criteria were baseline pain less than 3 on a VAS, age less than 18 yr, pregnancy, lactation, previous intraarticular corticosteroid or hyaluronic acid injections, NSAID allergy, congestive heart failure, kidney failure, liver failure, peptic ulceration or bleeding, coagulation disorders, previous use of glucosamine or chondroitin, and active dental disease. Patients taking an antidepressant or anxiolytic must have been taking it for at least 6 mo prior to enrolment, and use of any oral splint must have commenced at least 3 mo prior to enrolment. Forty-five subjects were enrolled. There was a 1-wk washout for all patients to eliminate any carryover effects from NSAID use.

Patients were randomized to one of the two treatment groups. Baseline patient characteristics were similar between groups. Subjects took the study medication every 8 h with food for 90 d. Acetaminophen 500 mg was supplied for use as a rescue medication. Use of rescue medication was assessed every 30 d by pill count. Four patients in the ibuprofen group and two patients in the gluosamine group dropped out. In the ibuprofen group, three dropouts did not complete the study because of stomach upset, and one dropped out because of lack of pain control. One of the dropouts in the glucosamine group experienced dizziness, and the other complained of stomach upset. Yates' corrected chi-square or Fisher's exact test, as appropriate, was used to compare frequency, and paired or independent sample *t*-tests were used for parametric data.

There was no significant difference in the number of patients in the two groups who met the primary endpoint ($p = 0.73$). For the subgroup of patients who experienced at least a 20% reduction in joint pain with function (i.e., patients who met the primary endpoint), between-group analysis showed a greater reduction in functional pain ($p = 0.017$) and effect of pain on quality of life ($p = 0.049$) in the glucosamine group. Use of rescue medication from days 90 to 120 (the 30 d following the supplementation period) was lower ($p = 0.009$) in the glucosamine group, suggesting glucosamine has a carryover effect after treatment is discontinued.

Of the glucosamine studies presented above, all but the study by Reginster and colleagues (2001) were of short duration and included a relatively small number of patients. All studies presented patient sex, age, and baseline symptom scores, and Houpt and colleagues (1999), Rindone and associates (2000), Reginster and colleagues (2001) explained the diagnostic criteria used to determine whether the study subjects were suffering from OA. In addition, Houpt and colleagues (1999) and Rindone and associates (2000) reported clinical and radiographic severity at baseline, weight, and disease duration. Thie and colleagues (2001) reported disease duration. Reginster and colleagues (2001) reported body mass index. Drovanti and colleagues (1980), Pujalte and colleagues (1980), Vaz (1982), Qiu and associates (1998), Houpt and colleagues (1999), Rindone and colleagues (2000), Reginster and associates (2001), and Thie and colleagues (2001) reported location of the affected joint. Such baseline data allows one to assess the similarity of the glucosamine-treated patients to the control patients and to compare the study patients with the OA population at large.

Some studies used inpatients (Drovanti et al., 1980; Crolle and D'Este 1980; D'Ambrosio et al., 1981; Müller-Faßbender et al., 1994) rather than outpatients (Pujalte et al., 1980; Vaz, 1982; Houpt et al., 1999; Qiu et al., 1998; Rindone et al., 2000; Reginster et al., 2001; Thie et al., 2001); the former might have benefited simply from inactivity or physical therapy provided in the hospital setting. Only Houpt and colleagues (1999) and Reginster and associates (2001) assessed compliance with the prescribed regimen. Although Pujalte and associates (1980) and Houpt and colleagues (1999) excluded patients taking other medications for OA, they did not confirm that patients were not taking other medications throughout the study period; Müller-Faßbender and associates (1994) appeared to do so. Reginster and colleagues (2001) excluded patients who had received coritcosteroids within the 3 mo prior to enrollment. A variety of rescue medications were allowed, although a washout of 5 half-lives was required prior to assessment. Thie and colleagues (2001) provided a 1-wk NSAID washout prior to beginning the study. Müller-Faßbender and colleagues (1994) excluded patients who had used NSAIDs habitually within the previous 2 mo but did not define habitual use. D'Ambrosio and colleagues (1981), Crolle and D'Este (1980), and Noack and associates (1994) excluded patients who had taken NSAIDs within the 2 wk prior to enrollment, but a 2-wk washout from corticosteroids use, as provided by D'Ambrosio and colleagues (1981) and Crolle and D'Este (1980), may not have been adequate for this drug class. These investigators did not report the number of previous corticosteroid users in each treatment group. Noack and associates (1994) and Müller-Faßbender and colleagues (1994) excluded patients who had received intraarticular corticosteroids within the 2 mo prior to enrollment.

Only Houpt and colleagues (1999), Reginster and associates (2001), and Thie and colleagues (2001) explained how the study subjects were recruited. Müller-Faßbender and colleagues (1994), Noack and associates (1994), Houpt and colleagues (1999), Rindone and associates (2000), Das and Hammad (2000), and Reginster and colleagues (2001) explained how they determined the number of subjects to include in the study.

Statistical treatment of data also contributes to difficulty in assessing these studies. Even though all studies used ordinal (e.g., symptom) scores, which cannot be averaged or manipulated mathematically, the statistical significance of the results was often assessed by comparing the mean scores of each group using Student's *t*-test (Drovanti et al., 1980; Pujalte et al., 1980; Vaz, 1981; Müller-Faßbender et al., 1994; Houpt et al., 1999; Thie et al., 2001), which should ideally be used only for parametric data (Kier, 1996). Pujalte and colleagues (1980), Rindone and associates (2000), and Reginster and colleagues (2001) used analysis of variance (a parametric test) to assess the significance of the change in mean symptom score (nonparametric data) (Kier, 1996). In the studies of Rindone et al. (2000), Reginster and colleagues (2001), and Thie and associates (2001), use of such parametric tests may have been justified because symptoms were assessed using a VAS, which is customarily treated as continuous data. Crolle and D'Este (1980) used the chi-square test to measure the difference in mean symptom scores in the glucosamine vs the control group at each assessment point, although the chi-square test is appropriate only for nominal data and is not appropriate for repeated measures (Kier, 1996). Appropriate tests for assessing ordinal data include the Mann-Whitney U-test for independent samples and the Wilcoxon signed rank tests for paired samples. These tests were correctly used in some studies (Drovanti et al., 1980; D'Ambrosio et al., 1981; Qiu et al., 1998; Houpt et al., 1999). Müller-Faßbender and associates (1994), Noack and colleagues (1994), Houpt and colleagues (1999), Reginster and colleagues (2001), and Thie and associates (2001) appropriately used Fisher's exact test for nominal data.

The intent-to-treat analysis, in which dropouts were included, was used by Müller-Faßbender and colleagues (1994), Noack and associates (1994), Houpt and associates (1998), and Reginster and colleagues (2001), whereas Vaz (1981), Pujalte and colleagues (1980), Qiu and associates (1998), and Rindone and colleagues (2000) excluded dropouts from the statistical analyses. The other investigators did not address treatment of dropouts.

Despite the statistical and design limitations of these studies, overall, the results suggest that glucosamine is effective in relieving pain and perhaps slowing disease progression. It is important to note that several studies used parenteral glucosamine or glucosamine products not commonly available in the United States, thus limiting the ability to extrapolate the results of these studies to most glucosamine supplements sold in the United States. As discussed under the Products Available, section above, glucosamine hydrochloride is more commonly found in U.S. products than is glucosamine sulfate, which was the form of glucosamine used in most published studies.

12.7.3. Chondroitin Sulfate for Osteoarthritis

In a 6-mo, double-blind, randomized study (Morreale et al., 1996), 146 patients with mono- or bilateral grade I or II OA of the knee were randomized to receive diclofenac 50-mg tablets tid plus placebo chrondroitin powder sachets for 1 mo, followed by a 1-mo treatment with placebo sachets alone, or placebo diclofenac tablets plus chondroitin sulfate powder 400 mg tid for 1 mo, followed by 1 mo of chondroitin sulfate 400 mg TID. Both groups were then treated with placebo sachets for 2 mo. Patients were allowed to take acetaminophen 500 mg as needed for pain and were instructed to record their acetaminophen use in a patient diary. Patients were assessed at baseline and at days 10, 20, 30, 45, 60, 90, 120, and 180. At each visit, the Lequesne index was used to assess treatment efficacy. Spontaneous pain was measured using the Huskisson VAS, and pain on loading was assessed on a 4-point VAS. The number of acetaminophen doses used was evaluated, and compliance was assessed by "pill counting" and rated on a 4-point ordinal scale. At the end of the study, the investigators were asked to make a global judgment of the patients' response to therapy. All adverse effects were recorded, regardless of causality. Analysis of variance with Bonferroni *t*-tests was used for analysis of the Lequesne index score, spontaneous pain, pain on loading, and intake of acetaminophen. In testing for intergroup differences, the Mann-Whitney U-test was used for categorical variables, and the two-tailed Student's *t*-test was used for continuous variables. At baseline, the two groups were similar in patient age, sex, disease severity, Lequesne index score, spontaneous pain, pain on loading, and acetaminophen use. Twenty patients withdrew from the study; 2 (1 from each group) withdrew owing to severe gastrointestinal side effects, 3 (1 from the chondroitin group and 2 from the diclofenac group) because of perceived lack of efficacy, and 15 for logistical reasons. Dropouts were not included in the data analysis.

At days 20 and 30, diclofenac was superior to chrondroitin sulfate in decreasing the Lequesne index score compared to baseline ($p < 0.01$). After the first month, the Lequense score stabilized, then worsened in the diclofenac group, but continued to improve in the chrondroitin group; on days 60 and 90, the Lequense score was significantly ($p < 0.01$) lower in the chondroitin group. Similar results were seen with pain on loading; during the first month of treatment, there was a greater reduction in pain on loading in the diclofenac group ($p < 0.01$), but the chondroitin group experienced a greater reduction at days 60 and 90 ($p < 0.01$). During the 3-mo placebo period, there was an increase in pain on loading in both groups, but the pain score remained higher in the diclofenac group during this period ($p < 0.01$). The chondroitin group experienced superior relief of spontaneous pain on days 120, 150, and 180 ($p < 0.01$). Acetaminophen intake paralleled the improvements in Lequesne index, pain on load, and spontaneous pain; intake was higher in the chondroitin group on days 10 ($p < 0.05$) and 20 ($p < 0.01$), but on days 30 and 60 there was no significant difference between the two groups. During 3-mo placebo phase, intake was significantly higher in the diclofenac group ($p < 0.01$). The authors concluded that although chondroitin sulfate was associated with a slow onset in effect, its therapeutic effects lasted even after suspension of treatment. The physicians' overall efficacy assessment was in favor of the chondroitin group ($p < 0.01$). In regard to adverse effects, three patients in the chondroitin group and two patients in the diclofenac group reported epigastric burning or pain, and one patient in the diclofenac group complained of nausea.

Chondroitin 4- and 6-sulfate [Chondrosulf, Institut Biochimique SA (IBSA), Lugano, Switzerland] in sachets of oral gel 1200 mg qd, 400-mg capsules tid, and placebo were compared in a 3-mo, double-blind, double-dummy study in 127 patients with OA of the knee (Bourgeois et al., 1998). Patients older than 45 yr with stage I–III OA taking an "authorized" NSAID at stable doses for at least 1 mo were eligible. Exclusion criteria included peptic ulcer disease, renal dysfunction, pregnancy, lactation, and "severe organic disease." Forty patients were enrolled in the daily chondroitin group, 43 in the thrice-daily group, and 44 in the placebo group. The three groups did not differ statistically in regard to age, weight, gender, baseline Lequesne index, baseline pain on VAS, duration of OA, and presence of unilateral or bilateral disease. Steroids, fluoride, biphosphonates, calcitonin, and hormone replacement were forbidden during in the study. Patients were assessed at days 0, 14, 42, and 91. Improvement in the Lequesne index was the primary outcome measure. Secondary outcome measures included spontaneous pain on a VAS, consumption of "authorized" NSAIDs (recorded daily by subjects), and overall judgment of treatment efficacy and tolerability by the physician and patient. The nonparametric Kruskall-Wallis test was used for comparison among groups in percent reduction of quantitative variables (e.g., Lequesne index, VAS, NSAID consumption), and chi-square was used for comparing efficacy and tolerance between the two chondroitin groups and placebo. To compare the Lequesne index, NSAID consumption, and VAS between days 0 and 91 (or the last known value for dropouts), a nonspecified nonparametric test was used. The Mantel-Haenzsel test was used to compare tolerance scores between day 0 and day 91. ANOVA for repeated measures was used in comparing the three groups in tolerance and efficacy judgments, with the Wilcoxon signed-rank test used to detect between-group differences.

The Wilcoxon signed-rank test was also used to test for a significant difference between groups in regard to the Lequesne index and VAS at days 0, 14, 42, and 91; differences were significant at days 42 and 91 for both the Lequesne index ($p < 0.00005$ and $p < 0.0001$) and the VAS ($p < 0.0009$ and $p < 0.0001$). The Lequesne index decreased in all three groups between days 0 and 91. The percent reduction in the Lequesne index became significantly different from placebo at day 14 in the chrondroitin 1200 mg qd group ($p < 0.05$) and significantly different in the 400 mg tid group at day 42 ($p < 0.001$). At day 91, the reduction in both treatment groups was significantly different from placebo ($p < 0001$) but was not different between treatment groups at days 42 or 91. At day 14, the percent reduction in the VAS for pain became significantly greater in the 1200 mg qd group than in the placebo group ($p < 0.01$) and became significant ($p < 0.005$) in the 400 mg tid group on day 42. At day 91, the difference was still significant for both groups ($p < 0.0001$ and $p < 0.0005$ for the qd and tid groups, respectively). Reduction in NSAID consumption between days 0 and 91 was significant in all three groups, but the reduction was not significantly greater in the treatment groups than in the placebo group ($p < 0.06$ for qd dosing and $p < 0.08$ for tid dosing), or between treatment groups.

In regard to overall treatment efficacy, the difference between the treatment groups and placebo was significant at days 42 ($p < 0.05$) and 91 ($p < 0.01$), but there was no difference between the two treatment groups. Tolerability was very good for both treatments as well as placebo, as judged by both the physician and patients; results of the statistical analysis were not reported. Twenty-one patients (11 in the chondroitin group) reported adverse gastrointestinal effects including gastralgia, nausea, swollen stomach, vomiting, and diarrhea leading to treatment discontinuation in 3 chondroitin patients and 3 placebo patients. There were also four reports of itching (two chondroitin, two placebo) and one report each of ankle edema, alopecia, and palpitations, all in chondroitin patients.

The ability of Chondrosulf powder 800 mg daily to influence the course of OA was assessed in a 1-yr, randomized, double-blind study (Uebelhart et al., 1998). Twenty-two men and 24 women ages 35–78 were enrolled. Some were inpatients. All suffered from uni- or bilateral OA of the knee with a minimum remaining medial femorotibial joint (MFTJ) space of 25%. Exclusion criteria included inflammatory or systemic diseases, other bone or joint conditions, lower limb axial deviation more than 5°, or use of steroids or drugs for bone disorders less than 3 mo prior to study enrollment. Acetaminophen was allowed as rescue medication, but consumption was not assessed.

The main outcome measure was spontaneous VAS at months 0, 3, 6, and 12. Secondary outcome measures included radiologic changes, serum osteocalcin (markers of bone formation), serum keratan sulfate (a marker of proteoglycan breakdown), and urine pyridinoline and deoxy-pyridinoline (markers of bone and connective tissue degradation). Knee radiographs were taken at months 0 and 12, and biochemical markers of bone and joint metabolism were measured at months 3, 6, and 12. Clinical tolerability was measured at months 1, 3, 6, and 12 on a 4-point scale. Analysis of variance (ANOVA) and covariance for repeated measures, Mann-Whitney U-test, Wilcoxon signed-rank test, and the t-test were used for quantitative assessments; chi-square was used for categorical variables. Two females in the chondroitin group and two males in the placebo group dropped out. At baseline, the two groups were similar in gender, age, weight, height, radiologic stage according to Kellgren and Lawrence, and VAS for pain and mobility.

At month 3, the percent decrease in joint pain was greater in the treatment group ($p < 0.05$, Mann-Whitney). The difference was even more marked at month 12 ($p < 0.01$). The difference in pain was significant between month 0 and month 12 in the chrondroitin group ($p < 0.01$, Wilcoxon). ANOVA results showed a difference between treatments ($p < 0.001$) and a time effect ($p < 0.05$). At months 6 and 12, there was a difference between groups in mobility ($p < 0.01$, Mann-Whitney) and an improvement between months 0 and 12 for the chondroitin group ($p < 0.01$, Wilcoxon). With ANOVA, there was a difference between times ($p < 0.001$) but not between treatments. Serial radiographs were available for only 14 chondroitin patients and 12 placebo patients. Compared with baseline, the MFTJ mean width decreased significantly in the placebo group ($p < 0.05$, paired t-test) but not in the chondroitin group. When percentage changes from baseline in MFTJ minimum width, mean width, and surface area in chondroitin patients were compared with placebo, a significant difference was found in favor of chondroitin ($p < 0.01$ t-test). The Kellgren and Lawrence radiologic score did not differ between months 0 and 12 in either group. Serum osteocalcin was measured in 21 chondroitin patients and 20 placebo patients. Between months 0 and 12, there was an increase in osteocalcin in the placebo group and a decrease in the chondroitin group ($p < 0.001$, ANOVA). A similar trend was seen with serum keratan sulfate, urinary pyridinoline, and urinary deoxy-pyridinoline ($p < 0.001$, Friedman two-way ANOVA). Overall tolerability was not significant between the two groups (chi-square).

Chondrosulf 800 mg QD was compared with placebo in a randomized, double-blind study in 85 patients with knee OA (Bucsi and Poor, 1998). Both inpatients and outpatients were included. All patients had Kellgren and Lawrence radiologic scores of I–III. Patients were excluded if they had other inflammatory disease or conditions affecting or possibly affecting the joints, or if they had secondary OA of the knee. Outcome variables assessed at months 1, 3, and 6 included spontaneous pain on a 10-cm VAS, acetaminophen consumption, time to walk 20 m, Lequesne index, and patient and physician judgment of global efficacy and tolerability on a scale of 0–4. Analysis of variance for repeated measures and the Bonferroni test were used for parametric variables. The Mann-Whitney test was used for nonparametric variables and data that were not normally distributed. Chi-square and Fisher's exact test were used to assess categorical variables. All results were computed as two-tailed. Eighty-five patients were enrolled in the study, 5 (2 placebo, 3 chondroitin) dropped out. The two groups were similar at baseline in radiographic score, presence of uni- vs bilateral disease, age, gender, weight, height, and spontaneous joint pain.

The difference in the groups in spontaneous joint pain was significant at months 3 and 6 (repeated-measures ANOVA with Bonferroni, $p < 0.01$). Acetaminophen consumption did not differ between groups at any time (Mann-Whitney test). Walking time was significantly different between the two groups at month 6 (repeated-measures ANOVA with Bonferroni, $p < 0.05$). Walking time differed from baseline in the chondroitin groups at months 3 ($p < 0.05$) and 6 ($p < 0.01$). The Lequesne index for the left knee differed between groups at months 3 (repeated-measures ANOVA and Bonferroni, $p < 0.05$) and 6 ($p > 0.001$) and between chondroitin and baseline at months 3 and 6 ($p < 0.01$). For the right knee, chondroitin and placebo differed at month 6 ($p < 0.01$). Both placebo and chondroitin differed from baseline at month 3 ($p < 0.01$), but only chondroitin differed from baseline at month 6 ($p < 0.01$). The patients and physician rated the efficacy of chondroitin to be superior to placebo (chi-square, $p < 0.01$). Only one patient (placebo) complained of gastrointestinal side effects.

Chondrosulf at a dose of 400 mg tid was compared with placebo in finger joint OA (Verbruggen et al., 1998). Thirty-four patients received chondroitin, 39 received placebo, and 46 received placebo as part of a previous clinical trial. The patients were followed for 3 yr. Each year, posteroanterior radiographs of the distal and proximal interphalangeal joints and the metacarpophalangeal (MCP) joints of the second, third, and fourth fingers. Joints were assessed as showing no OA (N), classical OA (S), loss of joint space (J), erosive OA (E), or remodeling, representing a continuum of anatomic phases of OA. The numbers of patients in the two treatment groups showing changes in their anatomic phase (e.g., progression from N to S, or S to J, and so on) were compared using the chi-square test. MCP joints did not benefit from chondroitin, a comparative number of chondroitin and placebo patients progressed from phase N to phase S. Chondroitin was beneficial in decreasing the number of patients with interphalangeal joints progressing from phases S or J to phase E. Additional details of the study design and results were not reported.

Problems that limit generalizability of the results of these studies include use of a supplement not available in the United States, small sample size, and short treatment duration. Although one study followed OA progression for 3 yr (Verbruggen et al., 1998), information on study subjects and other study details is lacking. Permissive use of acetaminophen (Morreale et al., 1996; Uebelhart et al., 1998, Busci and Poor, 1998) or NSAIDs (Bourgeois et al., 1998) may have confounded the results, particularly in the Uebelhart study, in which acetaminophen use was not assessed. In those studies in which inpatients were included as study subjects (Uebelhart et al., 1998; Busci and Poor, 1998), the authors did not state the number of inpatients in each treatment group; therefore, the treatment groups may not have been comparable in this regard.

Secondary outcome measures for one of the studies (Uebelhart et al., 1998), and the primary outcome measure for another study (Verbruggen et al., 1998) were radiographic joint changes. In addition, Uebelhart and colleagues (1998) assessed biochemical markers of cartilage breakdown as a a secondary outcome measure. Such measurements are more appropriate for studies of DMOADs than for SADOAs (Runkel and Cupp, 1999), although the results of these studies suggest that chondroitin may in fact have disease-modifying activity. Outcome measures were generally appropriate in other studies.

All studies treated VAS and the Lequesne index as continuous variables. Although it can be argued that such data should be treated as ordinal (nonparametric) data (Ascione et al., 1994), treatment of such scores as parametric data is widespread in the medical literature. In the study by Bourgeois and colleagues (1998), ANOVA for repeated measures and the Wilcoxon signed-rank test were used inappropriately, and the reason for choosing ANOVA to compare data between two treatment groups in the Uebelhart study is unclear. Failure to use intent-to-treat analysis (Morreale et al., 1996; Uebelhart et al., 1998; Busci and Poor, 1998) is another limitation of some of these studies.

Although financial support from the manufacturer is not always an indicator of bias, according to McAlinson and colleagues (2000) three of the studies (Bourgeois et al., 1998; Busci and Poor, 1998; Uebelhart et al., 1998) received such support, and in two (Busci and Poor, 1998; Uebelhart et al., 1998), the manufacturer conducted data collection, randomization, or statistical analysis. At least two additional studies reviewed here (Morreale et al., 1996; Pavelka et al., 2000) are known to have been funded by the product manufacturer. Three investigators in the Noack group (1994) and two working with Müller-Faßbender and colleagues (1994) were employed by the manufacturer.

12.7.4. Glucosamine and Chondroitin

A randomized, double-blind, 16-wk crossover study of Cosamin DS (glucosamine HCl 1500 mg/day, chondroitin sulfate 1200 mg/day, and manganese ascorbate 228 mg/day) vs placebo was undertaken in 34 males with chronic knee or low back pain recruited through fliers posted at U.S. Navy diving and special warfare commands (Leffler et al., 1999). Prospective study subjects were evaluated for inclusion based on duration of symptoms and degenerative changes on X-ray. Patients with no degenerative changes, patients with stage 4 disease, patients with inflammatory arthritis, and those referred for surgical intervention were excluded. After a 3-wk baseline run-in, subjects took Cosamin DS or placebo for 8 wk then and were crossed over to the alternate regimen. Acetaminophen use was allowed throughout the study. Outcome measures included the Lequesne index (for knee OA) or responses to the Roland questionnaire for back disability; patient's assessment of handicap (0–5); physician's overall assessment (0–3); 10-cm VAS for pain; tenderness with movement of the lower back or firm pressure on the knees (0–3); time to run 100 yards and to run up and down a tower of 80 stairs, touching every stair; physical exam parameters: tenderness with palpation in passive movements, decreased range of motion, warmth, crepitus, effusion, swelling, and muscle atrophy (0–3); knee active range of motion or lumbar flexion; and patient's assessment of treatment (–3 to +3). A summary score was obtained by adding the scores.

Outcomes were assessed after weeks 2 and 3 of the run-in period, and after weeks 7 and 8 of both 8-wk treatment periods. Patients recorded daily pain (0–7) and daily acetaminophen dose. Safety was assessed using a questionnaire, fecal occult blood testing, blood pressure, and pulse. Complete blood count (CBC) and coagulation studies were also performed in 21 patients. There were seven dropouts: two required NSAID use during the placebo phase, one required NSAID use during the treatment phase, three left the area, and one had no time to comply. Intent-to-treat analysis was used. The sign test was used to assess patient assessment of treatment result. From the limited information given by the investigators, it appears that the efficacy of glucosamine/chondroitin compared with placebo was done using the t-test as though the study was not a crossover study, but as though one group of patients received placebo and another group received glucosamine/chondroitin. Comparisons between placebo and baseline and glucosamine/chondroitin and baseline appear to have been performed using the paired t-test. Outcome measures (except patient assessment of treatment) were normalized by stating them as a percentage of the patient's mean score for the three study phases, such that patients with the same relative change would have the same score, regardless of the absolute change. If a patient had involvement of more than one knee, or both the knee and back, data were combined such that the unit of analysis was the patient, not the joint.

Based in the overall summary score, glucosamine/chondroitin was not significantly better than placebo ($p = 0.052$). Significantly greater improvement was seen with glucosamine/chondroitin in the patient assessment of treatment ($p = 0.02$), VAS for pain on exam ($p = 0.02$), and daily pain ($p = 0.02$). There was no significant benefit of glucosamine chondroitin on physical exam scores, acetaminophen use, Lequesne or Roland scores, patient assessment of handicap, physician assessment of severity, running times, or range of motion. When the knee data were separated from the back data, the overall summary score showed a greater change compared with placebo ($p = 0.049$), as did the physical exam score ($p = 0.01$), daily pain ($p = 0.02$), and pain on exam ($p = 0.048$). Glucosamine/chondroitin did not show a statistically significant benefit compared with baseline, and many outcome measures improved significantly during placebo treatment compared with baseline. No hematologic aberrations or other adverse effects were noted, despite the relatively large manganese dose (30 mg daily) provided by the product. Limitations of this study include small sample size, use of parametric tests for nonparametric data, mathematical treatment (i.e., calculation of mean, adding results of different scores) of ordinal data, and crossover design (not appropriate for OA, a disorder in which symptoms vary over time).

A higher dose of Cosamin DS (glucosamine HCl 2000 mg/d, chondroitin sulfate 1600 mg/d, and manganese ascorbate 304 mg/d) was studied in 93 patients with radiographically mild (grade 2), moderate (grade 3), or severe (grade 4) OA of the knee according to the criteria described by by Kellgren and Lawrence (Das and Hammad, 2000). In this randomized, placebo-controlled study, patients were evaluated every 2 mo for 6 mo. Efficacy was determined based on improvement in the Lequesne index and the WOMAC (visual analog version). The Lequesne index was used as the primary outcome measure because it was used in previous studies of glucosamine/chondroitin. Patients were also asked to make a global assessment of their OA using a VAS. In administering the assessment instruments, patients were instructed to consider their OA over the past 2 wk. At each visit, the principal investigator examined the patients, and the same interviewer was used throughout the study. Use of adjunct pain medication (e.g., nonprescription NSAIDs and acetaminophen) was assessed using a patient diary, and use for more than 3 d a wk was discouraged. Missing data were treated according to the intent-to-treat method; 16.6% of the data was modified in this manner.

Considering only patients with mild or moderate disease ($n = 72$), there was no difference in change from baseline in the Lequesne index between the placebo and intervention groups at month 2 ($p = 0.2$); however, the glucosamine/chondroitin group showed statistically greater improvement at month 4 ($p = 0.003$) and month 6 ($p = 0.04$). The WOMAC and global assessment showed a similar trend, but this was not statistically significant. As discussed previously, the authors suggest that the visual analog WOMAC might not be an appropriate assessment tool for efficacy of an slow-acting agent such as glucosamine/chondroitin, which provides subtle improvement over the course of several months, because there may be high intrapatient variability in rating over time, independent of disease severity, causing score variability and a resulting lack of statistically significant improvement. The 21 patients with severe OA randomized to glucosamine/chondroitin showed no greater improvement than placebo in the Lequesne index, WOMAC, or global assessment at any time point. At months 4 and 6, the changes from baseline in the mean Lequesne index were 3 and 2.8 points, respectively, for the mild-to-moderate OA patients in the treatment group. In patients with severe OA in the glucosamine/chondroitin group, the mean changes from baseline at months 4 and 6 were 1.7 and 1.5 points, respectively.

For comparison, an intervention is expected to cause an average decrease in 3 points in the Lequesne index. The sample size of 93 patients was calculated to be adequate to have an 80% power to detect a difference of 2 points in the Lequesne index between the placebo and glucosamine/chondrotin groups, but the sample was divided into mild/moderate and severe groups prior to analysis, limiting the power of the study. A larger sample size may have demonstrated improvement in additional assessment tools in the mild/moderate disease group; however, based on the relatively small improvement from baseline in the severe OA group, statistically significant improvement may not have been demonstrated in the severe group even with a larger sample. Response to treatment was defined as a 25% improvement in Lequesne index, WOMAC, or global assessment. In patients with mild or moderate disease, 52% of patients in the glucosamine/chondroitin group responded based on the Lequesne index, whereas 28% of the patients in the placebo groups responded ($p = 0.04$). Using the WOMAC, 58% of the treatment group responded vs 41% in the placebo group ($p = 0.2$) whereas 70% of the treatment group and 46% of the placebo group responded based on global assessment ($p = 0.04$). In patients with severe disease, there was no statistically significant difference in the percentage of responders in the treatment group compared with the placebo group regardless of assessment tool. Although there was a trend toward a reduction in adjunct medication use by 50% or more in both the mild/ moderate disease patients and the severe disease patients receiving glucosamine/chondroitin, it did not reach statistical significance.

Adverse effects occurred in 17% of the glucosamine/chondroitin patients and 19% of placebo patients, respectively. The most common adverse effects in the treatment group were gastrointestinal upset (constipation, indigestion, gas) [$n = 7$ ($n = 10$ placebo group)], bad taste [$n = 1$ ($n = 3$ placebo group)], fatigue ($n = 1$), diabetes ($n = 1$), and hypothyroidism ($n = 1$). One patient in each group dropped out owing to gastrointestinal effects. Cartilage deficiency may have been responsible for lack of response in the patients with severe disease, since existing cartilage is necessary for glucosamine/ chondroitin's action.

These studies, which suggest that Cosamin DS may have efficacy in patients with mild or moderate OA are particularly interesting because this product is widely available in the United States. Of further interest is that these are the only studies of glucosamine, chondroitin, or a combination thereof that have included patients with radiographically severe OA (Kellgren and Lawrence grade 4), with only Das and Hammad (2000) evaluating these patients' data separately. More study is needed on the efficacy of these products in severe OA.

12.8. PHARMACOKINETICS

Orally and intravenously administered [^{14}C]glucosamine sulfate were used to determine glucosamine pharmacokinetics in beagles (Setnikar et al., 1986). The investigators point out that glucosamine's pKa of 6.91 is favorable for absorption of glucosamine from the small intestine and diffusion across biologic membranes in the body. Based on fecal excretion of radioactivity in the dog, at least 87% of an orally administered dose is absorbed, whereas a comparison of the area under the plasma radioactivity/time curve (AUC) after intravenous and oral administration suggests that only 71.5% is absorbed.

The pharmacokinetic profile of glucosamine in plasma is complex because glucosamine is involved in the biosynthesis of the α- and β-globulins of plasma proteins. Thus, radioactivity in the plasma first decreases as glucosamine exits the vascular space, and then increases as the radiolabeled glucosamine becomes incorporated into plasma proteins. In dogs, the distribution half-life (α-half-life) after intravenous administration was 13 min, followed by a plasma elimination half-life (β-half-life) of 1.97 h. In this study, total radioactivity in the plasma decreased for approximately the first hour after injection, then increased, and by 8 h post injection reached the same level as 5 min after administration. Radioactivity then decreased with a half-life of 70 h, which is consistent with the half-life of plasma glycoproteins. After oral administration, the distribution half-life (α-half-life) was 15 min, followed by a plasma elimination half-life (β-half-life) of 4.62 h. Total radioactivity in the plasma peaked approx 24 h after oral dosing and disappeared from the plasma with a half-life of 60 h. Glucosamine was excreted mainly in the urine, with only small amounts excreted in the feces or metabolized to CO_2 and excreted in expired air. Two hours after intravenous administration, radiolabeled glucosamine concentrations were highest in the liver, ovaries, kidney, spleen, femoral head cartilage, uterus, and brain. Even 144 h after administration, glucosamine could still be detected in all organs; therefore, study use of radioactive glucosamine was deemed by the investigators to be unethical in humans.

For this reason, "cold" glucosamine was used to study the pharmacokinetics of glucosamine in humans. Dona 200-S (Opfermann Arzneimittel, Bergisch Gladbach, Germany) 6 g was administered to six healthy volunteers (three male, three female) aged 20–48. Blood was collected 15, 30, 45, 60, 90, 120, and 180 min after administration, and urine was collected 0–4, 4–8, and 12–24 h after administration. Glucosamine plasma concentrations were below the limits of detection (1–3 μg/mL) at all times; however, glucosamine was detected in the urine. Glucosamine (Dona) 800 mg was also administered intravenously to six healthy volunteers (three male, three female) aged 24–42. Blood samples were drawn 10, 20, 30, 45, 60, 90, 120, 180, and 240 min after administration, and urine was collected 0–2, 2–8, and 8–24 h after administration. The disappearance of glucosamine from the plasma compartment could be described using the equation for a two-compartment open model. Urinary excretion occurred mainly within the first 2 h of parenteral administration, with 38.3% of the administered dose recovered in the urine within 8 h of administration. These results were similar to those seen in the dog. The volume of distribution was calculated as 0.071 L/kg and the α-half-life (distribution half-life) was 6.1 min., with a terminal plasma half-life of 2.1 h. Although glucosamine is incorporated into plasma proteins, in vitro plasma protein binding studies revealed that glucosamine did not bind to plasma proteins in dogs or humans.

The same investigators undertook a subsequent study of the pharmacokinetics of glucosamine sulfate in humans (Setnikar et al., 1993). Although these authors had previously stated that the use of radiolabeled glucosamine sulfate would be unethical in humans (Setnikar et al., 1986), for regulatory reasons they were compelled to obtain more definitive human data than could be obtained using "cold" glucosamine. To limit exposure, only six male subjects were studied, and only a single dose of radiolabeled glucosamine sulfate was administered (iv in two subjects, im in two, and orally in two).

After iv administration, plasma radioactivity conferred by glucosamine decreased, with a distribution half-life (α-half-life) of 0.03 h and a plasma elimination half-life (β-half-life) of 1.82 h. These values were similar after im administration. The decrease in plasma radioactivity owing to radiolabeled glucosamine was followed by an increase in plasma radioactivity beginning 1–2 h post injection caused by incorporation of glucosamine and its metabolites into plasma proteins. This radioactivity peaked 10 h after iv administration, decreasing with a half-life of 70 h. This second wave of plasma radioactivity peaked 8 h after im or oral administration. With im administration, the terminal half-life was 57 h, and 68 h after oral administration, corresponding to the half-life of plasma proteins. After oral administration, radioactivity could be detected in plasma proteins within 1–2 h of administration. Bioavailability was 96% after administration, and 26% after oral administration. The authors attributed low bioavailability to first-pass metabolism by the liver, where glucosamine is metabolized into smaller molecules and ultimately into CO_2, water, and urea. In the feces, 11.3, 0.9, and 0.5% of the radioactivity was recovered over 120 h after oral, im, and iv administration, respectively. After oral administration, only about 10% of the radioactivity was recovered in the urine over 120 h. Radioactivity could be detected in plasma proteins for at least 5 d after administration by all routes.

N-acetyl-D-glucosamine (NAG) is a GAG component that is available in several glucosamine/chondroitin dietary supplements in the United States. Because NAG is hydrolyzed in vitro and in vivo to glucosamine, it was hypothesized that a polymeric form of NAG (chitin) could provide a long-lasting source of NAG (Talent and Gracy, 1996). A polymeric form of NAG, POLY-Nag® (Lescarden, New York, NY), was compared with NAG in a randomized, crossover pharmacokinetic study in 10 (5 males, 5 females) healthy volunteers, aged 36–50 yr, who were students and employees from the University of North Texas Health Sciences Center. Volunteers were randomized to receive either NAG or POLY-Nag by drawing names from two canisters, one for females and one for males. Between 8 AM and 9 AM on day 1 of the study, fasting blood samples were collected, and subjects then ingested 1 g of NAG or 1 g of POLY-Nag. On day 2, the subjects again took 1 g of the supplement before breakfast. On day 3, a fasting blood sample was drawn between 8 AM and 9 AM, and the subjects then ingested 1 g of the supplement. Blood samples (nonfasting) were drawn 1, 2, 4, 8, 24, and 48 h after ingestion. On day 8, the procedure was repeated, with subjects being crossed over to the alternate supplement. Compared with baseline, NAG levels measured 1 hour after the third dose increased in 8/10 subjects after NAG ingestion and 6/10 POLY-Nag after ingestion. Similar results are seen if the level taken prior to the third dose is compared with baseline; 13 of the 20 samples demonstrated increased serum NAG concentrations.

These results suggest that 1 g of NAG or POLY-Nag daily can increase serum NAG levels in most, but not all patients. Resulting NAG levels varied widely among study subjects. This variability was not discussed by the investigators, but it may have been caused by differences in body weight, bioavailability, or elimination among study subjects. Mean serum NAG levels 24 h after the last dose were higher after POLY-Nag ingestion than after NAG ingestion, but whether the difference was statistically significant was not reported. Mean serum NAG levels were above baseline even 48 h after the last dose, and serum glucosamine levels were elevated 10.2 and 12.8% over baseline at 48 h after NAG and POLY-Nag ingestion, respectively. Whether the difference between the two treatments was statistically significant was not reported. The results of this study suggest that compared with NAG, POLY-Nag may provide sustained levels of NAG and glucosamine and may provide a more pharmacokinetically useful source of glucosamine than NAG, but larger studies are needed, with discussion of the clinical and statistical significance of wide interindividual variation in NAG and glucosamine levels.

A pharmacokinetic study in eight human volunteers utilized intravenous chondroitin sulfate 500 mg (1:3 ratio of chondroitin sulfate A to chondroitin sulfate C) with a molecular weight of 16 kD. The mean elimination half-life was found to be 4.68 ± 0.53 h. The plasma level decreased according to a two-compartment model, with mean volumes of distribution of the central and tissue compartments of 6 and 22.9 L, respectively. More than 50% of the administered chondroitin was excreted in the urine within 24 h of administration as derivatives with various molecular weights. These derivatives were also detectable in the plasma. After oral administration of 3 g of chondroitin, a mean elimination half-life of 6.05 h was calculated. The bioavailability was calculated to be 13.2% based on the AUC (Conte et al., 1991).

Plasma levels and the metabolic fate of chondroitin sulfate [Chondrosulf, Institut Biochimique SA (IBSA), Lugano, Switzerland] derived from bovine trachea cartilage were studied in rats, beagles, and humans (Conte et al., 1995). Tritium-labeled chondrotin sulfate 16 mg/kg was administered to rats and dogs. Twelve healthy human volunteers (six male, six female), aged 24–56 yr, were administered a single dose of sodium chrondroitin sulfate 800 mg at 6 PM, or 400 mg at 6 PM and 400 mg at 6 AM. After a 7-d washout, volunteers were crossed over to the other dosing regimen.

For 3 d prior to chrondroitin ingestion and during blood sample collection, volunteers ate a consistent diet with meat intake limited to 150 g/d, and avoided meat containing visible connective tissue to minimize the effect of diet on study results. Volunteers were also instructed to avoid physical activity on blood collection days. Blood samples were collected on the day prior to chondroitin administration between 8 and 9 AM, between 11 and 12 AM, between 4 and 5 PM, and between 10 and 11 PM. Blood was also collected before dosing and at 2, 4, 6, 12, 14, 16, 18, and 24 h after chondroitin administration. In humans, the mean elimination half-life of chondroitin sulfate and its high molecular weight derivatives was 10.3 h (SD ± 6.8 for the 800-mg dose and ± 2.5 h for the 400-mg × 2 dose), with a mean C_{max} of 2.6 µg/mL occurring at a mean of 5 h after a single 800-mg dose, and a C_{max} of 1.2 µg/mL occurring at a mean of 5.2 h after a 400-mg dose.

Chondroitin plasma concentrations increased compared with baseline with both dosing regimens. Data from rats and dogs showed that more than 70% of the administered radioactivity was absorbed, with urine being the main route of excretion. Radioactive compounds of intermediate and low molecular weights were excreted in the urine. The relative amount of low molecular weight compounds detected in the plasma and urine increased over time. Part of this low molecular mass material found in the urine and plasma, as well as in the tissues, was tritiated water. These observations can be explained because chondroitin sulfate is radiolabeled at the reducing carbohydrate end of the molecule, and, in vivo, enzymatic degradation proceeds, step by step, from the nonreducing end. Thus, the low molecular weight species are produced after complete depolymerization of the molecule. In addition, tritiated water is produced from metabolism of the remaining radiolabeled sugar at the end of the molecule. Based on the molecular weight of the radioactive compounds excreted in the urine, the authors hypothesized that chondroitin sulfate is excreted as the parent compound and as compounds resulting from depolymerization of exogenously administered chondroitin. The authors subjected chondroitin sulfate to human gastric juice for 3 h at 37°C in vitro and found that desulfation and depolymerization can occur in this environment. They also hypothesized that because of their high molecular weight, GAGs are absorbed via pinocytosis, that chondroitin sulfates with low molecular weight and charge density are preferentially absorbed, or that desulfation and depolymerization occur during the pinocytotic process.

The presence of radiolabeled compounds with higher molecular weights than chondroitin sulfate in plasma and synovial fluid may be explained by binding of chondroitin and its depolymerized derivatives to plasma and tissue proteins. Twenty-four hours after administration in the rat, tissue/organ concentrations of radioactivity were highest in the small intestine, followed by the liver, kidney, synovial fluid, muscle, joint cartilage, trachea, lung, eye, brain, and adipose tissue.

Supporting the hypothesis of Conte and colleagues regarding the relationship of molecular weight to bioavailability, absorption of orally administered chondroitin sulfate was found to be inversely related to molecular weight based on studies using Caco-2 cell monolayers to simulate the gastrointestinal mucosa (F-D-C reports, 2000).

Wood and colleagues (1976) studied the metabolic fate of radiolabeled chondroitin 4-sulfate-peptide in rats. The chondroitin 4-sulfate-peptide was prepared using proteolytic enzymes to digest rat cartilage, producing proteoglycan degradation products similar to those normally released from cartilage in vivo; thus, the specifics of the investigators' results may not reflect the pharmacokinetics of commercially available chondroitin products. In general, their findings suggest that smaller molecular weight derivatives are likely to be excreted in the urine, whereas larger molecular weight species are taken up by the liver and broken down into smaller components for excretion in the urine.

12.9. ADVERSE EFFECTS AND TOXICITY

Glucosamine and chondroitin appear to be well tolerated compared with placebo based on information from clinical trials, and in some studies, no adverse effects were reported. Most of the adverse effects reported were gastrointestinal in nature. With the exception dermatologic reactions, other adverse effects reported in clinical trials of glucosamine and/or chondroitin may not be treatment-related (*see Clinical Studies* section). Although some review articles and tertiary references state bleeding may be problematic with chondroitin, owing to its similarity to heparin, no data from studies or case reports supports this contention.

12.9.1. Allergic Reactions

The manufacturer of one popular glucosamine/chondroitin product warns consumers who are allergic to shellfish to consult their healthcare professional before using the product (Nutramax Laboratories, 2000a); another manufacturer states that it is safe for patients allergic to shellfish to use their product (Nutrasense™ Company, 2000). Because shellfish allergies are usually reactions to shellfish proteins rather than chitin, from which glucosamine is produced, glucosamine should be safe for such patients (Conn et al., 1999); however, product contamination with shellfish proteins or allergy to glucosamine cannot be ruled out.

A 76-yr-old woman who was prescribed glucosamine sulfate one dose daily (brand and dose not specified) for OA experienced erythematous lesions and facial swelling within several hours of product ingestion. The next day, she presented to the emergency department with tongue, facial, and throat swelling that developed 5 min after taking the second dose. Treatment with corticosteroids and antihistamines led to symptom resolution within 4 h. A skin prick test with glucosamine sulfate was negative, but an intradermal test at a concentration of 1.5 mg/mL was positive, with a papule of 36 mm^3. A positive histamine control and negative saline control were also performed. Intrademal testing in 10 healthy volunteers was negative. Enzyme-linked immunosorbent assay (ELISA) for specific IgE against glucosamine sulfate was negative, although the authors of this case report attributed the patient's symptoms to an IgE-mediated mechanism.

They hypothesized that the negative ELISA was the result of a technical problem with the assay resulting from glucosamine's small molecular weight (Matheu et al., 1999).

12.9.2. Insulin Resistance

In vitro, glucosamine at a concentration of 5 mmol/L inhibited insulin secretion via inhibition of β-cell glucokinase activity in pancreatic islet cells obtained from 10 male Sprague-Dawley rats. In addition, intravenous infusion of glucosamine 200 mg/ mL lowered plasma insulin and resulted in an increase in blood glucose (Balkan and Dunning 1994). In another study, glucosamine infusion caused insulin resistance in normoglycemic Sprague-Dawley rats but not in 90% pancreatectomized rats with hyperglycemia (Rossetti et al., 1995). Normalization of glucose levels in the diabetic rats resulted in the ability to induce insulin resistance with glucosamine. Thus, the effect of glucosamine on insulin resistance is not additive with that of high glucose levels, suggesting that both high glucose levels and glucosamine may cause insulin resistance through a common pathway. Both glucosamine and to a lesser extent glucose are metabolized to glucosamine-6-phosphate, which enters the hexosamine biosynthetic pathway. In vitro, increased activity of this pathway is associated with insulin resistance. The terminal event may involve inhibition of glucose uptake or inhibition of glucose phosphorylation to glucose-6-phosphate such that glycolysis and glycogen synthesis cannot proceed normally. Glucosamine's effect on insulin resistance may be modest in comarison to that of high glucose levels, so that in the presence of high glucose concentrations glucosamine's effect is insignificant and an additive effect is not noted.

Anecdotally, individuals using glucosamine are reporting online that they are experiencing hyperlipidemia and hypertension, both of which are associated with insulin resistance (Anonymous, 2001a). In a 12-wk study, 15 patients with chronic low back pain were randomized to placebo ($n = 9$) or glucosamine sulfate (GS-500™) 500 mg ($n = 6$) three times daily. A trend toward increased fasting insulin levels was noted in the glucosamine group (Almada, 2000). One patient in the treatment group in a study of a glucosamine/chondroitin combination product (Das and Hammad, 2000) developed type 2 diabetes; however, the investigators did not have baseline glucose levels in this patient, so the onset of diabetes might have predated study enrollment. Adverse effects, including effects on blood glucose, did not differ from placebo in a 3-yr study (Reginster et al., 2001). Until more is known, fasting blood glucose should be checked periodically in patients taking glucosamine who are at risk for diabetes, and diabetic patients should be monitored for changes in glucose control.

12.9.3. Manganese Toxicity

Some glucosamine/chondroitin products contain manganese. In a study of one such product, adverse effects attributable to the manganese content of the product were not reported (Leffler et al., 2000). Manganese toxicity from excessive dietary intake has not been reported, and the American diet may actually predispose individuals to occult magnesium deficiency. Nevertheless, a definitive "toxic" level of dietary manganese intake has not been identified because several dietary factors affect body manganese stores (Das and Hammad, 2000). Manganese-containing glucosamine/chondroitin products should therefore be viewed with some degree of caution until more information is available.

12.10. INTERACTIONS

There are no published case reports of drug interactions with glucosamine or chondroitin, and no studies have been done to investigate their potential to interact with drugs. Only one study (Crolle and D'Este 1980) addressed the use of glucosamine in patients taking other medications and did so only in a very general fashion, so it is not possible to draw conclusions about glucosamine's ability to interact with medications. Product labels generally state that there are no known drug interactions. Owing to its similarity to heparin, some references state chondroitin should be used with caution with anticoagulants or antiplatelet agents.

12.11. REPRODUCTION

No studies have been done to assess the teratogenicity of glucosamine or chondroitin or their excretion into breast milk, and no case reports have been published in regard to their use in pregnancy. However, based on glucosamine's physical properties, some assumptions can be made. Glucosamine is a small (mol wt 179.17) water-soluble molecule that is unbound to plasma proteins. Glucosamine is a weak organic base with a pKa of 6.91. In the bloodstream, where the pH is 7.4, 25% of the glucosamine molecules are ionized and 75% are un-ionized (Setnikar et al., 1999). These factors favor passage of glucosamine into breast milk and across the placenta. In addition, because the pH of human breast milk is slightly more acidic (pH 7.1) than plasma, a greater percentage of glucosamine molecules become ionized when they enter the breast milk. The ionized molecules can become "trapped" in the milk because they move less readily through biologic membranes (Briggs, 1995).

12.12. CHEMICAL AND BIOFLUID ANALYSIS

A number of methods exist for measuring glucosamine, chondroitin, and other glycosaminoglycans, although methods for quantitating them in human serum or plasma are somewhat sparse. Campo and colleagues (2001) have recently published a sensitive and specific method for quantitating glucosamine in human plasma and serum. This method uses HPLC with amperometric detection of the analytes. First, glucosamine is isolated from plasma or serum (2 mL) by making the sample alkaline with 0.05 M NaOH and allowing it to incubate at 40°C for 16 h to release the glycosaminoglycan chains from the proteoglycans or peptoglycans. The samples are then filtered through an Ecteola-cellulose (chloride form) anion exchange column (4 × 0.7 cm). The resin is washed with 50 mL of 0.9% NaCl, and then the glucosamine is eluted with 4 mL of 2 M NaCl. This preparation is then desalted on a Bio-Gel P2 column (40 × 0.7 cm) and eluted with distilled water. To purify the samples further, they are then fractionated by placing the sample on a Dowex 1 × 2 column (4 × 0.7 cm), washing with 20 mL of 0.9% NaCl, and eluting with two-2 mL fractions of 2 M NaCl. The samples are then reduced in volume by placing them on a Rotavap under vacuum and desalting as described above. Glucosamine (monosaccharide) is derived from these purified glycosaminoglycan preparations by acid hydrolysis with 4 M HCl (4 h at 100°C). The

HCl is removed under vacuum at 37°C. Stock solutions (authentic standards) of glucosamine are prepared in 0.02 *M* NaOH.

Following injection onto the HPLC system, the analytes are separated with a CarboPac PA10 anion exchange column (250 × 4 mm). It should be noted that a carbonate trap is placed between the injector and column to limit carbonate interactions with the column, as this may shorten column life. The mobile phase consists of 0.02 *M* NaOH, and the flow rate is 1 mL/min. The amperometric detection system is equipped with a gold working electrode and a standard pH-Ag/AgCl reference electrode. The potentials are set as follows: t_1 (0.5s), E_1 (+0.1 V), t_2 (0.09s), E_2 (+0.6 V), t_3 (0.05s), E_3 (-0.6 V). Total run time for the assay is less than 15 minutes, and glucosamine is readily separated from the other glycosaminoglycans. Calibration curves for the assay are linear from 0.25 to 40 μ*M*.

Volpi (2000) has recently described a method for measuring chondroitin (nonsulfated) and the various sulfated forms of this glycosaminoglycan (including the trisulfated positional isomers). Samples are treated with chondroitinase ABC (25 mU) placed in 50 μL of 1 mM sodium phosphate (pH 7.0) and allowed to react for 3 h at 37°C. The reaction is then stopped by boiling the sample for 1 min, and the undigested glycosaminoglycans are precipitated with 200 mL of 98% ethanol at 4°C for 24 hours. Next, the ethanol supernatant is evaporated to dryness. The samples are then derivatized with dansylhydrazine to make them fluorescent and to allow for more specific and sensitive detection. Samples are reconstituted in 20 μL of 90% methanol and 20 μL of 0.75% (w/v) trichloroacetic acid in ethanol, and then 20 μL of 1.0% (w/v) dansylhydrazine are added. The mixture is reacted for 2 h at 40°C, diluted 1:10 with distilled water and injected onto the HPLC system. A μ-Bondapak NH_2 column (3.9 × 300 mm, 10 μm) is used for analyte separation. A mobile phase of acetonitrile/100 mM acetate (pH 5.6) (90:20, v/v) is pumped through the column at a flow rate of 2 mL/min. Fluorescence is monitored at an excitation wavelength of 350 nm and an emission wavelength of 530 nm. Total run time for the seven disaccharides is less than 50 minutes. The limit of detection is about 20 ng per sample.

Extraction and purification of chondroitin sulfate from bovine trachea cartilage has been described (Conte et al., 1995). Chromatographic determination of chondroitin sulfate in plasma using an ion exchange Ecteola-cellulose column has been performed (Conte et al., 1991). In this same study, the concentration of chondroitin sulfate degradation products in plasma and urine was also determined using the Multichrom Beckman (Palo Alto, CA) amino acid analyzer.

NAG and glucosamine have been identified and quantified in blood samples by HPLC using a Hewlett-Packard (Palo Alto, CA) 1090M liquid chromatograph/workstation with a diode array detector (Hewlett-Packard, Palo Alto, CA) optimized at 193 nm for maximum efficiency and minimum interference. Separation was performed using isocratic elution at 40°C from a 300 × 7.8 mm Rezex™ organic acid column (minimum efficiency > 7500 ppm) (Phenomenex, Torrance, CA) with 0.005 N H_2SO_4 at a flow rate of 0.6 mL/min. Limits of detection were 0.5 nmol (0.11 μg) for NAG and 10 mmol (1.8 μg) for glucosamine (Talent and Gracy, 1996).

Plasma and urine glucosamine concentration determination using ion-exchange chromatography has been described. The limit of detection is 5–15 nmol/L (1–3 μg/

mL) with this method (Setnikar et al., 1986). Reverse phase chromatography using precolumn derivitization with phenylisothiocyanate and ultraviolet detection at 254 nm was found to be specific and accurate for use in quantitating glycosamine in raw materials, dosage forms, and plasma (Liang et al., 1999)

12.13. REGULATORY STATUS

Glucosamine and chondroitin are regulated as dietary supplements in the United States. They are approved as a prescription treatment for OA in many European and other countries (Reginster et al., 2001). In Canada, they are regarded as a food supplement (Thie et al., 2001).

12.14. SUMMARY

- Glucosamine and chondroitin are cartilage components. Glucosamine and chondroitin supplements are made using crustacean shells and bovine trachea cartilage, respectively.
- Osteo Bi-flex and Cosamin DS are popular glucosamine/chondroitin products. Products for veterinary use are available as well.
- Studies of glucosamine/chondroitin in OA suggest that these products are effective and well tolerated and may affect disease progression as well as symptoms.
- Glucosamine and chondroitin are well absorbed and are widely distributed throughout the body. Both appear to undergo liver metabolism prior to excretion in the urine. Glucosamine may be excreted in breast milk.
- Adverse effects of glucosamine and chondroitin are mainly gastrointestinal.

REFERENCES

Almada AL, Harvey PW, Platt KJ. Effect of chronic oral glucosamine sulfate upon fasting insulin resistance index (FIRI) in nondiabetic individuals [abstract]. FASEB J 2000;14:A750.

American Nutraceutical Association. Dietary supplements containing glucosamine and chondroitin sulfate found in University of Maryland College of Pharmacy study to contain significantly less ingredients when compared with label claims. Available at: http://www.ana.jana.org/press.html. Accessed July 24, 2000.

Anonymous. Osteo-Bi-Flex success reflects traditional consumer branding approach. Dietary Suppl Market Review. August, 1999. p.1.

Anonymous. Supplements. Pharmacists Let 2001a;17:65.

Anonymous. Pharmacy Fax Monitor. Totowa, NJ:Healthcare News Monitor Inc. December 16, 2001b.

Anonymous. Questions and answers: NIH study on glucosamine/chondroitin sulfate for knee osteoarthritis. Available from: URL: http://www.altmed.od.nih.gov/nccam/ne/press-releases/gcs-facts.html. Accessed May 26, 2000.

Ascione FJ, Manifold CC, Parenti MA. Principles of drug information and scientific literature evaluation. Hamilton, IL: Drug Intelligence Publications, 1994.

Balkan B, Dunning BE. Glucosamine inhibits glucokinase in vitro and produces a glucose-specific impairment of in vivo insulin secretion in rats. Diabetes 1994;43:1173–9.

Bassleer C, Rovati L, Franchimont P. Stimulation of proteoglycan production by glucosamine sulfate in chondrocytes isolated from human osteoarthritic articular cartilage in vitro. Osteoarthritis Cartilage 1998;6:427–34.

Bodewes J. Glucosamine and chondroitin. Drs. Foaster and Smith, Inc. Veterinary Services Department. Available from: URL: http://peteducation.com/nutrition/glu_chond.htm. Accessed May 8, 2000.

Bourgeois P, Chales G, Dehais J, et al. Efficacy and tolerability of chondroitin sulfate 1200 mg/ day vs chondroitin sulfate 3 × 400 mg/day vs placebo. Osteoarthritis Cartilage 1998;6(suppl A):25–30.

Briggs GG. Teratogenicity and drug in breast milk. In: Young LY, Koda-Kimble MA, eds. Applied therapeutics; the clinical use of drugs. 6th edition. Vancouver, WA: Applied Therapeutics 1995; p. 45.1–39.

Bucsi L, Poor G. Efficacy and tolerability of oral chondroitin sulfate as a symptomatic slow-acting drug for osteoarthritis (SYSADOA) in the treatment of knee osteoarthritis. Osteoarthritis Cartilage 1998;6(suppl A): 31–6.

Campo GM, Campo S, Ferlazzo AM, Vinci R, Calatroni A. Improved high-performance liquid chromatographic method to estimate aminosugars and its application to glycosaminoglycan determination in plasma and serum. J Chromatogr B Biomed Sci Appl 2001;765:151–60.

Canapp SO, McLaughlin RM, Hoskinson JJ, Roush JK, Butine MD. Scintigraphic evaluation of dogs with acute synovitis after treatment with glucosamine hydrochloride and chondroitin sulfate. Am J Vet Res 1999;60:1552–7.

Conn DL, Arnold WJ, Hollister JR. Alternative treatments and rheumatic diseases. Bull Rheum Dis 1999;48:4.

ConsumerLab.com. News. Consumerlab.com finds many arthritis supplements lacking labeled ingredient. Glucosamine and chondroitin product review published today. Available at: http://www.consumerlabs.com/news/news_3700.html. Accessed September 26, 2000.

Conte A, de Bernardi M, Palmieri L, et al. Metabolic fate of exogenous chondroitin sulfate in man. Arzneimittelforschung 1991;41:768–72.

Conte A, Volpi N, Palmieri L, Bahous I, Ronca G. Biochemical and pharmacokinetic aspects of oral treatment with chondroitin sulfate. Arzneimittelforschung 1995;45: 918–25.

Crolle G, D'Este E. Glucosamine sulphate for the management of arthrosis: a controlled clinical investigation, Curr Med Res Opin 1980;7:104–9.

D'Ambrosio E, Casa B, Bompani R, Scali M. Glucosamine sulfate: a controlled clinical investigation in arthrosis. Pharmacotherapeutica 1981;2:504–8.

Das A, Hammad TA. Efficacy of a combination of FCHG49™ glucosamine hydrochloride, TRH122™ low molecular weight chondroitin sulfate and manganese ascorbate in the management of knee osteoarthritis. Osteoarthritis Cartilage 2000;8:343–50.

Donohoe M. Efficacy of glucosamine and chondroitin for treatment of osteoarthritis [letter]. JAMA 2000;284:1241.

Drovanti A, Bignamini AA, Rovati AL. Therapeutic activity of oral glucosamine sulfate in osteoarthritis: a placebo-controlled double-blind investigation. Clin Ther 1980:3:260–72.

F-D-C reports. Five of 32 chondroitin products tested met label claims—JANA study. The Tan Sheet 2000;8:19.

Horstman J, Wood C. Glucosamine and chondroitin. Arthritis Today 1998;12:46–9.

Houpt JB, McMillan R, Wein C, Paget-Dellio SD. Effect of glucosamine hydrochloride in the treatment of pain of osteoarthritis of the knee. J Rheumatol 1999;26:2423–30.

Hughes RA, Chertsey AJC. A randomized, double-blind, placebo-controlled trial of glucosamine to control pain in osteoarthritis of the knee [abstract]. Arthritis Rheum 2000;9(suppl):S384.

Kier KL. Clinical application of statistical analysis. In: Malone PM, Mosdell KW, Kier KL, Stanovich JE, eds. Drug information. A guide for pharmacists. Stamford, CT: Appleton and Lange; 1996.

Leeb BF, Schweitzer H, Montag K, Smolen JS. A metaanalysis of chondroitin sulfate in the treatment of osteoarthritis. J Rheumatol 2000;27:205–11.

Leffler CT, Philippi AF, Leffler SG, Mosure JC, Kim PD. Glucosamine, chondroitin, and manganese ascorbate for degenerative joint disease of the knee or low back: a randomized, double-blind, placebo-controlled pilot study. Mil Med 1999;164:85–91.

Liang Z, Leslie J, Adebowale A, Ashraf M, Eddington ND. Determination of the nutraceutical, glucosamine hydrochloride, in raw materials, dosage forms, and plasma using pre-column derivitization with ultraviolet HPLC. J Pharmaceut Biomed Anal 1999;20:807–14.

March LM. Osteoarthritis. Med J Aust 1997;166:98–103.

Matheu V, Garcia Bara MT, Pelta R, Vivas E, Rubio M. Immediate-hypersensitivity reaction to glucosamine sulfate. Allergy 1999;54:643–50.

McAlindon TE, LaValley MP, Gulin JP, Felson DT. Glucosamine and chondroitin for treatment of osteoarthritis. A systematic quality assessment and meta-analysis. JAMA 2000; 283:1469–75.

McCarty MF. The neglect of glucosamine as a treatment for osteoarthritis—a personal perspective. Med Hypotheses 1994;42:323–7.

Morreale P, Manopulo R, Galati M, et al. Comparison of the anti-inflammatory efficacy of chondroitin sulfate and diclofenac sodium in patients with knee osteoarthritis. J Rheumatol 1996; 23:1385–91.

Mosdell KW. Literature evaluation. In: Drug information: a guide for pharmacists. Stamford, CT: Appleton and Lange; 1996; p. 89–119.

Müller-Faßbender H, Bach GL, Haase W, Rovati LC, Setnikar I. Glucosamine sulfate compared with ibuprofen in osteoarthritis of the knee. Osteoarthritis Cartilage 1994;2:61–9.

Noack W, Fischer M, Förster KK, Rovati LC, Setnikar I. Glucosamine sulfate in osteoarthritis of the knee. Osteoarthritis Cartilage 1994;2:51–9.

Nutramax Laboratories, Inc. Cosequin®, Coseqin DS®. Available from: URL:http://www.cosamin.com/veterinary/products/cosequins.htm. Accesssed May 26, 2000a.

Nutramax Laboratories, Inc. Cosamin® DS FAQ. Available from:URL:http://www.cosamin.com/ human/cosaminfaq.htm. Accessed May 25, 2000b.

Nutramax Laboratories, Inc.. Cosequin® equine powder concentrate. Available from: URL: http://www.cosamin.com/veterinary/products/cosequine.htm. Accessed May 26, 2000c.

Nutramax Laboratories, Inc. Double Strength Cosamin® DS. Available from: URL:http://www.cosamin.com/human/cosamin.htm. Accessed May 13, 2000d.

Nutrasense™ Company. Glucosamine FAQ's. Available from: URL: http://www.nutrasense.com/glucfaq1.html. Accessed May 8, 2000e.

Pavelka K, Gatterova J, Olejarova M, et al. Glucosamine sulfate decreases progression of knee osteoarthritis in a long-term, randomized, placebo-controlled independent, confirmatory trial [abstract]. Arthritis Rheum 2000;9(suppl):S384.

Pinals RS. Mechanisms of joint destruction, pain and disability in osteoarthritis. Drugs 1996;52(suppl 3):14–20.

PhytoPharmica. Company news. Phytopharmica is the first to receive consumerlab.com seal of approval for glucosamine sulfate. Available from: URL: http://www.phytopharmica.com/consumer/new/conews.html. Accessed September 26, 2000.

Pujalte JM, Llavore EP, Ylescupidez FR. Double-blind clinical evaluation of oral glucosamine sulphate in the basic treatment of osteoarthritis. Curr Med Res Opin 1980;7:110–4.

Qiu GX, Gao SN, Giacovelli G, Rovati L, Setnikar I. Efficacy and safety of glucosamine sulfate versus ibuprofen in patients with knee osteoarthritis. Arzneimittelforschung 1998;48: 469–74.

Reginster JY, Deroisy R, Rovati LC, et al. Long-term effects of glucosamine sulphate on osteoarthritis progression: a randomised, placebo-controlled clinical trial. Lancet 2001;357:251–6.

Reichelt A, Forster KK, Fischer M, Rovati L, Setnikar I. Efficacy and safety of intramuscular glucosamine sulfate in osteoarthritis of the knee. Arzneim Forsch Drug Res 1994;44:75–80.

Rexall Sundown. Osteo Bi-Flex® glucosamine chondroitin. Frequently asked questions. Available from: URL: http://www.osteobiflex.com/pages/faq.htm. Accessed May 8, 2000a.

Rexall Sundown. Osteo Bi-Flex® glucosamine chondroitin. Available from: URL:// www.osteobiflex.com Accessed February 20, 2000b.

Rindone JP, Hiller D, Collacott E, Nordhaugen N, Arriola G. Randomized, controlled trial of glucosamine for treating osteoarthritis of the knee. West J Med 2000;172:91–4.

Rossetti L, Hawkins M, Chen W, Gindi J, Barzilai N. In vivo glucosamine infusion induces insulin resistance in normoglycemic but not in hyperglycemic conscious rats. Clin Invest 1995;96:132–40.

Runkel DR, Cupp MJ. Glucosamine sulfate use in osteoarthritis. Am J Health Syst Pharm 1999;56:267–9.

Setnikar I, Giacchetti C, Zanolo G. Pharmacokinetics of glucosamine in the dog and in man. Arzneimittelforschung 1986;36:729–35.

Setnikar I, Palumbo R, Canali S, Zanolo G. Pharmacokinetics of glucosamine in man. Arzneimittelforschung 1993;43:1109–13.

Talent JM, Gracy RW. Pilot study of oral polymeric *N*-acetyl-D-glucosamine as a potential treatment for patients with osteoarthritis. Clin Ther 1996;18:1184–90.

Thie NMR, Prasad NG, Major PW. Evaluation of glucosamine sulfate compared with ibuprofen for the treatment of temporomandibular joint osteoarthritis: a randomized double blind controlled 3 month trial. J Rheumatol 2001;28:1347–55.

Towheed TE, Hochberg MC. A systematic review of randomized controlled trials of pharmacologic therapy in osteoarthritis of the hip. J Rheumatol 1997;24:349–57.

Uebelhart D, Thonar EJMA, Delmas PD, et al. E. Effects of oral chondroitin sulfate on the progression of knee osteoarthrosis: a pilot study. Osteoarthritis Cartilage 1998;6(suppl A):39–46.

Vaz AL. Double-blind clinical evaluation of the relative efficacy of ibuprofen and glucosamine sulphate in the management of osteoarthrosis of the knee in outpatients. Curr Med Res Opin 1982;8:145–9.

Verbruggen G, Goemaere S, Veys EM. Chondroitin sulfate: S/DMOAD (structure/disease modifying anti-osteoarthritis drug) in the treatment of finger joint OA. Osteoarthritis Cartilage 1998;6 (suppl A):37–8.

Volpi N. Hyaluronic acid and chondroitin sulfate unsaturated disaccharides analysis by high-performance liquid chromatography and fluorimetric detection with dansylhydrazine. Anal Biochem 2000;277:19–24.

Wood KM, Curtis CG, Powell GM, Wusteman FS. The metabolic fate of intravenously injected peptide-bound chondroitin sulphate in the rat. Biochem J 1976;158:39–46.

Chapter 13

Huperzine

Arthur I. Jacknowitz and Timothy S. Tracy

13.1. HISTORY

For centuries, the rare Chinese club moss *Huperzia serrata* has been used in the preparation of the traditional Chinese medicine Qian Ceng Ta, a treatment for fever and inflammation (Skolnick, 1997). In 1986, an alkaloid, huperzine A was isolated from this herbal medicine and shown to be a potent inhibitor of the enzyme acetylcholinesterase (Bai et al., 2000). Acetylcholinesterase breaks down acetylcholine, an important neurotransmitter involved in thought, reasoning, and judgment. Scientists have long recognized that compounds with the ability to inhibit acetylcholinesterase can help improve memory and thus be used to treat the symptoms of Alzheimer's disease and other dementias.

Although the purified compound has been available as a prescription drug in China for the past decade to treat dementia, clinical trials in the United States have yet to be reported other than in abstract form.

13.2. CHEMICAL STRUCTURE

See Fig. 13-1 for the chemical structure of huperzine.

13.3. CURRENT PROMOTED USES

Results from several placebo-controlled, double-blind randomized controlled clinical trials in China show that huperzine A improved memory in older adults with age-associated memory decline, Alzheimer's disease, and vascular dementia, and it has been advocated as an ideal therapy "for people who are concerned about memory loss, cognitive decline, absent mindedness and increased forgetfulness" (Intlecs™, 2002).

From: *Forensic Science: Dietary Supplements: Toxicology and Clinical Pharmacology*
Edited by: M. J. Cupp and T. S. Tracy © Humana Press Inc., Totowa, New Jersey

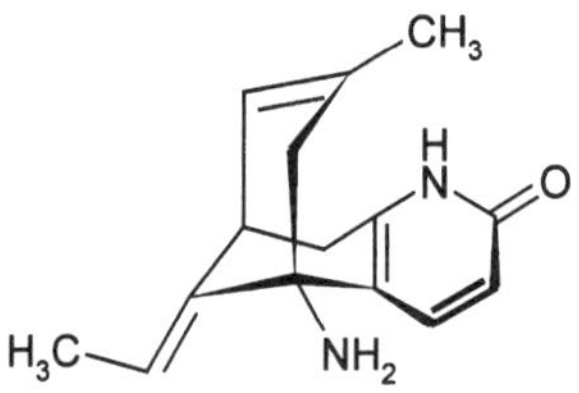

Fig. 1. Chemical Structure of huperzine.

13.4. SOURCES AND CLINICAL COMPOSITION

Huperzine A is an optically active stereoisomer isolated from the Chinese club moss *Huperzia serrata*. Only the levorotatory-isomer is pharmacologically active. It is a reversible, potent, and selective inhibitor of acetylcholinesterase, whose potency and duration of inhibition are comparable to those of physostigmine, tacrine, donepezil, and glantamine (Tang and Han, 1999). X-ray crystallography has shown that huperzine A "slides smoothly into the active site of acetylcholinesterase, where acetylocholine is broken down, and latches onto this site via a very larger number of subtle chemical links. This binding closes off the enzyme's 'cutting' machinery and keeps acetylcholine out of danger" (Raves et al., 1997).

Commercially available huperzine A is currently extracted and purified in China. However, because the moss from which huperzine A is derived is a rare Chinese herb, in the future chemical synthesis may be the most reliable source of this compound. In fact, a new and novel series of hybrids of huperzine A and other commercially available acetylcholinesterase inhibitors, known as huprines, may bind to the enzyme with significantly higher affinity than each of the individual components. These hybrids may overcome the adverse effects seen with each of the agents and would elicit higher levels of brain acetylcholine. The effects of these compounds on acetylcholinesterase have recently been reported (Ros et al., 2001).

13.5. PRODUCTS AVAILABLE

Huperzine A is available from various neutraceutical manufacturers as 50-µg capsules and tablets. Intlecs™ huperzine A tablets contain more than 98% pure alkaloid. The Cerebra™ brand name used for huperzine A has been confused with the prescription medications, Celebrex®, Celexa®, and Cerebyz®.

Huperzine A was initially thought to be structurally related to a substance isolated from *Lycopodium selago* named selagine. However, it was subsequently found to be identical. It is therefore important to avoid confusing this name with that of selegiline, which has also been advocated to halt the progression of Alzheimer's disease.

13.6. IN VITRO EFFECTS AND ANIMAL STUDIES

Huperzine A is a reversible, potent, and selective inhibitor of the enzyme acetylcholinesterase. In vitro, the inhibition of this enzyme by huperzine A is greater than that of physostigmine, tacrine, or galantamine but less than that of donepezil (Cheng et al., 1996). However, huperzine A had the highest specificity for acetylcholinest-erase of these agents.

In contrast to the inhibition of acetylcholinesterase in vitro, the relative inhibitory effect of oral huperzine A on cerebral cortex acetylcholinesterase was found to be about 24- and 180-fold, on an equimolar basis, as potent as donepezil and tacrine respectively (Wang and Tang, 1998a). In addition, as compared with donepezil and tacrine, huperzine A has greater bioavailability and more readily crosses the blood-brain barrier (Cheng and Tang, 1998). Of interest was the finding that repeated doses of huperzine A did not result in a decreased inhibition of acetylcholinesterase compared with a single dose, indicating that tolerance did not develop (Laganiere et al., 1991).

With regard to its effects on neurotransmitter levels, compared with tacrine and physostigmine, huperzine A shows the longest lasting increase in brain acetylcholine. Acetylcholine concentrations increased linearly from 10% at 5 min to 40% at 1 h following intramuscular administration. Not unexpectedly, the elevation of brain acetylcholine was slower than the onset of acetylcholinesterase inhibition (Tang et al., 1989).

There were significant differences in acetylcholine concentrations in various areas of the brain following huperzine A administration (Zhu and Giacobini, 1995). Maximal increases were observed at 1 h in the frontal and parietal cortex, intermediate increases at 30 min in the hippocampus and at 5 min in the medulla oblongata, and only slight increases at 30 min in the striatum. This regional specificity produced by huperzine A may prove valuable therapeutically, because the cerebral cortex shows a significant decline in acetylcholine in Alzheimer's disease.

Studies designed to determine whether the activity of choline acetyltransferase increased following administration of huperzine A showed no effect of huperzine A on this enzyme. Therefore, the increase in acetylcholine levels by huperzine is thought not to be mediated via an increase in the rate of acetylcholine synthesis or release (Laganiere et al., 1991).

It has been reported (Lipton and Rosenberg, 1994) that neuronal cell death caused by overexpression of glutamate receptors may be the final common pathway for various neurodegenerative diseases including Alzheimer's disease. Glutamate activates *N*-methyl-D aspartate (NMDA) receptors and increases the flow of calcium ions into nerve cells, which in large enough concentration can kill the cells. It has now been shown (Wang et al., 1999) that huperzine A acts as an inhibitor of NMDA receptors and may be effective in slowing down or blocking the pathogenesis of early-stage Alzheimer's disease.

It has been found that pretreatment of mice with huperzine A increased the 50% lethal dose (LD_{50}) of the nerve agent soman by twofold for more than 6 h compared with a 1.5-fold increase for only 1.5 h after physostigmine pretreatment (Grunwald et al., 1994). This finding followed an in vitro study in which a greater than 90% inhibition of acetylcholinesterase by huperzine A prevented irreversible phosphorylation of the enzyme by potent nerve toxins. Approximately 45 and 60% of active acetylcholinesterase sites were protected following 2 h of incubation with the agents soman and sarin. These findings suggest that huperzine A may provide a safe and long-lasting antidote against nerve agent toxicity in humans, a finding of particular interest in light of recent bioterrorism concerns.

Finally, huperzine A has been found to attenuate memory impairment in a variety of animal species. Studies in rodents have shown that huperzine A improves performance in a number of different tests including spatial memory tasks (Tang, 1996). Beneficial effects were observed not only in otherwise healthy adult rodents but also in aged rodents (Lu et al., 1988), those cognitively impaired (Lu et al., 1988), and those with cholinergic lesions (Xiong et al., 1998).

Huperzine A also significantly reversed memory deficits induced by scopolamine in young adult monkeys performing a delayed response task and increased choice accuracy in aged monkeys (Ye et al., 1999). The beneficial effects were long-lasting, with improvements remaining for about 24 h after a single injection, and were more pronounced in working memory than in reference memory (Wang and Tang, 1998b).

A recent report (Wang et al., 2001) exemplifies the potential benefit of huperzine A in Alzheimer's disease. In this study, the investigators infused the β-amyloid fragment (which is related to cognitive impairment, dysfunction of cholinergic neurons, and subsequent neuronal death characteristic of Alzheimer's neuropathology) into the cerebral ventricles of laboratory rodents. Daily intraperitoneal administration of huperzine A for 12 consecutive d produced significant reversals of the β-amyloid-induced neuronal degeneration and memory deficits and also reduced the loss of choline acetyltransferase activity in the cerebral cortex. Of great interest was the finding that huperzine A may attenuate apoptotic-like changes and neuronal losses by reversing the shift in the pattern of expression of apoptosis-related proteins induced by the β-amyloid fragment in the cerebral cortex and hippocampus.

Huperzine A has been compared with tacrine (Xiao et al., 2000) and donepezil (Zhou et al., 2001) in vitro in rodents. In the former study, pretreatment of cultured rat cortical neurons with huperzine A or tacrine prior to exposure with amyloid β-peptide significantly increased cell survival. Both drugs showed similar neuroprotective effects. When huperzine A was compared with donepezil for ability to alleviate injury from oxygen-glucose deprivation in an isolated rat pheochromocytoma cell line, once again there were no differences between these two agents in neuroprotective effect. The authors concluded that there are a number of different mechanisms by which huperzine A and donepezil could protect neurons against oxygen-glucose deprivation but indicated that the effect occurred specifically at the level of oxidative energy metabolism. With this in mind, the authors felt that these compounds would impact not only on Alzheimer's disease therapy, but also on vascular dementia and other neurodegenerative disorders with an ischemic pathogenesis.

13.7. CLINICAL STUDIES

Results from several clinical studies in China involving 447 patients suffering from age-related memory dysfunction or dementia have been summarized (Tang and Han, 1999). It should be noted however, that compared with clinical studies of prescription drugs conducted for approval by the Food and Drug Administration (FDA), the Chinese studies enrolled many fewer patients and were of shorter duration. Also, the criteria for assessing side effects may not have been identical to those used in clinical trials of the prescription drugs for Alzheimer's disease in the United States.

In one randomized, double-blind, placebo-controlled study, 103 patients who met Alzheimer's disease criteria received 0.2 mg of huperzine A twice daily and were evaluated using standardized instruments including the Mini Mental Status Examination (MMSE; Xu et al., 1995). Of the 50 huperzine A-treated patients, 29 (58%) showed significant improvement over baseline on tests of memory, cognition, and behavior compared with 19 (36%) of the 53 placebo recipients. Of note is that patients randomized to receive huperzine A had an average increase of 3 points on the MMSE scale compared with 0.5 points in the placebo group.

In a second study, the efficacy of huperzine A was evaluated in 34 pairs of junior high school students who complained of memory lapses and "inadequacy" by using a double-blind and matched-pair designed study (Sun et al., 1999). Huperzine A at a dose of 0.1 mg twice daily for a month increased the scores for Accumulation, Recognition, and Association factors but not Understanding.

Finally, an open-label, office-based study by practicing American neurologists sought to evaluate the safety and efficacy of huperzine A in 26 patients meeting established criteria for uncomplicated as well as possible or probable Alzheimer's disease (Mazurek, 1999). Patients were permitted to continue to receive concomitant therapies for their disease. They were given 50 or 100 µg of huperzine A twice daily for 12 wk. Efficacy was determined by changes in the MMSE. The mean change in the MMSE score at 1 mo was 0.5 point for those receiving the lower dosage and 1.5 points for those in the 100-µg group. At 2 mo, the change was 1.2 points for the former and 1.8 points for the later group. Finally, and notably at the end of the study each group's score increased approx 1 point over the previous month. The author concluded that even though both groups improved, those receiving the higher doses showed higher MMSE scores. No significant side effects were noted.

When evaluating the clinical studies reported to date, it is important to note that beneficial effects observed in small trials and in the research laboratory may turn out not to be clinically significant after large-scale, well-designed trials.

13.8. PHARMACOKINETICS

In the one published pharmacokinetic study (Qian et al., 1995), 0.99 mg of huperzine A was administered to six patients after an overnight fast and the pharmacokinetics measured for 10 h after dosing. The time to peak concentration (C_{max}) was approximately 80 min, and the mean plasma half-life was estimated to be 4.8 h. The apparent volume of distribution (Vd/F) was reported to be 0.11 L/kg, suggesting that it is distributed primarily in plasma water. Intersubject variability in plasma concentrations, and thus pharmacokinetic parameters, was not reported.

13.9. ADVERSE EFFECTS AND TOXICITY

Data from the published studies cited previously indicate that when huperzine A is administered for periods of 1–3 mo at therapeutic doses, mild adverse effects are seen that are primarily cholinergic (e.g., nausea, vomiting, diarrhea, hyperactivity, dizziness, and anorexia) (Xu et al., 1995). Clinically significant bradycardia was noted in the first study cited (Xu et al., 1995) and may result in a further decline in patients with preexisting cardiovascular disease. Nevertheless, the side effect profile of huperzine A appears to be similar to those acetylcholinesterase inhibitors currently marketed in the United States. Unlike tacrine, no hepatotoxicity has been noted (Xu et al., 1995).

A series of studies have been conducted to evaluate the toxicity of huperzine A in mice, rats, rabbits, and dogs (Yan et al., 1987). Dose-response curves for salivation indicate that huperzine A is less potent than other inhibitors of acetylcholinesterase. In addition, the characteristic symptoms of cholinergic hyperactivity was less severe for huperzine A in rats compared with donepezil and tacrine. The lethal (LD_{50}) doses of huperzine A in mice were 4.6 mg (po) 3.0 mg (sc) 1.8 mg (ip), and 0.63 mg (iv). In all cases, atropine exerted a significant antidotal effect on the toxicity induced by huperzine A (Tang and Han, 1999).

13.10. INTERACTIONS

No drug interactions involving huperzine A have been reported. However, theoretically, concurrent use of anticholinergic agents and huperzine A might decrease the effectiveness of huperzine A or the anticholinergic agent. Likewise, concurrent use of huperzine A and medications that increase acetylcholine levels in the brain or periphery might result in additive cholinergic effects.

Finally, because of the report of bradycardia following administration of huperzine A, additive cardiovascular effects may occur in the presence of β-blockers or other medications that can cause bradyarrhythmias.

13.11. REPRODUCTION

There is insufficient reliable information concerning the use of huperzine A in pregnancy; therefore its use should be avoided. No teratogenic effect was detected in mice or rabbits after the administration of huperzine A (Tang and Han, 1999).

13.12. CHEMICAL AND BIOFLUID ANALYSIS

Little analytical methodology exists for determining huperzine A concentrations, especially in human blood or urine. Felgenhauer and colleagues (2000) report a high-performance liquid chromatography (HPLC) method for quantitating huperzine A extracted from the fir club moss. This method could potentially be adapted for use with biologic fluids. In this procedure, 2 g of dried fir club moss is mortared with dichloromethane (40 mL) in the presence of dry ice. The resulting material is then refluxed for 1 h at 40°C in a Soxhlet apparatus, evaporated at reduced pressure, and extracted with 1 mL of water. Chromatographic conditions consist of a LiChrospher Select B column (3.9 × 15 cm) through which the mobile phase is pumped at a flow rate of 1 mL/min. The mobile phase consists of ammonium acetate (50 m*M*, pH 4.5)/ acetonitrile (90:10, v/v). Detection of the analytes is by ultraviolet absorbance at 308 nm. Samples are compared with absorbances obtained from authentic standards of huperzine A solution. The retention time for the assay is approximately 7 min.

An HPLC method has also been developed by Qian and associates (1995) that was used to estimate the pharmacokinetic parameters of huperzine A following an oral dose. The method appears to be sensitive enough to use for routine analysis. Briefly, to 2 mL of plasma is added 1 mL of $Na_2CO_3/NaHCO_3$ buffer (pH 11.9). To this is added chloroform (7.5 mL), and the samples are shaken for 2 min. Samples are then centrifuged for 10 min at 1000g, and the organic phase is removed and subsequently evaporated to dryness under nitrogen at 40°C. The resulting residue is then dissolved in 50 µL of mobile phase, and 20 µL is injected into the HPLC system. The mobile phase consists of methanol/water (45:55, v/v) pumped at 1 mL/min through a Spherisorb C18 column (150 × 5 mm, 5 µm) maintained at 30°C. Under these conditions, the retention times for dinor huperzine A is 3.5 min and for huperzine A the retention time is 8.3 min.

13.13. REGULATORY STATUS

Huperzine A is available as a dietary supplement. However, according to the Natural Medicines Comprehensive Database, "Huperzine A is a drug that stretches the guidelines of the Dietary Supplement Health and Education Act (DSHEA). Although derived from a plant, Huperzine A is a laboratory-manipulated, highly purified drug, unlike herbs, which typically contain hundreds of constituents."

13.14. SUMMARY

- Huperzine A is an acetylcholinesterase inhibitor that may be a safe and effective treatment for Alzheimer's disease based on small studies performed primarily in China.
- Huperzine's beneficial effects in Alzheimer's disease may also be a function of NMDA receptor inhibition or inhibition of neuronal apoptosis.
- Huperzine's adverse effects are cholinergic in nature. It may cause bradycardia, which could cause clinical decompensation in patients with heart failure.
- Although drug interactions have not been reported, huperzine may have additive effects with cholinergic drugs. Anticholinergic drugs may inhibit its efficacy. Its effect on heart rate may be additive with that of β-blockers.

REFERENCES

Bai DL, Tang XC, He XC. Huperzine A, a potential therapeutic agent for treatment of Alzheimer's disease. Curr Med Chem 2000;7:355–74.

Cheng DH, Ren H, Tang XC. Huperzine A, a novel promising acetylcholinesterase inhibitor. Neuroreport 1996;8:97–101.

Cheng DH, Tang XC. Comparative studies of huperzine A, E2020, and tacrine on behavior and cholinesterase activities. Pharmacol Biochem Behav 1998;60:377–86.

Felgenhauer N, Zilker T, Worek F, Eyer P. Intoxication with huperzine A, a potent anticholinesterase found in the fir club moss. J Toxicol Clin Toxicol 2000;38:803–808.

Grunwald J, Raveh L, Doctor BP, Ashani Y. Huperzine A as a pretreatment candidate drug against nerve agent toxicity. Life Sci 1994;54:991–97.

Intlecs, 2002. Huperzine A—product information. Available from: URL: http://store.yahoo.com/biomedisyn/index.html, Accessed February 6, 2002.

Laganiere S, Corey J, Tang XC, Wulfert E, Hanin I. Acute and chronic studies with the anticholinesterase huperzine A: effect on central nervous system cholinergic parameters. Neuropharmacology 1991;30:763–68.

Lipton SA, Rosenberg PA. Excitatory amino acids as a final common pathway for neurologic disorders. N Engl J Med 1994;330:613–22.

Lu WH, Shou J, Tang XC. Improving effect of huperzine A on discrimination performance in aged rats and adult rats with experimental cognitive impairment (Chinese). Acta Pharmacol Sin 1988;9:11–5.

Mazurek A. An open label trial of huperzine A in the treatment of Alzheimer's disease. Altern Ther Health Med 1999;5:97–8.

Qian BC, Wang M, Zhou ZF, et al. Pharmacokinetics of tablet huperzine A in six volunteers. Acta Pharmacol Sin 1995;16:396–98.

Raves ML, Harel M, Pang YP, et al. Structure of acetylcholinesterase complexed with the nootropic alkaloid, (-)-huperzine A. Nat Struct Biol 1997;4:57–63.

Ros E, Aleu J, Gomez DA, I, et al. The pharmacology of novel acetylcholinesterase inhibitors, (+/–)-huprines Y and X, on the *Torpedo* electric organ. Eur J Pharmacol 2001;421:77–84.

Skolnick AA. Old Chinese herbal medicine used for fever yields possible new Alzheimer disease therapy. JAMA 1997;277:776.

Sun QQ, Xu SS, Pan JL, Guo HM, Cao WQ. Huperzine-A capsules enhance memory and learning performance in 34 pairs of matched adolescent students. Acta Pharmacol Sin 1999;20:601–03.

Tang XC. Huperzine A (shuangyiping): a promising drug for Alzheimer's disease. Acta Pharmacol Sin 1996;17:481–484.

Tang XC, De Sarno P, Sugaya K, Giacobini E. Effect of huperzine A, a new cholinesterase inhibitor, on the central cholinergic system of the rat. J Neurosci Res 1989;24:276–85.

Tang XC, Han YF. Pharmacological profile of huperzine A, a novel acetylcholinesterase inhibitor from chinese herb. CNS Drug Rev 1999;5:281–300.

Wang H, Tang XC. Anticholinesterase effects of huperzine A, E2020, and tacrine in rats. Acta Pharmacol Sin 1998a;19:27–30.

Wang R, Zhang HY, Tang XC. Huperzine A attenuates cognitive dysfunction and neuronal degeneration caused by beta-amyloid protein-(1-40) in rat. Eur J Pharmacol 2001;421:149–56.

Wang T, Tang XC. Reversal of scopolamine-induced deficits in radial maze performance by (-)-huperzine A: comparison with E2020 and tacrine. Eur J Pharmacol 1998b;349:137–42.

Wang XD, Zhang JM, Yang HH, Hu GY. Modulation of NMDA receptor by huperzine A in rat cerebral cortex. Acta Pharmacol Sin 1999;20:31–5.

Xiao XQ, Wang R, Tang XC. Huperzine A and tacrine attenuate beta-amyloid peptide-induced oxidative injury. J Neurosci Res 2000;61:564–69.

Xiong ZQ, Cheng DH, Tang XC. Effects of huperzine A on nucleus basalis magnocellularis lesion-induced spatial working memory deficit. Acta Pharmacol Sin 1998;19:128–32.

Xu SS, Gao ZX, Weng Z, et al. Efficacy of tablet huperzine-A on memory, cognition, and behavior in Alzheimer's disease. Acta Pharmacol Sin 1995;16:391–95.

Yan XF, Lu WH, Lou WJ, Tang XC. Effects of huperzine A and B on skeletal muscle and the electroencephalogram (Chinese). Acta Pharmacol Sin 1987;8:117–23.

Ye JW, Cai JX, Wang LM, Tang XC. Improving effects of huperzine A on spatial working memory in aged monkeys and young adult monkeys with experimental cognitive impairment. J Pharmacol Exp Ther 1999;288:814–19.

Zhou J, Fu Y, Tang XC. Huperzine A and donepezil protect rat pheochromocytoma cells against oxygen-glucose deprivation. Neurosci Lett 2001;306:53–6.

Zhu XD, Giacobini E. Second generation cholinesterase inhibitors: effect of (L)-huperzine-A on cortical biogenic amines. J Neurosci Res 1995;41:828–35.

Chapter 14

Hydrazine Sulfate

Ona Dingess, Melanie Johns Cupp, and Timothy S. Tracy

14.1. HISTORY

Hydrazine sulfate is used industrially in metal refining, and in analytical tests for blood. It is used as an antioxidant agent in soldering flux and as a fungicide, although it is not registered as such in the United States (National Safety Council, 2000). Other chemicals in the hydrazine class include the antituberculosis drug isoniazid and the cancer chemotherapy drug procarbazine. Over 400 hydrazine compounds have been studied over the past century, and 7 have been identified as having anticancer activity in human tumors. One of these, methylhydrazine, showed activity in patients with Hodgkin's disease, melanoma, and lung cancer in the 1960s. Hydrazine sulfate was subsequently investigated because of its structural similarity to methylhydrazine (National Cancer Institute, 2000). In the early 1970s, hydrazine sulfate was studied in humans as a treatment for cancer by Dr. Joseph Gold of the Syracuse Cancer Research Institute (Gold, 1975). Russian investigators also began studying hydrazine sulfate at this time. Although tumor response was poor, nutritional status was thought to benefit (National Cancer Institute, 2000).

14.2. CHEMICAL STRUCTURE

See Fig. 14-1 for the chemical structure of hydrazine.

14.3. CURRENT PROMOTED USES

Hydrazine sulfate is currently being promoted as an alternative treatment regimen for cachexia and anorexia associated with cancer. Hydrazine sulfate is usually administered orally, with food or immediately before eating. The typical treatment cycle recommended by Internet web sites consists of 60 mg three times daily for 30–45 d followed by a resting period of 2–6 wk, repeated as many times as desirable; however, in published clinical trials, hydrazine was given continuously.

From: *Forensic Science: Dietary Supplements: Toxicology and Clinical Pharmacology*
Edited by: M. J. Cupp and T. S. Tracy © Humana Press Inc., Totowa, New Jersey

$$H_2N\!-\!NH_2$$

Fig. 1. Chemical structure of hydrazine.

14.4. SOURCES AND CHEMICAL COMPOSITION

Hydrazine sulfate is a white or colorless crystal (National Safety Council, 2000; Anonymous, 2000). Its molecular formula is $H_4N_2(H_2SO_4)$. It is water- and ethanol-soluble (National Safety Council, 2000). Although hydrazine sulfate is typically synthesized in a laboratory setting, natural sources of this compound include tobacco (National Cancer Institute, 2000), and poisonous mushrooms of the genus *Gyromitra* contain monomethylhydraine (Michelot and Toth, 1991). A popular hydrazine supplier, Life Energy Distributor, obtains hydrazine sulfate from US Pharmaceutical Grade, located in the United States (Life Energy Distributor, 2000).

14.5. PRODUCTS AVAILABLE

Hydrazine sulfate is available in 30- and 60-mg capsules. The capsules by Life Energy Distributor are white and gray and are packaged in bottles of 100. Hydrazine sulfate is available in Europe and Russia as Sehydrin.

14.6. IN VITRO EFFECTS AND ANIMAL DATA

Hydrazine has been studied as an antineoplastic in several rodent models, both as monotherapy and in combination with conventional chemotherapy, with variable results. NCE-sponsored studies performed in the 1980s showed little or no effect in any of the tumor models studied. These studies have been reviewed elsewhere (NCI, 2002).

It has been theorized that excessive gluconeogenesis might be responsible for cancer cachexia; the body is thought to expend energy-making glucose for use by the tumor. The enzyme phosphoenol pyruvate carboxykinase (PEP-CK) plays an important role in gluconeogenesis, specifically, the conversion of lactic acid into glucose. Tumors are thought to use this anaerobic pathway to obtain energy. Researchers have proposed that inhibition of PEP-CK would impair gluconeogenesis and reduce the severity of cachexia, as well as decrease the supply of glucose to the tumor, inhibiting tumor growth. Hydrazine sulfate has been found to be an effective inhibitor of PEP-CK. Hydrazine sulfate may also inhibit tumor necrosis factor-α (TNF-α), an inflammatory mediator released in infection in response to bacterial endotoxin and in malignancy. TNF-α may play a role in cancer cachexia.

Hydrazine sulfate has also been a recent topic of interest with respect to potential treatment of infectious disease in animal models. Hydrazine sulfate protected mice against the lethal effects of TNF-α at doses of 30–60 mg/kg (Jia et al, 1994).

A study was conducted to determine whether hydrazine sulfate can decrease the mortality of galactosamine-potentiated endotoxic shock in 10-d-old rats (Ravindranath et al., 1998). Administration of galactosamine, an amino sugar, increases TNF-α production, thus increasing the lethalality of endotoxin in adult animals. A previous study in mice demonstrated that the corticosteroid dexamethasone inhibits this effect by suppressing the expression of the TNF-α gene and increasing TNF-α binding protein production. Hydrazine sulfate provided similar protection in adult mice by stimulating endogenous glucocorticoid production. Because newborns are at increased risk of developing endotoxic shock owing to immaturity of the pituitary-adrenal axis, Ravindranath and colleagues (1998) hypothesized that hydrazine sulfate might provide protection against endotoxic shock in this population by stimulating the pituitary-adrenal axis and increasing glucocorticoid production.

In their first experiment, designed to determine the effect of hydrazine sulfate on mortality, newborn (10-d-old) rats were divided into 11 groups. Six groups received intraperitoneal injections of saline 0.2 mL with or without hydrazine sulfate 50 mg/kg, galactosamine 600 mg/kg with or without hydrazine sulfate 50 mg/kg, and *Salmonella enteritidis* lipopolysaccharide (LPS) 0.01 mL with or without hydrazine sulfate 50 mg/kg. Four groups received intraperitoneal injections of galactosamine, LPS, and hydrazine sulfate 0, 20, 50, or 80 mg/kg. One group received intraperitoneal injections of galactosamine, LPS, and dexamethasone 4 mg/kg.

In a second experiment, designed to examine the effect of hydrazine sulfate on plasma glucose and lactate concentrations, newborn rats were divided into nine groups. They received intraperitoneal injections of saline 0.2 mL with or without hydrazine sulfate, LPS 0.01 mg/kg with or without hydrazine sulfate, galactosamine 600 mg/kg plus LPS 0.01 mg/kg with or without hydrazine, and galactosamine 600 mg/kg plus LPS 0.01 mg/kg with dexamethasome 4 mg/kg. Statistical methods were not described. Dexamethasone, but not hydrazine sulfate, decreased mortality in galactosamine-sensitized endotoxic shock ($p < 0.05$). Hydrazine sulfate alone or in combination with galactosamine, LPS, or galactosamine plus LPS decreased plasma glucose concentration ($p < 0.05$). Plasma lactate was higher in the hydrazine sulfate-treated groups compared to groups receiving the same treatment without hydrazine sulfate ($p < 0.05$). Dexamethasone ameliorated both galactosamine-sensitized endotoxic shock-associated hypoglycemia and lactic acidemia ($p < 0.05$). The investigators concluded that hydrazine's lack of effect on mortality and effects on plasma glucose and lactate were owing to the immaturity of the newborns' pituitary-adrenal axis and hydrazine's ability to inhibit gluconeogenesis, which is an important mechanism by which newborns maintain glucose levels.

14.7. CLINICAL STUDIES

Several studies have been conducted to determine the efficacy of hydrazine sulfate in cancer. Loprinzi and colleagues (1994a) reviewed six open-label studies that reported positive results. They concluded that the subjective improvements reported in these trials were the result of a placebo effect and that the low tumor response rate was possibly owing to measurement error.

The first randomized, prospective, double-blind study of hydrazine sulfate was designed to evaluate its efficacy versus placebo on survival and nutritional status in patients with advanced non-small cell lung cancer (NSCLC) not amenable to surgery or radiation (International Staging System stage IIIb or IV disease) (Chlebowski et al, 1990). Patients were required to have an Eastern Cooperative Oncology (ECOG) performance status of 0, 1, or 2; adequate hematologic, renal, and hepatic function; and no prior chemotherapy. Patients with prior radiation therapy could be included only if there was evaluable disease outside the radiation field, the cancer had progressed, and the last radiation treatment was at least 3 mo prior to enrollment. Patients with central nervous system (CNS) metastasis requiring corticosteroid use were excluded. These inclusion/exclusion criteria were chosen because they resembled those used in the Cancer Cooperative Group NSCLC trials, and they provide a relatively homogenous patient population that oncologists would deem candidates for chemotherapy.

All patients received the same chemotherapy regimen, consisting of vinblastine 4 mg/m^2 on days 1 and 2; cisplatin 100 mg/m^2 on day 2; and bleomycin 10 mg/m^2 on days 1 (two doses) and 2. This induction regimen was repeated after 28 d. The maintenance regimen consisted of four cycles of cisplatin 50 mg/m^2 every 28 d, and vinblastine 5 mg/m^2 every 14 d. Dose reductions were permitted if necessary for toxicity. Patients were randomized to receive hydrazine sulfate 60 mg or placebo capsules. On the first 4 d of the study, one capsule was taken once daily before breakfast. On days 5–8, one capsule was taken before breakfast and before lunch. Thereafter, one capsule was taken three times daily, prior to breakfast, lunch, and dinner.

Hydrazine or placebo was continued after the six chemotherapy cycles were completed unless toxic effects occurred or cancer progressed. All patients received dietary counseling appropriate for their gender, height, and weight. Disease progression was assessed prior to each cycle of chemotherapy using clinical examination and chest X-ray. Weight, serum albumin, and 24-h calorie count were also measured prior to each cycle. Response frequency between the two groups was analyzed using chi-square analysis, and paired t-tests were used to identify differences over time in the same patient. Survival was calculated using the Kaplan-Meier method and was compared using the log-rank test. Based on prior studies showing that nutritional status is improved with hydrazine sulfate in approximately 70% of patients with NSCLC, and anticipating that half of the patients benefiting from hydrazine sulfate from a nutritional standpoint would also realize a survival benefit, a sample size of 60 was calculated to be adequate to detect a 35% difference in 1-yr survival with a power of 80% and significance accepted at p 0.05. Sixty-five patients were enrolled in the study. Baseline characteristics in the two treatment groups were comparable.

It was determined that after 28 d of therapy, hydrazine sulfate resulted in a significantly greater increase from baseline in serum albumin and caloric intake compared with placebo treatment ($p < 0.05$, paired t-tests). Survival was greater in the hydrazine sulfate group compared to the placebo group, but the difference did not reach statistical significance ($p = 0.11$). In patients with the most favorable performance status (0 or 1), survival was significantly prolonged in the hydrazine group (328 vs 209 d; $p < 0.05$). The authors attributed the increased survival to improvement in nutritional status as evidenced by albumin maintenance, which has been shown in previous studies to be correlated with survival. In addition, the improved survival with hydrazeine sulfate in patients with performance status 0 or 1 reflects findings in previous studies of chemotherapy.

Because subgroup analysis suggested that hydrazine sulfate may benefit patients with good performance status, another group of investigators performed a larger study to compare the effects of hydrazine sulfate with those of placebo on survival, quality of life, and toxicity in patients with advanced NSCLC not amenable to surgery or radiation (Loprinzi et al., 1994a). Patients were required to have an ECOG performance status of 0, 1, or 2; adequate hematologic, renal, and hepatic function; and no prior chemotherapy. Patients with prior radiation therapy could be included only if bone marrow function was not compromised as a result. Patients with CNS metastasis, severe infection, insulin-requiring diabetes, malabsorption, gastrointestinal obstruction, weight loss greater than 10% over the 3 mo prior to enrollment, or major sugery within the 3 wk prior to enrollment were excluded, as were patients with concurrent or planned use of corticosteroids, androgens, progestins, appetite stimulants, or tranquilizers. Although initially one alcoholic beverage was allowed per day, the protocol was modified to prohibit alcohol consumption after nine patients were enrolled. Prior to randomization, patients were stratified according to performance status, gender, number of metastatic sites, presence of liver involvement, stage, and presence of measurable disease.

All patients received cisplatin 30 mg/m^2/d and etoposide 100 mg/m^2/d for 3 d every 4 wk as tolerated, until disease progression. In the event of disease progression, patients were permitted to receive a second-line chemotherapy regimen, if desired. Patients were randomized to placebo or hydrazine sulfate, which was started on chemotherapy day 3 to minimize nausea and vomiting. On the first 4 d of the hydrazine sulfate/placebo administration, one capsule was taken once daily. On days 5–8, two capsules were taken, and then the dosage was advanced to three capsules daily for all patients weighing at least 50 kg. Hydrazine/placebo was continued indefinitely if tolerated, even in the event of disease progression. Each month, patient history, physical examination, tumor measurements, blood tests, and chest X-rays were performed. Patients completed a Functional Living Index-Cancer (FLIC) questionnaire, a measurement of quality of life, at baseline and at each visit. Survival was estimated using the Kaplan-Meier method, and log-rank statistics were used to compare survival curves. Cox's proportional hazards model was used to evaluate the effect of baseline characteristics on survival. The Wilcoxon rank-sum test was used to compare response rates and toxicities. One hundred nineteen patients were randomized to hydrazine sulfate and 118 patients were randomized to placebo. Baseline characteristics were similar.

Median time to progression was shorter in the hydrazine sulfate group compared to the placebo group (3.3 vs 4.2 mo; $p = 0.04$). Considering only patients with higher performance status (0 or 1), median time to progression was shorter in the hydrazine sulfate group than the placebo group ($p = 0.02$). Thus, the results of this trial do not support those of Chlebowski and colleagues (1990) suggesting that hydrazine sulfate can improve survival in patients with good performance status. There was a trend toward more dizziness and headache in the hydrazine sulfate group. There was also a trend toward poorer quality of life in the hydrazine sulfate group. The investigators concluded that their study failed to demonstrate any benefit from hydrazine sulfate.

Other investigators examined the effect of adding hydrazine sulfate to cisplatin and vinblastine in the treatment of unresectable NSCLC (Kosty et al., 1994). For study inclusion, patients were required to have a diagnosis of locally advanced NSCLC (stage T4), metastatic disease, or stage N3 disease by virtue of scalene or subclavicular node involvement. Patients were also required to have a performance status of 0 or 1; adequate hematologic, renal, and hepatic function; and a life expectancy of 2 mo or more. Patients with central nervous system metastasis, recurrent disease in the chest after surgery or radiation, prior chemotherapy or immunotherapy, serious medical or psychiatric illness, prior history of malignancy (except basal cell carcinoma of the skin or cervical cancer *in situ*), concomitant malignancy, edema, ascites, or condition precluding oral intake were excluded. Because hydrazine may affect glucose tolerance, patients with insulin-requiring diabetes were excluded, as were those taking corticosteroids, medroxyprogesterone, and other drugs that can stimulate appetite.

All patients received cisplatin 100 mg/m^2 iv every 28 days, plus vinblastine 5 mg/m^2 iv each week for 5 wk, and then every 2 wk. Doses were adjusted as appropriate for hematologic toxicity, renal or hepatic dysfunction, neurotoxicity, and gastrointestinal toxicity. Patients were randomized to receive either hydrazine sulfate 60 mg orally three times daily or placebo. After every two cycles, patients were evaluated for response according to the Cancer and Leukemia Group B (CALGB) criteria. The treatment regimen was continued indefinitely in patients showing response or stable disease. In patients with evidence of progressive disease, chemotherapy was discontinued, but hydrazine or placebo was continued. At baseline and every 2 mo, patients completed a quality-of-life questionnaire consisting of 52 questions that assessed physical functioning, physical symptoms, psychological functioning, perception of adequacy of social support, and a question about appetite. Two hundred sixty-six patients were enrolled in the study. This sample size was sufficient to detect a 50% increase in survival with 80% power using two-tailed tests and statistical significance accepted at p 0.05. Secondary outcome measures were weight change, serum albumin, and quality of life. Pearson chi-square and t-tests were used to examine differences in baseline characteristics and toxicity between the two groups. Survival was estimated using the Kaplan-Meier product-limit estimator, and the log-rank test was used to compare survival. Cox's proportional hazards model was used to evaluate the effect of baseline characteristics on survival. ANCOVA was used to compare change from baseline in quality of life between the two groups at each assessment.

The investigators found no difference between the two groups in any outcome measure. The incidence of sensory and motor neuropathy was significantly higher ($p = 0.013$ and $p = 0.045$, respectively) in patients receiving hydrazine sulfate. The results of this study suggest no benefit from the addition of hydrazine sulfate to an effective chemotherapeutic regimen.

Hydrazine's effect on survival and quality of life in colorectal cancer has also been examined (Loprinzi et al., 1994b). Patients enrolled in this study had advanced colorectal cancer resistant to fluorouracil (5-FU)-based chemotherapy, the standard treatment. Additional inclusion criteria were life expectancy of 4 mo or greater and ECOG performance score of 2 or less. Exlusion criteria were use or planned use of chemotherapy, severe infection, diabetes requiring insulin, malabsorption or gastrointestinal obstruction, greater than 10% weight loss in the previous month, major surgery in the previous 3 wk, pregnancy, lactation, CNS metastasis, or concurrent or planned use of corticosteroids, androgens, progestins, or appetite stimulants. Although the use of "tranquilizers" and alcohol was not allowed, patients could take antiemetics if needed. Prior to randomization, patients were stratified according to gender, weight, number of previous chemotherapy regimens, and presence of measurable disease.

Patients received either hydrazine sulfate 60 mg or placebo capsules. On the first 4 d of the study, one capsule was taken once daily before breakfast. On days 5–8, one capsule was taken before breakfast and before lunch. Thereafter, one capsule was taken three times daily, prior to breakfast, lunch, and dinner. Treatment was continued even if the disease progressed. Each month, patients were examined, a history was taken, and tumor measurements and blood tests were performed. Performance status, appetite, weight, and disease-associated symptoms were also recorded. Patients also completed a visual analog quality of life questionnaire each month. Survival was estimated using Kaplan-Meier survival curves, and the log-rank test was used to compare survival. Cox's proportional hazards model was used to evaluate the effect of baseline characteristics on survival. Least squares regression and generalized linear models for dependent data were used to analyze performance status and quality of life measurements over time. The Wilcoxon test was used to compare the slopes of these lines between the two groups, as well as the incidence of side effects. A sample size of 300 was calculated to be necessary to provide adequate power to detect a difference in the quality-of-life measures, and a sample size of 200 was necessary to detect a survival difference. Because routine semiannual patient safety monitoring noted increased mortality in one of the treatment arms, interim analysis was preformed using the Lan-DeMets spending function. It was found that after adjustment for the five baseline stratification characteristics, there was a higher mortality in the hydrazine sulfate group ($p = 0.013$). As a result of this finding, no further patients were enrolled in the study at that point. One hundred twenty-seven patients entered the study.

Tumor regression was not noted in any patient. Survival in the hydrazine sulfate group was less than that in the placebo group ($p = 0.034$). After adjustment for the five stratification factors, the p value was 0.012. After adjusting for age and life expectancy, the p value was 0.029. It decreased to 0.016 after adjustment for baseline quality-of-life scores plus the other seven baseline factors. The performance status of the hydrazine sulfate group decreased more quickly than that of the placebo group when comparing the slopes of the least squares lines ($p = 0.003$). Because the patients in the hydrazine sulfate group were dying faster than the patients in the placebo group, a performance score of 5 was assigned to each patient on the day of death, and slopes were recalculated. This maneuver resulted in there being no difference between the two groups ($p = 0.145$). Quality of life scores deteriorated more rapidly in the hydrazine sulfate group, but the difference from the placebo group was not statistically significant ($p = 0.371$). Again, to compensate for the number of deaths in the hydrazine sulfate group, a quality of life score of 0 was assigned to all patients on the day of death, and the slopes were recalculated, giving a p value of 0.074, suggesting a trend toward faster deterioration of quality of life in the hydrazine sulfate group. Rate of weight loss did not differ between the groups ($p = 0.381$). There was less dysguesia in the hydrazine sulfate group ($p = 0.04$) and trends toward less insomnia, more anorexia, and more lethargy in this group. The investigators concluded that based on the results of this and other randomized controlled trials, the use of hydrazine sulfate cannot be recommended at this time.

Overall, studies of the effect of hydrazine sulfate on survival, nutritional status, and quality of life in cancer patients suggest that its risks outweigh any small benefit. Perhaps certain subgroups of patients might benefit. Larger studies are needed but are unlikely to be performed.

14.8. PHARMACOKINETICS

The pharmacokinetics of hydrazine sulfate were determined in plasma and cerebrospinal fluid of 10 rabbits after separate intravenous and oral administration. The plasma concentrations of hydrazine were similar after either route, indicating that oral absorption was nearly complete (Walubo et al., 1991).

The tissue distribution of hydrazine in rats was determined by mass fragmentography using a gas chromatograph-mass spectrometer. A significantly high level of hydrazine was detected in the kidney. Free hydrazine was detected in both the tissues and the urine (Kaneo et al., 1984).

Animal studies have demonstrated that hydrazine appears to undergo *N*-acetylation to form acetylhydrazine (Colvin, 1969). Hydrazine-treated rats excrete greater quantities of hydrazine and acetylhydrazine with increasing dose over 24 h. However, the fraction of the original dose excreted as hydrazine (and acetylhydrazine) declined with increasing dose level (Preece et al., 1992b).

To date, no studies have been published on the pharmacokinetics of hydrazine following administration to humans. Two studies describe the formation of hydrazine from the antitubercular drug isoniazid, but data on hydrazine elimination rates were not calculated (Gent et al., 1992; Donald et al., 1994).

14.9. ADVERSE EFFECTS AND TOXICITY

Acute occupational exposure to hydrazine sulfate can irritate the eyes, nose, and throat and cause dizziness and lightheadedness, followed by tremors and seizures. Hydrazine sulfate can be absorbed through the skin or lungs. Chronic occupational exposure can cause nephrotoxicity, hepatotoxicity, anemia, methemoglobinemia, itching, and rash. When heated (as in a fire), hydrazine sulfate decomposes to toxic gaseous sulfur oxides and nitrogen oxides (Anonymous, 2001).

In animal studies, hydrazine sulfate and other related compounds have been shown to be carcinogens or cocarcinogens in some species (Kaegi, 1998). Hydrazine sulfate is classified by the U.S. Department of Health and Human Services' National Toxicology Program's Fifth Annual Report on Cacinogens as a substance that may reasonably be anticipated to be a carcinogen. The EPA's Toxic Release Inventory classifies hydrazine sulfate as a carcinogen (National Safety Council, 2000). Because hydrazine sulfate is classified as a carcinogen, there is no safe exposure level (Anonymous, 2000).

Although sensory and motor neuropathy (Kosty et al., 194), nausea and/or vomiting (NCI, 2002), dizziness, headache (Loprinzi et al., 1994a), anorexia, and lethargy (Loprinzi et al., 1994b) have been reported in randomized controlled trials of hydrazine, these symptoms are common in patients with cancer, making it difficult to attribute them to hydrazine sulfate (Loprinzi et al., 1994b).

In vitro cytotoxicity of hydrazine sulfate was assessed at five concentrations (200 nM, 400 nM, 600 nM, 800 nM, and 1 μM). For each treatment group, 2×10^5 trypsinized human and animal prostate cells were plated in three 25-cm² flasks in 5 mL of the culture medium RPMI. Cells were allowed to adhere for 48 hours and then were incubated in an appropriate amount of hydrazine sulfate dissolved in 5 mL of RPMI. Control flasks were only treated with RPMI. After 48 h of exposure, the cells were washed with phosphate-buffered saline and lysed. The cell nuclei were counted by using a

Coulter Z1 cell counter. It was concluded that in vitro, hydrazine sulfate demonstrated no growth inhibition of the cell lines examined (Kamradt and Pienta, 1998). These results may not reflect hydrazine's cytotoxicity in animal models or humans; the presence of drug-metabolizing enzymes in vivo could interact with hydrazine to increase its toxicity.

Hydrazine has been shown to inhibit gluconeogenesis irreversibly in animal models (Gold, 1987), and has been noted to decrease serum glucose in case series (NCI, 2002), but not in randomized, controlled trials.

Elevations of hepatic transaminase and alkaline phosphatase levels have also been noted in humans (Kosty et al., 1994). Indeed, hydrazine is a metabolite of isoniazid and is thought to be responsible for the hepatotoxicity of this antituberculosis drug (Sarich et al., 1996). Hydrazine's metabolite, acetylhydrazine, may also have a role in hepatotoxicity—it can be oxidized enzymatically in the liver to electrophilic intermediates that could covalently bind to hepatic macromolecules, thus resulting in liver damage (Woodward and Timbrell, 1984). Increased expression of CYP2E1 in the rat liver after intraperitoneal administration of hydrazine 100 mg/kg has been documented and may play a role in nephrotoxicity through the generation of organic free radicals (Runge-Morris et al., 1994; Runge-Morris et al., 1996).

A case of hepatorenal failure associated with use of hydrazine sulfate has been reported (Hainer et al., 2000). In this report, a 55-yr-old man was diagnosed with squamous cell carcinoma of the left maxillary sinus. He refused conventional treatment with surgery, radiation, and chemotherapy and instead opted to self-medicate with hydrazine sulfate 180 mg/d. He obtained the product and instructions for use via an Internet web site. He discontinued the product after developing a rash and presented 2 wk later with a pruritic macular rash on the chest and extremities, progressive malaise, palmar erythema, icteric sclera, and jaundice. Physical exam was otherwise unremarkable, with no hepatomegaly. Vitals were blood pressure 144/82 mmHg, respiratory rate 18 breaths per minute, and heart rate 76 beats per min. Abnormal lab values included blood urea nitrogen (BUN) 44 mg/dL, serum creatinine (SCr) 5.1 mg/dL, aspartate aminotransferase (AST) 770 U/L, alanine aminotransferase (ALT) 812 U/L, lactate dehydrogenase (LDH) 586 U/L, bilirubin 43.2 mg/dL, albumin 2.8 g/dL, prothrombin time (PT) 19.5 s, and white blood cell count 19.2×10^9 cells/L. Hemoglobin was 167 g/L, hematocrit was 49.7%, and platelet count was 111×10^9 cells/L. Electrocardiogram, chest X-ray, and abdominal ultrasound were normal.

The patient was admitted to the hospital. Because hydrazine sulfate is a pyridoxine (vitamin B6) antagonist, pyridoxine was administered intravenously. Tests for medications (acetaminophen) and infectious diseases (hepatitis A, hepatitis B, hepatitis C, and *Leptospira*) that can damage the liver were negative. Although upon initial presentation the patient was alert and conversant, on hospital day 3 he developed hepatic encephalopathy that did not respond to treatment with lactulose. His renal function worsened, and he required dialysis. Despite administration of vitamin K and blood transfusions, hematemesis occurred on hospital day 7. Esophagoduodenoscopy revealed erosive esophagitis and diffuse hemorrhagic gastritis. Life support was withdrawn per the family's request, and the patient expired. Autopsy revealed autolysis of the kidneys and submassive bridging necrosis of the centrilobular and midzonal areas of the liver. The absence of evidence of preexisiting liver disease or tumor metastasis and the temporal relationship between onset of hydrazine sulfate use and symptom development led to the conclusion that the cause of hepatorenal failure in this patient was hydrazine sulfate.

The rationale for administration of pyridoxine (vitamin B6) in the previous case report stems from hydrazine's role as a pyridoxine antagonist. Pyridoxine has been shown to protect rats from hydrazine toxicity, and it is a well-known antidote for isoniazid overdose. Pyridoxine 5 g iv was successful in treating hydrazine toxicity in a 76-yr-old man with esophageal cancer. After self-medicating with hydrazine sulfate 60 mg three times daily for 2 wk, followed by 120 mg three times daily for 5 wk, he presented to the hospital with confusion, irritability, and restlessness. Bilirubin was slightly elevated at 1.2 mg/dl. Over the first 12 h of the hospital course, mental status worsened, and the patient became combative. Babinski sign was noted. He was intubated after becoming unresponsive and unable to protect his airway. Cerebrospinal glucose and protein were elevated, with no evidence of infection. Pyridoxine was administered, and the patient improved markedly over the next 24 h. Hospital course was complicated by nosocomial pneumonia, but the patient survived to discharge and succumbed to esophageal cancer 9 mo later (Nagappan and Riddell, 2000).

In an accidental exposure, a 24-yr-old man swallowed a mouthful of hydrazine and quickly became confused, lethargic, and restless. Three days later, AST LDH, total bilirubin were elevated. Treatment with pyridoxine 10 g resulted in marked improvement of his mental status and liver function tests over the following 24 h, with complete normalization within 5 d. One week after discharge, the patient noted symptoms of sensory and motor neuropathy. Upon exam, diminished sensation in the distal extremities was noted. Weakness upon hand flexion and foot extension, absent ankle-jerk reflexes bilaterally, and ataxia were also documented. Although motor nerve conduction was normal, a muscle biopsy showed neurogenic atrophy and axonal degeneration. The neuropathy improved without treatment over the next 6 mo (Harati and Niakan, 1986).

14.10. INTERACTIONS

In vitro data suggests that hydrazine is a potent inhibitor of drug metabolism. It has been proposed that hydrazine inhibits drug access to the metabolizing enzyme's active site. Inhibition of the metabolism of chemotherapeutic agents by hydrazine was thought to be responsible for hydrazine's ability to enhance the efficacy of chemotherapeutic agents in vivo (Tretyakov and Filov, 1977).

Because published and unpublished data submitted to the National Cancer Institute indicated that hydrazine sulfate is a monoamine oxidase inhibitor (MAOI) (Gold, 1998), theoretically, one would expect similar interactions associated with other MAOIs. It is important to note that hydrazine's ability to inhibit monoamine oxidase, particularly in vivo, is not well characterized.

Coadministration of MAOIs and barbiturates can prolong the effect of barbiturates, perhaps because of inhibition of barbiturate metabolism (Hansten and Horn, 1999). Indeed, there is some evidence that hydrazine can potentiate the effects of CNS depressants. Sprague-Dawley rats with Walker 256 carcinoma given a combination of hydrazine sulfate 60 mg/kg/d and pentobarbital 25 mg/kg/d slept 331% longer than rats given pentobarbital alone ($p < 0.001$). Non-tumor-bearing rats slept 285% longer with the combination ($p < 0.001$). Some tumor-bearing rats that were administered pentobarbital and hydrazine in combination never woke up (Gold, 1977). A previous study (Seits et al., 1975) published in Russian also showed that the combination of hydrazine sulfate and barbiturates or ethanol resulted in increased sleep time and/or death in non-tumor-bearing mice (Gold, 1977).

Unpublished data supplied to the National Cancer Institute showed that concomitant use of benzodiazepines and hydrazine sulfate in murine models of cancer caused the animals to become comatose and resulted in a 50–60% increase in mortality (Gold, 1998).

Foods and alcoholic beverages containing tyramine (e.g., chianti wine) may induce a severe hypertensive crisis in patients taking a MAOI. In the presence of a MAOI, the normally rapid liver and intestinal metabolism of tyramine is impaired, resulting in an enhanced response to the pressor effects of tyramine (Hansten and Horn, 1999). Patients taking a MAOI should therefore avoid foods that are rich in tyramine (Kaegi, 1998). Monoamine oxidase inhibitors can interact with amphetamines, ephedrine, phenylpropanolamine, pseudoephedrine, dextromethorphan, meperidine, and antidepressants to increase peripheral and central catecholamine levels, leading to hypertension, postural hypotension, urinary retention, arrhythmias, nausea, vomiting, seizures, fever, sweating, flushing, shivering, movement disorders, and mood or mental status changes (Hansten and Horn, 1999).

Drugs that induce cytochrome P450 enzymes have been shown to decrease the hepatotoxicity of hydrazine in animal models, whereas cytochrome P450 inhibitors increase toxicity (Jenner and Timbrell, 1994). Thus, speeding up the metabolism of hydrazine sulfate appears to decrease its toxicity, whereas inhibition of metabolism increases its toxicity. These results imply that hydrazine is a direct hepatotoxin.

Animal data suggesting that alcohol, phenothiazines, and barbiturates decrease hydrazine efficacy, and that concomitant phenothiazine use results in synergistic toxicity, are purported to exist (Kosty et al., 1994). One author (Gold, 1998) expressed concerns that a phenothiazine [prochlorperazine (Compazine®)] was used by patients in one hydrazine study (Kosty et al., 1994). Gold (1998) implies that phenothiazine use may have contributed to the lack of efficacy and toxicities documented by these investigators. MAOIs can increase phenothiazine levels, increasing the risk of adverse effects (Hansten and Horn, 1999)

14.11. REPRODUCTION

Hydrazine administered parenterally to mice at doses of 4–40 mg/kg caused bone and soft tissue malformations. It was found to be embryotoxic when administered parenterally to rats at doses of up to 10 mg/kg. It has also been found to affect the morphology of sperm in the testes of rats and induce malformations in toads and chicks (Dabney, 2002). Hydrazine sulfate's effect on human reproduction has not been studied (Anonymous, 2000); nevertheless, it is recommended that pregnant women and women of child-bearing potential avoid hydrazine sulfate (Kaegi, 1998).

14.12. CHEMICAL AND BIOFLUID ANALYSIS

Measurement of hydrazine concentrations can be problematic in that the compound can rapidly autooxidize, making determinations difficult. Methods have been developed that rely on chemical derivatization of the hydrazine molecule for stabilization. Preece and associates (1992a) have developed a method for derivatization of hydrazine, permitting quantitation in biologic fluids by either nitrogen-sensitive or mass spectrometric detection. A discussion of the latter method is given here.

Immediately following collection of plasma or urine (0.9 mL), 0.1 mL of internal standard (0.02–0.5 mM [$^{15}N_2$]hydrazine sulfate) is added. Then, 0.2 mL of 1 M HCl and 2.3 mL of ammonium sulfate (5 M) are added, followed by vortex mixing. The samples are then centrifuged for 20 min at 1200g and the supernate is removed. An equal volume of citrate buffer (pH 5) is added to the supernate to keep the hydrazine dissolved in aqueous solution. Twenty milliliters of dichloromethane is added and the mixture vortexed (to extract away interfering lipids). Following separation of the layers, 20 µL of the pentafluorobenzaldehyde derivatizing agent (in excess) is added to the aqueous layer, and the solution is allowed to react for 30 min. The derivatives are then extracted with three 5 mL volumes of chloroform. If a nitrogen-phosphorous detector (NPD) is being used, then ethyl acetate is used as the extraction solvent to prevent undesired effects on the NPD detector. The resulting extractions are then combined and evaporated to dryness.

Chromatographic separation of the hydrazine is achieved with an OV-1 fused-silica column (0.25 µm, 12 m × 0.22 mm, i.d.). Following injection of 2 µL of sample (splitless mode), the column is maintained at 35°C for 3 minutes and then ramped to 180°C over the next 17 min (20-min total run time). Electron impact is used as the ionization method, and the samples are monitored in single-ion-monitoring mode. The resulting derivative, decafluorobenzalazine (DFBA), has a retention time of 10.8 min and is monitored at *m/z* 388, whereas the internal standard is monitored at *m/z* 390. It is important to use internal standard concentrations close to those expected in the plasma or urine samples since, 13C$_2$-labeled and ^{13}C/^{15}N-labeled isotopomers of DFBA can occur with an abundance approximately equal to 0.1% and thereby contribute to the *m/z* 390 molecular ion. Calibration curves appear to be linear when between 5 pg and 50 ng are injected onto the column. Slightly different chromatographic conditions are required for NPD detection, and the assay is approximately 1000 times less sensitive by this detection method (5 µg on column).

Seifart and associates (1995) have developed a liquid chromatography method for determining hydrazine concentrations in biologic fluids. This method involves derivatizing with cinnamaldehyde and detection of ultraviolet absorbance at 340 nm. The method is less sensitive than that of Preece and associates (1992a) above, but it does utilize more commonly available analytical equipment.

14.13. REGULATORY STATUS

Because controlled studies of hydrazine sulfate in various cancers have demonstrated lack of benefit and possible harm, the National Cancer Institute stopped funding studies of hydrazine sulfate, and the Division of Endocrine and Metabolic

Drug Products of the Food and Drug Administration (FDA) stopped issuing compassionate use Investigational New Drug Applications for hydrazine sulfate (Malozowski, 2001). The FDA views hydrazine sulfate as a new drug when it is labeled for cancer treatment, although it has been claimed to be a dietary supplement by one supplier because it is an "inorganic mineral salt...partially consisting of sulfur" (Michaelis, 2001).

14.14. SUMMARY

- Hydrazine was originally investigated as an anticancer agent, but it has been determined that the risks of hydrazine use in cancer treatment outweigh the benefits.
- Hydrazine can cause numerous toxicities including hepatic and renal dysfunction, tremors, and seizures and can irreversibly inhibit gluconeogenesis, leading to reductions in serum glucose.
- Because of its ability to inhibit monoamine oxidase, severe hypertensive crisis may occur when hydrazine is concurrently ingested with tyramine-containing foods and beverages.
- Hydrazine has been classified as a carcinogen, and thus there is no safe exposure level.

REFERENCES

Anonymous. Hydrazine sulfate. Available from: URL: http://www.ndcrt.org/data/ EPA_Chemical_Fact_ Sheets/Hydrazine-Sulfate-_16k_. Accessed July 13, 2000.

Chlebowski RT, Bulcavage L, Grosvenor M, et al. Hydrazine sulfate influence on nutritional status and survival in non-small cell lung cancer. J Clin Oncol 1990;8:9–15.

Colvin LB. Metabolic fate of hydrazine and hydrazides. J Pharm Sci 1969;58:1433–43.

Dabney, BJ. Hydrazine (REPROTEXT® Document). In: Heitland G, and Hurlbut KM (Eds.): REPROTEXT® Database. MICROMEDEX, Greenwood Village, Colorado (Edition expires 12/2002).

Donald PR, Seifart HI, Parkin DP, van Jaarsveld PP. Hydrazine production in children receiving isoniazid for the treatment of tuberculosis meningitis. Ann Pharmacother 1994;28:1340–3.

Gent WL, Seifart HI, Parkin DP, Donald PR, Lamprecht JH. Factors in hydrazine formation from isoniazid by paediatric and adult tuberculosis patients. Eur J Clin Pharmacol 1992;43:131–6.

Gold J. Use of hydrazine sulfate in terminal and preterminal cancer patients: results of investigational new drug (IND) study in 84 evaluable patients. Oncology 1975;32:1–10.

Gold J. Incompatibility of hydrazine sulfate and pentobarbital in the treatment of tumor bearing animals [abstract]. Proc Am Assoc Cancer Res 1977;8:250.

Gold J. Hydrazine sulfate: a current perspective. Nutr Cancer 1987;9:59–66.

Gold J. More about: the biology of cachexia [letter]. J Natl Cancer Inst 1998; 90:1101–2.

Hainer MI, Tsai N, Komura ST, Chiu CL. Fatal hepatorenal failure associated with hydrazine sulfate. Ann Intern Med 2000;133:877–80.

Hansten P, Horn J. Drug interactions analysis and management. St. Louis, MO: Facts and Comparisons, 1999.

Harati Y, Niakan E. Hydrazine toxicity, pyridoxine therapy, and peripheral neuropathy [letter]. Ann Intern Med 1986;104:728–9.

Jenner AM, Timbrell JA. Influence of inducers and inhibitors of cytochrome P450 on the hepatotoxicity of hydrazine in vivo. Arch Toxicol 1994;68:349–57.

Jia F, Morrison D, Silverstein R. Hydrazine sulfate selectivity modulates the tumor necrosis factor response to endotoxin in mouse macrophages. Circ Shock 1994;42:111–114.

Kaegi E. Unconventional therapies for cancer. CMAJ 1998;158:1327–30.

Kamradt J, Pienta K. The effect of hydrazine sulfate on prostate cancer. Oncol Rep 1998;5:919–21.

Kaneo Y, Iguchi S, Kubo H, et al. Tissue distribution of hydrazine and its metabolites in rats. J Pharmacobiodyn 1984;7:556–67.

Kosty MP, Fleishman SB, Herndon JE, et al. Cisplatin, vinblastine, and hydrazine sulfate in advanced, non-small-cell lung cancer: a randomized placebo controlled, double-blind phase III study of the Cancer and Leukemia Group B. J Clin Oncol 1994;12:1113–20.

Life Energy Distributor. Personal communication, Dr. Benjamin. PO Box 550, Abbotsford, B.C. V2S 5Z5, Canada. Tel: 1-604-856-0170.

Loprinzi CL, Goldberg RM, Su JQ, et al. Placebo controlled trial of hydrazine sulfate in patients with newly diagnosed non-small-cell lung cancer. J Clin Oncol 1994a;12:1126–9.

Loprinzi CL, Kuross SA, O'Fallon JR, et al. Randomized placebo-controlled evaluation of hydrazine sulfate in patients with advanced colorectal cancer. J Clin Oncol 1994b;12:1121–5.

Malozowski S. Hydrazine sulfate. Available from: URL: http://www.fda.gov/cder/pharmcomp/meeting/hydraz.ppt. Accessed August 2, 2001.

Michaelis K. News. Available from: URL: http://www.holisticalternatives.net/News.htm. Accessed August 2, 2001.

Michelot D, Toth B. Poisoning by *Gyromita esculenta*—a review. J Appl Toxicol 1991;11:235-43.

National Cancer Institute. Hydrazine sulfate. Available from: URL: http://www.cancer.gov/cancer_information. Accessed February 18, 2002.

Nagapappan R, Ridell T. Pyridoxine therapy in a patient with severe hydrazine sulfate toxicity. Crit Care Med 2000;28:2116–8.

National Safety Council. Environmental Health Center. Environment writer. Hydrazine (N2H4) and hydrazine sulfate (H4N2.H2O4S) chemical backgrounder. Available from: URL: http://www.nsc.org/ehc/ew/chems/hydrazine.htm. Accessed July 20, 2000.

Preece NE, Forrow S, Ghatineh S, Langley GJ, Timbrell JA. Determination of hydrazine in biofluids by capillary gas chromatography with nitrogen-sensitive or mass spectrometric detection. J Chromatogr 1992a;573:227–34.

Preece N, Ghatineh S, Timbrell J. Studies on the disposition and metabolism of hydrazine in rats in vivo. Hum Exp Toxicol 1992b;11:121–7.

Ravindranath T, Topaloglu AK, Goto M, Zeller WP. Effects of hydrazine sulfate on galactosamine-sensitized endotoxic shock in ten-day-old rats. Res Commun Mol Pathology 1998;99:233–9.

Runge-Morris M, Feng Y, Zangar RC, Noval RF. Effects of hydrazine, phenelzine, and hydralazine treatment on rat hepatic and renal drug-matabolizing enzyme expression. Drug Metab Dispos 1996;24:734-7.

Runge-Morris M, Wu N, Novak RF. Hydrazine-mediated DNA damage: role of hemoprotein, electron transport, and organic free radivcals. Toxicol Appl Pharmacol 1994; 125:123–32.

Sarich TC, Youssefi M, Zhou T, et al. Role of hydrazine in the mechanism of isoniazid hepatotoxicity in rabbits. Arch Toxicol 1996;70:835–40.

Seifart HI, Gent WL, Parkin DP, van Jaarsveld PP, Donald PR. High-performance liquid chromatographic determination of isoniazid, acetylisoniazid and hydrazine in biological fluids. J Chromatogr B Biomed Appl 1995;674:269–275.

Seits IF, Gershanovich ML, Filov VA, et al. Experimental and clinical data on antitumor action of hydrazine sulphate [Russian]. Vopr Onkol 1975;21:45–52.

Tretyakov AV, Filov VA. Concerning the mechanism of the enhancement of antitumor drugs effect by hydrazine sulphate. Vopr Onkol 1977;23:94–8.

Walubo A, Chan K, Wong C. The pharmacokinetics of isoniazid and hydrazine metabolite in plasma and cerebrospinal fluid of rabbits. Methods Find Exp Clin Pharmacol 1991;13:199–204.

Woodward KN, Timbrell JA. Acetylhydrazine hepatotoxicity: the role of covalent binding. Toxicology 1984;30:65–74.

Chapter 15

5-Hydroxytryptophan (5-Hydroxy-L-Tryptophan, L-5-Hydroxytryptophan, Oxitriptan)

Kerry Bowers, Melanie Johns Cupp, and Timothy S. Tracy

15.1. HISTORY

5-Hydroxytryptophan (5-HTP) has been used clinically for more than 30 yr (Birdsall, 1998). Sales and awareness of 5-HTP increased in 1989 after the Food and Drug Administration (FDA) banned its precursor, L-tryptophan, because of its association with eosinophilia-myalgia syndrome. Since then, 5-HTP has been marketed as a safe alternative to L-tryptophan.

15.2. CHEMICAL STRUCTURE

Refer to Fig. 15-1 for the chemical structure of 5-hydroxytryptophan.

15.3. CURRENT PROMOTED USES

5-HTP has been promoted to treat various conditions associated with serotinin deficiency. Manufacturers market 5-HTP to alleviate depression, reduce aggressiveness, balance mood, relieve pain, aid sleep, and promote weight loss.

15.4. PRODUCTS AVAILABLE

5-HTP is commonly available in 25-, 50-, or 100-mg capsules. Sublingual tablets supplying 5-HTP 25 mg are also available. Some products contain herbs such as St. John's wort, kava, gotu kola, and passion flower. Pyridoxine is added to some formulations, purportedly to enhance absorption.

From: *Forensic Science: Dietary Supplements: Toxicology and Clinical Pharmacology*
Edited by: M. J. Cupp and T. S. Tracy © Humana Press Inc., Totowa, New Jersey

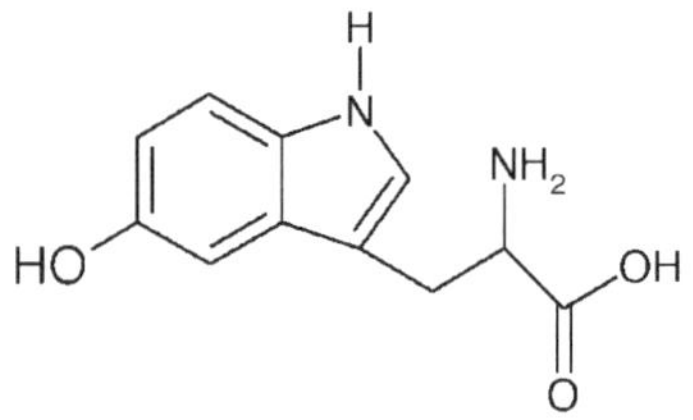

Fig. 1. Chemical structure of hydroxytrytophan.

Branded products available abroad include Lévotonine® in France, Levothym® Germany, Tript-OH® in Switzerland and Italy, Cincofarm® and Telesol® in Spain, and Oxyfan®, Serovit®, and Trimag® in Italy (Reynolds, 1996).

15.5. SOURCES AND CHEMICAL COMPOSITION

Some commercially available 5-HTP formulations are extracted from *Griffonia simplicifolia* seeds, and some are synthetic (Klarskov et al., 1999).

15.6. CLINICAL STUDIES

Shaw and colleagues (2001) systematically reviewed several studies of 5-HTP for treatment of depressive illness in adults to ascertain its safety and efficacy for that purpose. Only randomized, placebo-controlled studies in which efficacy was assessed using a depressive symptom scale were included in the analysis. Of the 16 references located, only 1 (Van Pragg et al., 1972) met the inclusion criteria. The reviewers concluded that although 5-HTP may be more effective than placebo, its association with EMS and the availability of other safe, effective antidepressants limit its clinical use until additional information is available.

Other uses of 5-HTP for which clinical studies have been performed include migraine (Nicoldi and Sicuteri, 1999), insomnia, and posthypoxic myoclonus (Reynolds, 1996). 5-HTP has been studied in a reasonable number of patients for treatment of fibromyalgia (Caruso et al., 1990) and anxiety disorders (Kahn et al., 1987), with promising results, and may it be effective for weight loss (Cangiano et al., 1998). Its use in chronic tension headache (Ribeiro, 2000), autism (Sverd et al., 1978), Down's syndrome (Pueschel et al., 1980), Alzheimer's disease, and multiinfarct dementia (Meyer et al., 1977) cannot be recommended based on the currently available data. 5-HTP may be effective for ataxia caused by degenerative cerebellar diseases, but results of well-designed studies are conflicting (Wessel et al., 1995; Trouillas et al., 1995).

15.7. PHARMACOKINETICS

Westenberg and colleagues (1982) studied the pharmacokinetics of both oral and intravenous administration of 5-HTP in humans. Oral administration of an enteric-coated product (Van Geuns, The Hague, The Netherlands) resulted in double peaks in plasma 5-HTP levels in three of five patients in one study. This double-peak phenomenon was documented in three previous studies, one of which used a simple gelatin capsule, suggesting that this absorption pattern is not a function of the dosage form, but rather biphasic stomach emptying or enterohepatic recirculation. 5-HTP is decarboxylated to serotonin by aromatic amino acid decarboxylase in the kidneys, liver, stomach, and small intestine. Although animal data suggest that 5-HTP is almost completely absorbed after oral administration, with only some metabolism in the intestinal mucosa, bioavailability was $49 \pm 19\%$ (mean $\pm$ SD) in this study. Approximately 25% of the dose is metabolized upon first pass through the liver. Incomplete absorption, metabolism in the intestinal mucosa, and degradation by gastrointestinal fluid also decreases bioavailability. Administration with carbidopa, an inhibitor of peripheral decarboxylase, has been shown to increase bioavailability to as much as 84%.

After intravenous infusion, the decrease in plasma 5-HTP levels can be described by a two-compartment open model. In this study, half-life after intravenous administration varied from 2.2 to 7.4 h [4.34 ± 2.80 h (mean $\pm$ SD)], with half-lives of approx 7 h in two patients and half-lives of approx 2 h in another two patients. The half-life of 5-HTP after oral administration was similar [4.4 ± 2.3 h (mean $\pm$ SD)]. In a previous study, a half-life of 5–7 h was documented. Thus, the elimination of 5-HTP exhibits wide interindividual variation. The volume of distribution of 5-HTP is 0.6 L/kg, reflecting distribution into tissues and organs. In animal studies using ^{14}C-labeled 5-HTP, organs with the highest radioactivity were the kidneys, stomach mucosa, pancreas, small intestine mucosa, and adrenal gland (Westenberg et al., 1982).

15.8. ADVERSE EFFECTS AND TOXICITY

Because of its gastrointestinal side effects, study blinding is a problem with 5-HTP, particularly at doses approaching 1 g/day or more (Currier, 1995). Indeed, the 1984 product information for Bolar Pharmaceuticals' 5-HTP product stated that the most common adverse effects were anorexia, nausea, diarrhea, and vomiting. To minimize adverse effects, the manufacturer recommended gradual dosage increases, treatment of diarrhea with diphenoxylate, and treatment of nausea and vomiting with prochlorperazine 5–10 mg or trimethobenzamide 250 mg four times daily. Adverse effects were said to diminish with time (Hermes, 2001).

In a pharmacokinetic study, adverse effects were experienced after oral, but not intravenous administration of 5-HTP. All adverse effects were gastrointestinal in nature. Nausea occurred with 4 of 21 administered doses. Vomiting and diarrhea were each reported by one of five study subjects. Adverse effects occurred only at 5-HTP concentrations greater than 1 mg/L, and severity was highest at t_{max} (Westenberg et al., 1982). Nausea, diarrhea, anorexia, heartburn, flatulence, dry mouth, fatigue, headache, vertigo, muscle pain, apathy, and orthostatic hypotension were reported in a subsequent study of 5-HTP in depression (Pöldinger et al., 1991).

In 1989, the 5-HTP precursor L-tryptophan was removed from the market by the FDA because of an epidemic outbreak of eosinophilia-myalgia syndrome (EMS) believed to be linked to this dietary supplement. Signs and symptoms of EMS included increased white blood cell count and severe muscle pain; *see* chapter 22 for detailed discussion). More than 1500 cases and at least 37 deaths were reported (FDA, 2001). A vast majority of the cases (95%) were traced to supplies from Showa Denko K.K. of Japan. Since then, episodes have occurred with L-tryptophan products from other supply sources (FDA, 2001). Although 5-HTP is marketed as a safe alternative to L-tryptophan, cases of EMS have also been associated with the use of 5-HTP. Therefore, the FDA, the Centers for disease Control and Prevention, and the National Institutes of Health continue to monitor 5-HTP (Health Source Plus, 1999). A product contaminant termed *peak X* (*see Chemical and Biofluid Analysis* section) may be associated with adverse reactions to 5-HTP (Klarskov et al., 1999)

EMS associated with 5-HTP exposure was reported in a 28-yr-old woman and her two sons, aged 13 and 33 mo (Michelson et al., 1994). The children had been receiving 5-HTP for treatment of GTP cyclohydrolase deficiency. Other medications included tetrahydrobiopterin 50 mg every other day, and levodopa/carbidopa 50 mg/5 mg/d. Both children received 5-HTP 5–7 mg/kg/d for approximately 1 yr. The children's mother did not take 5-HTP but did prepare the children's doses by mixing 5-HTP powder from commercially available capsules with juice or water. Eosinophilia was first noted in the children approximately 7 mo after beginning therapy. Leukocytosis with eosinophil counts of 800/mm^3 and 1100/mm^3 were documented. Soon after, the mother noticed that her legs were stiff and sore. Over the next month, her symptoms progressed to the upper extremities and included arthralgias and fatigue. She was found to have an eosinophil count of 3630/mm^3. Symptoms worsened over the following weeks, and ankle edema, painful induration of the calves, and dyspnea developed. Muscle biopsy revealed perivascular and interstitial infiltration with lymphocytes, macrophages, and (to a lesser extent) eosinophils and multinucleated giant cells. A ventilation/perfusion scan of the lungs showed only mild disease.

The children's father began preparing the children's medication, and the mother's symptoms resolved. Eosinophila persisted however, and the aldolase level was elevated at 12 U/L (normal 1–7 U/L). The children did not develop symptoms, but eosinophila and leukocytosis persisted, with thrombocytosis, elevated aldolase level (14 µ/L), elevated alkaline phosphatase (1252 U/L, upper limit of normal 423 U/L), and elevated creatine kinase (399 U/L, upper limit of nml 386 U/L) noted in the younger child. Although the mother was diagnosed with EMS the children did not meet the definition of EMS, and were diagnosed as having eosinophilia related to 5-HTP. Analysis of the 5-HTP product administered to the children revealed that it contained peak X. The children's eosinophil and leukocyte counts resolved within 3 wk when a 5-HTP product free of peak X was substituted. The father continued to assume responsibility for the children's dose preparation. The mother's symptoms improved only after prednisone 20 mg/d was prescribed.

Coleman (1971) reported development of seizures resembling infantile spasms in 15% of a series of patients with Down's syndrome receiving 5-HTP for treatment of hypotonia and buccolingual dyskinesias. This incidence was higher than would be expected in the general Down's syndrome population. Symptoms in these nine patients included staring spells, head nodding, flexion spasms, shaking of the extremities, eye blinking, and spasms or twitches during sleep or upon awakening. 5-HTP dosages ranged from 1.5–7 mg/kg/d when seizure activity was noted. Rapid dosage increases rather than a particular dose appeared to be associated with seizure development. Development of electroencephalogram (EEG) abnormalities (disorganized spikes and slow waves) was associated with seizures refractory to dosage decrease or discontinuation. Adrenocorticotropic hormone administration was successful in terminating seizures in one patient. Dosage decrease was useful in arresting clinical seizures in patients with normal EEGs. Administration of pyridoxine, a cofactor necessary for 5-HTP decarboxylation to serotonin, terminated seizures in one of the nine patients, despite continuation of 5-HTP. Diarrhea and hypertonia developed prior to seizure development in one infant receiving 5-HTP 1–1.4 mg/kg. Hyperactivity was also reported.

The authors suggest that development of such symptoms may be a prodrome heralding seizure onset and serving as a sign that a patient is particularly susceptible to 5-HTP effects. In addition, low baseline levels of 5-hydroxyindoleacetic acid, a serotonin metabolite, were associated with seizure development. The authors also noted that seizures occurred less often in patients receiving a racemic mixture of -D,L-5-HTP compared with those receiving pure L-5-HTP, suggesting that the L-isomer is responsible, although the difference was not statistically significant (chi-square analysis). Because seizures developed only after months of treatment with 5-HTP, the authors hypothesized that 5-HTP loading might, over a period of time, cause an imbalance in neurotransmitters that leads to seizures.

A report from the ASPCA National Animal Poison Control Center in Urbana, IL described the clinical signs, treatment, and outcome of accidental ingestion of 5-HTP 2.5–573 mg/kg in 21 dogs. The minimum lethal dose was 128 mg/kg, and the miniumum dose resulting in clinical signs was 23.6 mg/kg. Clinical signs resembling serotonin syndrome developed in 19 dogs 10 min to 4 h post ingestion and lasted for up to a day and a half. Clinical signs included seizures ($n = 9$), depression ($n = 6$), tremors ($n = 5$), hyperesthesia ($n = 5$), ataxia ($n = 4$), vomiting or diarrhea ($n = 12$), signs of abdominal pain ($n = 3$), hypersalivation ($n = 2$), hyperthermia ($n = 7$), reversible blindness ($n = 3$), and death ($n = 3$). Seventeen dogs received treatment, 16 of which survived. Treatment was supportive in nature and included gastrointestinal evacuation, seizure control, cooling, and administration of fluids (Gwaltney-Brant et al., 2000).

15.9. INTERACTIONS

Sternberg and colleagues (1980) described a 70-yr-old man who developed a scleroderma-like illness 20 mo after beginning a regimen of 5-HTP plus carbidopa 150 mg/d for treatment of intention myoclonus. The rationale for combining carbidopa or other peripheral decarboxylase inhibitor with 5-HTP is to prevent the peripheral conversion of 5-HTP to serotonin, which cannot cross the blood-brain barrier, thus increasing the amount of 5-HTP available for conversion to serotonin in the central nervous system (Westenberg et al., 1982). Patient complaints and physical findings at presentation included proximal muscle weakness, edema and pain of the extremities with synovitis of the ankles and wrists, a 7-kg weight loss, widespread itchy macular skin discoloration, pale purple discoloration of the periorbital area, and a patchy papulosquamous eruption on his back. Skin biopsy revealed pervascular dermatitis. Muscle biopsy revealed type II muscle fiber atrophy consistent with carcinoid myopathy. Muscle enzymes were normal. Nerve conduction studies showed impaired sensory and motor nerve conduction. Eosinophil count was elevated at 1885/mm^3. Antinuclear antibody titer was positive at 1:1024.

Five months later, the patient presented again with difficulty walking and severe pain and edema of the hands and feet, despite discontinuation of both 5-HTP and carbidopa. The skin of the arms, legs, shoulders, and hips was now thickened and tight. He had flexion contractures of the elbows and knees. Skin biopsy revealed scleroderma. Two months later the patient was treated with pyridoxine 100 mg/d and showed improvement in pain, skin thickness, and contractures. He exhibited elevated kynurenine levels, which increased with a 4-d rechallenge with 5-HTP 800 mg and carbidopa 200 mg/d. Eight other patients treated with 5-HTP and either carbidopa or benserazide who did not develop scleroderma did not have increased kynurenine levels; however, 7 of 15 patients with idiopathic scleroderma had elevated levels.

The authors hypothesized that scleroderma in this patient was caused by worsening of an underlying deficiency or functional impairment of a pyridoxine-dependent enzyme involved in kynurenine metabolism (i.e., kynureninase). Because kynurenine levels decreased when 5-HTP was discontinued despite continuation of carbidopa, carbidopa alone cannot be blamed for the patient's symptoms. In addition, the patient's scleroderma cannot be attributed to carbidopa-induced pyridoxine deficiency because the patient's pyridoxine levels were normal and because carbidopa is not known to decrease pyridoxine levels. The combination of 5-HTP and carbidopa might somehow interfere with kynureninase's binding of its cofactor, pyridoxine, causing decreased enzyme activity. Because carbidopa inhibition of peripheral conversion of 5-HTP to serotonin is not complete, elevated serotonin levels may also be involved (Sternberg et al., 1980).Years later, contaminants were identified in the 5-HTP product taken by the patient described by Sternberg and colleagues (1980) that could have some as yet unidentified role in the patient's pathology (Klarskov et al., 1999).

A similar case occurred in 1985 (Joly et al., 1991). The patient, who began taking 5-HTP 750 mg/d in 1983, developed itching and burning of the skin 2 yr later. He presented 4 wk after symptom onset, at which time edema of the upper extremities, pseudobullous morphea-like lesions on the legs, and tight skin on the torso, abdomen, and lower extremities were noted. Other medications included carbidopa and flunitrazepam. He had a history of Parkinson's disease and depression. Abnormal laboratory values included a WBC count of 8700/mm^3 with 19% eosinophils, an erythrocyte sedimentation rate of 20 mm/h, and an antinuclear antibody titer of 1:250. Skin biopsy showed several pertinent dermal findings, including edema resulting in pseudobullae, thickening and hyalinization of collagen, and an inflammatory infiltrate extending to the fatty tissue. Mucin deposits were revealed using Alcian blue. After discontinuation of 5-HTP, the patient was treated with prednisone with improvement of skin tightness and painful edema.

The authors hypothesized that the patient's symptoms were caused by genetic susceptibility to scleroderma in combination with a carbidopa-induced abnormality of tryptophan metabolism. The authors point out that this patient was taking a benzodiazepine. Some patients who developed L-tryptophan-associated EMS (which is similar to this patient's symptomatology in that it has been associated with scleroderma-like skin abnormalities of the limbs and trunk, induration of subcutaneous tissues, and morphea-like lesions) had also taken benzodiazepines. Increased serotonin levels, which could result from concomitant administration of carbidopa and 5-HTP as described in the previous case, are associated with the morphea-like lesions seen in carcinoid syndrome (Medsger, 1990).

The 1984 product information for 5-HTP produced by Bolar Pharmaceuticals recommended discontinuing reserpine or monoamine oxidase inhibitors at least 2 wk prior to initiation of 5-HTP/carbidopa therapy (Hermes, 2001).

15.10. REPRODUCTION

Contaminants linked to the development of EMS have been found in 5-HTP preparations (FDA, 1998) Therefore use of 5-HTP products during pregnancy and lactation is not advised.

15.11. CHEMICAL AND BIOFLUID ANALYSIS

Also *see Chemical and Biofluid Analysis* section in chapter 22.

Klarskov and colleagues (1999) identified a five-member family of contaminants in 5-HTP associated with a scleroderma-like reaction and described by Sternberg and colleagues (1980) (*see Interaction* section); they tested six commercially available 5-HTP products; and two analytical grade products. All products tested contained at least three of the contaminants. All contaminants had a molecular weight of approximately 234 and comparable retention times and were collectively termed peak X. The two major constituents of peak X were termed X_1 and X_2. Both had an empiric formula of $C_{11}H_{11}N_2O_4$ and have seven unsaturated bonds. They are thought to be regioisomers of oxidized L-tryptophan. Peak X_3 has the same empiric formula as peaks X_1 and X_2, but X_4 has a slightly higher molecular weight (234.1085), corresponding to an empiric formula of $C_{12}H_{15}N_2O_3$, and may be 6-hydroxy-hexahydo-β-carboline-3-carboxylic acid. Peak X_5 has an empiric formula of $C_{10}H_{11}N_4O_3$. Peak X_1 was the major contaminant of the case-associated 5-HTP, representing 94% of the peak X family present, with peak X_2 and X_3 representing approx 5 and 1%, respectively. Peaks X_4 and X_5 were not detectable. The eight commercial products contained between 0.1 and 10.3% of the peak X_1 content of the case-implicated products. Despite these low levels, daily intake of 300–900 mg of these 5-HTP products would provide case-associated levels of peak X. In one sample, peak X_1 was not detectable. This product contained the highest amounts of peaks X_4 and X_5. All five contaminants were present in one of the analytical grade products.

To establish the identity of these components of peak X, Klarskov et al. (1999) employed high-performance liquid chromatography with mass spectrometric detection. Using a Primesphere HC, C18, 5 μm (150 × 3.2 mm) column, a mobile phase flow rate of 350 μL/min, and a gradient elution profile, the components were separated and identified. The mobile phase elution conditions consisted of 98:1:1 (v/v/v) H_2O/CH_3CN/acetic acid [solvent A] for 35 min, followed by a rapid ramp over the next 10 min from 100% solvent A to 5% solvent A and from 0% solvent B [90:9:1 (v/v/v) CH_3CN/MeOH/acetic acid] to 95% solvent B. The eluent is split (20%, 70 μL/min) into the mass spectrometer. For exact mass determinations, a reference solution consisting of tetrabutyl ammonium acetate and cetyl trimethyl ammonium bromide at concentrations of 500 pg/µL in 2-propanol/water/acetic acid (50:49:1, v/v/v) is used. The reference solution is introduced into the ESI source at a flow rate of 20 µL/min. For the first 11 min, the scan range is from m/z 218 to m/z 245 at 30 s per mass decade. After 11 min, the scan range is from m/z 282 to m/z 340 at 20 s per mass decade.

15.12. REGULATORY STATUS

5-HTP is regulated as a dietary supplement in the United States.

15.13. SUMMARY

- 5-Hydroxytryptophan has been used for the treatment of depressive illness, aggressiveness, pain, and insomnia and for weight loss. Only studies of its use for fibromyalgia and anxiety disorders have included enough patients to provide credible data on positive results.
- The primary side effects of 5-HTP therapy are gastrointestinal symptoms including anorexia, nausea, vomiting, and diarrhea. These side effects are thought to diminish with time.
- Contamination of some 5-HTP formulations has been found, with patients reporting development of an eosinophilia-myalgia syndrome similar to that seen with contaminated batches of L-tryptophan.
- Scleroderma development has been associated with concomitant administration of 5-HTP and the decarboxylase inhibitor carbidopa. Careful monitoring should be undertaken when these agents are used in combination.

REFERENCES

Birdstall TC. 5-hydroxytryptophan: a clinically-effective serotonin precursor. Alt Med Rev 1998;3:271–80.

Cangiano C, Laviano A, Del Ben M, et al. Effects of oral 5-hydroxy-tryptophan on energy intake and macronutrient selection in non-insulin dependent diabetic patients. Int J Obes 1998;22:648–54.

Caruso I, Sarzi Puttini P, Cazzola M, Azzolini V. Double-blind study of 5-hydroxytryptophan versus placebo in the treatment of primary fibromyalgia syndrome. J Int Med Res 1990;18:201–9.

Coleman M. Infantile spasms associated with 5-hydroxytryptophan administration in patients with Down's syndrome. Neurology 1971;21:911–9.

Currier RD. A treatment for ataxia [editorial]. Arch Neurol 1995;52:449.

FDA. FDA talk paper: Impurities confirmed in dietary supplement 5-hydroxy-L-tryptophan. August 31, 1998. Available from: URL: http://vm.cfsan.fda.gov/~lrd/tp5htp/html. Accessed February 12, 2002.

Gwaltney-Brant SM, Albretsen JC, Khan SA. 5-Hydroxytryptophan toxicosis in dogs: 21 cases (1989–1999). J Am Vet Med Assoc 2000;15:1937–40.

Health Source Plus. Possible link found between supplements and serious illness. NCRHI newsletter 1999;22:1–2.

Hermes AE. Hydroxytryptophan (drug evaluation): In: Hutchinson TA, Shahan DR, Eds. DRUGDEX ® System. Greenwood Village, CO: MICROMEDEX (edition expires December, 2001).

Joly P, Lampert A, Thomine E, Lauret P. Development of psuedobullous morphea and sclerodema-like illness during therapy with L-5-hydroxytryptophan and carbidopa. J Am Acad Dermatol 1991;25:332–3.

Kahn RS, Westenberg HG, Verhoeven WM, et al. Effect of a serotonin precursor and uptake inhibitor in anxiety disorders: a double-blind comparison of 5-hydroxytryptophan, clomipramine and placebo. Int Clin Psychopharmacol 1987;2:33–45.

Klarskov K, Johnson KL, Benson LM, et al. Eosinophilia-myalgia syndrome case-associated contaiminants in commercially available 5-hydroxytryptophan. Adv Exp Med Biol 1999; 467:461–8.

Medsger TA Jr. Tryptophan-induced eosinophilia-myalgia syndrome. N Engl J Med 1990;322:926–8.

Meyer JS, Welch KM, Deshmukh VD, et al. Neurotransmitter precursor amino acids in the treatment of multi-infarct dementia and Alzheimer's disease. JAGS 1977;25:289–98.

Michelson D, Page SW, Casey R, Trucksess MW, Love LA, Milstien S, et al. An eosinophilia-myalgia syndrome related disorder associated with exposure to L-5-hydroxyryptophan. J Rheumatol 1994;21:2261–5.

Nicolodi M, Sicuteri F. L-5-hydroxytryptophan can prevent nociceptive disorders in man. Adv Exp Biol 1999;467:177–82.

Pueschel SM, Reed RB, Cronk CE, Goldstein BI. 5-Hydroxytryptophan and pyridoxine. Their effects in young children with Down's syndrome. Am J Dis Child 1980;134:838–44.

Pöldinger W, Calanchini B, Schwarz W. A functional-dimensional approach to depression: serotonin deficiency as a target syndrome in a comparison of 5-hydroxytryptophan and fluvoxamine. Psychopathology 1991;24:53–81

Reynolds JEF, ed. Martindale: the extra pharmacopoeia, 31st ed. London: Royal Pharmaceutical Society; 1996. p. 328.

Ribeiro CA, For the Portugese Head Society. L-5-hydroxytryptophan in the prophylaxis of chronic tension-type headache: a double-blind, randomized, placebo-controlled study. Headache 2000;40:451–6.

Shaw K, Turner J, Del Mar C. Tryptophan and 5-hydroxytryptophan for depression (Cochrane Review). In: The Cochrane Library, Issue 3, 2001. Oxford: Update Software.

Sternberg EM, Van Woert MH, Young SN, et al. Development of a scleroderma-like illness during therapy with L-5-hydrxytryptophan and carbidopa. N Engl J Med 1980;303:782–7.

Sverd J, Kupietz SS, Winsberg BG, et al. Effects of L-5-hydroxytryptophan in autistic children. J Autism Child Schizophr 1978;8:171–80.

Trouillas P, Serratrice G, Laplane D, et al. Levorotatory form of 5-hydroxytryptophan in Friedrich's ataxia: results of a double-blind drug-placebo cooperative study. Arch Neurol 1995;52:456–60.

Van Praag J, Korf J, Dols L, Schut T. A pilot study of the predictive value of the probenecid test in application of 5-hydroxytryptophan as antidepressant Psychopharm 1972;25:14–21.

Wessel K, Hermsdörfer, Deger K, et al. Double-blind crossover study with levorotatory form of hydroxytryptophan in patients with degenerative cerebellar diseases. Arch Neurol 1995;52:451–5.

Westenberg HGM, Gerritsen TW, Meijer BA, van Praag HM. Kinetics of L-5-hydroxytryptophan in healthy subjects. Psychiatry Res 1982;7:373–85.

Chapter 16

Melatonin (N-acetyl-5-Methoxytryptamine)

Ann Sullivan, Melanie Johns Cupp, and Timothy S. Tracy

16.1. HISTORY

Melatonin was isolated in the late 1950s and had been administered intravenously by 1960. Studies of its sedative/hypnotic effects soon followed (Dawson and Encel, 1993). Melatonin promotion to the public began in the mid-1990s.

16.2. CHEMICAL STRUCTURE

Refer to Fig. 16-1 for the chemical structure of melatonin.

16.3. CURRENT PROMOTED USES

Melatonin is promoted as a sleep aid, stress reliever, jet lag remedy, antioxidant, immunostimulant, age-fighting substance, and aphrodisiac.

16.4. PHYSIOLOGIC ROLE

Melatonin controls sleep onset and other circadian activities (i.e., biologic functions that repeat on a daily cycle). The suprachiasmatic nucleus, an area of the hypothalamus, controls the rhythmic secretion of melatonin by the pineal gland in response to information about the light/dark cycle conveyed through the eyes and the retinohypothalamic tract. Melatonin is produced and secreted by the pineal gland during darkness, and its secretion is "turned off" by exposure to bright light; thus, the duration of melatonin secretion is directly proportional to the length of night (Monti and Cardinali, 2000). Peak melatonin levels normally occur between 2 AM and 6 AM (Arendt, 2000). Light exposure during the first part of the night delays sleep onset, whereas light exposure during the early morning hours advances the circadian cycle.

From: *Forensic Science: Dietary Supplements: Toxicology and Clinical Pharmacology*
Edited by: M. J. Cupp and T. S. Tracy © Humana Press Inc., Totowa, New Jersey

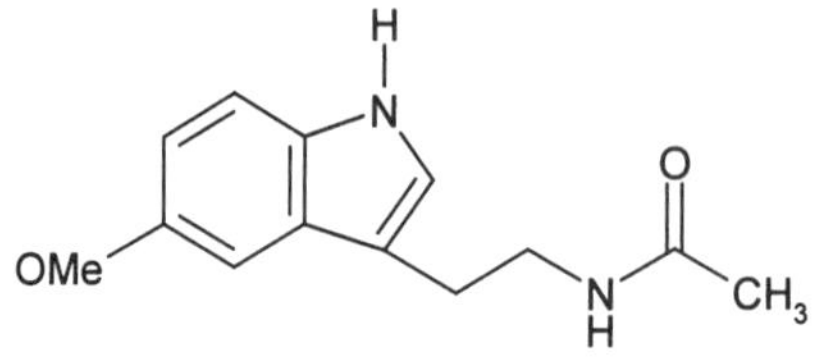

Fig. 1. Chemical structure of melatonin.

Melatonin can thus be viewed as a hormone that communicates information about the day/night cycle to the body, creating changes in physiology and behavior that reflect the time of day (Monti and Cardinali, 2000).

16.5. PRODUCTS AVAILABLE

Melatonin marketed as a dietary supplement is either synthetic or extracted from bovine pineal glands (Shaughnessy, 1996).

Investigators examined the quality of nine immediate-release and three controlled-release melatonin products using United States Pharmacopeia (USP) tests and other tests for weight variation, friability, hardness, disintegration, and dissolution (Hahm et al., 1999). Two products exhibited excessive friability. Four of the immediate-release products did not meet USP standards for disintegration and dissolution, and one showed a high variation in hardness. Such product problems make findings of clinical studies difficult to extrapolate to the melatonin products used by consumers because bioavailability of these products is uncertain.

Impurities unable to be identified by the laboratory were discovered in four of six melatonin products in one study (Anonymous, 1995). In another study (Williamson et al., 1998), "peak E" and "peak C," contaminants of L-tryptophan products associated in 1989 with the disabling and sometimes fatal eosinophilia-myalgia syndrome (*see* Chapter 22), were identified in three over-the-counter melatonin products.

16.6. IN VITRO AND ANIMAL STUDIES

In birds and reptiles, melatonin is known to be important in setting the sleep/wake cycle, and removal of the pineal gland disrupts circadian rhythms. In contrast, pinealectomy has little effect on circadian rhythm in mammals, and studies in humans show that melatonin administration does not appear to alter circadian phase. Because of the difficulty of studying humans in a controlled environment for long periods, a study was undertaken in baboons to determine whether melatonin can cause circadian phase shift in primates (Hao, 2000). Three baboons were housed in rooms where they were exposed to 12 h of light and 12 h of dark for at least 2 wk. Circadian phases were determined based on activity. Melatonin solution was administered in food at a dose of 0.5, 3, 5, and 10 mg. Each dose was administered twice daily for 3 consecutive days, before activity offset (late day) and after activity onset (early day). No circadian phase shifts were detected; however, activity levels decreased after the evening doses of melatonin 5 and 10 mg. To ensure that melatonin was absorbed, levels were assessed 1 h after administration of 0.5 mg in two baboons. Melatonin levels were 108 and 168 pg/mL in these two animals, compared with 1.5 and 1.3 pg/mL in two control animals that did not receive melatonin.

Melatonin has been shown to function as a free radical scavenger in vitro and in animal models. It has been shown in rats to protect against liver injury caused by endotoxic shock and reperfusion injury. Melatonin 50–100 mg/kg administered intraperitoneally 6 h after injection of carbon tetrachloride (CCl_4) minimized liver injury in a dose-dependent manner, as evidenced by amelioration of the increased aspartate aminotransferase (AST) and alanine aminotransferase (ALT) levels, increased liver lipid peroxide content, and reduction in glutathione content seen with CCl_4 (Ohta et al., 1999).

16.7. CLINICAL STUDIES

16.7.1. Sleep

Oral doses of melatonin taken during the day increase sleep susceptibility and decrease body temperature in a dose-dependent manner. Melatonin's effects may be centrally or peripherally mediated, or both; for example, melatonin's ability to increase sleep propensity may be triggered by peripheral heat dissipation. Melatonin administration can also shift circadian rhythms. When melatonin is taken in the afternoon or early evening, the circadian clock is advanced, as evidenced by changes in endogenous melatonin concentrations, core body temperature, and the sleep/wake cycle. Conversely, there is some evidence that melatonin taken in the early morning hours can cause a delay in the sleep/wake cycle. Melatonin's effects on sleep are probably owing to a combination of its hypnotic effect and its effect on the circadian clock (Arendt, 2000).

Studies of melatonin in the treatment of insomnia in the geriatric population have shown conflicting results (Arendt, 2000). This may be related to differences in dose, dosage form, administration times, underlying cause of insomnia, and method of assessing efficacy. For example, studies using polysomnography have generally shown less impressive results than studies using wrist actigraphy or patient questionanaires to assess sleep parameters (Monti and Cardinali, 2000). One study (Haimov et al., 1995) in elderly insomniacs showed that melatonin 2 mg administered as a sustained-release preparation improved sleep maintenance (sleep as a percentage of time in bed and activity during sleep), whereas an immediate-release preparation decreased sleep latency (time required to fall asleep). In a double-blind, placebo-controlled crossover study (Garfinkel et al., 1995) of 12 elderly subjects complaining of long-term insomnia, 2 mg of sustained-release melatonin taken 2 h before bedtime reduced sleep latency, increased total sleep time, improved sleep efficiency (sleep time as a percentage of time in bed), and decreased nocturnal awakenings as measured using wrist actigraphy. Melatonin was not found to decrease sleep latency or to increase total sleep time.

It should be noted that the patients enrolled in these studies (Garfinkel et al., 1995; Haimov et al., 1995) exhibited significantly lower melatonin levels than those in elderly patients without sleep disturbances. Melatonin deficiency might be associated with medication use or health status. Although most elderly patients have melatonin levels that are similar to those of younger patients, those with "normal" melatonin levels could have problems with timing of melatonin release leading to sleep disorders (Arendt, 200). However, efficacy is not consistently related to baseline melatonin levels, and studies have shown benefit in geriatric patients with insomnia and Alzheiemer's disease regardless of baseline melatonin levels. Doses as low as 0.3 mg have been effective in middle-aged and elderly patients with insomnia, although doses as high as 75 mg have been studied (Monti and Cardinali, 2000).

Based on a case report in which melatonin was successfully used to facilitate the discontinuation of long-standing benzodiazepine use (Dagan et al., 1997), Garfinkel and associates (1999) performed a placebo-controlled trial to further assess melatonin's utility in this regard. Thirty-four subjects with at least a 6-mo history of daily benzodiazepine use were randomized to controlled-release melatonin 2 mg (Circadin, Neurim Pharmaceuticals, Tel Aviv, Israel) or placebo 2 h prior to bedtime for six wk. A benzodiazepine taper was also implemented. Subsquently, all patients were administered melatonin in single-blind fashion for an additional 6 wk. Outcome measures were benzodiazepine discontinuation rate and sleep quality questionnaire score reported each morning on a scale of 1 to 10 (poor to excellent). This ordinal scale was treated as continuous data, with mean scores of the groups compared using t-tests. At week 6, the discontinuation rate in the melatonin group (14 of 18 subjects) was higher than that of the placebo group (4 of 16 subjects) ($p = 0.002$, chi-square). At week 6, mean sleep score was higher in the melatonin group ($p = 0.04$, t-test). The investigators suggest that this may reflect tolerance to the benzodiazepine with accompanying poor sleep quality. Fifteen subjects in each group participated in the single-blind portion of the study. By the end of this treatment period, an additional six patients, all from the original placebo group, had discontinued benzodiazepine therapy. These 30 patients chose to continue melatonin therapy as part of a 6-mo open-label follow-up. By the end of the open-label portion of the study, almost 80% of the subjects who had discontinued benzodiazpine use continued to be benzodiazepine-free. The mean sleep quality score for these patients was significantly lower than their mean baseline sleep score ($p = 0.002$).

The investigators noted no difference in discontinuation rates among the various benzodiazepines used by study participants; however, statistical analysis was not performed with this data. It appears as though discontinuation was particularly difficult in patients taking alprazolam and flunitrazepam; only one patient in each group was able to discontinue benzodiazepine therapy. In an accompanying editorial (Bursztajn, 1999), it is suggested that patients who were unable to discontinue benzodiazepine therapy may have had underlying conditions that were particularly amenable to the amnestic properties of benzodiazepines, such as disturbing memories or unpleasant dreams. The editorialist also comments that patient motivation to discontinue benzodiazepines may have affected the study results.

Patients with schizophrenia have been reported to have low melatonin levels, and sleep disturbances are common in this population. Especially during the acute phase of the illness, prolonged sleep latency is commonly reported, and nocturnal awakenings and decreased stage 2 sleep have also been documented. One group of investigators hypothesized that insomnia in schizophrenia is at least partly caused by decreased melatonin production and thus designed a randomized, double-blind, crossover study to assess the effects of melatonin administration on sleep efficiency in schizophrenic patients with insomnia (Shamir et al., 2000). An additional primary objective of this study was to measure urinary 6-sulfatoxymelatonin (6-SMT) excretion in these patients.

Twenty-seven patients meeting DSM-IV criteria for both schizophrenia (paranoid schizophrenia, disorganized schizophrenia, or schizoaffective disorder) and insomnia were enrolled. Patients with liver disease, renal disease (serum creatinine >1.5 mg/dL), other psychiatric disorders, or major medical illness were excluded. Before commencement of the study, urine samples were collected every 3 h from 9 PM to 9 AM. Each patient took melatonin 2 mg (Circadin) or placebo 2 h before bedtime for 3 wk, with a 1-wk placebo washout between the two treatments. On three consecutive nights during the last week of each of the two treatment periods, sleep was assessed using a wrist actigraphy device in the patients' homes. Four patients dropped out owing to noncompliance, and data for four additional patients were incomplete because of technical difficulties. The mean amount of 6-SMT excreted was lower than expected for healthy young or elderly subjects with good sleep quality. Sleep efficiency was improved with melatonin compared with placebo ($p = 0.038$, paired t-test) and was most improved in patients with sleep efficiency while taking placebo that was lower than the median ($p < 0.0014$, repeated-measures ANOVA).

There has been interest in using melatonin in shift workers to "reset" their circadian clocks to ensure that sleep onset occurs at a time appropriate to their work schedule. Using a randomized, double-blind, placebo-controlled crossover design, Wright and colleagues (1998) investigated the effects of melatonin supplementation in 15 emergency room physicians after they had completed night shift duty. Seven physicians received melatonin 5 mg during the first study period, and eight received placebo. Subjects worked two 8-h night shifts in a row, with the second shift ending at 7 AM on study day 1. Subjects took the study drug at bedtime on days 1, 2, and 3. The regimen was later repeated with the alternate intervention. Melatonin showed no benefit using a visual analog scale (VAS) for subjects' global assessment of recovery from night shift work, duration of sleep, sleep latency, alertness/tiredness, mood, study drug tolerability, cognitive function, or motor function. Problems with this study acknowledged by the investigators include small sample size, questionable bioavailability of the melatonin product, lack of objective outcome measures, and inability to extrapolate the results to individuals who work longer shifts or who work several consecutive shifts.

In a double-blind, randomized, crossover study in 23 emergency medical personnel working rotating night shifts, subjects (mean age 29 ± 8 yr) were randomized to receive melatonin 6 mg (Vitamin Research Products, Carson City, NV) or placebo 30 min prior to sleep for 4–6 consecutive d. Each volunteer underwent four "cycles" of melatonin or placebo treatment in randomized fashion, such that each subject took melatonin for two cycles and placebo for two cycles. Exclusion criteria were history of sleep disorder, intolerance to melatonin, pregnancy, thyroid disease, diabetes, heart disease, neurologic disease, and use of "minor tranquilizers," narcotics, antidepressants, or sleeping pills. Sleep variables (sleep latency, number of awakenings, sleep efficiency, and duration of daytime naps) were measured using a sleep diary. Use of alcohol and caffeinated beverages was also reported. Sleep quality, mood, and job performance were measured daily using a 10-point VAS. The only statistically significant difference between melatonin and placebo was significantly fewer awakenings during day sleep with melatonin. The authors suggested that, like benzodiazepines, melatonin acts as a hypnotic and that its inability to improve sleep duration or sleep efficiency is caused by its relatively short half-life (James et al., 1998).

When individuals travel rapidly across several time zones, internal circadian rhythms are out of sync with time of day at the destination, causing a certain constellation of symptoms commonly referred to as "jet lag." These symptoms include fatigue, sleep disturbances, irritability, and cognitive difficulties. Westward travel is less problematic than eastward travel because it is easier to lengthen than shorten the circadian cycle. It has been proposed that melatonin can prevent and treat jet lag symptoms by synchronizing the sleep-wake cycle with the night/day cycle at the destination. Nine randomized trials of the effect of oral melatonin vs placebo or medication on subjective ratings of jet lag symptoms, time for symptom resolution, or indicators of circadian rhythms were analyzed (Herxheimer and Petrie, 2001). Only one study found no effect of melatonin compared with placebo, but these results were attributed to the study population, which were physicians traveling from New York to Oslo after staying in New York for only 5 d. These travelers would not have spent sufficient time in New York for their circadian clocks to adjust to New York time; therefore, melatonin would not have been expected to be effective on the return trip.

Based on the results of the remaining studies, the reviewers concluded that melatonin 0.5–5 mg taken at the destination bedtime on the day of arrival and for up to 4 additional days minimized jet lag caused by crossing five or more time zones. Individuals crossing two to four time zones may also benefit. Doses of 5 mg were associated with a greater hypnotic effect (faster sleep onset and better sleep quality) than 0.5 mg, but doses higher than 5 mg were not more effective. The reviewers suggested that a dose of 2–3 mg is reasonable for most individuals. One study demonstrated that sustained-release melatonin products are less effective than rapid-release products, which are therefore preferable. Dosing of melatonin prior to arrival requires more study, but is inconvenient and may actually worsen symptoms.

Blind individuals often suffer from sleep disturbances because their melatonin secretion is "free-running" and does not produce a 24-h sleep/wake cycle (Arendt, 2000). This is because melatonin secretion by the pineal gland is controlled by light perception (Gordon, 2000). This may result in daytime fatigue or nighttime insomnia. Administration of melatonin 5–10 mg before bedtime is effective in entraining the free-running circadian rhythms in blind persons, as evidenced by cortisol levels, core body temperature, endogenous melatonin secretion, and improved sleep. It appears to be most effective when timing of melatonin administration is individualized based on the patient's circadian rhythms (Sack et al., 2000; Lockley et al., 2000).

A focus group of sleep researchers, assembled to delineate the role of melatonin in sleep disorders, stated that the use of melatonin in the treatment of sleep disorders of unknown origin is inappropriate (Arendt, 200). Other clinicians (Bursztajn, 1999) have alluded to the importance of a thorough diagnostic workup as well. Zisapel (1999) suggests that melatonin use is appropriate in patients with insomnia caused by benzodiazepine discontinuation, jet lag, blindness, and melatonin deficiency. In the latter case, the sustained-release formulation is recommended.

16.7.2. Neurological Disease

It has been demonstrated that melatonin can ameliorate levodopa-induced movement disorders in mice, and two groups of investigators have reported at least some improvement in parkinsonian symptoms in humans administered melatonin. However, in a subsequent study, melatonin 3–6.6 g/d had no effect on parkinsonian symptoms, levodopa efficacy, or levodopa-induced adventitious movements in a small, single-blind, placebo-controlled study (Papavasiliou et al., 1972).

16.7.3. Cancer

Melatonin appears to have a role in the prevention and treatment of cancer, the treatment of cancer-related symptoms such as cachexia and fatigue, and protection of normal cells from the effects of chemotherapy.

Lissoni and colleagues (1994) have studied the ability of melatonin to augment the action of interleukin-2 (IL-2) on solid tumors not normally responsive to IL-2. In their first randomized study examining this combination, 80 patients who either refused chemotherapy or who had advanced solid tumors not previously responsive to chemotherapy were randomized to subcutaneous IL-2 (Euro-Cetus, Amsterdam, Holland) with or without oral melatonin (Medea Research, Milan, Italy) 40 mg/d, beginning 7 d prior to the first IL-2 injection.

Each treatment cycle consisted of an evening injection of IL-2 6 d each week for 4 wk, with or without melatonin. After a 3-wk rest, the cycle was repeated. Thereafter, treatment was administered for 1 wk each month until cancer progression or the development of toxicity (maintenance phase). Patients who received at least one treatment cycle were considered evaluable. Tumor types investigated included non-small cell lung cancer (NSCLC) ($n = 9$), colorectal cancer ($n = 11$), liver cancer ($n = 5$), gastric cancer ($n = 5$), pancreatic cancer ($n = 5$), and breast cancer ($n = 4$). Disease was assessed radiologically at baseline, after each treatment cycle, and every 2 mo. Complete response, partial response, stable disease, and progressive disease were defined using the World Health Organization (WHO) criteria. Complete response was defined as absence of disease for at least 1 mo, and partial response was a decrease by at least 50% in lesion size for at least 1 mo. Stable disease was defined as no increase in lesion size or increase of up to 25%. Progressive disease was defined as an increase in lesion size by 25% or more or the appearance of new lesions. Leukocyte count, other laboratory tests, and electrocardiographs (ECGs) were performed at baseline weekly during each immunotherapy cycle and every 15 d during the maintenance phase. Weekly serum neopterin levels were measured to evaluate macrophage activity. Minimum follow-up was 13 mo, and the median follow-up was 18 mo. Chi-square, *t*-tests, and ANOVA with the Newman-Keuls test for multiple comparisons were used to analyze data, as appropriate. The log-rank test was used to compare 1-yr survival between the two groups.

Tumor response was higher in the melatonin group ($p < 0.005$), as were progression-free survival ($p < 0.05$) and 1-yr survival ($p < 0.05$). The mean increases from baseline in lymphocyte count ($p < 0.05$) and eosinophil count ($p < 0.001$) were higher in the melatonin group. The increase in neopterin levels was higher in the group that did not receive melatonin ($p < 0.05$), suggesting that melatonin suppresses macrophages, which inhibit cytotoxic lymphocytes. Although some adverse effects appeared to be lower in the melatonin group, there were no significant differences between groups in regard to toxicities. Placebo-controlled studies are necessary to confirm these promising results, particularly since IL-2 is not a standard treatment for solid tumors other than melanoma and renal cell carcinoma.

Melatonin's ability to enhance the efficacy of tamoxifen in breast cancer was also studied by Lissoni and associates (1995). Fourteen consecutive patients with metastatic cancer that had not responded to tamoxifen alone ($n = 3$) or progressed after intial stabilization ($n = 11$) were enrolled. Eight patients had estrogen receptor-positive disease. Patients with estrogen receptor-negative disease had been prescribed tamoxifen because they were unable to tolerate chemotherapy owing to advanced age, low performance status, or concomitant diseases. All patients had been off tamoxifen for at least 1 mo. Patients were given melatonin (Medea Research, Milan, Italy) 20 mg/d starting 7 d before beginning a regimen of tamoxifen 20 mg/d. Patients who were treated for at least 2 mo were considered evaluable. Radiologic examinations were made at baseline, after each month of therapy for the first 3 mo, and every 3 mo thereafter. Response was defined using the WHO criteria described above. Performance status was assessed using Karnofsky's score. Blood was drawn for routine lab tests weekly during the first 3 mo and then once monthly thereafter. Serum levels of insulin-like growth factor-1 (IGF-1) and prolactin, purported breast cancer growth factors, were determined monthly for the first 3 mo. Chi-square, Student's t-test, and ANOVA were used to analyze the data.

All patients were evaluable. Partial response was achieved in four patients; two were estrogen receptor-positive. Ten patients survived for more than 1 yr. Two patients experienced an increase in Karnofsky score and quality of life. IGF-1 levels decreased significantly compared with baseline after 1 mo of therapy ($p < 0.05$) as well as after months 2 and 3 ($p < 0.01$). IGF-1 levels were significantly lower in patients with partial response than in the other patients ($p < 0.05$). Prolactin levels also decreased with treatment ($p < 0.05$), but there was no significant difference in levels between reponders and nonresponders. The investigators concluded that this preliminary study suggests that melatonin may enhance the efficacy of tamoxifen by augmenting its inhibitory effect on IGF-1 secretion, but the small sample size prohibits definitive conclusions. The investigators call for larger, randomized studies comparing melatonin and tamoxifen, individually and in combination, with investigation of the role of melatonin receptor expression in predicting melatonin responders.

Lissoni and colleagues (1999) evaluated the effect of melatonin 20 mg/d on clinical response, survival, and toxicity of chemotherapy in 250 patients with solid tumors, including metastatic NSCLC, breast cancer, gastrointestinal (GI) cancer, or head and neck cancer. Patients admitted to a radiation oncology unit were enrolled consecutively. Patients with brain metastases, advanced age, poor performance status, serious medical illness other than cancer, and extensive prior chemotherapy were excluded. Patients were stratified based on type of cancer and chemotherapy regimen prior to randomization. No placebo control was used; patients were randomized to melatonin (Helsinn Chemicals, Breganzona, Switzwerland) or no melatonin. Patients with NSCLC were treated with three cycles of etoposide plus cisplatin, or with gemcitabine if they had been previously treated with a cisplatin-containing regimen. Breast cancer patients were treated with eight cycles of doxorubicin, or three cycles of mitoxantrone or paclitaxel, depending on previous chemotherapy. Patients with GI cancers were treated with five cycles of 5-fluorouracil (5-FU) plus folinic acid. Head and neck cancer patients were treated with three cycles of cisplatin plus 5-FU.

Melatonin was administered each evening beginning 7 d prior to chemotherapy and continued until disease progression was noted. Radiologic examination was made at baseline and every 2 mo thereafter. Clinical response was evaluated using the WHO criteria described above. Chi-square or *t*-tests were used to analyze data, as appropriate. Survival was calculated using the Kaplan-Meier method and compared using the log-rank test. The melatonin and no-melatonin groups were similar in age, cancer type, prognostic variables, previous chemotherapy, and performance status.

Five percent of the melatonin patients achieved a complete response, whereas none of the patients receiving placebo attained a complete response ($p < 0.02$). A partial response was achieved in 29% of the melatonin patients and in only 15% of the patients who did not receive melatonin ($p < 0.01$). Accordingly, the regression rate (complete plus partial response) was higher in the melatonin group ($p < 0.001$). For individual chemotherapy regimens, the regression rate was statistically higher in patients receiving cisplatin, etoposide, and melatonin for NSCLC than in NSCLC patients receiving etoposide and cisplatin without melatonin ($p < 0.001$). The regression rate was also higher in melatonin-treated patients receiving 5-FU plus folinic acid for GI cancers ($p < 0.05$) and doxorubicin for breast cancer ($p < 0.05$) than in patients receiving these regimens without melatonin.

For other chemotherapy regimens, there was a nonsignificant trend toward a higher regression rate in melatonin-treated patients. The exception was mitoxantrone, for which the regression rate was lower for melatonin-treated patients. The median time to progression was 9 mo in the melatonin group and 4 mo in the group that did not receive melatonin ($p < 0.05$). One-year survival ($p < 0.001$) and overall survival ($p < 0.05$) were higher in the melatonin group than in patients who did not receive melatonin. For individual chemotherapy regimens, 1-yr survival was higher for melatonin patients receiving cisplatin plus etoposide ($p < 0.001$), 5-FU plus folinic acid ($p < 0.05$), 5-FU plus cisplatin ($p < 0.02$), gemcitabine ($p < 0.05$), doxorubicin ($p < 0.05$), and paclitaxel ($p < 0.05$). The melatonin group experienced significantly less chemotherapy-associated adverse effects, including less myelosuppression, ($p < 0.001$), thrombocytopenia ($p < 0.05$), neurotoxicity ($p < 0.05$), cardiotoxicity ($p < 0.05$), stomatitis ($p < 0.05$), and asthenia ($p < 0.05$). A larger, placebo-controlled trial is needed to confirm these promising results suggesting that melatonin may be a useful adjunct to certain chemotherapy regimens.

Other investigators (Ghielmini et al., 1999) randomized 20 chemotherapy-naïve patients with NSCLC or SCLC not amenable to surgery to melatonin 40 mg/d or placebo for 21 d beginning 2 d prior to treatment with a 4-wk cycle of carboplatin and etopoide. Patients received the alternate treatment with the second cycle. Melatonin did not ameliorate the myelotoxicity of this chemotherapy regimen as measured by hemoglobin, platelets, absolute neutrophil count (ANC), ANC nadir, or duration of neutropenia. Differences in the results of this study from Lissoni and colleagues (1999) may have stemmed from differences in chemotherapy doses; doses were not stated in the larger study. In addition, Lissoni and colleagues (1999) did not analyze the myelotoxicity data separately for carboplatin/etoposide. Also, in contrast to the findings of Lissoni's group in patients with solid tumors, melatonin 20 mg/d was unable to protect patients with aggressive B-cell lymphomas from the myelosuppressive effects of the CHOP (cyclophosphamide, doxorubicin, vincristine, prednisone) chemotherapy regimen, but it may enhance cellular immunity by binding to melatonin receptors on T-lymphocytes (Rodriguez et al., 2000).

16.7.4. Other Uses

An open-label study suggests that melatonin 3 mg at bedtime might benefit fibromyalgia symptoms, including sleep, number of trigger points, and pain (Citera et al., 2000). Data from double-blind, placebo-controlled studies are needed before melatonin can be recommended for this purpose.

Melatonin may prove to be effective as a preoperative sedative. In a randomized, double-blind study in 84 women, melatonin at a dose as low as 0.05 mg/kg decreased preoperative anxiety and increased sedation compared with placebo, but without the cognitive and motor impairment and postoperative sedation associated with midazolam premedication (Naguib and Samarkandi, 2000).

Prompted by anecdotal reports by patients that their tinnitus improved while taking melatonin supplements, Rosenberg and associates (1998) performed a double-blind, randomized crossover study of melatonin 3 mg vs placebo in 30 patients. The results suggest that the supplement may benefit patients who have difficulty sleeping owing to their tinnitus, patients with more severe tinnitus, and patients with bilateral tinnitus.

In a pilot study of melatonin for treatment of winter depression, 10 patients received melatonin 0.125 mg or placebo twice each afternoon, with 4 h between doses (Lewy et al., 1998). The low dose was chosen to minimize melatonin's hypnotic effects. The investigators theorized that afternoon melatonin administration followed by nocturnal melatonin secretion would lead to a relative reduction in melatonin levels the following morning. This would induce a phase advance, which may have an antidepressant effect, as evidenced by the antidepressant and phase advance effects of exposure to bright light in the morning. Efficacy was assessed using the Structured Interview Guide for the Hamilton Depression Rating Scale-Seasonal Affective Disorder Version (SIGH-SAD). All five melatonin patients experienced a decrease in the SIGH-SAD of 39% or more after 2 wk of therapy, compared with only one of the five placebo patients ($p = 0.476$, Fisher's exact test). Because of the small sample size and marginally significant difference between treatments, further trials are needed.

16.8. PHARMACOKINETICS

There is much interindividual variation in the pharmacokinetics of oral immediate-release melatonin products. Doses greater than 0.5 mg are generally considered "pharmacologic" rather than "physiologic," producing plasma melatonin levels that are higher than usual nocturnal levels (Arendt, 2000). Peak blood levels produced by a 5-mg dose are on the order of 25 times normal (Shaughnessy, 1996) and occur within 20 min (James et al., 1998).

The bioavailability of melatonin is poor, because of either poor absorption, high (85%) first-pass hepatic metabolism, or both (DeMuro et al., 2000). In one study, 12 healthy subjects with normal sleep cycles received melatonin 2 mg intravenously, melatonin 2 mg orally, and melatonin 4 mg orally. Each treatment was separated by a 1-mo washout. Oral doses were taken on an empty stomach. Blood samples were taken prior to each dose and periodically thereafter. The area under the curve (AUC) and C_{max} for the two oral doses were similar ($p = 0.07$, one-way ANOVA) but were significantly lower than after intravenous dosing ($p < 0.0001$, one-way ANOVA). The bioavailability of melatonin was calculated to be approximately 15%, with little intersubject variability. Total body clearance and half-life did not differ between doses or administration routes. Clearly, the bioavailability of melatonin is low and may affect efficacy. Studies of the effect of food or higher dosages on bioavailability are needed.

The plasma half-life of melatonin is approximately 40 min (Shaughnessy, 1996). The half-life is relatively short because 90% of circulating melatonin is cleared by a single pass through the liver (Sanders et al., 1999). Distribution is postulated to follow a two-compartment model, with the first compartment being the plasma and the second compartment the cerebrospinal fluid, corresponding to its effects on peripheral organs and the central nervous system (Monti and Cardinali, 2000).

Clearance is hepatic via oxidative metabolism to 6-hydroxymelatonin, followed by glucuronic acid conjugation (20–30%) or sulfate conjugation (60–70%) (Sanders et al., 1999; Hartter et al., 2000) to form 6-sulfatoxymelatonin (6-SMT; Shamir et al., 2000). There is evidence that the oxidative metabolism of melatonin is achieved through CYP1A2 and/or CYP2C19 (von Bahr et al., 2000). Because of the great reliance upon the liver for elimination of melatonin, clearance is impaired in individuals with liver disease. A small percentage is metabolized to N-γ-acetyl-5-methoxykynurenamine in the brain (Sanders et al, 1999).

16.9. ADVERSE EFFECTS AND TOXICITY

Melatonin has been generally well tolerated in clinical studies (Lissoni et al., 1999), although treatment-emergent adverse effects were not often methodically evaluated.

In mice, the median lethal dose (LD_{50}) is more than 800 mg/kg. This dose was not lethal, and testing of higher doses was limited by melatonin's water solubility (James et al., 1998).

Eosinophilia was reported in two studies in which melatonin 15 mg/d was used as an immunostimulant in cancer patients. These observations are of particular concern because two chemicals associated with the development of eosinophilia-myalgia syndrome (EMS) in individuals consuming contaminated L-tryptophan products have also been identified as contaminants in commercially available melatonin products (*see* Chapter 22 for a more detailed discussion of EMS). Despite this concern, daily doses of melatonin are on the order of several milligrams, compared with several grams of L-tryptophan, thus limiting the amount of contaminants consumed. This may explain why EMS has not been associated with melatonin use despite the presence of these contaminants (Williamson et al., 1998).

Melatonin 3–6.6 g/d administered to 11 patients with Parkinson's disease for 15–35 d was associated with migraine-like headache (4 patients), scotoma lucidum, abdominal cramps (4 patients), diarrhea (4 patients), cutaneous flushing, and daytime somnolence (6 patients) (Papavasiliou et al., 1972). Doses of 200–1200 mg/d for 3–24 d caused weight gain, average reduction in total sleep time of 2 h/night, and exacerbation of dysphoric symptoms in six patients with moderate to severe depression (Carman et al., 1976). These doses are higher than are typically used.

In a study of night shift workers (James et al., 1998), one subject reported feeling "tired and not very motivated" the first night after taking melatonin 6 mg for day sleep. The patient did not report these symptoms with subsequent melatonin doses.

In a review of nine studies of melatonin in the treatment and prevention of jet lag, reported symptoms that were possibly associated with melatonin include headache, "heavy head," disorientation, nausea, and other GI complaints. Sleepiness was reported in five of the studies and affected approximately 10% of the patients. One patient experienced dysphagia and dyspnea within 20 min after taking 0.5 mg of melatonin. These symptoms resolved after 45 min and recurred with rechallenge but were not as severe (Herxheimer and Petrie, 2001).

Other adverse effects reported in clinical studies of melatonin include headache and "odd" taste in mouth in 2 patients in an insomnia study (Ellis et al., 1995), headache in 2 of 18 patients receiving melatonin for benzodiazepine discontinuation (Garfinkel et al., 1999), and a mixed affective state in a patient in a study of melatonin in treatment-resistant depression (Dalton et al., 2000).

Adverse events associated with melatonin use in 13 patients have been reported to the WHO Uppsala Monitoring Center. Symptoms included hallucinations, paranoia, confusion, "abnormal thinking," insomnia, ataxia, dizziness (two patients), headache (two patients), hypertonia, tremor, paresthesia (two patients), paresis, seizure, ventricular arrhythmia, atrial fibrillation, arrhythmia (not specified), tachycardia (four patients), palpitations, chest pain (three patients), hypotension, dyspnea (two patients), fatigue (two patients), and syncope. Duration of use was reported in seven patients and ranged from 1 (four patients) to 8 d. Symptoms commonly resolved with discontinuation. Two patients were rechallenged, with recurrence of seizures in one patient and confusion, insomnia, tachycardia, and insomnia in another (Herxheimer and Petrie, 2001).

A case report described a fixed drug eruption associated with melatonin use in two men, aged 35 and 42 yr (Bardazzi et al., 1998). One patient presented with pruritic, burning, well-demarcated, erythematous, vesicular plaques and erosions on the glans and shaft of the penis. The 2–3-cm lesions occurred after taking Nature's Bounty Natural melatonin to prevent jet lag. Product ingredients included melatonin 3 mg, magnesium stearate, stearic acid, and silica. The patient reported that 4 mo previously, he had experienced a similar episode after taking this same product. A second patient presented with a 4-cm round, erosive plaque on the shaft of the penis after use of the same product. Both patients were rechallenged with melatonin 1 mg, and within 6–8 h, burning plaques recurred in both patients at the previously affected location. A 10% solution of melatonin in ethanol was applied to the backs of both patients, with negative results. Both patients refused application of the solution to the site of the reaction.

A case of acute melatonin overdose was reported to the Southern Poison Center in Memphis Tennessee (Holliman and Chyka, 1997). A 66-yr-old man who regularly took lisinopril and diltiazem for hypertension, and melatonin (Melatone®) 6 mg and chlor-diazepoxide/amitiptyline for sleep ingested 24 mg of meltaonin at 9 PM the night before prostate surgery to enhance sleep and ease anxiety. He became lethargic and disoriented within 20 min of taking melatonin and called the Poison Center. He was coherent, and his only complaints were somnolence and fatigue. He denied taking alcohol or any other drugs in addition to his prescribed medication. Upon follow-up by the Poison Center 1.5 h later, he was sitting up reading and reported feeling sleepy. After sleeping for 5 h, he awoke and reported feeling "drugged," per his spouse. The Poison Center staff advised him to inform the anesthesiologist about his melatonin use. Surgery was performed under spinal anesthesia, with no complications and a normal recovery.

In a study of the efficacy of melatonin in children with neurologic disabilities and chronic severe sleep disturbances, four of six children enrolled experienced increased or new seizure activity. One patient was a 9-yr-old with spastic quadriplegia, cortical blindness, obstructive sleep apnea, and generalized tonic/clonic and generalized myoclonic seizures. This child experienced generalized myoclonic activity 45 min after taking melatonin. The patient was dechallenged and rechallenged with similar results. A similar patient, an 8-yr-old with a history of generalized tonic/clonic seizures and spastic quadriplegia, experienced generalized tonic/clonic activity after sleep onset following melatonin administration. Seizures abated on melatonin discontinuation and recurred with rechallenge. A 9-mo-old infant with cystic encephalomalacia and history of intrauterine cerebrovascular accident experienced an increase in generalized myoclonic activity to 150 epidoses/d after taking melatonin. Frequency of myoclonic activity decreased to 30/d upon discontinuing melatonin and increased with rechallenge. The fourth patient was a 7-yr-old with developmental delay, delayed myelination of the corpus callosum, growth hormone deficiency, and generalized tonic/clonic seizures. This patient developed complex partial seizures that resolved with melatonin discontinuation. The patient was not rechalleged. The investigator points to several studies suggesting that melatonin has *anticonvulsant* activity but cautions against its use in children with neurologic disabilities pending further investigation (Sheldon, 1998).

Evaluation of a cause–effect relationship between melatonin use and treatment-emergent symptoms is complicated because some symptoms may be caused by the disorder for which melatonin is being used, other disease states, medications, or an interaction between melatonin and a medication taken by the patient. Most melatonin studies have not been designed to identify treatment-emergent symptoms systematically, and case reports are often incomplete, leaving out details concerning patient health, concomitant medications, specific melatonin product used, and duration of use prior to symptom onset. Timing of melatonin use might also affect symptom occurrence. Based on the available information, headache, psychosis, somnolence, GI disturbances, allergic reactions, cardiac stimulation, and seizures are likely adverse effects of melatonin.

16.10. Interactions

In a study in which fluvoxamine's effect on melatonin levels was studied, five healthy volunteers aged 34–55 yr were given melatonin 5 mg (Horizon Natural Products, Santa Cruz, CA) at 10 AM. Blood samples of melatonin were taken 1, 2, 3, 4, 5, 6, 7, 24, 26, and 28 h after administration. One week later, the study subjects took fluvoxamine 50 mg at 7 AM, followed by melatonin 5 mg at 10 AM. Blood samples for both melatonin and fluvoxamine were taken as before. Fluvoxamine administration was associated with a mean 17-fold higher AUC ($p < 0.05$, paired one-tailed t-test) and on average a 12-fold higher peak (C_{max}) melatonin concentration ($p < 0.01$, paired one-tailed t-test). Half-life was not affected. There was a significant correlation between fluvoxamine and melatonin concentrations ($r = 0.63$, $p < 0.01$, Spearman rank correlation test). All patients reported excessive drowsiness after melatonin administration, which inceased with concurrent fluvoxamine administration. One study subject was known to lack the enzyme CYP2D6. In this subject, fluvoxamine AUC and C_{max} were threefold higher than in the other subjects, and fluvoxamine half-life was twice as long. This is explained by fluvoxamine's dependence on CYP2D6 for metabolism. In accord with this patient's high fluvoxamine concentrations, melatonin concentrations at each time point and melatonin AUC and C_{max} were higher in this patient than in the other patients. Fluvoxamine is known to inhibit CYP1A2 and, to a lesser extent, CYP2C19, CYP3A4, and possibly CYP2D6. This suggests that the oxidative metabolism of melatonin is mediated by by CYP1A2 and that fluvoxamine increases melatonin concentrations by inhibiting its hepatic metabolism. However, because melatonin half-life was not affected, it is possible that fluvoxamine affects the synthesis of endogenous melatonin or the intestinal transport of melatonin (Hartter et al., 2000).

In another study (von Bahr et al., 2000), the effects of fluvoxamine on melatonin levels was compared with that of citalopram, which, like fluvoxamine, is a selective serotonin reuptake inhibitor, but does not affect the cytochrome P450 drug metabolizing enzymes in a clinically significant manner. A placebo control was also administered in one arm of this crossover study. Fluvoxamine increased melatonin AUC 2.8-fold over placebo, but citalopam had no significant effect. With fluvoxamine administration, more melatonin was eliminated renally than after placebo administration. These results suggest that melatonin levels are increased via inhibition of one or more drug-metabolizing enzymes (von Bahr et al., 2000). Patients taking melatonin along with drugs known to be inhibitors of CYP1A2 (and perhaps of CYP3A4, CYP2C19, and CYP2D6) should be monitored for excessive melatonin effects.

A case report described psychosis in a 73-yr-old woman taking melatonin and fluoxetine 10 mg/d (Force et al., 1997). The patient had a history of depression and anxiety and was also taking conjugated estrogens 1.25 mg/d for osteoporosis prevention, beclomethasone nasal spray as needed for allergic rhinitis, and mulitvitamins. She took melatonin 3–6 mg in the morning or whenever she wanted to sleep. She also smoked half a pack of cigarettes each day and occasionally drank alcohol. The patient was admitted to the hospital with confusion, delusions, and paranoia. Although a neighbor who had seen the patient 2 d prior to admission reported that she was acting normally at that time, another friend noted that the night before admission, she had been acting strangely and had not slept. Upon admission the patient reported that she had taken about 10 melatonin tablets that morning. After admission, the patient slept through the night, and her mental status was normal the next morning. At that time, she denied ever taking more than one to two melatonin tablets. The authors of the case report suggest that the patient's psychotic episode may have been caused by an interaction between fluoxetine and melatonin.

Six cases reported to the WHO Uppsala Monitoring Center suggest that melatonin can interact with warfarin. Prothrombin levels were reduced in four of the patients, who experienced eye hemorrhage, purpura, and a nosebleed. One patient was also taking digoxin, furosemide, and diclofenac. In two other patients taking warfarin, prothrombin was "affected," but the report did not say whether it was increased or decreased (Herxheimer and Petrie, 2001).

Melatonin was shown to antgonize the antihypertensive effects of nifedipine GITS, a special sustained-release nifedipine product available in the United States as Procardia XL® and its generic equivalent. Forty-seven hypertensive patients whose blood pressure had been controlled with nifedipine GITS 30–60 mg/d for 3 mo or longer received melatonin (Sigma Aldrich, Milan, Italy) 5 mg or placebo at 10:30 PM for 4 wk in crossover fashion. Study subjects were instructed to take their nifedipine at 8:30 AM and to sleep from 11 PM to 7 AM. At the end of each treatment phase, subjects underwent 24-hour blood pressure monitoring. Systolic blood pressure, diastolic blood pressure, and heart rate were all significantly higher after melatonin administration ($p < 0.01$, paired t-tests). Mean 24-h systolic blood pressure was approximately 6 mmHg higher, diastolic blood pressure was approximately 4 mmHg higher with melatonin, and heart rate was approximately 4 beats per min higher. The mechanism of the interaction is unknown. Experimental evidence suggests that it may involve a direct effect of melatonin on calcium channels, an increase in sensitivity of arteries to norepinephrine, and/or increased sensitivity of compensatory sympathetic activity in response to calcium channel blocker-mediated vasodilation. Melatonin should be used with caution in patients taking calcium channel blockers (Lusardi et al., 2000).

16.11. REPRODUCTION

It has been suggested that high doses of melatonin (oral or parenteral) may have a contraceptive effect (Pierce, 1999); however, in one study, a subject became pregnant after taking melatonin 6 mg for 4–6 nights (James et al., 1998). It is unknown whether lower doses produce the same effect. Insufficient data exists to evaluate the safety of supraphysiologic doses of melatonin in pregnant or lactating women. One source has listed melatonin as Category C with regard to its use in pregnancy (Anonymous, 2001) based on adverse effects noted in female rat fetuses.

16.12. CHEMICAL AND BIOFLUID ANALYSIS

A number of methods have been developed for the measurement of melatonin concentrations in plasma and other tissues. In addition to radioimmunoassay (RIA; Wurzburger et al., 1976) and enzyme-linked immunosorbent assay (ELISA; Yie et al., 1993), gas chromatography-mass spectrometry, and high-performance liquid chromatography (HPLC) with either fluorescent or electrochemical detection have been used for the analysis of melatonin concentrations. The chromatographic methods have been discussed in a recent review by Harumi and Matsushima (2000). Because of the low endogenous concentrations of melatonin, extremely sensitive analytical methods are required. To this end, Iinuma and associates (1999) recently published an HPLC method with fluorescent detection that was capable of measuring melatonin in the amol range

(10^{-18} mol). The method involves derivatization of melatonin with Na_2CO_3 and H_2O_2, to enhance its fluorescence.

To a 100-μL sample placed in a glass vial, 10 μL of 300 mM Na_2CO_3 and 10 μL of H_2O_2, both in water are added. The vial is then tightly capped and heated at 90°C for 30 min. Twenty microliters of this reaction mixture is then injected onto the HPLC system. A J'sphere ODS-H80 reversed phase column (150 × 4.6 mm, i.d.) maintained at 40°C is used for chromatographic separation. The mobile phase consists of 100 mM sodium phosphate (pH 7.0)-acetonitrile (88:12, v/v) pumped at a flow rate of 0.5 mL/min. Fluorescence detection is carried out using an excitation wavelength of 245 nm and an emission wavelength of 380 nm. This method has been shown to detect accurately and reproducibly melatonin amounts of 500 amol–5 pmol injected on the column, which would correspond to concentrations of 5 fmol–50 pmol per milliliter of sample. Since endogenous melatonin concentrations typically range from 0.04 to 0.48 pmol/mL (Waldhauser and Dietzel, 1985), this method is not only adequate for measurement of endogenous melatonin concentrations but could also be adapted for measurement of plasma concentrations after exogenous administration of melatonin, which would produce much higher concentrations.

Since melatonin is an indoleamine, similar to tryptophan, it could potentially suffer from contaminant issues analogous to those seen with tryptophan, which led to a number of cases of EMS (*see* Chapter 22). To this end, Williamson and colleagues (1998) utilized electrospray ionization-tandem mass spectrometry combined with nuclear magnetic resonance to identify several contaminants in commercial melatonin preparations. These contaminants were close structural analogs to the case-associated contaminants of tryptophan, namely, indoline products. These authors describe some case reports of eosinophilia (not EMS) in persons taking large doses of melatonin, but the number of cases is less than reported for tryptophan. This method described by Williamson and colleagues (1998) is definitive in its structural identification and thus could be used to identify contaminants in melatonin products if necessary.

16.13. Regulatory Status

In the United States, melatonin is regulated as a dietary supplement and is thus available without a prescription. Sale of melatonin is more restricted in Switzerland, the United Kingdom, France, and Italy (Bardazzi et al., 1998).

16.14. Summary

- Melatonin is a naturally occurring endogenous hormone that controls sleep onset and various circadian functions. It appears to have some value in the treatment of insomnia and jet lag, although conflicting results have been reported.
- Due to formulation variances among products, bioavailability among melatonin preparations is highly variable and may impact on outcomes seen in clinical studies.
- Melatonin may have value as an adjunct to cancer chemotherapy regimens, but larger, randomized, controlled trials are needed to validate these findings.
- Adverse effects associated with melatonin therapy are generally mild (drowsiness, diarrhea, and so on) and generally resolve on discontinuation.
- Patients taking melatonin along with drugs known to be inhibitors of CYP1A2 or CYP2C19 (and perhaps of CYP3A4 and CYP2D6) should be monitored for excessive melatonin effects

since inhibition of melatonin metabolism may occur with these inhibitors. Additionally, melatonin should be used with caution in patients receiving calcium channel blockers, as melatonin may antagonize the antihypertensive effects of these agents.

REFERENCES

Anonymous. Melatonin. Briggs Update-Drugs in Pregnancy and lactation. 2002;14:28–9.

Anonymous. Melatonin. Med Lett Drugs Ther 1995;37:111–2.

Arendt J. In what circumstances is melatonin a useful sleep therapy? Consensus statement, WFSRS Focus Group, Dresden, November 1999. J Sleep Res 2000;9:397–8.

Bardazzi F, Placucci F, Neri I, et al. Fixed drug eruption due to melatonin. Acta Derm-Venereol 1998;78:69–70.

Bursztajn HJ. Melatonin therapy: from benzodiazepine-dependent insomnia to authenticity and autonomy [editorial]. Arch Intern Med 1999;159:2393–4.

Carman JS, Post RM, Buswell R, Goodwin FK. Negative effects of melatonin on depression. Am J Psychiatry 1976;133:1181–6.

Citera G, Arias MA, Maldonado-Cocco JA, et al., The effect of melatonin in patients with fibromyalgia: a pilot study. Clin Rheumatol 2000;19:9–13.

Dagan Y, Zisapel N, Nof D, et al. Rapid reversal of tolerance to benzodiazepine hypnotics by treatment with oral melatonin: a case report. Eur Neuropsychopharmacol 1997;7:157–69.

Dalton EJ, Rotondi D, Levitan RD, et al. Use of slow-release melatonin in treatment-resistant depression. J Psychiatry Neurosci 2000;25:48–52.

Dawson D, Encel N. Melatonin and sleep in humans. J Pineal Res 1993;15:1–12.

DeMuro RL, Nafziger AN, Blask DE, et al. The absolute bioavailability of oral melatonin. J Clin Pharmacol 2000;40:781–4.

Ellis CM, Lemmens G, Parkes JD. Melatonin and insomnia. J Sleep Res 1996;5:61#-35.

Force RW, Hansen L, Bedell M. Psychotic episode after melatonin [letter]. Ann Pharmacother 1997;31:1408.

Garfinkel D, Laudon M, Nof D, Zisapel N. Improvement of sleep quality in elderly people by controlled-release melatonin. Lancet 1995;346:541–4.

Garfinkel D, Zisapel N, Wainstein J, Laudon M. Facilitation of benzodiazepine disontinuation by melatonin. Arch Intern Med 1999;159:2456–60.

Ghielmini M, Pagani O, de Jong J, et al. Double-blind randomized study on the myeloprotective effect of melatonin in combination with carboplatin and etoposide in advanced lung cancer. Br J Cancer 1999;80:1058–61.

Gordon N. The therapeutics of melatonin: a paediatric perspective. Brain Dev 2000;22:213–7.

Hahm H, Kujawa J, Augsburger L. Comparison of melatonin products against USP nutritional supplements standards and other criteria. J Am Pharm Assoc 1999;39:27–31.

Haimov I, Lavie P, Laudon M, et al. Melatonin replacement therapy of elderly insomniacs. Sleep 1995;18:598–603.

Hao H. Melatonin does not shift circadian phase in baboons. J Clin Endocrinol Metab 2000;85:3618–22.

Hartter S, Grozinger M, Weigmann H, et al. Increased bioavailability of oral melatonin after fluvoxamine coadministration. Clin Pharmacol Ther 2000;67:1–6.

Harumi T, Matsushima S. Separation and assay methods for melatonin and its precursors. J Chromatogr B Biomed Sci Appl 2000;747:95–110.

Herxheimer A, Petrie KJ. Melatonin for preventing and treating jet lag (Cochrane Review). In: The Cochrane Library, Issue 2. Oxford: Update Software, 2001.

Holliman BJ, Chyka PA. Problems in assessment of acute melatonin overdose. South Med J 1997;90:451–3.

Iinuma F, Hamase K, Matsubayashi S, et al. Sensitive determination of melatonin by precolumn derivatization and reversed-phase high-performance liquid chromatography. J Chromatogr A 1999;835:67–72.

James M, Trema MO, Jones JS, Krohmer JR. Can melatonin improve adaptation to night shift? Am J Emerg Med 1998;16:367–70.

Lewy AJ, Bauer VK, Cutler NL, Sack RL. Melatonin treatment of winter depression: a pilot study. Psychiatry Res 1998;77:57–61.

Lissoni P, Barni S, Mandala M, et al. Decreased toxicity and increased efficacy of cancer chemotherapy using the pineal hormone melatonin in metastatic solid tumor patients with poor clinical status. Eur J Cancer 1999;35:1688–92.

Lissoni P, Barni S, Meregalli S, et al. Modulation of cancer endocrine therapy by melatonin: a phase II study of tamoxifen plus melatonin in metastatic breast cancer patients progressing under tamoxifen alone. BJM 1995;71:854–6.

Lissoni P, Barni S, Tancini G, et al., A randomized study with subcutaneous low-dose interleukin 2 alone v interleukin 2 plus the pineal hormone melatonin in advanced solid neoplasms other than renal cancer and melanoma. Br J Cancer 1994;69:196–9.

Lockley SW, Skeene DJ, James K, et al. Melatonin administration can entrain the free-running circadian system of blind subjects. J Endocrinol 2000;164:R1–6.

Lusardi P, Piazza E, Fogari R. Cardiovascular effects of melatonin in hypertensive patients well controlled by nifedipine: a 24-hour study. Br J Clin Pharmacol 2000;49:423–7.

Monti JM, Cardinali DP. A critical assessment of the melatonin effect on sleep in humans. Biol Signals Recept 2000;9:328–39.

Naguib M, Samarkandi AH. The comparative dose-response effects of melatonin and midazolam for premedication of adult patients: a double-blinded, placebo-controlled study. Anesth Analg 2000;91:473–9.

Ohta Y, Kongo M, Sasaki E, et al. Preventive effect of melatonin on the progression of carbon tetrachloride-induced acute liver injury in rats. Adv Exp Med Biol 1999;467:327–32.

Pierce A. The American Pharmaceutical Association practical guide to natural medicines. New York: The Stonesong Press; 1999. p. 19.

Papavasiliou PS, Cotzias GC, Duby SE, et al. Melatonin and parkinsonism [letter]. JAMA 1972;221:88–9.

Rodriguez MA, Cabanillas F, Dang NH, et al. Lymphocyte changes in lymphoma patients receiving melatonin plus CHOP chemotherapy. Proc Ann Meet Am Soc Clin Oncol 2000;19:Abstract 72.

Rosenberg SI, Silverstein H, Rowan PT, Olds MJ. Effect of melatonin on tinnitus. Laryngoscope 1998;108:305–10.

Sack RL, Brandes RW, Kendall AR, Lewy AJ. Entrainment of free-running circadian rhythms by melatonin in blind people. N Engl J Med 2000;343:1070–7.

Sanders DC, Chaturvedi AK, Hordinsky JR. Melatonin: aeromedical, toxicopharmacologial, and analytic aspects. J Anal Toxicol 1999;23:159–67.

Shamir E, Laudon M, Barak Y, et al. Melatonin improves sleep quality of patients with chronic schizophrenia. J Clin Psychiatry 2000;61:373–7.

Shaughnessy AF. Melatonin: miracle or not? Fam Pract Recert 1996;18:46–8.

Sheldon SH. Pro-convulsant effects of oral melatonin in neurologically disabled children. Lancet 1998;351:1254.

von Bahr C, Ursing C, Yasui N, et al. Fluvoxamine but not citalopram increases serum melatonin in healthy subjects—an indication that cytochrome P450 CYP1A2 and CYP2C19 hydroxylate melatonin. Eur J Clin Pharmacol 2000; 56:123–7.

Waldhauser F, Dietzel M. Daily and annual rhythms in human melatonin secretion: role in puberty control. Ann NY Acad Sci 1985; 453:205–14.

Williamson BL, Tomlinson AJ, Mishra PK, et al. Structural characterization of contaminants found in commercial preparations of melatonin: similarities to case-related compounds from l-tryptophan associated with eosinophilia-myalgia syndrome. Chem Res Toxicol 1998;11:234–40.

Wright SW, Lawrence LM, Wrenn KD, et al. Randomized clinical trial of melatonin after night-shift work: efficacy and neuropsychologic effects. Ann Emerg Med 1998;32:334–40.

Wurzburger RJ, Kawashima K, Miller RL, Spector S. Determination of rat pineal gland melatonin content by a radioimmunoassay. Life Sci 1976;18:867–77.

Yie SM, Johansson E, Brown GM. Competitive solid-phase enzyme immunoassay for melatonin in human and rat serum and rat pineal gland. Clin Chem 1993;39:2322–5.

Zisapel N. The use of melatonin for the treatment of insomnia. Biol Signals Recept 1999;8:84–9.

Chapter 17

Methylsulfonylmethane (Dimethylsulfone)

Timothy S. Tracy and Melanie Johns Cupp

17.1. HISTORY

Methylsulfonylmethane (dimethylsulfone; MSM) is a natural product whose primary use has been as a high-temperature solvent in the chemical industry. Early therapeutic uses included its application as an antiinflammatory agent (Merck Index, 1996).

17.2. CHEMICAL STRUCTURE

See Fig. 17-1 for the chemical structure of MSM (dimethylsulfone).

17.3. CURRENT PROMOTED USES

MSM is used both orally and topically for a variety of ailments, particularly those involving inflammation (Natural Medicines Database, 2002). It is used for such conditions as chronic pain, arthritis (both rheumatoid and osteo-), joint inflammation, tendonitis, and musculoskeletal pain.

MSM is also used to treat a variety of other conditions such as abrasions/cuts, allergies, gastrointestinal maladies, hypertension, premenstrual syndrome, mood elevation, diabetes mellitus (type 2), interstitial cystitis, Alzheimer's disease, autoimmune disorders, HIV/AIDS, cancer, migraines, and *Trichomonas vaginalis*, *Giardia*, *Candida albicans* infections, and as an immunostimulant (Natural Medicines Database, 2002).

17.4. SOURCES AND CHEMICAL COMPOSITION

MSM can be found in primitive plants such as *Equisetum arvense* and Equisetaceae (Pearson et al., 1981) as well as in the adrenal cortex of cattle, milk from both bovines and humans, and human urine (Hucker et al., 1966; Williams et al., 1966a, b). It is most easily prepared through the oxidation of dimethyl sulfoxide (Merck Index, 1996).

From: *Forensic Science: Dietary Supplements: Toxicology and Clinical Pharmacology*
Edited by: M. J. Cupp and T. S. Tracy © Humana Press Inc., Totowa, New Jersey

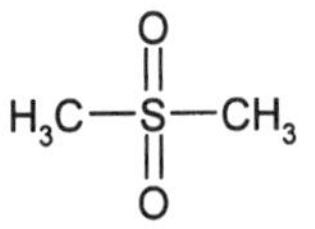

$$H_3C-\overset{\overset{\displaystyle O}{\|}}{\underset{\underset{\displaystyle O}{\|}}{S}}-CH_3$$

Fig. 1. Chemical structure of methylsulfonylmethane (MSM).

17.5. PRODUCTS AVAILABLE

MSM is available alone and in combination with other ingredients, most notably glucosmaine and chondroitin. MSM itself is available under a variety of names including crystalline DMSO, dimethyl sulfone, $DMSO_2$, MSM, methylsulfonylmethane, OptiMSM and sulfonyl sulfur. The independent laboratory ConsumerLab.com has released their results of potency testing of 17 brands of MSM and MSM-containing products commonly available through catalogs, retail stores, multilevel marketing companies, and online. Two products failed to meet ConsumerLab.com's standards because they contained only 85–88% of the labeled amount of MSM. One of these products also contained small amounts of DMSO, an indicator of poor manufacturing quality (ConsumerLab.com 2002). A list of MSM products that passed testing, as well as details about testing methodology, is available at the web site www.consumerlabs.com.

17.6. IN VITRO EFFECTS AND ANIMAL STUDIES

MSM serves as a precursor source of sulfur for the amino acids cysteine and methionine. Richmond (1986) studied the incorporation of sulfur from MSM into serum proteins of guinea pigs. Radiolabeled ^{35}S-MSM was administered to guinea pigs via intubation, and blood, urine, and fecal samples were collected. Most of the radioactivity was excreted in the urine (chemical species not reported), none in the feces, and approximately 1% in serum proteins. Serum methionine and cysteine residues were found to be radioactive, suggesting incorporation of sulfur from ^{35}S-MSM.

Studies in animals have also been conducted to assess the role of MSM as a chemopreventive agent. O'Dwyer et al. (1988) studied the ability of oral MSM (added to drinking water) to prevent 1,2-dimethylhydrazine-induced colon cancer. Animals were injected subcutaneously with 1,2-dimethylhydrazine every week for 20 wk. The animals were given MSM for 1 wk prior to the injections and throughout the course of the experiment. Animals receiving MSM had a significantly longer time to tumor onset ($p = 0.04$) than animals in the control group. In addition, fewer poorly differentiated tumors were noted in the MSM treatment group. However, there were no differences in the number of tumors noted between the groups.

These same researchers also studied the ability of MSM to prevent dimethylbenzanthracene-induced mammary tumors (O'Dwyer et al., 1988). Animals were given either 1 or 4% MSM in drinking water beginning 1 wk prior to the initiation of the experiment and continuing through the observation period. Animals were treated with 15 mg of dimethylbenzanthracene in 1 mL of sesame oil via gastric intubation. Time to first tumor, tumor size, and number of tumors were recorded. Only 4% MSM (1% MSM had no effect on any measured parameters) produced a statistical lengthening of time to first tumor and times to all tumors compared with control animals. However, it did not affect the mean growth rate of all tumors. With respect to toxic reactions, none were noted with 1% MSM treatment, but three unusual tumors (one liver lymphoma, one kidney cancer, and one abdominal wall sarcoma) were noted in the 4% MSM treatment group. Thus, it appears that in rats, a dose of 4% MSM is required for chemopreventive effects of mammary tumors but that other tumors may occur in response to treatment.

It has also been proposed that MSM may be used as a treatment for diabetic conditions. Klandorf et al. (1989), using spontaneously diabetic and control mice, studied the ability of MSM to prevent the expression of diabetes in the spontaneously diabetic mice. MSM (2.5%) was added to the animals' drinking water immediately after weaning, and the animals were monitored until they became glycosuric or they were 240 d of age. MSM treatment had no effect on the development of diabetes.

17.7. CLINICAL STUDIES

Two clinical studies of the effects of MSM have been conducted in humans. Unfortunately, both studies were unblinded and neither involved placebo control. Childs (1994) reported the administration of MSM to six patients for the treatment of interstitial cystitis. All the patients had failed standard treatment therapies. The dose of MSM was 30–50 mL given intravesically. Five of the six patients responded to the treatment (four became asymptomatic and one had a moderate response). In two of the responders, no further treatment was necessary, and the symptoms did not recur. The patient in whom a moderate response was noted was lost to follow up.

Barrager and colleagues (2002) studied the effects of MSM for the treatment of seasonal allergic rhinitis. Fifty subjects were given 2600 mg of methylsulfonylmethane oral for 30 d. Again, control subjects receiving placebo were not employed. At baseline and days 7, 14, 21, and 30, subjects were evaluated for symptom relief by use of questionnaire. Additionally, plasma IgE and C-reactive protein were measured at baseline and day 30. Total and upper respiratory symptoms were reported relieved by day 7 and lower respiratory symptoms by day 21. All respiratory improvements were reported as being maintained throughout the 30-d study period. No changes in plasma IgE levels were observed. The authors reported that few side effects were observed. It was concluded that MSM might be a useful agent in the treatment of seasonal allergic rhinitis. However, a larger, randomized, double-blind, placebo-controlled trial is needed to confirm these findings.

17.8. PHARMACOKINETICS

There have been no studies of MSM pharmacokinetics in humans. In the rhesus monkey, MSM was observed as a metabolite of dimethyl sulfoxide administration (Layman and Jacob, 1985). MSM was detectable in the blood within 2 h of dimethyl sulfoxide administration, and a half-life of 38 h was observed.

17.9. ADVERSE EFFECTS AND TOXICITY

MSM Eye Drops and MSM Eye and Nasal Drops by Ultra Botanicals, were recalled in the summer of 2001 owing to contamination with the bacteria *Pseudomo-*

nas mendocina and *Klebsiella pneumoniae*, infection with which could potentially cause blindness (Anonymous, 2001). The predominant adverse effects associated with MSM administration are nausea, diarrhea, and headache (Natural Medicines Database, 2002). Comprehensive studies of adverse effects in humans have not been conducted.

17.10. INTERACTIONS

To our knowledge, no drug interactions have been reported. However, owing to the paucity of studies involving MSM use, definitive conclusions cannot be made as to whether interactions with this agent may occur.

17.11. REPRODUCTION

Insufficient reliable information exists to determine the safety of MSM in pregnant or lactating women. Therefore, it is suggested that the product be avoided in these patients (Natural Medicines Database, 2002). In a nematode (*Caenorhabditis elegans*) model of developmental and reproductive genetics, MSM was found to cause chromosome abnormalities and a decrease in fertility (Goldstein et al., 1992). Effects on X-chromosome nondisjunction were noted along with senescent morphology of meiotic prophase nuclei. As the concentration of MSM was increased, a decrease in fertility and an increase in the production of abnormal gametes was observed. It should be noted that the relevance of these findings to the human situation is unclear.

17.12. CHEMICAL AND BIOFLUID ANALYSIS

Only one assay has been published specifically for the quantitation of MSM (dimethylsulfone) (Mehta et al., 1986); most assays are for polychlorinated biphenyl methylsulfones. Mehta and colleagues (1986) used gas chromatography with flame ionization detection to measure plasma or urine concentrations of MSM. Briefly, 0.2 mL of plasma or urine is spiked with 0.8 mL of internal standard (0.02% toluene in acetone, v/v) and the sample is vortexed for 30 s. Following centrifugation (750g for 5 min), the supernatant is collected, and 1 µL is injected onto the chromatograph. The chromatographic system consists of a gas chromatograph with a flame ionization detector and glass column (2 mm × 3 mm, i.d.) packed with Porapak Q. (A more contemporary capillary column, e.g., DB-1, would work equally well but modifications of the chromatographic conditions would be required.) The column temperature is set to 240°C, the injection port to 250°C, and the detector to 275°C. The nitrogen flow rate is 25 mL/min, the hydrogen flow rate is 33 mL/min, and the air flow rate is 390 mL/min. Total run time is less than 11 min. The method appears to be accurate and reproducible with a limit of detection of 0.1 µg/mL.

17.13. REGULATORY STATUS

MSM is regulated as a dietary supplement by the Food and Drug Adminstration.

17.14. Summary

- MSM is a source of sulfur in the body's synthesis of cysteine and methionine. It has been used for the treatment of various inflammatory disorders. Animal studies have suggested it may be effective as a chemopreventive agent.
- No controlled clinical studies exist on the use of MSM but reports suggest it may have value in the treatment of interstitial cystitis and seasonal allergies.
- Adverse effects of MSM administration appear to be mild and include nausea, diarrhea, and headache.

References

Anonymous. Pharmacy fax monitor. July 18, 2001.

Barrager E, Veltmann JR Jr, Schauss AG, Schiller RN. A multicentered, open-label trial on the safety and efficacy of methylsulfonylmethane in the treatment of seasonal allergic rhinitis. J Altern Complement Med 2002;3:167–73.

Childs SJ. Dimethyl sulfone (DMSO$_2$) in the treatment of interstitial cystitis. Urol Clin North Am 1994;21:85–8.

ConsumerLab.com. News. Consumerlab.com reports test results of arthritis supplement—MSM. Quality found higher than for most supplements, but room for improvement remains. Available from: www.consumerlabs.com/news/news_060410.asp. Accessed January 25, 2002.

Goldstein P, Magnano L, Rojo J. Effects of dimethyl sulfone (DMSO$_2$) on early gametogenesis in *Caenorhabditis elegans*: ultrastructural aberrations and loss of synaptonemal complexes from pachytene nuclei. Reprod Toxicol 1992;6:149–59.

Hucker HB, Ahmad PM, Miller EA, Brobyn R. Metabolism of dimethyl sulphoxide to dimethyl sulphone in the rat and man. Nature 1966;209:619–20.

Klandorf H, Chirra AR, DeGruccio A, Girman DJ. Dimethyl sulfoxide modulation of diabetes onset in NOD mice. Diabetes 1989;38:194–7.

Layman DL, Jacob SW. The absorption, metabolism and excretion of dimethyl sulfoxide by rhesus monkeys. Life Sci 1985;37:2431–7.

Mehta AC, Peaker S, Acomb C, Calvert RT. Rapid gas chromatographic determination of dimethyl sulphoxide and its metabolite dimethyl sulphone in plasma and urine. J Chromatogr 1986;383:400–4.

Natural Medicines Database. Methylsulfonylmethane. In: Jellin, JM, ed. Natural medicines comprehensive database, 2002, Therapeutic Research Faculty. Available from: http://www.naturaldatabase.com/monograph.asp?mono_id=522&hilite=1, Accessed January 16, 2002.

O'Dwyer PJ, McCabe DP, Sickle-Santanello BJ, et al. Use of polar solvents in chemoprevention of 1,2-dimethylhydrazine-induced colon cancer. Cancer 1988;62:944–8.

Pearson TW, Dawson HJ, Lackey HB Natural occurring levels of dimethyl sulfoxide in selected fruits, vegetables, grains, and beverages. J Agric Food Chem 1981;29:1089–91.

Richmond VL. Incorporation of methylsulfonylmethane sulfur into guinea pig serum proteins. Life Sci 1986;39:263–8.

The Merck Index. Whitehouse Station: Merck Research Laboratories, 1996.

Williams KI, Burstein SH, Layne DS. Dimethyl sulfone: isolation from cows' milk. Proc Soc Exp Biol Med 1966a;122:865–6.

Williams KI, Burstein SH, Layne DS. Dimethyl sulfone: isolation from human urine. Arch Biochem Biophys 1966b;113:251–2.

Chapter 18

Pyruvate

Melanie Johns Cupp and Timothy S. Tracy

18.1. HISTORY

Pyruvate is the final three-carbon fragment produced during glycolysis, the metabolic breakdown of glucose (Wolfe, 1993). Results of studies of the effect of pyruvate supplementation on ethanol-induced hepatic steatosis in rats led to additional studies suggesting that pyruvate has an inhibitory effect on lipid synthesis and weight gain (Stanko and Adibi, 1986). Human studies soon followed, and pyruvate-containing supplements appeared on the Internet in the late 1990s.

18.2. CHEMICAL STRUCTURE

Refer to Fig. 18-1 for the chemical structure of pyruvate.

18.3. CURRENT PROMOTED USES

Pyruvate supplements are purported to promote fat loss, inhibit fat deposition, and improve exercise endurance and performance.

18.4. PRODUCTS AVAILABLE

Most pyruvate products contain 500 mg of calcium pyruvate in capsule form. Tablet and powder formulations are also available. Pyruvate is also found in combination products. Pyruvex is a combination product containing 250 mg calcium pyruvate (supplying 45 mg calcium), 250 mg potassium pyruvate (supplying 75 mg of potassium), 8 mg of dihydroxyacetone, 50 mg of L-carnitine, and 20 mg of chromium picolinate. Pyruvate HCA contains 500 mg calcium pyruvate and 10 mg of *Garcinia cambogia* per capsule. Advertisements for pyruvate products often imply that their products have shown a 48% fat loss or that they help the body lose fat 48% faster. These numbers apparently come from a study in which pyruvate was substituted for a portion of the carbohydrate calories in a liquid diet, described in the *Clinical Studies*

From: *Forensic Science: Dietary Supplements: Toxicology and Clinical Pharmacology*
Edited by: M. J. Cupp and T. S. Tracy © Humana Press Inc., Totowa, New Jersey

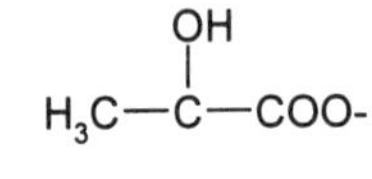

$$OH$$
$$H_3C-\overset{|}{C}-COO-$$

Fig. 1. Chemical structure of pyruvate.

section (Stanko et al., 1992b). The results of this study may not apply to pyruvate products promoted to consumers because the dosage form is different and the manufacturers' recommended dosages are much lower than those used in this and similar studies.

18.5. IN VITRO EFFECTS AND ANIMAL STUDIES

The exact mechanism responsible for pyruvate's favorable effects on body composition is unclear, but one theory suggests that pyruvate supplementation may activate and/or enhance the pyruvate-phosphoenolpyruvate futile cycle and increase energy expenditure, promoting maintenance of body weight. Another hypothesis is that pyruvate promotes fat oxidation over glucose oxidation, inhibiting fat deposition (Stanko and Arch, 1996).

Study of the effects of pyruvate on body composition and weight loss in humans was triggered by the results of investigations into the effect of compounds known to be hydrogen acceptors and/or intermediates in oxidative metabolism on the development of hepatic steatosis in ethanol-fed rats (Stanko and Adibi, 1986). In the first of these studies (Stanko et al., 1978) ethanol-fed rats consuming a diet supplemented with pyruvate and dihydroxyacetone (DHA) (a six-carbon intermediate in glycolysis) gained less weight than rats fed ethanol alone (not statistically significant) and produced fewer liver triglycerides ($p < 0.05$). This observation suggested that fat storage was inhibited by the combination and was supported by earlier data showing that hydrogen produced by liver oxidation of alcohol reduces certain intermediates involved in oxidative metabolism, favoring fat storage rather than fat oxidation. During the course of subsequent study, it was observed that rats supplemented with pyruvate and DHA had less abdominal fat than control rats, further supporting the combination's inhibitory effect on lipid synthesis (Stanko and Adibi, 1986).

A subsequent investigation (Stanko and Adibi, 1986) examined the effects of pyruvate and DHA on lipid accumulation and energy expenditure in two groups of rats fed isocaloric diets. The groups were fed identical liquid diets, but part of the carbohydrate in the experimental group was supplied as pyruvate and DHA. Energy expenditure, measured by oxygen consumption and carbon dioxide production, was greater, whereas lipid synthesis, measured by incorporation of tritiated water into adipose tissue, was lower in the experimental group. After 112 d, the rats were sacrificed, and body composition was measured. The experimental group exhibited 32% less body fat and had gained less weight than the control group ($p < 0.01$, t-test). The rates of energy expenditure and carbon dioxide production were significantly greater in rats receiving the experimental diet vs the control diet ($p < 0.05$, t-test). These results suggest that inhibition of weight gain associated with substitution of pyruvate and DHA in the diet is the result of increased energy expenditure and decreased lipid synthesis.

The effects documented in rats were shown to be applicable to other species in a study in which 24 swine were pair-fed, in littermate pairs of the same sex, a diet containing 4% by weight polyglucose or triose (Polycose®), a 3:1 mixture of DHA and pyruvate (Stanko et al., 1989). Average backfat depth was less in the triose group compared with the control (Polycose; $p < 0.01$, paired t-test).

A subsequent study in genetically obese Zucker rats (Cortez et al., 1991) showed that rats fed a diet containing 6% pyruvate substituted for a portion of the carbohydrate calories consumed less food than rats with free access to a control diet. Whether this was owing to taste or appetite suppression is unknown. When compared with pair-fed controls, rats fed the pyruvate-containing diet had a lower net weight gain than the pair-fed controls ($p < 0.05$, one-way ANOVA). Oxygen consumption and caloric expenditure per kg body weight were also greater in the pyruvate group than in the pair-fed controls ($p < 0.05$, one-way ANOVA).

18.6. CLINICAL STUDIES

18.6.1. Weight Loss/Maintenance and Body Composition

Based on these favorable animal data, body composition, energy expenditure, and nitrogen balance were studied in 13 obese women [mean body mass index (BMI) 38.4 kg/m² placebo group, 39.4 kg/m² experimental group]. Subjects were prescribed a calorically restricted diet in which pyruvate and dihydroxyacetone (DHAP) were substituted for glucose calorie-for-calorie (Stanko et al., 1992c). Pregnant women and women with heart, liver, kidney, intestinal, or pulmonary diseases were excluded. Patients were confined to bed except to walk to the bathroom or metabolic kitchen, where they were closely observed to ensure the diet was completely consumed. All subjects consumed a 500-kcals liquid diet for 21 d. Subjects were randomly assigned to receive either DHA 12 g and pyruvate 16 g (10 g sodium pyruvate and 9 g calcium pyruvate; Chemical Dynamics Company, South Plainfield, NJ) or 26 g polyglucose (Polycose) substituted for a portion of the diet's carbohydrate content.

Total weight and fat loss (measured by bioelectrical impedence) and weight and fat loss per 1000 kcal energy deficit were significantly greater in the pyruvate group ($p < 0.05$, Mann-Whitney two-tailed t-test). The absolute difference in weight loss and fat loss between the two groups was less than 1 kg. No statistically significant difference was found between the two groups in resting energy expenditure as measured by metabolic cart, or in weekly or cumulative nitrogen balance. Although this study showed that pyruvate and DHA substituted for part of the carbohydrate content of a liquid hypocaloric diet can enhance weight and fat loss compared with a glucose-based diet, the difference in weight and fat loss between the two groups was of minimal clinical significance. The liquid hypocaloric diet containing less than 1 g of fat used in this study is not suitable for unsupervised use by consumers.

A subsequent study was undertaken in which 14 obese (mean BMI 37.4 kg/m² placebo group, 42.4 kg/m² experimental group) women were randomly assigned to a liquid diet providing 1000 kcals with pyruvate 30 g (20 g sodium pyruvate plus 16 g calcium pyruvate; Chemical Dynamics Company) or Polycose 22 g substituted for a portion of the carbohydrate calories for 21 d (Stanko et al., 1992b). Exclusion criteria were the same as for the previous study by Stanko and colleagues (1992c). Although two patients had hypertension controlled with "mild" diuretics, these were discontinued 3 d prior to the study. Patients were confined to bed except for trips to the bathroom and metabolic kitchen, and compliance with the prescribed diet was monitored.

The pyruvate group demonstrated a 37% greater weight loss and a 48% greater fat loss than the control group, as measured by bioelectrical impedance ($p < 0.05$, Mann-Whitney one-tailed *t*-test). The total energy deficit was similar in the two groups during the study period; however, weight and fat loss per 1000 kilocalorie energy deficit were significantly greater in the pyruvate group ($p < 0.05$, Mann-Whitney one-tailed *t*-test). Weight loss as a percentage of initial body weight was 29% greater, and fat loss as a percentage of initial body fat was 37% greater in the pyruvate group ($p <$ 0.05, Mann-Whitney one-tailed *t*-test). Decrease in body mass index was 47% greater in the pyruvate group ($p < 0.05$, Mann-Whitney one-tailed *t*-test). As in the previous study, the actual difference between the two groups in total weight and fat loss was slight—patients in the pyruvate group lost an average of 5.9 kg vs 4.3 in the polyglucose group, whereas fat loss was 4 kg and 2.7 kg in the pyruvate and polyglucose groups, respectively ($p < 0.05$, Mann-Whitney one-tailed *t*-test). The two groups had comparable weekly and cumulative nitrogen balances, as well as resting metabolic rates.

These studies suggest that a severely calorie-restricted liquid diet containing pyruvate is superior to a liquid diet containing the same number of calories without pyruvate in regard to weight loss and body composition. Pyruvate supplements are advertised for use *in addition* to a normal diet; however, the findings of these studies may be applicable only to medically supervised liquid diets in which pyruvate is *substituted for* a portion of the carbohydrate calories. Although no studies have examined the ability of pyruvate supplementation to promote weight loss when used in addition to a normal diet, studies have examined the ability of pyruvate to minimize weight regain when used in addition to a hypercaloric diet.

Because obese patients who lose weight on a calorie-restricted diet usually regain the lost weight when they resume normal diets, 17 obese females were enrolled in a study to investigate the ability of pyruvate and DHA to inhibit weight regain with hyperenergetic feeding after weight loss (Stanko and Arch, 1996). After a 3-d run-in during which subjects consumed a normal diet, all subjects were fed a hypoenergetic diet of fruits, vegetables, and eggs for 21 d. Subsequently, subjects were fed diets providing calories equal to 150% of resting energy expenditure. At that time, subjects were randomized to receive either pyruvate 15 g and DHA 75 g or Polycose five times daily. These isocaloric liquid supplements comprised approx 20% of caloric intake. Patients were confined to bed except for travel to the lavatory and metabolic kitchen, and compliance was closely monitored. Weight gain was noted in both groups as a result of the hypercaloric diet; however, weight gain was 36% (1.1. kg) less in patients receiving the pyruvate and DHA supplement ($p < 0.05$, ANOVA with Bonferoni's *post hoc* test). This group also gained 55% (1 kg) less body fat than the placebo group ($p < 0.05$, ANOVA with Bonferoni's *post hoc* test). There was no difference between the two groups in regard to nitrogen balance. These data suggest that pyruvate provides a statistically significant but clinically negligible benefit for patients eating regular diets. The results remain to be confirmed with the pyruvate products marketed to consumers, as the closely monitored inpatient setting used in this study limits the generalizability of the results.

18.6.2. Antilipemic Effects

In studies of the effect of pyruvate on weight loss and body composition, choles-terol and triglycerides did not significantly differ between the pyruvate and control groups (Stanko et al., 1992b, c). Although in one study (Stanko et al., 1992c), both cholesterol and triglycerides decreased in both the pyruvate and control groups, there was no significant difference between the two groups. These investigators subsequently perfomed studies designed spccifically to evaluate the effects of pyruvate on plasma lipid levels. In one such study (Stanko et al., 1992a), pyruvate 36–53 g or polyglucose (Polycose) 21–37 g was substituted for a portion of the carbohydrate calories supplied by a high cholesterol (560–620 mg), high fat (45–47% of total calories), anabolic (approx 27 kcal/kg) diet. This diet was chosen because it reflected that consumed in most developed countries. Forty hyperlipidemic subjects were enrolled in the study. The Mann-Whitney t-test was used to determine differences between groups. Total cholesterol and low-density lipoprotein (LDL) were unchanged in the polyglucose group but decreased by 4 and 5%, respectively, in the pyruvate group ($p < 0.05$). High-density lipoprotein (HDL) and trigycerides were similar in the two groups. Rest-ing heart rate, diastolic blood pressure, and rate-pressure product decreased by 9, 6, and 12%, respectively, in the pyruvate group but did not change in the polyglucose group. The difference between the two groups was statistically significant ($p < 0.05$).

In a subsequent study (Stanko et al., 1994), 34 hyperlipidemic outpatients received a low-cholesterol (approx 165 mg), low-fat (approx 24% of calories) diet providing approx 21 kcal/kg/d based on the American Diabetes Association exchange system. After 4 wk, subjects were randomized to a liquid diet supplement containing pyruvate 22–44 g (14–28 g sodium pyruvate plus 13–25 g calcium pyruvate) or polyglucose (Polycose) 18–35 g. The liquid supplement was consumed daily in three divided por-tions in addition to solid food for 6 wk. The liquid supplement provided approx 7% of total calories, which had been shown to affect plasma lipids in the previous study (Stanko et al., 1992a). Alcohol consumption, medication use, and duration of exercise were similar between the two groups. After 6 wk, changes in plasma cholesterol, LDL, HDL and triglycerides were not statistically different between the two groups; how-ever, the decrease in body weight and body fat was significantly greater in the pyru-vate group compared with the control group ($p < 0.05$, one-tailed nonpaired t-test). Actual mean weight loss was 0.7 kg in the pyruvate group and 0.1 kg in the polyglucose group, and mean fat loss was 0.5 and 0.1 kg in the pyruvate and polyglucose groups, respectively.

18.6.3. Exercise

Another finding of the rat study by Stanko and Adibi (1986) described previ-ously was an increase in the percentage of carcass glycogen in the pyruvate group. Because carbohydrate depletion is associated with muscle fatigue, this observation led to studies of pyruvate's effect on exercise endurance in humans.

The effect of supplementation using pyruvate with DHA on endurance and meta-bolic response to arm exercise was studied (Stanko et al., 1990b). Ten untrained males (mean age 23.3 yr) consumed a diet consisting of 55% carbohydrate, 30% fat, and 15% protein with 100 g of either polycose (Polycose) or a 3 to 1 mixture of DHA and pyruvate (DHAP; Chemical Dynamics, South Plainfield, NJ) substituted for a portion of the carbohydrate calories. The diet provided 35 kcal/kg body weight and was similar to the subjects' normal diets, based on diet history. DHAP or placebo was administred three times daily, with meals, in Jello Instant Pudding with sugar-free fiber to promote congealment. After 7 d of diet therapy, subjects performed arm ergometer exercise to exhaustion at 60% peak oxygen consumption. The triceps muscle was biopsied before and after exercise, and arterial and venous blood samples were drawn before, during, and after exercise. After a 7–14-d washout, subjects received the alternate diet for 7 d, and the experimental protocol was repeated. Paired t-tests were used to analyze differences in endurance, and two-way repeated measures ANOVA with the Scheffe *post hoc* test was used to evaluate changes in blood chemistry, glycogen stores, and cardiorespiratory responses.

Arm endurance increased with DHAP ($p < 0.01$), and triceps glycogen was greater at rest with DHAP ($p < 0.05$). Arteriovenous glucose difference was greater after DHAP both before and after 60 min of exercise ($p < 0.05$), but not at exhaustion. No differences were found between the two treatments in respiratory exchange ratio, respiratory quotient, plasma free fatty acids, glycerol, β-hydroxybutyrate, catecholamines, or insulin at any time. The investigators concluded that DHAP improved exercise endurance by improving muscle glucose extraction.

In another study, the effects of DHAP on metabolic response and endurance capacity during leg exercise were studied in eight physically active but untrained males with a mean age of 23.6 yr (Stanko et al., 1990a). At baseline, peak oxygen consumption (VO$_2$max) was determined using cyle ergometry. All subjects were then given a high (70%) carbohydrate, low fat (12%) diet providing 35 kcal/kg to consume at home. Subjects were randomized to Polycose 100 g or DHA 75 g and sodium pyruvate (DHAP) 25 g substituted for a portion of the carbohydrate calories. After 7 d, subjects performed cycle ergometer exercise to exhaustion at 70% maximum oxygen consumption. The vastus lateralis was biopsied before and after exercise. Blood samples were obtained before, during, and after exercise. After a 7–14-d washout, subjects consumed the alternative diet, and the experimental methods were repeated. Leg endurance was increased with DHAP compared with Polycose ($p < 0.01$, paired t-test). Difference in arteriovenous glucose concentration was greater after DHAP than after Polycose® at rest, and after 30 min of exercise, but not at exhaustion ($p < 0.05$, 2-way ANOVA). Estimated glucose oxidation was greater after DHAP than Polycose ($p < 0.05$, paired t-test). The authors concluded that DHAP in addition to a high carbohydrate diet increased leg exercise endurance by increasing muscle glucose extraction. Another study (Robertson et al., 1990) demonstrated that DHAP-associated improvement in glucose extraction decreases perceived exertion in the exercised limb. Although these studies demonstrate that DHAP improves muscle glucose extraction, it does not improve muscle amino acid extraction (Stanko et al., 1993).

18.6.4. Diabetes

After a 7-d washout from antidiabetic medications, seven women (mean age 49 yr, mean BMI 42.1 kg/m^2) were randomized to a 1500 kcal/d diet supplying 13% of calories as either DHAP or Polycose (Stanko et al., 1990a). Subjects consumed this diet for 7 d. On the last 3 d of the diet, subjects were housed in the metabolic unit. On day 8, after an overnight fast, subjects received a continuous infusion of radiolabeled glucose, followed by an oral 3-h glucose tolerance test. After a 2-wk washout, subjects were crossed over to the alternate diet and the study was repeated. Paired *t*-tests were used to identify differences between the two diets.

DHP significantly decreased both glucose turnover and plasma glucose ($p < 0.05$) without affecting plasma insulin, glucagon, or C-peptide concentration, suggesting inhibition of hepatic gluconeogenesis and possibly increased muscle glucose extraction. DHAP did not affect plasma glucose levels in non-diabetic men (Stanko et al., 1990c), reflecting the importance of an abnormally high rate of gluoneogenesis as a cause of increased plasma glucose levels in diabetic persons.

18.7. PHARMACOKINETICS

Limited data exist on the pharmacokinetics of pyruvate following the administration of the compound. Wu (Wu, 1997a, b, 1998, 1999) conducted a series of studies on the effect of ethanol administration on pyruvate pharmacokinetics in mice. $1\text{-}^{14}C$-labeled sodium pyruvate was administered into the hind limb of mice and the elimination of $^{14}C\text{-}CO_2$ expired in air and ^{14}C-labeled material eliminated in urine and feces were measured. Approximately 30% of the injected pyruvate was eliminated as $^{14}C\text{-}CO_2$ in expired air and 50% of the labeled products were eliminated in the urine. Because a closed pharmacokinetic model was used for data analysis, it is difficult to extrapolate the findings to elimination rates from the body. Interestingly, ethanol intake significantly increased expiration of $^{14}C\text{-}CO_2$, suggesting a potential interaction of ethanol with pyruvate in subjects consuming both products simultaneously.

18.8. ADVERSE EFFECTS AND TOXICITY

Adverse effects associated with pyruvate-containing liquid diets include diarrhea and/or borborygmus in three to four pyruvate patients in each study (Stanko et al., 1992b, c; Stanko and Arch, 1996). In another study (Stanko et al., 1994), loose stool (24% pyruvate vs 12 % placebo), diarrhea (pyruvate 35% vs 0% placebo), and gas and bloating (65% pyruvate vs 46% placebo) were reported.

The potential for sodium overload exists with sodium pyruvate use. In one study, the maximum daily sodium pyruvate consumption was limited to 25 g to avoid excess sodium intake (Stanko et al., 1990a).

18.9. INTERACTIONS

No known interactions of pyruvate-containing supplements with drugs, food, or lab tests have been reported.

18.10. REPRODUCTION

Insufficient evidence exists to determine the safety of pyruvate in pregnant or lactating women. Therefore, it is recommended that pyruvate usage be avoided in these patients.

18.11. CHEMICAL AND BIOFLUID ANALYSIS

Early methods of analyzing pyruvate in biologic tissues (including blood) utilized an enzyme-based assay (Bücher et al., 1965). Commercial kits are available, and these methods are still used in some clinical laboratories today. However, recent advances in mass spectrometric detection have afforded investigators more specific and sensitive means of measuring pyruvate concentrations in biologic fluids.

Dias and collegues (1990) report a gas chromatography-mass spectrometry (GC-MS) assay for the determination of pyruvate along with a number of other organic acids, amino acids, ketone bodies and medium-chain dicarboxylic acids. Urine samples (4 mL) are spiked with succinic acid-d6 (internal standard) and then made strongly alkaline with 30% sodium hydroxide. In the case of plasma samples, proteins are first precipitated by addition of an equal volume of 95% ethanol and then treated in the same manner as the urine samples. The samples are then extracted three times with equal volumes of diethyl ether and the ether extract discarded. To the remaining aqueous phase is added 25 mg of hydroxylamine hydrochloride (with further sodium hydroxide added if necessary to maintain a basic pH). The mixture is then heated at 60°C for 30 min, and allowed to cool. Samples are acidified with 5 N HCl, saturated with NaCl, and extracted three times with diethyl ether (1:1, v/v). The diethyl ether layer is dried over sodium sulfate and evaporated to dryness. Samples are then silylated with Tri-Sil/Sylon BFT for 15 min at 60°C. The resulting derivatives are subjected to gas chromatography using an HP ultra-2 capillary column (25 m × 0.31 mm). The initial oven temperature is 50°C and is increased at a rate of 4°C/min to a final temperature of 300°C. Injection port temperature is set to 250°C and the detector port temperature to 280°C. Helium (36 cm/s) is used as the carrier gas. Samples are monitored with the mass spectrometer in positive ion mode set for m/z 247. Peak areas from unknown samples are compared with those obtained from a calibration curve using authentic standards.

As mentioned earlier, commercial kits based on the method of Bücher and colleagues (1965) for enzymatic assay of pyruvate in biologic fluids are available. However, one must run appropriate controls and background samples since this is a colorimetric assay, and background signal and interferences can be problematic.

18.12. REGULATORY STATUS

Pyruvate is regulated as a dietary supplement by the Food and Drug Administration.

18.13. SUMMARY

- Pyruvate is the final three-carbon product of glycolysis. Studies in humans have shown that substitution of pyruvate for carbohydrate calories can result in modest weight loss compared with a diet in which pyruvate was not substituted for carbohydrates. Doses used in these studies were substantially larger than those recommended by the manufacturer and the liquid diets used are probably not suitable for use by consumers.
- Pyruvate does not appear to produce a clinically significant effect on plasma lipids or cholesterol.
- A combination of DHA/pyruvate substituted for a portion of dietary carbohydrates may have a positive effect on exercise performance.

- The primary adverse effects associated with pyruvate therapy are gastrointestinal symptoms (e.g., diarrhea).

REFERENCES

Bücher T, Czok R, Lamprecht W, Latzko E. Pyruvate. In: Bergmeyer HU, ed. Methods of Enzymatic Analysis. New York: Academic Press, 1965:253–259.

Cortez MY, Torgan CE, Brozinick JT, et al. Effects of pyruvate and DHA consumption on the growth and metabolic state of obese Zucker rats. Am J Clin Nutr 1991;53:847–53.

Dias VC, Fung E, Snyder FF, et al. Effects of medium-chain triglyceride feeding on energy balance in adult humans. Metabolism 1990;39:887–91.

Robertson RJ, Stanko RT, Goss FL, et al. Blood glucose extraction as a mediator of perceived exertion during prolonged exercise. Eur J Appl Physiol 1990;61:100–5.

Stanko RT, Adibi SA. Inhibition of lipid accumulation and enhancement of energy expenditure by the addition of pyruvate and dihydroxyacetone to a rat diet. Metabolism 1986;35:182–6.

Stanko RT, Arch JE. Inhibition of regain in body weight and fat with addition of 3-carbon compounds to the diet with hyperenergetic refeeding after weight reduction. Int J Obes Rel Metab 1996;20:925–30.

Stanko RT, Diven WF, Robertson RJ, et al. Amino acid arterial concentration and muscle exchange during submaximal arm and leg exercise: the effect of DHA and pyruvate. J Sports Sci 1993;11:17–23.

Stanko RT, Ferguson TL, Newman CW, Newman RK. Reduction of carcass fat in swine with dietary addition of diydroxyacetone and pyruvate. J Anim Sci 1989;67:1272–8.

Stanko RT, Mendelow H, Shinozuka H, Adibi SA. Prevention of alcohol-induced fatty liver by natural metabolites and riboflavin. J Lab Clin Med 1978;91:228–35.

Stanko RT, Reynolds HR, Hoyson R, et al. Pyruvate supplementation of a low-cholesterol, low-fat diet: effects on plasma lipid concentration and body composition in hyperlipidemic patients. Am J Clin Nutr 1994;59:423–7.

Stanko RT, Reynolds HR, Lonchar KD, Arch JE. Plasma lipid concentrations in hyperlipidemic patients consuming a high-fat diet supplemented with pyruvate for 6 wk. Am J Clin Nutr 1992a;56:950–4.

Stanko RT, Tietze DL, Arch JE. Body composition, energy utilization, and nitrogen metabolism with a 4.25-MJ/d low-energy diet supplemented with pyruvate. Am J Clin Nutr 1992b;56:630–5.

Stanko RT, Tietze DL, Arch JE. Body composition, energy utilization, and nitrogen metabolism with a severely restricted diet supplemented with DHA and pyruvate. Am J Clin Nutr 1992c;55:771–6.

Stanko RT, Mitrakou A, Greenawalt K, Gerich J. Effect of dihydroxyacetone and pyruvate on plasma glucose concentration and turnover in noninsulin-dependent diabetes mellitus. Clin Physiol Biochem 1990a;8:283–8.

Stanko RT, Robertson RJ, Galbreath RW, et al. Enhanced leg exercise endurance with high-carbohydrate diet and DHA and pyruvate. J Appl Physiol 1990b;69:1651-6.

Stanko RT, Robertson RJ, Spina RJ, et al. Enhancement of arm exercise endurance capacity with DHA and pyruvate. J Appl Physiol 1990c;68:119–24.

Wolf RR. Carbohydrate metabolism and requirements. In: Rombeau JL, Caldwell, eds. Clinical nutrition: parenteral nutrition, 2nd ed. Philadelphia, PA: WB Saunders: 1993.

Wu G. Use of a fiev compartment closed model to describe the effects of ethanol inhalation on the transport and elimination of injected pyruvate in the rat. Alcohol 1997a;32:555–61.

Wu G. Using a four-compartment closed model to describe inhalation of vaporised ethanol on 1-^{14}C-pyruvate kinetics in mice. Arch Toxicol 1997b;71:501–07.

Wu G. Effect of vaporized ethanol on [1-^{14}C]pyruvate kinetics in mice using a four-compartment closed model. Pharmacol Res 1998;37:49–55.

Wu G. Ethanol inhalation in 1-[^{14}C]-pyruvate kinetic in mice using a six-compartment closed model. Eur J Drug Metab Pharmacokinet 1999;24:113–19.

Chapter 19

Red Yeast Rice Extract

Tim Berry, Melanie Johns Cupp, and Timothy S. Tracy

19.1. HISTORY

Red yeast rice extract is a Chinese remedy known as Hongqu that has been used for centuries (Reeder, 1998). Its use was first documented in China during the Tang Dynasty in 800 AD. It has been used for making rice wine and to preserve and enhance the taste and color of foods, including meat, fish, and soybean products (Herber et al., 1999; Ma et al., 2000). Li Shizhen, a pharmacologist of the Ming Dynasty (1368–1644), reported that red yeast rice promotes "digestion and blood circulation, can strengthen the spleen and dry the stomach" (Ma et al., 2000). Red yeast rice extract has been sold commercially in the United States since the late 1990s.

19.2. CHEMICAL STRUCTURE

See Fig. 19-1 for chemical structures of the monacolins. Note that red yeast rice is thought to contain varying amounts of these monacolins depending on the method of preparation. Some products may not contain detectable levels of some monacolins.

19.3. CURRENT PROMOTED USES

Recent clinical observations in animals and humans indicate that red yeast rice is useful in lowering blood lipid levels (Ma et al., 2000). Red yeast rice extract is claimed to promote and maintain healthy cholesterol levels and inhibit cholesterol production (Reeder, 1998).

19.4. SOURCES AND CHEMICAL COMPOSITION

Rice (*Oryzae sativa* L. Gramineae) is a food source throughout the world, especially in Asian countries. Rice is cultivated in areas with a warm climate, with China being one of the largest producers. Red yeast rice extract is the food fungus Went yeast (*Monascus purpureus*) fermented on premium rice plus the byproducts of the

From: *Forensic Science: Dietary Supplements: Toxicology and Clinical Pharmacology*
Edited by: M. J. Cupp and T. S. Tracy © Humana Press Inc., Totowa, New Jersey

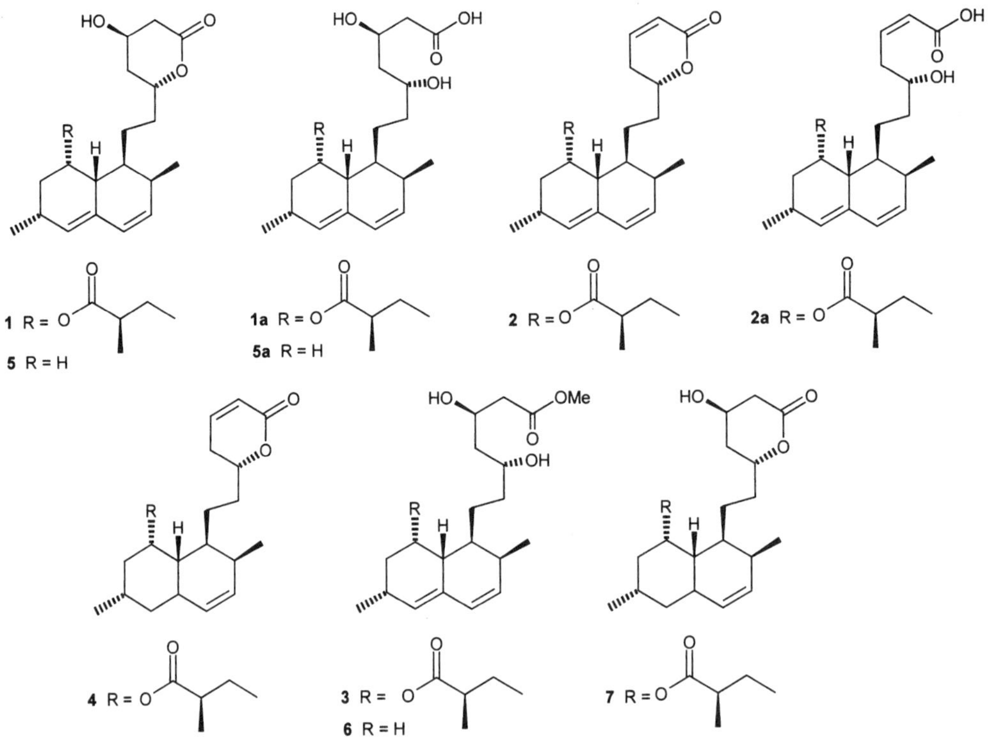

Fig. 1. Chemical structure of the monacolins found in red yeast rice in varying amounts.

fermentation process (Reeder, 1998; Ma et al., 2000). The traditional method of making red yeast rice involves fermentation of cooked nonglutinous whole rice kernel in red wine mash, polygonum grass juice, and alum water (Li et al., 1998).

Monacolins, one constituent of red yeast rice, are 3-hydroxy-3-methylglutaryl coenzyme A (HMG-CoA) reductase inhibitors, as are statin drugs (Havel, 1999a), highly effective low-density lipoprotein (LDL)-cholesterol lowering medications. Cholestin® was once a popular red yeast rice supplement that was reformulated in 2001 and now contains policosanol (beeswax extract) instead of red yeast rice. The manufacturer of Cholestin used a production process specifically designed to maximize the production of a specific monacolin, monacolin K, also known as lovastatin, which is sold as a prescription statin drug, Mevacor®. Whereas the traditional method of preparing red yeast rice extract uses a mixture of yeast strains, not all of which produce lovastatin, the Cholestin manufacturer used a specific strain of *M. purpureus* known to produce lovastatin. The yeast's ability to produce lovastatin is inversely related to its ability to produce red pigment; thus, the resulting product, unlike the product of the traditional method, is not suitable as a food colorant. The temperature must be held at approximately 25°C in order for the special strain of *M. purpureus* to produce lovastatin, but no such temperature controls are used with the traditionally produced product (Havel, 1999b). Thus, Cholestin, as well as Xuezhikang, a Chinese product that has been shown in clinical trials to lower cholesterol, differed from the traditional red yeast rice in method of preparation and lovatatin content (Havel, 1999a). Of the total monacolins in Cholestin, approximately 50% was lovastatin and 25% was its active hydroxy acid form (Heber et al., 1999).

In addition to monacolin K (lovastatin) and its ring-opened hydroxy acid form (which is actually the pharmacologically active form), other monacolins have been identified in products prepared by fermentation on moist rice, including the methyl ester of the ring-opened hydroxy acid form of monacolin K, dihydromonacolin K, dehydromonacolin K and its hydroxy acid form, monacolin L and its hydroxy acid form, dihydrodehydromonacolin K, and the methyl ester of the ring-opened hydroxy acid form of monacolin L (Ma et al., 2000; Heber et al., 2001). Heber and colleagues (2001) assayed the monacolin content of nine red yeast rice products commercially available in the United States (*see* Products Available section below for list). These investigators found that the total monacolin content ranged from 0 to 0.58% wt/wt. Because of these significant differences among product content, results of studies performed using one product cannot be extrapolated to other red yeast rice products.

Together, the monacolins comprised 0.4% wt/wt of Cholestin (Havel, 1999a,b) and a similar Chinese preparation made by the WPU Company (Beijing, China) by fermenting moist rice with a proprietary strain of *M. purpureus* for 9 d at 25°C and a pH of 5–6, followed by air-drying. Other constituents of the Chinese product include sugars (73.4%), protein (14.7%), moisture (6%), fatty acids (2.8%), ash (2.45%), fiber (0.8%), monacolins (0.4%), phosphorus (0.4%), pigments (0.3%), vitamin C (0.03%), organic phosphorus (0.02%), vitamin A less than 70 IU/100 g, Na 2370 µg/g, Mg 1092 µg/g, Ca 352 µg/g, Al 78 µg/g, Fe 36 µg/g, Mn 19 µg/g , Zn 12 µg/g, Cu 8 µg/g, and Se less than 0.25 µg/g (Ma et al., 2000).

An important constituent of red yeast rice created under certain production conditions is citrinin, a food colorant. All but two (Cholestin and Beyond Cholesterol®) of the nine products tested by Heber and associates (2001) contained citrinin, at 0.47–67.7 µg/capsule (*see* Adverse Effects and Toxicity section below for more discussion of citrinin).

19.5. PRODUCTS AVAILABLE

Cholesterex® (Oralabs, Englewood, CO), Cholestene® (HPP, LLC, Hatboro, PA), Cholactive® (Herbscience, Windmill Health Products, West Caldwell, NJ), Cholester-Reg® (Nature's Sunshine, Provo, UT), Beyond Cholesterol® (TwinLab, Hauppauge, NY), Hongqu (Nature's Sunshine, Provo UT), Cholesterol Powder® (Nature's Herbs, Hauppauge, NY), and RYR® (Solaray, Park City, UT) are red yeast rice products available in the United States (Heber et al., 2001). In addition to these products, which have been independently analyzed, other products, including Choleste-Care™ and products sold simply as "red yeast rice," "red yeast rice extract,"or "red rice yeast" are available in retail outlets and via the Internet.

19.6. IN VITRO EFFECTS AND ANIMAL STUDIES

Li and colleagues (1998) studied the effects of red yeast rice on blood lipids in three animal models. Rabbits were fed a control diet for 5 d, and after a 12-h fast, baseline lipid levels were obtained. The rabbits were then divided into six groups and fed a control diet, casein diet, casein diet plus *M. purpureus* 0.2 g/kg/d, casein diet plus *M. purpureus* 0.4 g/kg/d, casein diet plus *M. purpureus* 0.8 g/kg/d, or casein diet plus lovastatin 8 mg/kg/d for 60 d. The purpose of using casein was to simulate endogenous hyperlipidemia. Rabbits fed a 25% casein diet showed a fourfold increase in total cholesterol and LDL cholesterol. High-density lipoproteins (HDLs) and triglycerides were not affected. Treatment with *M. purpureus* for 30 d after 60 d of the casein diet resulted in a dose-related decrease in total cholesterol. Compared with the total cholesterol levels on day 60, the levels on day 90 were reduced by 45% ($p < 0.05$, *t*-test), 43% ($p < 0.05$, *t*-test), and 59% ($p < 0.01$, *t*-test) at doses of 0.2, 0.4, and 0.8 g/kg/d respectively. Lovastatin reduced total cholesterol by 52% ($p < 0.05$) at a dose of 8 mg/kg.

The second animal model utilized rabbits fed fatty diets for 2 mo to stimulate hyperlipidemia. This fatty diet produced a ninefold increase in total cholesterol, a threefold increase in triglycerides, and a twofold increase in both HDL and LDL cholesterol. Supplementation of the fat-rich diet with red yeast rice 0.4 and 0.8 g/kg/d beginning on day 40 reduced the increase in total cholesterol and triglycerides by 33.2 and 43.2%, respectively. Lovastatin at 8 mg/kg/d decreased total cholesterol by a similar amount. HDL increased and LDL decreased, but the change was not statistically significant. The addition of red yeast rice also reduced the increase in liver-to-body weight ratio, which was increased by the fatty diet. The mean liver-to-body weight ratios for the control diet, hyperlipidemic diet, hyperlipidemic diet plus red yeast rice 0.4 g/kg/d, hyperlipidemic diet plus red yeast rice 0.8 g/kg/d, and hyperlipidemic diet plus lovastatin 8 mg/kg/d were 0.029, 0.048, 0.040, 0.035, and 0.038, respectively ($p < 0.01$ compared with hyperlipidemic diet alone, *t*-test). The diet and treatment also affected the severity of aortic atheromatous plaques, a sequela of long-term elevation of cholesterol.

The third animal model utilized a high-fat diet in quail to stimulate exogenous hyperlipidemia. Total cholesterol, triglycerides, and LDL cholesterol increased five-to ninefold after 2 wk of the high-fat diet. Addition of red yeast rice 0.2 g/kg/d, 0.4 g/kg/d, 0.8 g/kg/d and lovastatin 4 mg/kg/d all decreased the negative effect of this diet on total cholesterol ($p < 0.05$, *t*-test) and triglycerides ($p < 0.05$, *t*-test).

19.7. Clinical Studies

Wang and colleagues (1997) compared the effects of Cholestin™ to those of Jiaogulan (Gynostemma pentaphylla), a Chinese herbal hypolipemic agent. Cholestin™ was compared to this preparation rather than to placebo due to a requirement of the Chinese Ministry of Public Health that a positive control be used. Exclusion criteria were heart attack, stroke, trauma, or major surgery within the past 6 mo, diabetes, liver disease, gout, allergies, or psychosis. Inclusion criteria were total cholesterol of at least 230 mg/dL, triglyceride of a least 200–400 mg/dL, LDL of a least 130 mg/dL, HDL of 40 mg/dL or lower for men, and 45 mg/dL or lower for women. In this open-label, multicenter study, 502 patients diagnosed with primary hyperlipidemia were first divided into groups based on triglyceride levels, then randomized to Cholestin™ or to the herbal product. Patients were required to discontinue any antilipemic agents at least 4 wk prior to randomization. Other medications were not addressed. Patients also received instruction in lifestyle modifications 2–4 wk prior to the start of the study. Lipids were measured at baseline, and at weeks 4 and 8. Two patients dropped out of the study due to stomachache, and seven were excluded due to noncompliance. Data for these nine patients was not included in the statistical analysis. Compared to baseline, in the red yeast rice extract group, triglycerides had decreased by 19.8% ($p < 0.001$) by week 4, and by 34.1% ($p < 0.001$) by wk 8. Total cholesterol had decreased by 17.1% ($p < 0.001$) by week 4, and 22.7% ($p < 0.001$) by week 8, while LDL had decreased by 24.6% ($p < 0.001$) by week 4, and by 30.9% ($p < 0.001$) by week 8. HDL increased by 19.9% by week 8 ($p < 0.001$). Lipid profiles also improved in the positive control group, but to a lesser extent. The open label design and lack of placebo group are limitations of this study.

Herber and associates (1999) conducted a double-blind, placebo-controlled study of red yeast rice extract (Cholestin). Eighty-three white subjects (46 men and 37 women) aged 34–78 yr with hyperlipidemia completed the study. Subjects were randomized to receive either red yeast rice (Pharmanex, Simi Valley, CA) 2.4 g/d (10 mg monacolins) or rice powder placebo for 12 wk, and were instructed to consume the American Heart Association Step I diet. The main outcome measures were total cholesterol, triglycerides, HDLs, and LDLs. There were no significant differences in the baseline lipid, demographic, or dietary variables. Baseline total cholesterol was 254 ± 29 mg/dL in the control group and 250 ± 30 mg/dL in the treatment group. Baseline triglycerides were 143 ± 46 mg/dL in the control group and 133 ± 48 mg/dL in the treatment group. Baseline HDL cholesterol was 46 ±10 mg/dL in the control group and 50 ± 13 mg/dL in the treatment group.

Total cholesterol concentrations decreased significantly from baseline in the treatment group compared with the placebo group at week 8 ($p < 0.05$, t-test). Total cholesterol was significantly different between treatment and placebo groups for both weeks 8 and 12 ($p < 0.05$, t-test), as were LDL ($p < 0.01$, t-test) and triglyceride concentrations ($p = 0.05$, t-test for independent samples). At week 8, the mean total cholesterol concentration was 208 mg/dL in the treatment group and 254 mg/dL in the placebo group. This was a significant decrease from baseline in the treatment group ($p < 0.05$, paired t-test). HDL concentrations did not differ significantly within or between the two groups at either week 8 or 12. At week 12, the mean LDL concentration in the treatment group was 135 mg/dL compared with 175 mg/dL in the placebo group. At week 12, the mean triglyceride concentrations in the treatment group were 124 mg/dL compared with 146 mg/dL in the placebo group. Red yeast rice showed a dose-dependent lowering of total cholesterol, LDL cholesterol, and triglycerides.

19.8. PHARMACOKINETICS

Pharmacokinetic data are not available for red yeast rice monacolins, and differences would be expected among the various products owing to differences in production processes and monacolin content. The pharmacokinetics of the lovastatin component of red yeast rice may be similar to the pharmacokinetic parameters reported in the literature for prescription lovastatin; however, components of red yeast rice not found in prescription lovastatin may affect its absorption, distribution, or elimination.

In vivo, lovastatin is hydrolyzed to its active β-hydroxy acid form; the parent lactone is inactive. Approximately 30% of an oral dose of lovastatin (Mevacor) is absorbed after oral administration, but it subsequently undergoes extensive first-pass metabolism by the cytochrome P450 isoenzyme CYP3A4, and thus less than 5% of an oral dose reaches systemic circulation. Lovastatin and its β-hydroxyacid are more than 95% protein bound. Approximately 83% of the dose is eliminated in the feces, either as unabsorbed drug or as metabolites eliminated in the bile (Merck & Co., 2001).

19.9. ADVERSE EFFECTS AND TOXICITY

There has been one published case report of an anaphylactic reaction to red yeast rice (Wigger-Alberti et al., 1999). This was an occupational exposure in a 26-yr-old butcher who experienced sneezing, red and watery eyes, itching, urticaria, angioedema, and dyspnea requiring treatment with intravenous glucocorticoids, theophylline, antihistamines, and inhaled bronchodilators minutes after handling red yeast rice used to color sausages. Skin prick testing for red yeast rice and *M. purpureus* were strongly positive, but the prick test to rice was negative. Ten control subjects did not react to any of the three test substances. CAST (cellular allergen stimulation test) was positive to both red yeast rice and the fungus, and RAST (radioallergosorbent test) showed IgE antibodies to the fungus. Serologic tests also revealed the presence of specific IgE antibodies to *M. purpureus*.

Adverse effects of the marketed statins might also be expected from red yeast rice. Adverse effects reported with prescription lovastatin include gastrointestinal disturbances, headache, myalgias, weakness, elevated liver enzymes, elevated creatine kinase, and (very rarely) rhabdomyolysis (Merck & Co., 2001). Herber and associates (1999) reported that the only adverse events observed during their study were headaches and a rash that responded to prednisone and antihistamine. Although several tertiary references list elevated liver function tests as a side effect of red yeast rice, there were no significant differences in liver function tests between groups at either baseline or week 12. Similarly, Wang and colleagues (1997) found that no patient in their study developed an ALT greater than twice the upper limit of normal, but did not report whether or how much ALT actually increased. Other adverse effects noted in this study included a mean 46% increase in creatine kinase form baseline, heartburn (1.9%), gas (0.9%), and dizzinesses (0.3%). These studies were not conducted over an adequate time or in sufficient numbers of patients to determine a true adverse events profile.

Citrinin, a mycotoxin produced by Monascus species, is found in some red yeast rice products; it is a mutagen and nephrotoxin with a median lethal dose (LD_{50}) of 35 mg/kg in animal models (Heber et al., 2001).

19.10. INTERACTIONS

Certain azole antifungals (itraconazole, ketoconazole), some macrolide antibiotics (erythromycin, clarithromycin), nefazodone, HIV protease inhibitors, and grapefruit juice from concentrate may increase monacolin levels based on interactions with prescription lovastatin. Increased lovastatin levels are a risk factor for myopathy and rhabdomylolysis. Cyclosporine, niacin, and gemfibrozil increase the risk of myopathy and rhabdomyolysis, particularly in patients receiving doses of lovastatin greater than 20 mg/d. Whether lovastatin increases warfarin levels is unclear (Merck & Co., 2001).

19.11. REPRODUCTION

Lovastatin is in pregnancy category X, meaning it should not be used during pregnancy. Skeletal muscle deformities have been seen in the offspring of mice and rats exposed to lovastatin, and there is a three- to fourfold increase in congenital abnormalities in human offspring exposed *in utero* to lovastatin (Merck & Co., 2001).

19.12. CHEMICAL AND BIOFLUID ANALYSIS

To date, no assays for measurement of the various monacolins in biologic fluids have been developed. However, Ma and colleagues (2000) have developed excellent methods for evaluating and quantitating the constituents present in red yeast rice formulations. For the analysis of monacolins, red yeast powder (0.5 g) is dissolved in 75% aqueous alcohol (10 mL) and sonicated for 60 minutes. The sample is then centrifuged for 10 minutes to pellet any undissolved materials, and the supernatant is filtered with a 0.45-μm filter. Individual monacolins are quantitated using high-performance liquid chromatography (HPLC) with ultraviolet detection (237 and 218 nm). Chromatographic separation is achieved on a Nova-Pak C18 (3.9 × 150 mm, 5 μm) column at a mobile phase flow rate of 1 mL/min. The mobile phase consists of acetonitrile (A) and 0.04% phosphoric acid (B) pumped through the column in a linear gradient fashion. The gradient conditions are: 0–20 min (20% A to 60% A), 20–30 min (60% A to 80% A), and 30–32 min (80% A to 90%A).

Additional confirmation of identification can be made using HPLC-mass spectrometry. Samples are prepared in the same manner, but the column is a Zorbax C18 (4.6 × 75 mm, 3.5 μm), and an isocratic mobile phase of methanol-water (70:30, v/v) is pumped at a flow rate of 0.5 mL/min. The column temperature is maintained at 30°C. Masses are monitored over the range of 150–900 mass units. The quadrapole temperature is set to 140°C, and the electron multiplier voltage at 2173 V, and spectra are acquired in positive ion mode.

The potentially toxic component citrinin can also be measured using related conditions. For citrinin analysis, 2.5 g of red yeast powder is dissolved in 20 mL of absolute alcohol and sonicated for 30 min. The sample is then centrifuged for 10 min at 3000 rpm. The resulting supernatant is then evaporated to dryness and reconstituted in 1 mL of methanol. The same HPLC column (Nova Pak) is used, but the mobile phase consists of acetonitrile (A) and 0.2% phosphoric acid (B). The gradient profile is as follows: 0–10 min (10% A to 55% A), 10–15 min hold at 55% A, and 15–20 min (90% A to 10% A).

Recently, Heber and colleagues (2001) have also published methods for identifying the monacolin products in red yeast rice and found that only one of nine commercial preparations contained the full complement of 10 monacolins. This alternative method could also be used for assessing the formulations of red yeast rice preparations.

19.13. REGULATORY STATUS

There has been much debate on the regulatory status of red yeast rice extract Cholestin. On May 20, 1998, the Food and Drug Administration (FDA) announced that Cholestin was not a dietary supplement, but rather "an unapproved drug under the terms of the Federal Food, Drug and Cosmetic Act" (FDA, 1998). The FDA based this decision in part on Cholestin-containing lovastatin, the active ingredient in the cholesterol-lowering medication Mevacor manufactured by Merck Research Labs of Whitehouse Station, NJ. Merck took exception to the marketing of lovastatin as a dietary supplement. Originally, Cholestin's label stated that the product reduced LDL and triglycerides and increased HDL; however, these claims were removed when Merck complained to the FDA (Reeder, 1998). The FDA argued that even though red yeast rice had been previously used as a food product, it was not marketed as a dietary supplement prior to the approval of Mevacor by the FDA. Pharmanex, the manufacturer of Cholestin, challenged the FDA ruling in federal court. A federal judge subsequently lifted the ban imposed by the FDA on Cholestin (Havel, 1999a). Cholestin has since been reformulated to contain policosanol (beeswax extract). Red yeast rice products are regulated as dietary supplements.

19.14. SUMMARY

- Red yeast rice contains several monacolins, but the quantities of each vary depending on the method of preparation. Thus, results of studies using different preparations may not be directly comparable.
- Red yeast rice has been shown to lower plasma lipids and cholesterol in human clinical studies. Adverse effects of red yeast rice include rash and headaches. Gastrointestinal disturbances, myalgias, elevated liver enzymes, and (in rare cases) rhabdomyolysis might be expected since red yeast rice may contain statin-type antilipemic compounds. Some red yeast products contain citrinin, which is a mutagen and nephrotoxin.
- CYP3A enzyme inhibitors may increase monacolin levels, potentially leading to an increased incidence of adverse effects.
- Since lovastatin (monacolin K) is labeled as pregnancy category X, red yeast rice products should not be used during pregnancy.

REFERENCES

Cenedella RJ. Cholesterol and cataracts. Surv Ophthalmol 1996;40:320–37.
FDA. FDA Talk paper. FDA home page Available from: URL: http://www.fda.gov/bbs/topics/ANSWERS/ANS00871.html. Accessed October 17, 2001.
Havel RJ. Dietary supplement or drug? The case of Cholestin. Am J Clin Nutr 1999a;69:175–6.
Havel R. Reply to D Heber [letter]. Am J Clin Nutr 1999b;70:107.
Heber D. Herbs and Atherosclerosis. Curr Atheroclerosis Rep 2001;3:93–6.
Heber D, Lembertas A, Lu QY, Bowerman S, Go VL. An analysis of nine proprietary Chinese red yeast rice dietary supplements: implications of variability in chemical profile and contents. J Altern Complement Med 2001;7:133–9.
Heber D, Yip I, Ashley JM, et al., Cholesterol-lowering effects of a proprietary Chinese red-yeast-rice dietary supplement. Am J Clin Nutr 1999;69:231–6.
Li C, Zhu Y, Wang Y, et al., *Monascus purpureus*-fermented rice (red yeast rice): a natural food product that lowers blood cholesterol in animal models of hypercholesterolemia. Nutr Res 1998;18:71–81.
Ma J, Li Y, Ye Q, et al., Constituents of red yeast rice, a traditional Chinese food and medicine. J Agric Food Chem 2000;48:5220–5.
Merck & Co. Mevacor® (lovastatin) package insert. Whitehouse Station, NJ, April, 2001.
Reeder G. Drug or dietary supplement? The Cholestin™ question. Natural Pharm 1998;2:1,18–20.
Wigger-Alberti W, Bauer A, Hipler UC, et al., Anaphylaxis due to *Monascus purpureus*-fermented rice (red yeast rice). Allergy 1999;54:1330–1.

Chapter 20

SAMe (S-adenosyl-L-methionine)

Michele Brula, Melanie Johns Cupp, and Timothy S. Tracy

20.1. HISTORY

Because of its instability, SAMe was not investigated as a therapeutic agent until the 1970s, when Stramentinoli and colleagues developed a stable *p*-toluene-sulfonate complex of SAMe-sulfate (Stramentinoli and Catto, 1976). This preparation was administered parenterally. Its antidepressant effects were first described in 1970 (DeVanna and Rigamoni, 1992). An enteric-coated oral formulation was then developed, but bioavailability was poor, necessitating dosing on the order of 1 g/d compared with several hundred mg/d with the parenteral formulation (Baldessarini, 1987). More stable formulations were subsequently developed (Franzese, 2001). SAMe did not appear on the shelves of retail outlets in the United States until February 1999 (Chamberlain, 2001).

20.2. CHEMICAL STRUCTURE

Refer to Fig. 20-1 for the chemical structure of S-adenosyl-L-methionine.

20.3. CURRENT PROMOTED USES

SAMe products are generally advertised to improve mood, promote emotional well-being, improve mobility, promote joint health, maintain cartilage, provide joint comfort, and enhance liver health.

20.4. SOURCES AND CHEMICAL COMPOSITION

SAMe is synthesized in vivo from methionine and ATP in a reaction catalyzed by the enzyme methionine adenosyltransferase. Dietary sources alone are inadequate to supply the amount of methionine necessary to produce SAMe; thus, additional methionine is synthesized in reactions in which vitamin B12 and folate are cofactors. Sufficient supplies of these vitamins are thus necessary for adequate SAMe production (Bottiglieri et al., 1994).

From: *Forensic Science: Dietary Supplements: Toxicology and Clinical Pharmacology*
Edited by: M. J. Cupp and T. S. Tracy © Humana Press Inc., Totowa, New Jersey

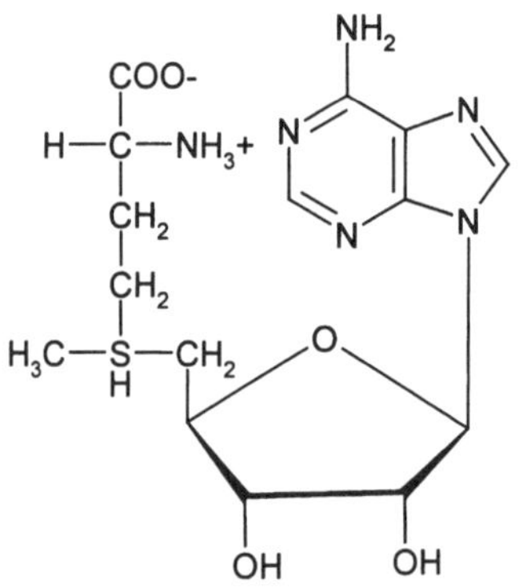

Fig. 1. Chemical structure of S-adenosylmethionine.

20.5. PRODUCTS AVAILABLE

The most stable form of SAMe is purportedly 1,4-butane-disulfone, or Actimet SAMe, manufactured by BASF Pharma in (Milan, Italy). Its shelf life is said to be 3 yr; a competing product, Tosylat SAMe, is allegedly more heat-labile, with a shelf-life of only 1 yr. SAMe products sold in the United States containing Actimet SAMe include Puritan's Pride, Vitamin Shoppe, GNC, and Nature Made brands. These products are available at Wal-Mart, CVS, Costco, and Internet outlets (Franzese, 2001). Most SAMe products sold in the United States are supplied as 200-mg tablets. The manufacturer's suggested dosing is often lower than doses shown to be effective in clinical studies for various indications.

Potency is obviously a problem with SAMe supplements. The Good Houskeeping Institute found that three of eight SAMe products tested contained less than the labeled amount of SAMe, with one product containing no SAMe. This problem has purportedly been corrected by the company, which now claims to use a more stable form of SAMe. Five products contained 10–86 mg in excess of the labeled amount (F-D-C Reports, 2000). Likewise, the independent laboratory ConsumerLab.com released their results of potency testing of 13 brands of SAMe commonly available through catalogs, retail stores, multilevel marketing companies, and on-line. Six products failed to meet ConsumerLab.com's standards, with several failing because they included the weight of inactive ingredients in the labeled amount of SAMe (ConsumerLab.com, 2002). A list of SAMe products that passed testing, as well as details about testing methodology, is available at the web site www.consumerlabs.com.

20.6. PHYSIOLOGIC ROLE

SAMe is a the main source of methyl groups for biochemical reactions including the synthesis and regulation of neurotransmitter production (Berlanga et al., 1992), and the synthesis of nucleic acids, phospholipids, and proteins (Bottiglieri et al., 1994). It may aid neurotransmission by increasing cell membrane fluidity, increasing the number of receptors, or facilitating binding of neurotransmitters to receptors (Bressa, 1994). SAMe is also involved in the production of glutathione (Mato et al., 1999). Although SAMe is found in every cell; its highest concentrations are in the brain and liver (Baldessarini, 1987).

20.7. In Vitro Effects and Animal Data

SAMe administration causes increases in serotonin, norepinephrine, and dopamine brain concentrations in rats. It also appears to inhibit neuronal reuptake of neurotransmitters via a mechanism that differs from that of conventional antidepressants. SAMe administration has been noted to increase as well as decrease monoamine oxidase (MAO) activity. In vivo and in vitro, SAMe administration increases the number of muscarinic cholinergic receptors and β-receptors in the brains of aged rats, perhaps by increasing phospholipid synthesis, thus increasing neuronal cell membrane fluidity. SAMe-enhanced receptor binding of γ-aminobutyric acid (GABA) and diazepam has been shown to be associated with increased methylation of cell membrane phospholipids (Bottiglieri et al., 1994).

20.8. Clinical Studies

The focus of this section will be studies in which oral SAMe was utilized.

20.8.1. Depression

Most of the controlled trials of SAMe have utilized the parenteral product, comparing it with oral or parenteral tricyclic antidepressants (Baldessarini, 1987; Bressa, 1994). SAMe has been found to be more effective than placebo and at least as effective as tricyclics, with a faster onset of action and a better side effect profile (Baldessarini, 1987; Bell et al., 1988; Bressa, 1994). Sample size is small in all studies (<100 patients).

Ten men and ten women, mean age 43.1 yr, with a DSM-III diagnosis of major depression and a Hamilton Depression (HAM-D) scale score of 18 or higher were enrolled in an uncontrolled, open study to assess the efficacy, safety, and pharmacologic effects of various dosages of SAMe in major depression (Rosenbaum et al., 1990). Nine of the subjects were characterized as having treatment-resistant depression, defined as having at least one prior 4-wk course of imipramine 150 mg or its equivalent without benefit. A 1-wk washout was followed by a 1-wk single-blind placebo run-in. Subjects then received SAMe (p-toluene-sulfonate salt, BioResearch, Milan, Italy) 200 mg twice daily. On day 3, the dose was increased to 1000 mg. By day 12, the dose had been increased to 1200 mg/d, and to 1600 mg by day 19. Efficacy and side effects were assessed weekly using the HAM-D, the Clinician's Global Impression (CGI) Severity Scale, and the Kupfer-Detre Scale for Side-Effect Scale. At the screening visit and at weeks 3 and 6, complete blood count, urinalysis, electrocardiogram (EKG), and routine blood chemistries were obtained. At the end of the placebo run-in and at week 6, the dexamethasone suppression test, the thyrotropin-releasing hormone test, and a test for platelet membrane fluidity were performed. Complete responders were defined as patients with a decrease in the CGI score by at least 2 points from baseline, a final CGI score of 1 or 2, and a 50% decrease in HAM-D. Six of the 11 of the patients without a history of treatment-resistant depression were complete responders, while only one patient with a history of treatment-resistant depression responded. Overall, HAM-D improved significantly compared with baseline ($p < 0.001$, paired t-test). Lack of placebo control and funding from the supplement manufacturer are the limitations of this study.

In a double-blind study, 18 consecutive male inpatients diagnosed with major depression per the DSM-III criteria were randomly assigned to SAMe (BioResearch, Milan, Italy) or placebo for 21 d (Kagan et al., 1990). All patients had HAM-D scores higher than 20. Patients were excluded if they were suicidal or bipolar, were substance abusers, or had psychotic symptoms. Biochemistry, urinalysis, complete blood count, thyroid function tests, ECG, and physical exam were performed to rule out serious medical disorders. In the first 5 patients, the dose of SAMe or identical placebo was gradually increased from 200 mg on day 1 to 800 mg twice daily on days 8–21. The remaining 13 patients were given 800 mg twice daily beginning on day 1. Fifteen patients completed the study. One dropout was a placebo-treated patient who required electroshock therapy, one was a placebo patient who was found to be hypothyroid, and one was a SAMe patient who was non-adherent. Depression was assessed using the HAM-D and the Carroll self-rating depression scale on days 0, 3, 7, 14, and 21. ANOVA with Tukey's test for multiple comparisons was used to analyze mean scores. At days 14 and 21, the mean HAM-D score was lower in the SAMe group than in the placebo group ($p < 0.05$). The HAM-D score was significantly lower than baseline in the placebo group on day 14, whereas the mean score in the SAMe group was significantly different from baseline by day 7 ($p < 0.01$). The Carroll score was lower in the SAMe group than the placebo group on day 21 ($p < 0.05$). Compared with baseline, the Carroll score was lower in the SAMe group by day 7 ($p < 0.05$).

A double-blind study was undertaken to assess the ability of SAMe to hasten the onset of action of imipramine (DeVanna and Rigamonti, 1992). Thirty subjects with major depression per the DSM-IIIR criteria with a HAM-D score or at least 18 were included. Exclusion criteria were suicidal ideation, psychosis, pregnancy or lactation, alcohol or drug abuse, and severe hepatic, renal, endocrine, cardiovascular, or neurologic disease. After a 7-d placebo run-in to identify placebo responders, defined as a 20% or greater improvement in the HAM-D, subjects were randomized to imipramine 140 mg/d or SAMe 1600 mg/d for 6 wk. The only concomitant medication allowed was triazolam 0.25 mg for sleep up to twice weekly. Prior to the placebo run-in, before starting the double-blind phase, and 10, 20, and 42 d after the start of the double-blind phase, patients were assessed using the Montgomery-Asberg Rating Scale for Depression (MADRS), HAM-D, Hamilton Rating Scale for Anxiety (HAM-A), and the Zung Self-Rating Scale for Depression. At baseline and at study completion, blood was drawn for determination of complete blood count, electrolytes, liver function tests, and renal function. Urinalysis was also performed. Chi-square, Fisher's exact test, ANOVA with Tukey's test, and Mann-Whitney's nonparametric test were used as appropriate to analyze data. Five patients in the imipramine group and three patients in the SAMe group dropped out owing to side effects. Statistical treatment of data from dropouts was not discussed. Patient demographics between the two groups were similar.

At day 10, the MADRS ($p < 0.001$), HAM-D ($p < 0.01$), and HAM-A ($p < 0.05$) scores were significantly better than baseline in the SAMe group, but in the imipramine group, only the HAM-D had improved ($p < 0.01$). On day 20, MADRS, HAM-D, and HAM-A were again better than baseline in the SAMe group, whereas the imipramine group showed improvement from baseline in both the MADRS and HAM-D ($p < 0.01$). On day 42, both groups showed a significant improvement from baseline in all efficacy measures ($p < 0.01$). Neither treatment affected any laboratory test or urinalysis. These results suggest that SAMe has a faster onset of action than imipramine. Blinding may have been a problem in this study owing to the anticholinergic effects of imipramine.

SAMe was compared with placebo in a double-blind study in 80 women who were 6–36 mo post natural or surgical menopause (Salmaggi et al., 1993). All women had been diagnosed with major depressive disorder or dysthymia according to the DSM-III-R criteria, had a HAM-D score of at least 17, and a Rome Depression Inventory (RDI) score of at least 40. After a 1-wk washout from their antidepressant, subjects underwent a single-blind placebo washout to rule out placebo responders. Eligible subjects were then randomized to SAMe (BioResearch, Milan, Italy) 1600 mg or placebo for 30 d. Efficacy was assessed using the HAM-D and RDI administered at baseline and at days 10 and 30. At the end of the study, the CGI-I was used to assess overall improvement. HAM-D and RDI decreased significantly in the treatment group both compared with placebo and compared with baseline beginning at day 10 ($p < 0.01$, ANOVA). The investigators concluded that additional study of the efficacy of SAMe in this population is needed, particularly in comparison with traditional antidepressants.

Bressa (1994) performed a metaanalysis of randomized, double-blind, controlled trials of oral or parenteral SAMe for treatment of patients with a diagnosis of depression based on DSM-III or DSM-III-R criteria. Only short-term studies (12 wk or less) in which the HAM-D was used to assess efficacy and that utilized a parenteral dose of SAMe of at least 200 mg/d or an oral dose of SAMe of at least 1600 mg/d were included. Of the studies described above, only the studies by DeVanna and Rigamonti (1992), Kagan and associates (1990), and Salmaggi and colleagues (1993) met the inclusion criteria. Full response was defined as an increase in the HAM-D by at least 50% from baseline. Patients with an increase of at least 25% were classified as partial to full responders. Five of six studies in which SAMe was compared with placebo showed a higher partial to full response rate, with 70% response in the SAMe group vs a 30% response in placebo-treated patients ($p < 0.00001$). Full response rate was 38% for SAMe and 22% for placebo ($p < 0.05$). Data from six studies of SAMe vs tricyclic antidepressants were analyzed. There was no difference in response between tricyclics and SAMe. The investigators comment on the significant heterogeneity of these studies and the high placebo response rate in one study of SAMe 1600 mg/d vs placebo, which might explain the slightly higher response rate with the parenteral SAMe vs oral SAMe. Based on the study results, the efficacy of SAMe compared with placebo is 17–38%, which is a larger effect size than in studies of tricyclic antidepressants. This difference might be explained by the recognizable side effects of tricyclics that compromise blinding.

20.8.2. Alzheimer's Disease

Bottiglieri and colleagues (1994) reviewed studies in which SAMe, both oral and parenteral, was used in various neurologic diseases. Two small ($n = 7$) studies, one uncontrolled, suggest that SAMe 400 mg orally three times daily for 3–5 mo may improve both mood and cognitive function in Alzheimer's patients. At least one author of the review was a coinvestigator in both studies. More study is needed.

20.8.3. Fibromyalgia

Orally administered SAMe was compared with placebo in patients with fibromyalgia (Jacobsen et al., 1991). Patients were selected at random from a patient database at the Department of Rheumatology at Hvidovre Hospital in Copenhagen. All patients had been referred for evaluation of chronic muscle pain. Patients were eligible for study inclusion if they had had aches, pain, and stiffness in three or more areas for at least 3 mo, at least four trigger points, and at least three of the following: change in symptoms with physical activity; change in symptoms by weather, stress, or anxiety; sleep disturbance; fatigue or tiredness; headaches; swelling or numbness; or irritable bowel. Patients who were allergic to SAMe or acetaminophen, patients with other illnesses that could be responsible for their symptoms, patients unable to cooperate with measurement of quadriceps strength, patients who were pregnant or lactating, and patients not using reliable contraception or who could be pregnant were excluded. Twenty-two patients were randomly assigned to each study group. This sample size was calculated to be adequate to provide 90% power to detect a difference between the treatments.

The SAMe product used was an enteric-coated tablet containing sulfo-adenosyl-L-methionine sulfate-p-toluensulfonate 768 mg, providing SAMe 400 mg. Subjects were instructed to take one tablet twice daily 1/2 h before meals. Outcome measures were pain at each of 14 trigger points rated on a scale of 0 to 3; quadriceps muscle strength; pain at rest, pain with movement, fatigue, sleep quality, and well-being on a 10-cm visual analog scale (VAS); duration of morning stiffness; and mood, assessed using the Beck Depression Inventory (BDI) and the Face Scale, consisting of 20 drawings depicting a range of moods from happy to sad. Patients were assessed at baseline and at weeks 3 and 6. Patients also rated disease activity as much better, better, no change, or worse compared with baseline at weeks 3 and 6. Analgesics, antiinflammatory agents, and antidepressants were not to be taken during the study, but there was no washout period prior to study. Physical therapy was also prohibited. Acetaminophen 500 mg every 4 h was permitted for pain, and acetaminophen use was documented by patients. Statistical significance was accepted at the 0.05 level. Dropouts were handled using intent-to-treat analysis.

Results were difficult to interpret owing to discrepancies between data reported in tabular form vs text. There was a significant difference in disease activity between groups at week 6 ($p = 0.04$; Mann-Whitney rank sum test). Although the text stated that morning stiffness decreased in the SAMe patients and increased in the placebo group ($p = 0.03$, significant interaction between time and treatment, repeated-measures MANOVA), examination of the data presented in tabular form revealed that median duration of stiffness appeared to increase in both groups over time, but that stiffness was less in the treatment group even at baseline. Pain at rest improved in the treatment group and worsened in the placebo group ($p = 0.002$, significant interaction between time and treatment, repeated-measures MANOVA). Fatigue improved significantly in the treatment group compared with the placebo group, with a p value of 0.04 (as reported in table) or 0.02 (as reported in text; interactions significant between time and treatment, repeated-measures MANOVA). Depression improved per the Face Scale ($p < 0.006$, interaction significant between time and treatment, repeated-measures MANOVA). Although the text stated that depression did not improve per the BDI, it appeared to improve significantly per the data presented in tabular form ($p = 0.04$, significant interaction between time and treatment repeated-measures MANOVA). Acetaminophen use was not different between the two groups. Although patients were discouraged from using other pain medications, three SAMe patients used narcotics, and two used nonprescription analgesics. Three placebo patients also required narcotics. Although SAMe appeared to improve subjective measurements, it did not improve objective measures, and use of rescue pain medications may have confounded the results.

The mechanism of SAMe's effect in fibromyalgia is unknown, but it may be related to its antidepressant or analgesic effect (Tavoni et al., 1987; Jacobsen et al., 1991). Although the results of these studies suggest that SAMe may be an effective treatment for some fibromyalgia symptoms, studies of longer duration with larger numbers of patients are necessary.

20.8.4. Osteoarthritis

Di Padova (1987), a clinical researcher for BioResearch, a SAMe manufacturer, reviewed 12 studies in which oral SAMe was studied in the treatment of osteoarthritis. Four of the studies were open-label, six compared SAMe with nonsteroidal antiinflammatory drugs (NSAIDs) [ibuprofen ($n = 4$), piroxicam, indomethacin], one compared SAMe with placebo, and one compared SAMe with both placebo and naproxen. Study duration ranged from 21 to 730 d, and dosages ranged from 400 mg/d to 400 mg three times per day. SAMe was superior to placebo and comparable to NSAIDs in improving subjective and objective outcome measures. Onset of action may be slower with SAMe than with NSAIDs, with the two treatments being similar in efficacy after 4, but not 2, wk of treatment. SAMe was well tolerated in these trials.

A subsequent randomized, double-blind, placebo-controlled study was performed to assess the effectiveness and onset of action of SAMe 400 mg/d for 5 d followed by 200 mg three times/d for 23 d (Bradley et al., 1994). Eighty-one patients 40–85 yr of age meeting the American College of Rheumatology diagnostic criteria for osteoarthritis were recruited at two university communities (study centers A and B). Exclusion criteria included fibromyalgia, bursitis, tendonitis, neurologic or vascular disease affecting the legs, inflammatory rheumatic disease, need for assistive devices for ambulation, BDI score grater than 18, and knee surgery, trauma, or corticosteroid injection within the preceding 3 mo. Patients meeting the inclusion/exclusion criteria were randomized only if they had at least mild pain on one of three pain scales and at least mild global knee arthritis activity after a 7-d washout. During the washout and the remainder of the study, only acetaminophen at a dose of up to 3900 mg/d was allowed for breakthrough pain. Outcome measures included patient and physician assessment of overall arthritis activity (inactive, mild, moderate, severe), BDI, Face Scale, range of motion, swelling, tenderness, time to walk 50 feet, analgesic use, duration of morning stiffness, and the disability and pain scales of the Stanford Health Assessment Questionnaire (HAQ) expanded to include VAS for pain at rest, pain on walking, and tolerable walking distance. Patients were also asked about any adverse effects.

Patients were assessed at baseline, at the end of the washout, after the second and fourth injections, and at days 9 and 23 of oral therapy. Pill counts were used to confirm adherence to the study protocol and to assess acetaminophen use after the washout, on the day of the fifth injection, and on days 9 and 23 of oral therapy. Complete blood cell count, liver function tests, urinalysis, serum creatinine, and testing for occult blood in the stool was performed at baseline, after the fifth parenteral injection, and at the end of oral therapy. Baseline characteristics were compared using t-tests and chi-square tests. Differences between placebo and SAMe in change from baseline in the various outcome measures were identified using repeated-measures ANOVA with the Bonferoni procedure for multiple comparisons. Paired t-tests were also used to compare each measurement with baseline. There were several differences in treatment groups at baseline. At study center A, duration of osteoarthritis symptoms in years was greater in the placebo group, and the time to walk 50 ft in seconds was greater in the treatment group at baseline ($p = 0.05$, t-test). At study center B, the mean HAQ disability score, walking pain, and time to walk 50 ft were greater in the SAMe group than in the placebo group ($p = 0.006$, $p = 0.019$, and $p = 0.05$, respectively; t-test). Patient-estimated tolerable walking distance was less in the SAMe group ($p = 0.015$; t-test). Differences also existed between study populations at the two centers. Patients at study center A were mostly women with mild osteoarthritis, whereas the subjects from study center B were mainly men with moderate to severe disease. Because the study populations at the two study centers were different in disease severity and baseline characteristics, the data were reported separately for each study center. Compliance was more than 95% in both groups.

At study center A, SAMe significantly improved HAQ pain score, knee pain at rest, and walking pain compared with placebo after 9 d of oral treatment, but only rest pain remained significantly different at day 23 ($p < 0.05$). At site B, patient's estimate of tolerable walking distance significantly improved in the SAMe group ($p = 0.05$). When the data from the two centers were combined, there were no differenes in outcome between treatment groups. These results suggest that SAMe may improve symptoms in patients with mild osteoarthritis, but not more severe disease. Another possible reason for these results is limited power to detect significant differences resulting from analysis of data from the two centers separately.

20.8.5. Liver Disease

Based on studies showing that SAMe administration can increase liver glutathione stores in patients with liver disease, 123 subjects with alcoholic liver disease were randomized to AdoMet® (Knoll Farmaceutici, Liscate MI, Spain) 400 mg or three times daily for 2 yr to determine the effect of SAMe on mortality and need for liver transplantation (Mato et al., 1999). Eight of the patients enrolled were in Child class C. When these patients with more severe disease were excluded from the analysis, the percentage of patients in the SAMe group who died or needed a liver transplant was lower than in the placebo group ($p = 0.025$, chi-square test). Time to death or liver transplant was also longer in the SAMe group, but again, only when patients with more severe disease were excluded ($p = 0.046$, log rank test). Statistical significance held even when the two patients in the placebo group who died of causes unrelated to liver disease were excluded ($p = 0.05$).

The results of a small uncontrolled study (Frezza et al., 1988) suggest that oral SAMe 800 mg/d might protect against estrogen-induced cholestasis, such as that seen in pregnancy or as a result of oral contraceptive use. However, more study is needed to assess its usefulness in this regard.

20.9. PHARMACOKINETICS

Stramentinoli and Catto (1976) first described the pharmacokinetics following intravenous and intramuscular administration of SAMe in humans. SAMe was rapidly eliminated from the bloodstream with a half-life of 80 min. Upon intramuscular administration, the bioavailability was estimated to be 80–90% and absorption was complete within 1–2 h. In a more complete study, these same investigators (Guilidori et al., 1984) examined the pharmacokinetics of intravenously administered SAMe following either a 100-mg or 500-mg dose to six healthy volunteers. Data were best described by a two-compartment model. Following the 100-mg dose, the volume of distribution was estimated to be 407 ± 27 mL/kg and the terminal half-life 81 ± 8 min. After the 500-mg dose, the volume of distribution and half-life estimates were comparable to those seen after 100 mg of SAMe, 443 ± 36 mL/kg and 101 ± 7 min, respectively. At either dosing level, the percentage of the dose excreted in the urine was between 34 and 40%. These investigators also reported that binding to plasma proteins was negligible. Thus, it appears that iv administered SAMe is both metabolized and excreted unchanged and probably distributes to tissues beyond the plasma space, as evidenced by the estimated volume of distribution.

These same investigators later studied the pharmacokinetics of SAMe after oral administration of an enteric-coated tablet (Stramentinoli, 1987). Subjects were given one of two formulations of a 200-mg enteric coated tablet containing [methyl-^{14}C]SAMe. Approximately 16% of the radioactivity was excreted in the urine in 48 h, whereas approx 24% of the radioactivity was measured in the feces over a 72-h collection interval. These investigators speculate from these findings that approximately 60% of the dose is incorporated into stable endogenous sulfur pools. In a separate experiment, 50 mg of SAMe ([methyl-^{14}C]SAMe) was given either orally or intravenously and plasma concentrations measured over 48 h. Peak plasma radioactivity concentrations were achieved between 8 and 24 h. Furthermore, plasma radioactivity was higher after oral dosing, which the author speculated was owing to metabolism, causing it to be incorporated into the endogenous pools more completely.

20.10. ADVERSE EFFECTS

In an open study (Carney et al., 1989) of both oral and intravenous SAMe, 9 of 11 bipolar subjects switched from depression to hypomania, mania, or euphoria. Two of the nine patients received two courses each of SAMe. These two patients switched each time they received SAMe, for a total of 11 switches. One of the 11 switches occurred immediately, 9 occurred after a mean of 3.5 d (range a few hours to 6 d), and one occurred on day 42 of oral SAMe. Based on the 6-mo switch rate reported in the literature, the probabililty that the switches that occurred within 6 d of starting SAMe happened because of chance alone was small ($p < 0.001$, Poisson). SAMe was the most likely cause based on temporal association. None of the 14 unipolar patients in the study switched. The difference in the incidence of switching was significant between bipolar and unipolar patients ($p < 0.001$, Fisher's exact test). The patients who switched tended to be younger and tended to have higher Newcastle Diagnostic Scale scores. Bipolar patients who did not switch had a higher number of previous affective episodes and higher scores on the HAM-D and BDI. There was no difference between oral and intravenous SAMe administration in regard to switching. With oral dosing, switching occurred only at doses greater than 800 mg (as did clinical response).

Elevated mood associated with SAMe administraion is not isolated to patients with bipolar disorder. Hypomania was reported in 1 of 20 patients taking SAMe 1600 mg/d in a study of patients with major depression. He reported a 5-d episode of hyperactivity, including bursts of energy resulting in a need to talk or dance, as well as decreased sleep requirement (Rosenbaum et al., 1990). Kagan and collegues (1990) and DeVanna and Rigamonti (1992) also noted mania in one patient each in their studies of major depression.

Less serious, albeit bothersome, side effects, particularly gastrointestinal disturbances, have been reported in several studies of oral SAMe. Jacobsen and colleagues (1991) reported adverse gastrointestinal effects in 7 of 22 patients treated with SAMe 800 mg/d, leading to withdrawal from the study of 3 patients. For comparison, only three patients in the placebo group experienced gastrointestinal effects. Another patient withdrew owing to dizziness. Routine biochemical testing and urinalysis were normal. Similarly, DeVanna and Rigmonti (1992) reported nausea and vomiting in 6 of 15 patients treated with SAMe 1600 mg/d, prompting 3 patients to discontinue treatment. One patient reported dry mouth. In another study (Kagan et al., 1990), a patient receiving oral SAMe complained of arm soreness, hot and itching ear, and a crawling sensation in the skin. Another patient reported headache. These side effects resolved spontaneously and could not be definitely attributed to SAMe. Mild adverse effects including nausea, bloating, dyspepsia, dizziness, drowsiness, and headache were among the adverse effects associated with SAMe 600 mg/d (Bradley et al., 1994). In a study of patients with alcoholic liver disease, 3 of 57 patients in the SAMe group and 1 of 58 in the placebo group dropped out because of nausea, and 2 patients receiving SAMe experienced heartburn severe enough to prompt them to discontinue therapy (Mato et al., 1999). SAMe's propensity to cause nausea and vomiting have been attributed to its being an acid (DeVanna and Rigamonti, 1992).

Because SAMe is involved in homocysteine metabolism, it has been suggested that it might exacerbate elevated homocysteine levels in susceptible individuals (Fetrow and Avila, 2001). Such patients include those with deficiencies of vitamin B12, folic acid, or pyridoxine (vitamin B6), co-factors necessary for the metabolism of homocysteine via various pathways, and those with a genetic absence of cystathionine β-synthase or inherited defects in the remethylation pathways. Hyperhomocysteinemia is undesirable because it causes thrombosis and atherosclerosis, putting the patient at risk for cardiovascular events (Schafer, 2000).

20.11. INTERACTIONS

A 71-yr-old woman had been receiving SAMe 100 mg/d IM plus clomipramine 25 mg/d without incident. Within 72 h after an increase in the clomipramine dose to

75 mg/d, the patient experienced anxiety, agitation, and confusion. On admission she was stuporous and verbally unresponsive. Other findings included diarrhea, myoclonus, tremors, rigidity, hyperreflexia, shivering, sweating, and dehydration. Heart rate was 130 beats per min, respiratory rate was 30 breaths per minute, and temperature was 40.5°C, which later increased to 43°C. Labs included a white blood cell count of 13,040/mm^3, lactate dehydrogenase 662 U/L, creatine kinase (CK) 8920 U/L, potassium 2.7 mEq/L, and hyperosmolarity. After ruling out other etiologies, the patient was diagnosed with serotonin syndrome. The patient was rehydrated, and rigidity responded to treatment with dantrolene 50 mg intravenously every 6 h for 48 h. The level of consciousness did not improve for more than 2 d. Complete recovery, including normalization of CK, took approximately 15 d. The authors attributed serotonin syndrome in this patient to a synergistic action of clomipramine and SAMe on central nervous system serotonin levels (Iruela et al., 1993).

20.12. REPRODUCTION

Eighteen women were randomized to SAMe (p-toluene-sulfonate salt; BioResearch, Milan, Italy) 200 mg, SAMe 800 mg, or saline placebo intravenously each day for 20 days for treatment of cholestasis of pregnancy (Frezza et al., 1984). All subjects were between 28 and 32 wk gestation when treatment was initiated. All newborns had Apgar scores of 7–10 at 5 min. No adverse outcomes were reported. Similarly, in a subsequent study of intravenous SAMe 900 mg or placebo for 20 d in 18 women with cholestasis of pregnancy, all newborns had Apgar scores greater than 7 and normal postnatal development (Ribalta et al., 1991).

20.13. CHEMICAL AND BIOFLUID ANALYSIS

A number of methods have been developed for the detection of SAMe in various biologic fluids using techniques such as liquid chromatography with ultraviolet detection (Delabar et al., 1999), capillary zone electrophoresis (Panak et al., 1997), and liquid chromatography with detection of fluorescent derivatives (Capdevila and Wagner, 1998). One difficulty in measuring SAMe concentrations in plasma is the relatively low concentrations observed under physiologic conditions (obviously, they would be higher if SAMe was administered exogenously).

Capdevila and Wagner (1998) have developed a method involving the measurement of SAMe as its fluorescent isoindole derivative that is sensitive enough to measure SAMe concentrations under physiologic conditions as well as following administration of exogenous compound. To 0.5 mL of plasma is added 50 μL of 100% trichloroacetic acid to precipitate the proteins. The samples are then centrifuged at 13,000g for 8 min (5°C) and the supernate removed. The trichloroacetic acid is then removed by addition of 0.55 mL freon-trioctylamine (This mixture is made by adding 180 μL of 0.5 *M* trioctylamine to 820 μL of freon kept on ice.) The resulting upper layer is then introduced onto a C-8 (25 × 0.4 cm) column previously equilibrated with 50 m*M* NaH$_2$PO$_4$/10 m*M* heptane sulfonic acid (pH 3.2), containing 4% acetonitrile. Elution is accomplished with a linear gradient from 4 to 20% acetonitrile over 15 min. SAMe elutes at 11 min, and a fraction is collected around this retention time. The fraction is desalted by dilution with 4 volumes of water and absorption onto a 1 mL HLB extraction cartridge. The extraction cartridge (prior to introduction of the sample) is treated with methanol and then equilibrated with 10 mM NaH$_2$PO$_4$/2 mM heptane sulfonic acid, pH 3.2, containing 3% acetonitrile.

After sample introduction, the extraction cartridge is washed with water (1 mL), and the sample is eluted with 50% acetonitrile/10 mM formic acid (1 mL). The samples are then evaporated to dryness and redissolved in water (50 µL) just prior to derivatization. Samples are derivatized by the addition of 30 µL of sodium borate (0.4 M, pH 9.0), 4 µL of 5 mM sodium cyanide in sodium borate (pH 9.0) and 10–25 mL of the sample. Four mL of 5 mM naphthalene dialdehyde in 50% methanol is then added to start the reaction. The samples are allowed to incubate at room temperature for 10 minutes and then injected onto the liquid chromatography column. The analytes are separated with a Hi-Chrom ODS II C18 column through which the mobile phase is pumped. Mobile phase A consists of 15% acetonitrile in 50 mM potassium phosphate (pH 7.0), and mobile phase B consists of 40% acetonitrile in 50 mM potassium phosphate (pH 7.0). A linear gradient of 0–50% B is run over 2 min and held at 50% B until SAMe is eluted at approx 7 min. The samples are detected with a fluorescence detector set to an excitation wavelength of 400 nm and an emission wavelength of 490 nm. The limit of detection for SAMe is less than 50 nM.

Delabar and colleagues (1999) also report a liquid chromatography method for determining SAMe concentrations, although the method has only been applied to urine samples. This method utilizes ultraviolet detection following separation by ion pair chromatography and a gradient elution system. The method has a sensitivity to 250 nM and does not require derivatization of the samples.

20.14. REGULATORY STATUS

SAMe is marketed as a dietary supplement in the United States but is a prescription medication for depression, arthritis, and cholestasis in Italy, Spain, Germany, and other countries (Anonymous, 1999).

20.15. SUMMARY

- In small studies, SAMe administration has been demonstrated to be superior to placebo and at least as effective as tricyclic antidepressants in the treatment of depression. Its efficacy in fibromyalgia appears to be limited only to symptoms that can be measured subjectively, such as pain and mood. It also appears to be effective in mild osteoarthritis, alcoholic liver disease, and estrogen-associated cholestasis. Its efficacy in improving cognitive function in Alzheimer's disease is equivocal.
- SAMe has been given to pregnant women for the treatment of cholestasis of pregnancy, and no adverse events were noted.
  Adverse effects include mood elevation, gastrointestinal side effects, and dizziness.

REFERENCES

Anonymous. SAMe for depression. Med Lett Drugs Ther 1999;41:107–8.
Baldessarini RJ. Neuropharmacology of S-adenosyl-L-methionine. Am J Med 1987;83(suppl 5A):95–103.

Bell KM, Plon L, Bunney WE, Potkin SG. S-adenosylmethionine treatment of depression: a controlled clinical trial. Am J Psychiatry 1988;145:1110–4.

Berlanga C, Ortega-Soto HA, Ontiveros M, Senties H. Efficacy of S-adenosyl-L-methionine in speeding onset of action of imipramine. Psychiatry Res 1992;44:257–62.

Bottiglieri T, Hyland K, Reynolds EH. The clinical potential of ademetionine (S-adenosylmethionine) in neurological disorders. Drugs 1994;48:137–52.

Bradley JD, Flusser D, Katz BP, et al. A randomized, double blind, placebo controlled trial of intravenous loading with S-adenosylmethionine (SAM) followed by oral SAM therapy in patients with knee osteoarthritis. J Rhemumatol 1994;21:905–11.

Bressa GM. S-adenosyl-methionine (SAMe) as antidepressant: meta-analysis of clinical studies. Acta Neurol 1994;154:7–14.

Capdevila A, Wagner C. Measurement of plasma S-adenosylmethionine and S-adenosylhomocysteine as their fluorescent isoindoles. Anal Biochem 1998;264:180–4.

Carney MWP, Chary TKN, Bottiglieri T, Reynolds EH. The switch mechanism and the bipolar/unipolar dichotomy. Br J Psychiatry 1989;154:48–51.

Chamberlain C. Happy to meet 'Sammy.' Available from: URL: http://more.abcnews.go.com/sections/living/inyourhead/allinyourhead_36.html. Accessed July 31, 2001.

ConsumerLab.com. Product review: SAMe. Available from: URL: http://www.consumerlabs.com/results/same/asp. Accessed January 25, 2002.

Delabar U, Kloor D, Luippold G, Muhlbauer B. Simultaneous determination of adenosine, S-adenosylhomocysteine and S-adenosylmethionine in biological samples using solid-phase extraction and high-performance liquid chromatography. J Chromatogr B Biomed Sci Appl 1999;724:231–8.

DeVanna M, Rigamonti R. Oral S-adenosyl-L-methionine in depression. Curr Ther Res 1992;52:478–85.

Di Padova C. S-adenosylmethionine in the treatment of osteoarthritis. Review of the clinical studies. Am J Med 1987;83(suppl 5A):60–5.

F-D-C Reports. SAM-e labeling tests. The Tan Sheet. February 21, 2000.

Fetrow CW, Avila JR. Efficacy of the dietary supplement S-adenosyl-L-methionine. Ann Pharmacother 2001;135:1414–25.

Franzese TA. The facts on the nutritional supplement SAM-e. Available from:URL: http://content.health.msn.com/content/article/1700.50735. Accessed July 31, 2001.

Frezza M, Pozzato G, Chiesa L, et al. Reversal of intrahepatic cholestatis of pregnancy in women after high dose S-adenosyl-L-methionine administration. Hepatology 1984;4:274–8.

Frezza M, Tritapepe R, Pozzato G, Di Padova C. Prevention by S-adenosylmethionine of estrogen-induced hepatobiliary toxicity in women. Am J Gastoenterol 1988;83:1098–102.

Guilidori P, Cortellaro M, Moreo G, Stramentinoli G. Pharmacokinetics of S-adenosyl-L-methionine in healthy volunteers. Eur J Clin Pharmacol 1984;27:119–21.

Iruela LM, Minguez L, Merino J, Monedero G. Toxic interaction of S-adenosylmethinine and clomipramine [letter]. Am J Psychiatry 1993;150:522.

Jacobsen S, Danneskiold-Samsoe B, Andersen RB. Oral S-adenosylmethionine in primary fibromyalgia. Double-blind clinical evaluation. Scand J Rheumatol 1991;20:294–302.

Kagan BL, Sultzer DL, Rosenlicht N, Gerner RH. Oral S-adenosylmethionine in depression: a randomized, double-blind, placebo-controlled trial. Am J Psychiatry 1990;147:591–5.

Mato JM, Camara J, de Paz JF, et al. S-adenosylmethionine in alcoholic liver cirrhosis: a randomized, placebo-controlled, double-blind, multicenter clinical trial. J Hepatol 1999;30:1081–9.

Panak KC, Giorgieri SA, Diaz LE, Ruiz OA. Simultaneous determination of S-adenosylmethionine and S-adenosylhomocysteine by capillary zone electrophoresis. Electrophoresis 1997;18:2047–9.

Ribalta J, Reyes H, Gonzalez MC, et al. S-adenosyl-L-methionine in the treatment of patients with intrahepatic cholestasis of pregnancy: a randomized, double-blind, placebo-controlled study with negative results. Hepatology 1991;13:1084–9.

Rosenbaum JF, Fava M, Falk WE, et al. The antidepressant potential of oral S-adenosyl-l-methionine. Acta Psychiatr Scand 1990;81:432–6.

Salmaggi P, Bressa GM, Nicchia G, et al. Double-blind, placebo-controlled study of S-adenosyl-L-methionine in depressed postmenopausal women. Psychother Psychosom 1993;59:34–40.

Schafer AI. Thrombotic disorders: hypercoagulable states. In: Goldman L, Bennett JC, eds. Cecil textbook of medicine, 21st ed. Philadelphia: WB Saunders, 2000. p. 1016–21.

Stramentinoli G, Catto E. Pharmacokinetic studies of S-adenosyl-L-methionine (SAMe) in several animal species. Pharmacol Res Commun 1976;8:211–8.

Stramentinoli G. Pharmacologic aspects of S-adenosylmethionine: pharmacokinetics and pharmacodynamics. Am J Med 1987;83(suppl 5A):35–42.

Tavoni A, Vitali C, Bombardieri S, Pasero G. Evaluation of S-adenosylmethionine in primary fibromyalgia. Am J Med 1987;83(suppl 5A):107–10.

Chapter 21

Shark Cartilage

Kerri J. Pettrey, Melanie Johns Cupp, and Timothy S. Tracy

21.1. HISTORY

Hammerhead sharks of the Sphyridae family have inhabited oceans for over 300 million years (Pettit and Ode, 1977), and the Chinese have been consuming shark cartilage in the form of shark fin soup for hundreds of years (Lane and Comac, 1991). Shark cartilage has been used medicinally since the 1950s for treatment of many conditions, including the pain and swelling associated with osteoarthritis and rheumatoid arthritis, and for arthritis prevention (Miller et al., 1998). Squalene, which is isolated from shark stomachs, has been used in skin therapy, wrinkle prevention, and scar healing. It is also believed to have antibiotic activity against protozoa, fungi, and gram-positive and gram-negative bacteria (Marshall, 1996).

21.2. CHEMICAL STRUCTURE

See Fig. 21-1 for the chemical structure of shark cartilage components.

21.3. CURRENT PROMOTED USES

Angiogenesis, "the formation of new capillary blood vessels from pre-existing ones" (Berbari et al., 1999), is required for solid tumors to grow. Inhibition of angiogenesis may either decrease the size or totally eliminate the tumor. Since cartilage is avascular tissue, and because the shark endoskeleton is composed almost entirely of cartilage, it is believed to be a potent angiogenesis inhibitor and therefore a potential agent in the treatment of cancer (Lee and Langer, 1983).

21.4. SOURCES AND CHEMICAL COMPOSITION

Shark cartilage is "obtained from freshly caught sharks, and then cleaned, shredded, and dried. It is ground to a fine powder, sterilized, and encapsulated" (Marshall,

From: *Forensic Science: Dietary Supplements: Toxicology and Clinical Pharmacology*
Edited by: M. J. Cupp and T. S. Tracy © Humana Press Inc., Totowa, New Jersey

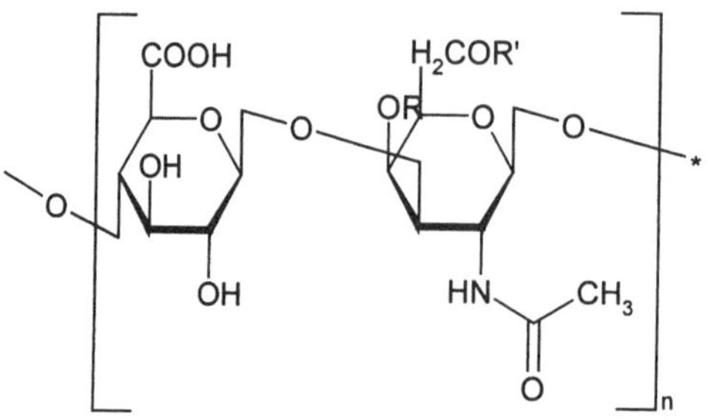

Fig. 1. Chemical structure of shark cartilage components: chondroitin sulfate, with R = H or SO₃H and R′ = H or SO₃H.

1996). Chondroitin sulfates are the primary constituents of shark cartilage (Cockin et al., 1986). According to one distributor, dry shark cartilage is approx 41% ash, 39% protein, 12% carbohydrates, 7% water, less than 1% fiber, and less than 0.3% fat. The ash is 60% calcium and phosphorus (Real Life, 2000).

21.5. PRODUCTS AVAILABLE

Cartilade®, a 100% pure shark cartilage product, has been manufactured and sold for the past 7 yr by BioTherapies. It is "the first shark cartilage product ever sold with consistent proprietary manufacturing and is the world's leading brand of shark cartilage" (Real Life, 2000). There is a patent pending for Cartilage LED, which is under development by BioTherapies. Cartilage LED is a liquid shark extract currently available as a dietary supplement (Real Life, 2000).

Benefin® is a brand of shark cartilage manufactured by Lane Labs, it is available as a dietary supplement. BeneJoint® is also manufactured by Lane Labs and is a topical analgesic made with shark cartilage and capsaicin (Havlick, 1999).

21.6. IN VITRO EFFECTS AND ANIMAL STUDIES

The use of shark cartilage as an antineoplastic agent is based on its antiangiogenic effects. One study evaluated the antiangiogenic activity of shark cartilage, tumor necrosis factor-α (TNF-α), and a combination of the two using a human umbilical vein endothelial cell proliferation assay. Although shark cartilage does not seem to be directly cytotoxic to tumor cells, use of TNF-α is limited because of severe toxicity with systemic administration; thus the two were tested in combination because of possible synergic effects related to different mechanisms of action. The study showed that shark cartilage had no effect on astrocytoma or fibroblast cell cultures. At a concentration of 500 µg/mL, shark cartilage reduced endothelial cell proliferation by 32%; TNF-α, at a concentration of 10 ng/mL, reduced endothelial cell proliferation by 29%. The combination of shark cartilage and TNF-α reduced endothelial cell proliferation by 44%. These results suggest that the antiangiogenic effect of shark cartilage is specific for endothelial cells. It is believed that specific compounds of shark cartilage directly inhibit endothelial cell proliferation, but the active ingredient(s) have yet to be identified (McGuire et al., 1996).

Other investigators tested the effects of shark cartilage on the efficacy of boron neutron capture therapy (BNCT). It is believed that some angiogenesis inhibitors can enhance the effectiveness of chemotherapy and radiation therapy by "increasing the permeability of tumor vasculature and reducing hypoxia" (Morris et al., 2000). BNCT depends on the tumor vasculature for delivery of boron-targeting agents, and thus its effects could be enhanced by shark cartilage. The tumor model used in this study was the rat 9L gliosarcoma, which was implanted intracerebrally. Shark cartilage was administered orally as an aqueous suspension at a daily dose of approx 2000 mg/kg of body weight. Of the rats receiving no treatment, the mean survival time was 20.7 ± 0.5 d post intracranial tumor implantation. Administration of shark cartilage alone extended survival times, and two of the rats were healthy and fully active at the end of the evaluation period (43 d post implantation). The rats that received BNCT (with or without shark cartilage) had an increased survival time approximately twice that of controls. Approximately 20% of the rats were healthy 1 yr after BNCT. The authors' conclusions were that shark cartilage, when given alone, increased the survival time of tumor-bearing rats, presumably because of its antiangiogenic effects but that BNCT's effects were not enhanced by shark cartilage administration (Morris et al., 2000).

21.7. CLINICAL STUDIES

A prospective, randomized controlled, double blind trial was performed in 29 healthy male subjects to study the antiangiogenic effects of the oral administration of liquid shark cartilage extract in humans. The subjects were randomized to receive liquid shark extract (LCE) 7 mL ($n = 10$), LCE 21 mL ($n = 10$), or placebo (7 mL of water) for 23 days. To measure angiogenesis, a polyvinyl alcohol sponge threaded in perforated silicone tubing was inserted subcutaneously on the anterior side of the arm on day 12. No toxicity or side effects related to LCE were reported, and no differences were reported between the three groups in blood chemistry, urine analysis, and bleeding times (data not shown). There was a significant reduction of endothelial cell density in the groups receiving the LCE compared with the placebo group ($p < 0.01$). There was no significant difference between the two LCE dosages ($p > 0.1$). According to the authors, the results demonstrate that LCE contains an antiangiogenic component that is orally absorbed in humans, but they did not identify a dose-response relationship (Berbari et al., 1999).

Miller and colleagues (1998) published an uncontrolled phase I/II trial designed to determine the safety and efficacy of shark cartilage in the treatment of advanced cancer. Only patients whose disease was resistant to conventional treatment, patients who had not recently undergone chemotherapy, patients with a life expectancy was at least 12 weeks, and patients with an Eastern Cooperative Oncology Group (ECOG) performance status of 0–2 were included. Sixty adult patients were enrolled. The patients had stage III or IV cancers, including lung cancer ($n = 16$), breast cancer ($n = 16$), colorectal cancer ($n = 16$), prostate cancer ($n = 8$), brain neoplasm ($n = 1$), non-Hodgkin's lymphoma ($n = 3$), and unknown primary ($n = 2$). Ninety-seven percent (58) of the patients had stage IV cancer. Patients took shark cartilage 1 g/kg/day in three divided doses for 12 wk. Patients were evaluated at weeks 6 and 12. The dose was increased to 1.3 g/d if there was no response after 6 wk.

A complete response was defined as the complete disappearance of lesions and normalization of all cancer-related clinical and laboratory signs and symptoms. A partial response was defined as no new lesions with a 50% or greater decrease in the diameter(s) of the sentinel lesion(s). Stable disease was defined as no new lesions and a 25% or less increase in the cross-sectional area of any lesion. Progressive disease was the appearance of new lesions and/or an increase in the cross-sectional area of any lesion by more than 25%. Ten patients were lost to follow-up or refused further therapy before 6 wk of treatment. Three patients with stable disease at 6 wk were lost to follow-up or refused thereapy thereafter. Progressive disease had occurred in five patients by week 12. Five patients died of progressive disease during the study, and no complete remissions or partial remissions were reported. Median time to tumor progression was 7 ± 9.7 wk. Twenty percent of the 50 evaluable patients had stable disease for 12 wk or more. Of these 10 patients, median time to disease progression was 28.8 wk. Shark cartilage also provided no effect on quality of life, as measured using the Functional Assessment of Cancer Therapy-General (FACT-G) scale. It should be noted that this was not a placebo-controlled trial, no historical controls were used, and various cancer types were included.

AE 941-Neovastat® is a liquid shark cartilage extract being developed by AEterna Laboratories in Canada for the treatment of cancer. This product has been studied in phase I/II studies in more than 450 patients with lung and prostate cancer (Anonymous, 1999a). National Cancer Institute (NCI)-sponsored phase III clinical trials of this product, in combination with platinum-based chemotherapy and radiotherapy in stage III non-small cell lung cancer (NSCLC), and in comparison with placebo in metastatic kidney cancer, are under way. Benefin is also being used in an NCI-sponsored study as an adjunct to standard therapy in patients with advanced colorectal or breast cancer (NCI, 2002).

21.8. PHARMACOKINETICS

See Chapter 12, Glucosamine and Chondroitin, for the pharmacokinetics of chondroitin sulfate, the primary constituent of shark cartilage.

21.9. ADVERSE EFFECTS AND TOXICITY

In the study conducted by Miller and colleagues (1998), shark cartilage was not associated with any laboratory test abnormality or hepatitis. Toxicity was graded on a scale of 1 to 3, with 1 being generally mild. There were six episodes of grade 3 toxicities reported (two reports of nausea, one report of hyperglycemia, one report of decreased motor strength, one report of decreased sensation, and one report of decreased performance).

A 57-yr-old man presented with a 3-wk history of nausea, vomiting, diarrhea, and anorexia after taking shark cartilage for 10 wk (no dose or indication given). The patient was not known to be taking prescription medications. The patient had a history of cigarette smoking [one pack per day (number of years not given)], and denied any alcohol, drug use, or blood transfusions. He stopped taking the shark cartilage a few days before his symptoms began because he noticed a change in the odor of the supplements. The patient's physical exam revealed low-grade fever and jaundiced skin. Notable laboratory values included an aspartate aminotransferase level of 319 U/L (normal, 0–45 U/L), an alanine aminotransferase level of 404 U/L (normal, 3–36 U/L), an alkaline phosphatase level of 430 U/L (normal, 30–125 U/L), a total bilirubin level of 12.9 mg/dL, and a direct bilirubin level of 6.8 mg/dL. The patient was discharged with a diagnosis of drug-induced hepatitis (Ashar and Vargo, 1996).

21.10. INTERACTIONS

It has been theorized that concomitant use of shark cartilage preparations with calcium supplements could lead to hypercalcemia (Miller et al., 1998). Caution should be exercised when these two preparations are taken together. The potency of shark cartilage preparations may be reduced over time if they are mixed with acidic fruit juices (Lane and Comac, 1992). It is recommended that if shark cartilage is to be mixed with fruit juice, the preparation be made immediately prior to use.

21.11. REPRODUCTION

Because shark cartilage inhibits angiogenesis in vitro, it has been suggested that pregnant women should not take shark cartilage (Anonymous, 1999b).

21.12. CHEMICAL AND BIOFLUID ANALYSIS

Chondroitin sulfates are thought to be the primary constituents of shark cartilage, although a number of glycosaminoglycans are thought to be present, and keratan sulfates have been identified (Cockin et al., 1986). The methods of Volpi (2000) described in Chapter 12 are adequate to measure the chondroitin sulfates. An alternate method has been developed by Kinoshita and Sugahara (1999) for identifying and quantifying several of the chondroitin sulfates, as well as heparin/heparin sulfate disaccharides. The method uses enzymatic digestion of the glycosaminoglycans, derivatization and subsequent high-performance liquid chromatography (HPLC) separation with fluorescence detection. Cartilage is first digested with hyaluronidase and then, to digest the chondroitin sulfate-derived oligosaccharides, 5 mIU of chondroitinase AC-II is added to the sample in 50 mM sodium acetate, pH 6. The samples are incubated at 37°C for 50 min, and then the reaction is terminated by immersing the sample tubes in boiling water for 1 min. Derivatization is accomplished by adding 5 μL of the derivatization reagent mixture [0.35 M 2-aminobenzamide/1.0 M NaCNBH$_4$ / 30% (v/v) acetic acid in dimethyl sulfoxide] to each sample and allowing it to incubate for 2 h at 65°C. The derivatized mixture is then separated by paper chromatography (Whatman 3MM paper) with a solvent system of butanol/ethanol/water (4:1:1, v/v). Chromatographic separation via HPLC is accomplished using a PA03 column (4.6 × 250 mm) through which the mobile phase is pumped at a rate of 1 mL/min. The mobile phase consists of NaH$_2$PO$_4$, and analytes are monitored with fluorescence detection set at an excitation wavelength of 330 nm and an emission wavelength of 420 nm.

21.13. REGULATORY STATUS

Shark cartilage is currently available as a dietary supplement in the United States (Anonymous, 1999b).

21.14. SUMMARY

- Shark cartilage has been shown to inhibit angiogenesis in vitro and in rats and thus is promoted for use in the treatment of cancer. In a human, experimental in vivo model of angiongenesis, shark cartilage did appear to exhibit an antiangiogenic effect.
- Human clinical trials to date have not demonstrated a positive effect of shark cartilage in patients with cancer. Additional trials are under way to study potential efficacy.
- Adverse effects of shark cartilage therapy are generally mild and usually involve gastrointestinal symptoms. A case of hepatitis has been reported.
- Shark cartilage is regulated as a dietary supplement.

REFERENCES

Anonymous. AE 941—Neovastat. Drugs R D 1999a;1:135–6.

Anonymous. Shark cartilage costly last resort for cancer patients. Alt Med Alert 1999b;2:24.

Ashar B, Vargo E. Shark cartilage-induced hepatitis. Ann Intern Med 1996;125:780–1.

Berbari P, Thibodeau A, Germain L, et al. Anti-angiogenic effects of the oral administration of liquid shark cartilage extract in humans. J Surg Res 1999;87:108–13.

Cockin GH, Huckerby TN, Nieduszynski IA. High-field N.M.R. studies of keratan sulphates. ^{1}H and ^{13}C assignments of keratan sulphate from shark cartilage. Biochem J 1986;236:921–4.

Havlick, HD. Looking at Lane Labs: compassion, quality, solutions. Natural Pharmacy 1999;3:1,12–3.

Kinoshita A, Sugahara K. Microanalysis of glycosaminoglycan-derived oligosaccharides labeled with a fluorophore 2-aminobenzamide by high-performance liquid chromatography: application to disaccharide composition analysis and exosequencing of oligosaccharides. Anal Biochem 1999;269:367–78.

Lane IW, Comac L. Sharks don't get cancer. Garden City, NY: Avery Publishing Group, 1992.

Lee A, Langer R. Shark cartilage contains inhibitors of tumor angiogenesis. Science 1983;221:1185–7.

Marshall J. Shark cartilage for cancer treatment? P&T Newslett Exchange 1996;21:159–60.

McGuire TR, Kazakoff PW, Hoie EB, et al. Antiproliferative activity of shark cartilage with and without tumor necrosis factor-alpha in human umbilical vein endothelium. Pharmacotherapy 1996;16:237–44.

Miller DR, Anderson GT, Stark JJ, et al. Phase I/II trial of the safety and efficacy of shark cartilage in the treatment of advanced cancer. J Clin Oncol 1998;16:3649–55.

Morris GM, Coderre JA, Micca PL, et al. Boron neutron capture therapy of the rat 9L gliosarcoma: evaluation of the effects of shark cartilage. Br J Radiol 2000;73:429–34.

NCI. Office of Cancer Complementary and Alternative Medicine. Available from:URL: www3.cancer.gov/occam/trials.html. Accessed January 31, 2002.

Pettit GR, Ode RH. Antineoplastic agents I: isolation and characterization of sphyrnastatins 1 and 2 from the hammerhead shark *Sphyma lewini*. J Pharm Sci 1977;66:757–8.

Real Life. What is shark cartilage. Available from: URL: http://www.realife.com. Accessed October 9, 2000.

Volpi N. Hyaluronic acid and chondroitin sulfate unsaturated disaccharides analysis by high-performance liquid chromatography and fluorimetric detection with dansylhydrazine. Anal Biochem 2000;277:19–24.

Chapter 22

L-Tryptophan

Beth McDermitt Knapp, Melanie Johns Cupp, and Timothy S. Tracy

22.1. HISTORY

Tryptophan was first isolated in 1901 by the English biochemists Hopkins and Cole from an enzymatic digest of casein. In 1954, L-tryptophan was shown by Rose and colleagues to be an essential amino acid (i.e., one that must be obtained from exogenous sources) in humans (Sidransky, 1997). L-Tryptophan was once a very popular dietary supplement. However, in 1989, the Food and Drug Administration (FDA) requested a recall of L-tryptophan products and took steps to limit the availability of L-tryptophan supplements because of an association between consumption of the supplement and a serious blood disorder known as eosinophilia-myalgia syndrome (Nightingale, 1990).

22.2. CHEMICAL STRUCTURE

Refer to Fig. 22-1 for the chemical structure of L-tryptophan.

22.3. CURRENT PROMOTED USES

L-Tryptophan has been promoted for the treatment of insomnia, depression, premenstrual symptoms (Medsger, 1990), and stress (Archer, 1991).

22.4. SOURCES AND CHEMICAL COMPOSITION

The daily requirement for L-tryptophan is 3.5 mg/kg for adults (Wildman and Medeiros, 2000), and the average daily diet in the United States supplies 0.7–1 g of L-tryptophan daily (Brody, 1999). The average L-tryptophan content of dietary proteins is 1%. Proteins found in milk, eggs, and other animal products contain up to 1.5%

From: *Forensic Science: Dietary Supplements: Toxicology and Clinical Pharmacology*
Edited by: M. J. Cupp and T. S. Tracy © Humana Press Inc., Totowa, New Jersey

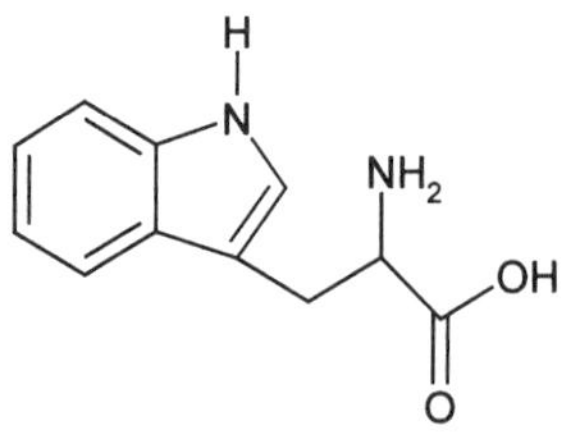

Fig. 1. Chemical structure of tryptophan.

L-tryptophan, whereas corn protein is approximately 0.6% (McCormick, 2000). L-Tryptophan is synthesized commercially by fermentation of various nutrients using mutant bacteria (Medsger, 1990).

Synonyms for L-tryptophan include tryptophan and and tryptophanum. The chemical name is L-2-amino-3-(indol-3-yl)propionic acid. The molecular formula for L-tryptophan is $C_{11}H_{12}N_2O_2$, and its molecular weight is 204.2. A 1% aqueous solution has a pH of 5.5–7.0 (Parfitt, 1999). Tryptophan is slightly bitter (Hartmann et al., 1974) and purportedly imparts an aftertaste similar to that of saccharin (Coppen et al., 1963).

22.5. PRODUCTS AVAILABLE

In 1989, the FDA requested a recall of all commercial forms of L-tryptophan because of its association with eosinophilia-myalgia syndrome. There were more than 300 manufacturers, repackers, and distributors of L-tryptophan products at that time. Examples of L-tryptophan supplements that were commercially available in the United States include Tryptophan P.R.N. 350 mg capsules, L-tryptophan 500 mg capsules, Free Aminos 750 mg capsules, and Free Aminos powder, sold under the Allergy Research Group and NutriCology labels (Nightingale, 1990). Despite the recall of L-tryptophan in the United States, L-tryptophan is discussed here because of its availability abroad, the potential for individuals in the United States to obtain it by prescription through "compounding pharmacies" (California Pharmacy, 2000), and the possibility that it may be marketed as a dietary supplement in the future (Nightingale, 1990).

L-Tryptophan trade name products currently available abroad include Tryptan® in Canada (Parfitt, 1999; Steinberg et al., 1999); Ardeytropin®, Kalma®, and Lyphan® in Germany (Faurie and Fries, 1999; Parfitt, 1999); and Optimax® in the United Kingdom (Parfitt, 1999).

22.6. IN VITRO EFFECTS AND ANIMAL STUDIES

Studies have demonstrated that L-tryptophan administered to rats or mice shortly before sacrifice induces a shift in hepatic polyribosomes toward heavier aggregates accompanied by enhanced hepatic protein synthesis (Sidransky et al., 1971; Sarma et al., 1971; Murty and Sidransky, 1972). Murty and Sidransky (1972) demonstrated that compared with control (distilled water), administration of L-tryptophan 4 mg to fasted mice 1 h prior to sacrifice increased incorporation of radioactive orotic acid into messenger RNA (mRNA). This suggests that L-tryptophan administration increases mRNA synthesis. In rats pretreated with actinomycin D, an inhibitor of RNA synthesis, tryptophan administration did not result in an increase in incorporation of radioactivity into mRNA; however, compared with control animals, livers of L-tryptophan-treated rats nonetheless showed a shift toward heavier polyribosomes. This observation led to an additional experiments in which RNA was radiolabeled prior to actinomycin D treatment. Tryptophan or distilled water was then administered, and the rats were sacrificed. This experiment demonstrated that even with inhibition of RNA synthesis, tryptophan administration caused an increase in cytoplasmic RNA, most likely secondary to increased transfer of newly synthesized mRNA from the nucleus to the cytoplasm. Subsequent studies confirmed that tryptophan stimulates hepatic polyribosomes and protein synthesis both by increasing mRNA synthesis and by increasing transfer of mRNA from the nucleus to the cytoplasm (Murty et al., 1979).

22.7. CLINICAL STUDIES

22.7.1. Premenstrual Dysphoric Disorder

L-Tryptophan's role as a serotonin precursor has stimulated research into psychiatric applications of L-tryptophan. To provide an appreciation for the benefit vs risk of L-tryptphan, clinical studies of L-tryptophan for these disorders will be discussed in some detail. L-Tryptophan was found to be effective in the treatment of mood symptoms of premenstrual dysphoric disorder (PMDD) in a double-blind placebo-controlled trial (Steinberg et al., 1999). All subjects included in this study met DSM-III-R criteria for late luteal dysphoric disorder (currently known as PMDD). Thirty-seven women were treated with L-tryptophan (Tryptan, ICN Canada) 2 g three times daily with meals, and 34 women were given placebo. Patients were treated for 3 mo, 17 d each month, from the time of ovulation to the third day of menstruation. The mean of a combined Visual Analogue Mood Scale (VAMS) score rating depression, mood swings, tension, and irritability showed a significant difference favoring L-tryptophan ($p = 0.004$; ANCOVA). The mean reduction from baseline in the combined VAMS score was 34.5% for L-tryptophan, but only 10.4% for placebo. No significant differences or trends were seen between treatments for the physical symptoms (e.g., headache) of PMDD. Adverse effects reported were of mild or moderate intensity. The only adverse effect that was seen significantly more frequently in the L-tryptophan group than in placebo was dizziness ($p = 0.03$; Fisher's exact test).

22.7.2. Seasonal Affective Disorder

The efficacy of L-tryptophan in the treatment of seasonal affective disorder (SAD) has been evaluated. In one study (Lam et al., 1997), 16 patients meeting DSM-IV criteria for recurrent major depressive disorder with a seasonal (winter) pattern were treated for 2 wk with light therapy. Partial or nonresponders to light therapy were then supplemented with L-tryptophan 1 g 3 times daily with a carbohydrate snack for 2 wk in an open-label fashion. Light therapy was continued. The specific L-tryptophan product used was not stated, but the study was funded in part by ICN Canada, makers of Tryptan. Two patients discontinued L-tryptophan after the first few days of therapy because of nausea, gastrointestinal distress, and headache. The 14 patients who completed the trial had mild side effects including headache ($n = 3$), nausea or gastrointestinal distress ($n = 2$), and flushing or sweating ($n = 2$). Compared with baseline, L-tryptophan supplementation produced responses in 9 of the 14 patients, as measured using the Structured Interview Guide for the Hamilton Depression Rating Scale, SAD version (SIGH-SAD) ($p < 0.001$; paired t-test). Eight of the 14 patients experienced a clinical remission with L-tryptophan, defined as a more than 50% decrease in score from baseline as well as a posttreatment score of less than 15. In addition, 9 of the 14 patients were rated much improved or very much improved on the Clinical Global Impression (CGI) scale compared with baseline. Weaknesses of this study include open-label design, lack of a placebo control, small number of patients, and use of a parametric test (i.e., the t-test) to evaluate a symptom score.

A second study evaluated the effects of light vs L-tryptophan on 13 patients diagnosed with SAD per DSM-III-R criteria (Ghadirian et al., 1998). Inclusion criteria also included a SIGH-SAD of 18 or higher. Patients were required to be medication-free for at least 2 wk (or 5 wk if taking fluoxetine, because of its long half-life). Patients in group 1 ($n = 6$) received light therapy for 2 wk followed by L-tryptophan 2 g twice daily for 4 wk, separated by a 1-wk washout. Group 2 patients ($n = 7$) received tryptophan for 4 wk followed by light therapy for 2 wk, with a 1-wk washout between. During the 4-wk treatment with L-tryptophan, the dose was increased if no improvement was seen by week 2. Improvement was defined as a 50% or greater decrease in the SIGH-SAD score.

Four patients (31%) did not respond to either light or L-tryptophan treatment. The same number of patients responded to light, but not to L-tryptophan, while one patient responded to L-tryptophan, but not to light. The remaining four patients responded to both treatments. Eight patients responded to or maintained improvement with light, and five with tryptophan. There was a significant response, with 7 (54%) patients responding ($p = 0.012$ for light before tryptophan and $p = 0.014$ for tryptophan before light; paired t-test). By the end of 7 weeks there was no significant difference between the two treatment sequences $p = 0.59$). The Hamilton Depression Scale (HAM-D) score increased after stopping light therapy during the washout $p = 0.05$) but fell slightly after stopping tryptophan (NS). The weaknesses of this study are similar to those of the study by Lam and colleagues (1997). In addition, the reason for use of the HAM-D score during the washout rather than the SIGH-SAD was not explained, nor was timing of patient follow-up.

22.7.3. Smoking Cessation

Other investigators have studied L-tryptophan supplementation as an adjunct to counseling for smoking cessation (Bowen et al., 1991). Subjects were recruited from the local community using posters and media advertisements. Subjects were required to be healthy, to be 18–60 yr, to have smoked at least 15 cigarettes daily for 2 yr, and to be less than 140% of ideal weight. Exclusion criteria were chronic medication use or past history of a major physical illness. Thirty-one subjects were randomly assigned to either L-tryptophan 50 mg/kg/d plus a high-carbohydrate diet (7/1 ratio of carbohydrates to protein) or placebo plus a low-carbohydrate diet (1/1 ratio of carbohydrate to protein). The rationale for the high-carbohydrate diet was based on research suggesting that such a diet may improve mood by increasing the influx of L-tryptophan into the brain for use in serotonin synthesis.

Smoking cessation counseling was identical for the experimental and control groups and consisted of four 2-h weekly sessions of multicomponent group therapy that included motivational assessment, identification of triggers, identification of substitute activities, precessation planning and self-management strategies, support after cessation, and relapse prevention. The treatment goal was complete smoking abstinence. Subjects stopped smoking immediately after the second counseling session and began their pills and diets the same evening. Smoking abstinence was measured by self-report and measurement of exhaled carbon monoxide; symptoms of nicotine withdrawal were measured using the Multiple Affect Adjective Checklist (MAAC) with anxiety, depression, and hostility subscales, as well as the Smoker Complaint Scale (SCS), which rates 14 symptoms. Assessments were made during the 3 d after the first group session (baseline while still smoking), during the first 3 d following the second group session (after smoking cessation), and for three days during the second week of smoking cessation. Nutrient intake was recorded in a food diary. Data collected during each 3-d assessment period were averaged, and analysis of covariance was done for each cessation time point to account for differences in baseline variables. Comparisons using multiple *t*-tests failed to detect differences between the two groups at baseline in the MAAC anxiety and SCS withdrawal symptom scores at baseline. Chi-square test was used to compare the proportion of patients abstinent in each group at week 2.

The proportion of tryptophan-treated subjects abstinent at week 2 (12 of 16) exceeded that of placebo (7 of 15) but failed to reach statistical significance. L-Tryptophan-treated subjects who could not fully abstain were noted to smoke fewer daily cigarettes than nonabstaining placebo patients. The MAAC anxiety score was lower in the tryptophan group during cessation week 1 compared with the placebo group ($p < 0.001$) and was lower during week 2 as well, although not statistically different ($p < 0.1$). SCS withdrawal symptoms were lower in the tryptophan group compared with control subjects during week 1 ($p < 0.001$) and week 2 ($p < 0.01$). L-Tryptophan did not improve the MAAC hostility score, and there was a trend toward more depression in the L-tryptophan group. This study suggests that L-tryptophan plus a high-carbohydrate diet decreases anxiety and other withdrawal symptoms associated with smoking cessation. The contribution of diet alone was not assessed. Other study weaknesses include use of statistical tests inappropriate for ordinal data and lack of follow-up for assessment of long-term abstinence.

22.7.4. Depression (Unipolar and Bipolar)

In one double-blind study performed at two National Institutes of Mental Health research units, patients diagnosed as manic-depressive or psychotic-depressive were given L-tryptophan titrated to an average maximum dose of 8 g daily for an average of 16 d (Bunney et al., 1971). Patients were evaluated twice daily by trained research nurses using a 15-point multi-item scale designed to evaluate depression, psychosis, and mania. Improvement was defined as a change of more than 2 points during the 5 d at maximum dose compared with the 5 d prior to beginning L-tryptophan or placebo. Placebo substitution was used to evaluate drug effects in light of the frequency of spontaneous remissions and exacerbations in depressive illness. Eight patients received

L-tryptophan. It was not stated whether these patients were taking other medications. Two showed a decrease in psychosis rating on L-tryptophan followed by an increase when placebo was substituted. One of these patients also showed a decrease in depression rating, which increased with placebo substitution. L-Tryptophan was unable to produce a lasting clinical remission in any patient. Urinary 5-HIAA, the major metabolite of serotonin, increased in seven of the eight patients.

Murphy and colleagues (1974) found that L-tryptophan (average dose and duration of therapy 9.6 g and 20 d, respectively) in combination with pyridoxine 50 mg and ascorbic acid 100 mg was somewhat effective in 10 patients in the manic phase of bipolar depression. A double-blind, "placebo substitution" design was used. Patients were evaluated twice daily by a trained nursing research team using a 15-point, multiitem scale developed by Bunney and Hamberg. Seven patients exhibited a statistically significant decrease in manic behavior, and three of these relapsed with placebo substitution. Three of four patients with ratings in the upper manic range (4.0–6.0 on the manic scale) exhibited a complete recovery. Six more severely manic patients had only partial improvement. Modest antidepressant effects were noted in the manic patients.

An additional crossover study of bipolar depression in manic phase showed that L-tryptophan 6 g plus pyridoxine 100 mg daily acts rapidly to reduce hyperactivity, but despite a trend toward superiority, its advantage over chlorpromazine 400 mg/d was not statistically significant (Prange et al., 1974). Limitations of this study include small sample size ($n = 10$) and relatively small chlorpromazine dose.

In an additional double-blind, placebo-controlled trial (Mendels et al., 1975), patients in a psychiatric research ward with either bipolar disorder or recurrent depressive illness were assigned to receive L-tryptophan dose titration ($n = 6$) or placebo ($n = 3$), as well as pyridoxine 50 mg for 42 d. L-Tryptophan was dissolved in Metrecal® (Mead Johnson, Evansville, IN), and placebo patients received Metrecal without L-tryptophan. The dose of L-tryptophan was increased as quickly as possible based on patient tolerance. Baseline patient characteristics were similar, including age, sex, severity of depression, and whether the illness was unipolar or bipolar. Patients were evaluated by two nurses twice daily with the scale developed by Bunney and Hamberg. There was a high degree of interrater reliability. The mean maximum daily dosage of L-tryptophan was 14 g, with a range of 11.6–16 g/d. Two patients in the L-tryptophan group were bipolar, and one in the placebo group was bipolar. Only one patient showed any improvement. After the study, all patients required inpatient treatment with antidepressant therapy.

The effect of L-tryptophan vs placebo was evaluated using the "placebo substitution" design in six patients with primary bipolar or unipolar affective disorder at the New York State Psychiatric Insititute (Dunner and Fieve, 1975). All patients were in the depressive phase of their illness. In the double-blind portion of the study, a 10-d drug-free period was followed by 3–7 d of placebo, after which L-tryptophan (8.4–9 g/d) was administered for 10–18 d, followed by placebo substitution. During both the placebo and treatment periods, pyridoxine 150 mg and ascorbic acid 900 mg were administered daily. Patients received a diet low in biogenic amine precursors throughout the study. Vital signs were monitored several times daily, and lab tests were usually checked weekly. Assessments were performed by a trained nursing team three times daily using a global mood rating scale and twice weekly using a structured interview for manic and depressive symptoms. Four patients failed to have an antidepressant response, meaning that there was no improvement in depression rating during the last days of L-tryptophan treatment. These patients subsequently responded to a monoamine oxidase inhibitor. The only patient in the study who was bipolar demonstrated an equivocal response, meaning that the patient improved during L-tryptophan treatment but did not relapse and in fact continued to improve with placebo substitution. Her response was attributed to spontaneous remission rather than to L-tryptophan, and she was subsequently discharged on lithium. An additional patient had a good antidepressant response to L-tryptophan therapy. No side effects were reported.

L-Tryptophan has been compared with the tricyclic antidepressants in several double-blind trials. Unlike the previously described trials in which L-tryptophan was compared with placebo, efficacy was evaluated using the HAM-D, which is considered the gold standard assessment tool for screening patients for inclusion into drug studies, evaluating symptom severity, and assessing treatment outcome (Marken and Schneiderhan, 1997). In a trial lasting for 4 wk (Coppen et al., 1972), eight patients who met criteria for major depression were treated with L-tryptophan 9 g/d (Cambrian Chemicals, Beddington Farm, Croyden, England), and another eight patients were treated with imipramine 150 mg/d. The L-tryptophan tablets also contained ascorbic acid and pyridoxine, cofactors necessary for functioning of the enzyme responsible for decarboxylating L-tryptophan to serotonin. Subjects assigned to the L-tryptophan group received imipramine placebo, and subjects assigned to the imipramine group received L-tryptophan placebo. Although all subjects were euthyroid, liothyronine sodium (T3) 25 µg or placebo was also administered for the first 14 d of the study, based on previous studies suggesting that a longer duration of therapy is unnecessary. Subjects were fed the standard hospital diet.

The same two investigators rated patients twice weekly using the HAM-D, with raters alternately interviewing each patient. In addition, on the evening before the trial began, each patient was interviewed by one rater while the other listened. Both raters then individually completed the HAM-D. Although all subscales were completed at baseline and at subsequent twice weekly interviews, only subscales 1–16 were used to determine efficacy because there was poor correlation between the raters for these sections. Twice weekly, patients also completed the Beck Depressive Inventory (BDI). Today, the BDI is considered the standard for self-rating scales and provides an objective measure of change in symptoms owing to treatment (Marken and Schneiderhan, 1997). At the end of the study, patients were asked if they had experienced any side effects and also rated 21 symptoms on a scale of 0 to 4. Statistical analysis of efficacy measures was performed using a modified analysis of covariance technique, with gender being one of the covariates.

Patients responded equally well to both imipramine and L-tryptophan. In men, there was a nonsignificant trend toward greater improvement in the HAM-D with imipramine. Although the imipramine/liothyronine group showed a greater change from baseline in the HAM-D than the other three groups, this finding was statistically significant at the $p < 0.05$ level only when the data for the other three groups were combined. Patients in the imipramine/liothyronine group also improved more ($p < 0.05$)

on the BDI than patients in the other groups. In both the imipramine and L-tryptophan groups, there was a nonsignificant trend toward greater change from baseline in the HAM-D in women who received liothyronine compared with those who received placebo, and the response curve suggested that longer duration of treatment with liothyronine might have shown benefit. In analyzing the subscales of the HAM-D, there were no significant differences among treatments in regard to improvement in any particular symptom; however, trends suggested that whereas L-tryptohan did not improve sleep more than other treatments, it might be of particular benefit in improving motor retardation. This finding might be explained by imipramine's tendency to cause sedation and at least temporarily worsen motor retardation, rather than an actual benefit of L-tryptophan. Of the three bipolar patients in the study, one was assigned to the L-tryptophan/liothyronine group, and two received imipramine/liothyronine. The latter two patients experienced manic symptoms during treatment, and the former showed no improvement.

Student's *t*-test was used to analyze side effect data. It was found that L-tryptophan produced more side effects than imipramine ($p < 0.05$). The investigators suggested that the mean side effect score for L-tryptophan might have been elevated by one patient, described as a "persistently hypochondriacal woman," who rated 14 of 21 side effects as a "2" or "3" in severity. Addition of liothyronine appeared to decrease side effects compared with imipramine ($p < 0.025$) or L-tryptophan ($p < 0.001$) alone, a finding that the investigators could not adequately explain.

This study, although limited by small sample size and uncertain statistics (analysis of nonparametric data with parametric tests), showed that patients respond equally well to imipramine and L-tryptophan, a finding mirroring that of previous unblinded trials (Broadhurst, 1970; Kline and Shah, 1973). Coppen and colleagues (1972) made the additional suggestion that imipramine might be a better choice than L-tryptophan in men. Their results also suggest that L-tryptophan has no specific effect on sleep in depressed patients, improving all symptoms equally. Liothyronine potentiated the efficacy of imipramine in this study, a finding that supported previous reports, with women appearing to benefit most from this combination. Data from this study also suggest that in women, addition of liothyronine to L-tryptophan may be beneficial.

A double-blind study (Jensen et al., 1975) compared the use of L-tryptophan and imipramine in 42 patients with endogenous depression, either unipolar or bipolar, with a total score of 5 or greater on items 1, 2, and 8 of the HAM-D. Patients with psychosis or a depressive episode of more than 6 mo duration were excluded. All patients were treated for 3 wk according to a fixed-dose schedule starting with half of the dose during the first 3 d of treatment followed by either 6 g of tryptophan (Cambrian) or 150 mg of imipramine beginning on the fourth day. The only other drugs allowed were diazepam and chloral hydrate. Patients were evaluated using the HAM-D. Both the imipramine ($n = 20$) and the L-tryptophan groups ($n = 22$) showed improvement compared with baseline ($p < 0.01$ at week 3 for both groups). However, the reduction of symptoms was more rapid in the imipramine group. A side effect rating scale previously described by other authors was also used. Side effects in the L-tryptophan group were less frequent than in the imipramine group. The authors attributed the difference in their findings compared with previous studies to larger sample size and more homogeneous patient sample.

Another double-blind study (Rao and Broadhurst, 1976) comparing L-tryptophan with imipramine produced similar results. Sixteen patients with depressive illness received six 25-mg imipramine tablets plus 12 L-tryptophan placebo tablets, or six tablets of imipramine placebo plus 12-500 mg L-tryptophan tablets. Each L-tryptophan tablet also contained 5 mg of pyridoxine and 10 mg of ascorbic acid. Thus, each patient received 6 tablets three times daily. Patients were evaluated using the HAM-D at baseline and after 4 wk of treatment. Because imipramine has anticholinergic side effects that might jeopardize the double-blind nature of the study, patients were instructed to discuss any possible side effects with a staff member other than the rater. Compared with baseline, both imipramine and L-tryptophan were equally effective in the treatment of depression ($p < 0.01$ for both treatments).

L-Tryptophan was compared with amitriptyline in a double-blind trial (Herrington et al., 1976) in patients with a primary diagnosis of depression per the Medical Research Council (MRC) criteria published in 1965. Patients with mild depression or severe social problems, and those requiring electroconvulsive therapy (ECT) were excluded. Treatment consisted of 4 wk of either amitriptyline ($n = 20$) or L-tryptophan ($n = 20$). Diazepam was the only other medication allowed. Patients receiving L-tyrptophan were administered 6 g daily for 2 wk and then 8 g/d for the next 2 wk. All patients were also given pyridoxine 100 mg/d. Amitriptyline patients received 75 mg daily for 1 wk and 150 mg/d for the remainder of the study. To preserve blinding, L-tryptophan patients were given amitriptyline placebo, and amitriptyline patients were given L-tryptophan placebo. Hypnotic placebo (lactose) was administered to patients who requested a sleeping pill, although nitrazepam 5 mg (a benzodiazepine) was allowed if insomnia was a problem after 10 d.

Patients were evaluated at baseline and weekly for 4 wk. The MRC depression scale, items 1–17 of the HAM-D, and an overall rating of depression severity was completed by an investigator. In the first and final assessments, the HAM-D was completed by a second designated investigator to confirm rater reliability. The BDI and the Taylor Manifest Anxiety Scale were completed by the patient. In an attempt to preserve blinding, adverse effects were not discussed with the patients. *t*-tests and chi-square tests were used to confirm that the two groups did not differ at baseline in regard to gender, age, family history of depression, duration of present episode, HAM-D scores, MRC scale, overall score, and BDI. At baseline, the amitriptyline group was found to have a higher Taylor Anxiety Scale score ($p < 0.01$, *t*-test). ANOVA was carried out on the pre-treatment and weekly scores. The only significant differences between the two groups over the course of 4 wk were MRC insomnia scale ($p < 0.01$) and somatic symptoms ($p < 0.05$); the severity of these symptoms appeared to increase in patients treated with L-tryptophan.

L-Tryptophan has also been studied in combination with monoamine oxidase inhibitors (MAOIs) for depression. One study (Coppen et al., 1963) involved 41 patients with severe depressive illness who had had no ECT for at least 1 mo and no drug therapy for at least 2 wk. Patients with cardiovascular disease were also excluded. The diagnosis of severe depression was based on a history of profound depression with symptoms such as feelings of worthlessness, guilt, hopelessness, or unreality; thoughts or intent of suicide; or loss of interest, concentration, appetite, or energy. All patients were fed the standard hospital diet. All patients received tranylcypromine (Parnate®)

30 mg (weight < 50 kg), 40 mg (weight 50–70 kg), or 50 mg (weight > 70 kg) daily for 4 wk. For those patients randomized to tryptophan, a suspension containing D,L-tryptophan 214 mg/kg, cocoa 5 g, and milk to a total volume of 340 mL was added to the treatment regimen during the second week of therapy for 1 wk. Placebo was identical to the tryptophan suspension, except that kaolin 20 g was added in place of tryptophan, and saccharin was added to mimic the sweet aftertaste of tryptophan. Response to therapy was evaluated using the HAM-D. Blood pressure, deep tendon reflexes, and side effects were noted daily. One patient was withdrawn from the study on day 2 owing to urgent need for ECT.

Patients treated with combination therapy improved significantly more ($p < 0.001$, statistical tests not described) than the control group during the second week. During the last 2 wk of the study, the tryptophan group continued to show greater improvement than the control group, even though the rate of improvement slowed. This finding suggests that tryptophan potentiates the action of MAOIs and that the benefits are not lost even after tryptophan discontinuation. The authors did not recommend routine tryptophan supplementation in patients taking MAOIs owing to the risk of adverse effects (*see Drug Interactions* section).

Other investigators (Glassman and Platman, 1969) subsequently attempted to duplicate the results of Coppen and colleagues (1963). This double-blind study involved 20 hospitalized patients categorized as "involutional manic depressive or endogenous depressives." All had been depressed for 2–6 mo. Patients with chronic unremitting depression, those with acute situational depression, and those with schizophrenia, schizoaffective disorder, or delusional thinking were excluded. Phenelzine sulfate 30 mg twice daily was prescribed, and patients were reevaluated 48–72 h later. Those with no improvement were given either D,L-tryptophan 4, 5, or 6 g plus 26 g malt three times daily, depending on weight, or placebo, which consisted of gum arabic, saccharin, and malt. Patients were given only one-third of the daily dose on day 1, two-thirds of the dose on day 2, and, if there were no serious side effects, the total dose on days 3–14. Patients also received pyridoxine and a barbiturate hypnotic at bedtime. Efficacy was evaluated on days 7, 14, 28, and 60 using a "slightly modified" version of the HAM-D designed to measure self-esteem and decrease the weight carried by somatic complaints. Six of 10 tryptophan and 2 of 10 placebo patients were discharged at the end of week 3. The other patients were either switched to a tricyclic antidepressant or underwent ECT. Fisher's exact test revealed $p = 0.055$ for the difference between the two treatments in regard to discharge at week 3; the authors deemed this difference to be statically significant.

At baseline, the two groups were similar in their scores on the modified HAM-D, but at the end of week 3, the tryptophan group had responded better than the placebo group per the Mann Whitney U-test ($0.05 < p < 0.1$) and t-test ($p < 0.05$) calculated using the percent change. The tryptophan group responded better than the placebo group in 16 of 18 items ($p < 0.01$, sign test), with the largest differences occurring in concentration ($p < 0.05$) and early awakening ($p < 0.1$). These investigators pointed out that 30–40 patients were originally to have been studied, but owing to a change in study site, the number of suitable patients was limited. They felt that with only 20 patients, the level of statistical significance reached (approx $p = 0.05$) suggests a moderately strong benefit of tryptophan. They also suggested that the use of tranylcypromine instead of phenelzine might have produced more favorable results, perhaps following the rationale of Coppen and colleagues (1963) that it is more selective for MAO in the central nervous system.

Results from studies involving L-tryptophan and ECT are conflicting. In the first study comparing ECT with L-tryptophan (Coppen et al., 1967), D,L-tryptophan 5–7 g daily plus pyridoxine 100 mg/d was found to be as effective as ECT in severely depressed hospitalized patients. Subsequently, Carroll and colleagues (1970) and Herrington and associates (1974) showed that ECT was superior to L-tryptophan. In the more recent study, consecutive patients admitted to the hospital with a primary diagnosis of depression according to the MRC criteria were allocated randomly to treatment with ECT ($n = 21$) twice weekly for 6–8 wk, or with L-tryptophan ($n = 22$) 6 g/d for 2 wk, then 8 g/d for 2 wk. Patients in both groups received pyridxine 100 mg/ d. If no improvement was seen after 2 wk, patients were given a trial of the other therapy. If a hypnotic was requested, lactose was administered, although nitrazepam 5 mg was allowed if insomnia was a "considerable" problem. Diazepam 15–30 mg/d was also administered for "severe" agitation. Although nitrazepam was administered to four of the tryptophan patients, none of the ECT patients required nitrazepam. Five ECT patients and six tryptophan patients required diazepam.

Patients were assessed at baseline and weekly for 4 wk by one of the investigators using the MRC depression scale, the HAM-D, and an overall severity of depression. At the first and final ratings, a second investigator completed the HAM-D as a reliability indicator. In addition, patients who were capable of doing so completed the Taylor Anxiety Scale and the BDI. At baseline, the treatment groups were similar in regard to sex, age, family history of depression, number of previous episodes of depression, duration of present episode, duration of hospital stay prior to randomization, and scores on assessment instruments (one-way AVOVA, $p < 0.05$). Two patients in the L-tryptophan group and one patient in the ECT group were switched to the other treatment after 2 wk; these patients were not included in the data analysis.

Using ANCOVA, both groups were shown to improve significantly after 2 and 4 wk of therapy compared with baseline. There were no differences between groups at week 2. However, the ECT group continued to improve after week 2 whereas the L-tryptophan group showed little further improvement; at week 4, all assessments in the ECT group showed more improvement than in the L-tryptophan group ($p < 0.05$ for the Taylor Manifest Anxiety Scale, $p < 0.001$ for all others). Using two-way ANOVA, the investigators found that women responded better to ECT, whereas men responded better to L-tryptophan. The investigators concluded that ECT was superior to L-tryptophan in severely depressed patients (i.e., patients requiring hospitalization).

The investigators compared their study with that of Coppen et al. (1967), which favored D,L-tryptophan, and with that of Carroll et al. (1970), which had findings similar to those of their own study. Coppen and colleagues (1967) used D,L-tryptophan, such that the daily dose of L-tryptophan was less than 4 g, whereas Herrington and associates (1974) and Carroll and colleagues (1970) used 7 g. They suggested that perhaps the optimum dose of L-tryptophan is 4 g/d, with larger doses stimulating L-tryptophan metabolism, and/or that the dose of pyridoxine used in the studies favoring

ECT were not sufficient given the relatively large dose of L-tryptophan administered. The Coppen et al. study (1967) was not randomized and there was no placebo group, so the results could have been influenced by a change in ward atmosphere or admissions policies. Herrington et al.'s study (1974) included a higher percentage of women, who appear to respond better than men to ECT, and who have higher tryptophan pyrrolase activity than men; however, even men responded better to ECT than L-tryptophan in their study. Furthermore, both the Coppen et al. study (1967) and the Carroll study (1970) enrolled equal numbers of men and women but had different results.

Because it is possible that bipolar patients respond differently to L-tryptophan than unipolar patients, inclusion of bipolar patients in some studies might have attributed to varying study results. Although no patients in the Herrington et al. study (1974) had a personal or family history of manic episodes, this information is not available for the Coppen et al. (1967) or Carroll et al. (1970) studies. Coppen et al.'s patients appeared to have had less severe depression, based on the BDI, than the Herrington et al.'s study patients (1974); moderately depressed patients might respond better to L-tryptophan and/or be less responsive to ECT than more severely depressed patients. Because studies comparing a pharmacologic treatment to ECT cannot be blinded, bias on the part of the investigators or patients may influence the results. Use of both objective clinician rating scales and self-rating scales might minimize the influence of bias. In the Coppen et al. study (1967), the BDI was the main outcome measure. Although such self-rating scales may be unreliable in severely depressed patients, in the Herrington et al. study (1974) there was good correlation (0.62) between BDI scores and HAM-D scores, and within-patient correlation was as high as 0.90. On the strength of these correlations, the investigators felt that differences in rating procedures were an unlikely source of the discrepant results. Finally, because both groups had improved to the same extent by week 2, followed by additional improvement in the ECT group alone, the investigators suggested that the initial improvement may have been a nonspecific effect rather than a treatment effect. A placebo group would be needed to explore this possibility further.

Another unblinded study examined the effect of L-tryptophan (Optimax) 3 g plus nicotinamide 1 g daily vs ECT in 27 patients with severe depression (MacSweeney, 1975). Only patients with unipolar depression were included in the study; those with a personal or family history of hypomania or mania were excluded. Patients were randomly assigned to one of the two treatments. Patients randomized to ECT received treatment twice weekly for a maximum of eight treatments. To eliminate observer bias, the BDI was used to evaluate patient response to treatment, as in the Coppen et al. study (1967). The BDI was completed at baseline and on days 3, 7, 10, 14, 17, 21, 24, and 28. One patient randomized to the ECT group refused ECT, and one patient in the L-tryptophan group underwent ECT due to worsening depression. There was a trend toward earlier improvement in the L-tryptophan group, and this group achieved a significantly ($p < 0.05$, statistical test not described) lower rating of depression at day 21 than those receiving ECT. However, by day 28 of the trial, depression ratings were almost identical in both groups.

The author concluded that L-tryptophan was superior to twice weekly ECT. Because L-tryptophan induces its own metabolism, the author hypothesized that the results reported by Herrington and colleagues (1974) described above, i.e., improvement during the first 2 wk of L-tryptophan use followed by a plateau in effect coinciding with a dosage increase from 6 g daily to 8 g daily, could be attributed to induction of tryptophan pyrrolase, an enzyme in the metabolic pathway of L-tryptophan.

Oral adminstration of L-tryptophan was found to be ineffective for the potentiation of the antidepressant effect of ECT in a double-blind trial (D'Elia et al., 1977). Thirty-one depressed patients received L-tryptophan 6 g/daily, whereas 30 depressed patients received placebo and ECT. Efficacy was assessed using the Cronholm-Ottosson depression scale (CODS), the nurses' rating scale (NRS), and a physician's global assessment on a scale of 0 to 3. Assessments were made by the same two doctors. Simultaneous assessments were done at several sessions to test rater reliability. The Zung Self-Rating Scale was also used as an assessment tool. All assessments were performed before ECT, 4 d after ECT, and 1 mo after ECT. At baseline, the only statistically significant difference between the two treatment groups was on the Zung Self-Rating Scale; more placebo patients reported weight loss (Mann-Whitney U-test, $p < 0.05$). After using analysis of covariance to adjust for baseline differences between the groups in the CODS, there were no differences between the two groups 4 d and 1 mo after ECT. Global assessment did not differ between groups at any time point measured. The L-tryptophan group exhibited lower scores for depressive symptoms, slowness of speech, psychomotor retardation, and retardation syndrome (a composite of slowness of speech, psychomotor retardation, and inactivity) on the NRS ($p < 0.05$, analysis of covariance). On the Zung Self-Rating Scale, the L-tryptophan group exhibited a lower constipation score 4 d after ECT than the placebo group (Mann-Whitney U-test, $p < 0.05$). The authors concluded that L-tryptophan provided only a marginal benefit over ECT alone.

The results of these studies suggest that L-tryptophan has at least modest antidepressive activity, and may be as effective as the tricyclic antidepressants. It should be noted, however, that the results of these studies, performed in the 1960s and 1970s, are difficult to interpret and apply today in light of present diagnostic criteria for psychiatric illnesses (DSM IV-R), standardized patient assessment tools currently in use, and modern pharmacotherapy. In addition, the "placebo substitution" study design used by Murphy and colleagues (1974), Bunney and associates (1971), and Dunner and Fieve (1975) is not used today.

To establish whether L-tryptophan is safe and effective in the treatment of depression in adults, Shaw and colleagues (2001) systematically reviewed randomized placebo-controlled studies in patients with unipolar depression or dysthymia in which efficacy was assessed using a depressive symptom scale. Only one study met the inclusion criteria (Thomas et al., 1982), and hence it was the only study of L-tryptophan selected for review. Several of the studies described above (Glassman and Platman, 1969; Carroll et al., 1970; Coppen et al., 1972; Prange et al., 1974; Dunner and Fieve, 1975; Jensen et al., 1975; Mendels et al., 1975; MacSweeney, 1975; Herrington et al., 1976; Rao and Broadhurst, 1976; D'Elia et al., 1977) were among those excluded from the review. The investigators concluded that L-tryptophan may be superior to placebo for this purpose, but until further research is available, its clinical utility is limited, given its association with eosinophilia-myalgia syndrome and the availability of safe, effective antidepressants.

22.7.5. Insomnia

In one study (Hartmann et al., 1974), the hypnotic effects of L-tryptophan at a dosage range of 1–15 g were observed. Study subjects were 10 males ages 21–35 yr who were otherwise free of medical or psychiatric disorders but who reported sleep latencies of 15 min or more. Each subject slept in a sleep laboratory for an all-night recording on 10 occasions approximately once weekly. To become accustomed to sleeping in the laboratory, subjects slept there on two occasions prior to the 10 study nights. Twenty minutes prior to bedtime on each of the 10 study nights, subjects received, in a random fashion, placebo (on three occasions) or L-tryptophan 1, 2, 3, 4, 5, 10, and 15 g. The placebo (methylcellulose and sucrose) or L-tryptophan was administered in a milkshake. The milkshake itself provided tryptophan 40 mg, so even the placebo shake contained a relatively small amount of L-tryptophan. The placebo shake and the L-tryptophan shake were indistinguishable. Throughout each study night, continuous electroencephalogram (EEG), rapid eye movement (REM), and electromyogram recordings were made. Each morning, subjects completed a questionnaire regarding sleep, side effects, and how they felt in the morning.

Sleep latency, defined as time from "lights out" to stage 1 sleep, was decreased compared with placebo at all L-tryptophan dosages ($p < 0.001$, Wilcoxon signed rank test). The investigators attributed the effect of L-tryptophan on sleep latency to its role in serotonin metabolism. They considered the flat dose-response curve to be a result of saturation of enzymes or transport mechanisms involved in serotonin synthesis with as little as 1 g of L-tryptophan. There was a nonstatistically significant trend toward better sleep ratings with L-tryptophan. Only relatively high doses of L-tryptophan appeared to affect sleep architecture; L-tryptophan 10 g produced a significant increase in slow-wave sleep (stages 3 and 4 sleep), and REM sleep was decreased by approx 30% with L-tryptophan 10 and 15 g. These changes, noted only with higher L-tryptophan doses, suggest, according to the investigators, that the previously mentioned saturation is short lived. Interestingly, the investigators noted that increases in slow-wave sleep have been noted in animal studies with serotonin. The authors also suggested that the decrease in REM sleep associated with larger L-tryptophan doses might have been caused by an unreported but sleep-disrupting side effect such as nausea, although they also point out that reports of REM sleep disruption with large L-tryptophan doses differ among studies. Side effects did not differ between placebo and L-tryptophan.

It is important to note that L-tryptophan does not appear to improve sleep in patients with depression (Mendels et al., 1975; Coppen et al., 1972), possibly because of decreased serotonin receptors sensitivity in these patients.

22.7.6. Pain

L-Tryptophan supplementation was found to be ineffective in the treatment of patients with chronic myofascial pain (Stockstill et al., 1989). Patients with chronic facial or jaw pain that had lasted for at least 6 mo and that had been diagnosed (the exact diagnosis was not specified) by a dentist or physician were recruited for the study via public announcement. Two hundred fifteen people responded to the announcement, and 104 were examined for study inclusion. Inclusion criteria consisted of pain on palpation of two or more muscles of mastication or referred pain from the head and neck areas to the temporomandibular joint (TMJ) and facial areas. Exclusion criteria included joint derangements, cancer, pulpitis, pericoronitis, history of pain for less than 6 mo, and use of prescription pain medication.

Thirty-five patients were randomly assigned to one of four groups: L-tryptophan 50 mg/kg body weight daily for 5 wk and diet instruction; placebo (lactose) daily for 5 wk and diet instruction; L-tryptophan 50 mg/kg daily for 5 wk without diet instruction; and placebo daily for 5 wk without diet instruction. The purpose of the diet instruction was to control for the effect of a high-carbohydrate, low-fat (15%), low protein (15%) diet, which enhances the uptake and conversion of L-tryptophan to serotonin. The diet included soft foods to promote compliance by patients who suffer pain from chewing harder foods and was designed specifically for each patient by a registered dietician (RD), taking into account patient height, weight, and age. The RD instructed patients in the diet and emphasized the importance of diet in the study design.

At baseline and at the end of each of the 5 study weeks, pain on masticatory muscle palpation (scale of 0 to 3), Tursky Pain Perception questionnaire, maximal jaw opening in millimeters, deviation of at least 2 mm on opening or closing (present or absent), and joint sounds (present or absent) were assessed. These data were obtained by two clinicians, and the interrater masticatory muscle palpation technique was evaluated and standardized. Beginning the week following the baseline evaluation and during the 5-wk intervention, patients kept a pain dairy in which they recorded pain in the morning, afternoon, and evening on a scale of 0 to 5. Patients also noted any medications taken. Other measurements, taken before and after the 5-wk intervention, included the Taylor Manifest Anxiety Scale and the Center for Epidemiological Studies-Depression Scale. Three patients dropped out of the L-tryptophan/diet group and the placebo/no diet group, respectively, and two dropped out of the placebo/diet group. Data analysis was performed using one-way ANOVA, with statistical significane accepted at $p < 0.05$.

All patients, regardless of treatment group, improved significantly from pretreatment to posttreatment on the pain measures (muscle palpation scores, pain diary scores, Tursky intensity scores) and maximal jaw opening. Patients did not improve based on anxiety or depression scores. Statistical analysis did reveal evidence for benefit of diet in improving pain diary scores and maximal jaw opening. These findings did not support the investigators' hypothesis that patients receiving both L-tryptophan and diet instruction would improve the most.

Although a previous study found benefit for L-tryptophan in patients with chronic maxillofacial pain, the investigators in this study controlled better for diet instruction. The investigators suggested that the favorable results of previous studies of L-tryptophan for pain, including migraine headache, pain tolerance threshold in normal volunteers, and facial pain, might have been the result of concomitant treatments, lack of diet control, or choice of pain measurement instruments. The authors felt that their study was of adequate duration to show a benefit for L-tryptophan supplementation, if one did exist, and pointed out that the dose used in their study was larger than in previous pain studies.

22.7.7. Fatigue

Results of research on the efficacy of L-tryptophan supplementation to improve running performance has been conflicting. In a randomized, placebo-controlled cross-over trial, Segura and Ventura (1988) evaluated the effects of L-tryptophan on endurance and perceived exertion. The rationale for studying L-tryptophan in this setting was based on studies suggesting that serotonin and 5-hydroxytryptamine, for which L-tryptophan is a precursor, might alter perception of pain and discomfort. After a graded exercise test to establish maximal oxygen consumption (VO$_2$ max), 12 healthy athletes ran on a treadmill at a rate corresponding to 80% of their VO$_2$ max on two separate occasions: after receiving placebo and after receiving four doses of L-tryptophan 300 mg. L-Tryptophan or identical placebo was administered in capsules the night before the test, at breakfast and lunch on the day of the test, and 1 h prior to the test. The total exercise time was 49.4% greater after receiving L-tryptophan than after receiving placebo ($p < 0.05$; Wilcoxon signed rank test). Individual results varied greatly. A lower rate of perceived exertion using a perceived exertion scale was exhibited with L-tryptophan, although the differences from the control group were not statistically significant.

In a subsequent investigation, Stensrund and colleagues (1992) evaluated the effect of L-tryptophan on running performance in 45 well-trained male runners. After two trials, which served as a learning experience and to establish VO$_2$max and anaerobic threshold, participants ran to exhaustion at a speed corresponding to 100% of their VO$_2$max and then repeated the run after receiving a total of 1.2 g of L-tryptophan or placebo over the 24-h period prior to the run. Treatment was assigned in a randomized, double-blind fashion. Appropriate statistical tests were used. Baseline characteristics (age, height, weight, VO$_2$max, anaerobic threshold, and running speed) were not different between the two groups. No significant difference in improvement from baseline in the L-tryptophan and placebo groups could be demonstrated in regard to running speed or heart rate. The investigators concluded that L-tryptophan supplementation does not enhance running performance. They also hypothesized that the difference between their results and those of Segura and Ventura (1988) could be explained by greater variation in the degree of training (and thus greater variation in individual results) of the subjects in the previous study, whereas the subjects in their study were more alike and were more highly trained.

Conversely, it has also been hypothesized that L-tryptophan, through its ability to increase brain serotonin synthesis, can increase fatigue, and diet-induced increases in plasma tryptophan have been associated with fatigue. In a study designed to assess the effect of L-tryptophan 30 mg/kg on plasma amino acids and fatigue (Cunliffe et al., 1998), six subjects (staff and students) recruited from Queen Mary and Westfield College in London were administered, in a crossover fashion, diet Coke or diet Coke plus L-tryptophan after at least a 1-wk washout. After consuming the beverage, subjects performed light office work or studied. Prior to and hourly for 4 h after drinking the beverage, fatigue was assessed using a 13-item visual analog scale; Flicker Fusion Frequency (FFF; test of central fatigue in which flicker rate is started at 200 Hz and reduced until the subject perceives the flicker; the greater the fatigue, the lower the frequency at which the flicker is seen); Simple Visual Reaction Time (reaction time to color change on a computer screen); grip strength measured using a hand dynamometer; and wrist ergometry.

The mean percentage change from baseline in subjective fatigue scores was greater with L-tryptophan compared with placebo ($p < 0.002$, two-way ANOVA). Likewise, the mean percentage change from baseline in the FFF score was significantly greater with L-tryptophan than with placebo ($p < 0.001$, two-way ANOVA), indicating increasing fatigue with L-tryptophan. The mean percentage change in reaction time from baseline also indicated increasing fatigue with L-tryptophan vs placebo ($p < 0.001$, two-way ANOVA). There was no difference between L-tryptophan and placebo in regard to grip strength, and L-tryptophan actually increased work output as measured by wrist ergometry compared with placebo ($p < 0.001$, two-way ANOVA). These results suggest that L-tryptophan supplementation increases central fatigue measured both objectively and subjectively but may increase tolerance to physical discomfort, as suggested by improvements in wrist ergometry compared with placebo and supported by the findings of Segura and Ventura (1988) described above.

22.8. PHARMACOKINETICS

L-Tryptophan is 65–78% bound to plasma albumin (Pakes, 1979). This binding is saturable, with approximately one binding site per albumin molecule; thus, the unbound (free) fraction increases with increasing dose. With chronic treatment, the binding affinity increases, but the number of binding sites does not change (Green et al., 1985).

The plasma half-life of L-tryptophan is 2.65 h in depressed patients, 2.7 h in healthy persons, and 2.85 hours in schizophrenic patients (Pakes, 1979). Although half-life is not dose-dependent, clearance decreases with increasing dose. Decreased clearance may be caused by saturable systemic metabolism or saturable first-pass hepatic metabolism, which has been demonstrated in the isolated perfused rat liver. Volume of distribution also decreases with increasing dose and is directly proportional to change in clearance. Because the decrease in volume of distribution is larger than would be expected if the change in clearance were caused solely by saturable systemic metabolism, the decreases in clearance and volume of distribution are probably the result of saturable first-pass metabolism (Green et al., 1985).

Tryptophan is extensively metabolized. Important metabolites include the neurotransmitter serotonin as well as niacin (nicotinic acid), a vitamin that participates in the biosynthesis of nicotinamide-adenine dinucleotide (NAD^+) and its phosphate ($NADP^+$), which are electron carriers essential for biologic redox reactions (Halkerston, 1988). The main tryptophan metabolic pathway involves tryptophan pyrrolase (tryptophan dioxygenase), a hepatic enyme that biotransforms tryptophan into kynurenine metabolites that are excreted in the urine (Pakes, 1979; Sidransky, 1997). The product of the first step in the hepatic metabolism of L-tryptophan is *N*-formylkynurenine. This product is also formed in the lung, intestine, brain, and monocytes by the action of indoleamine-2,3-dioxygenase (Sidransky, 1997). The liver kynurenine pathway then forms a series of intermediates (including kynurenine, 3-hydroxykynurenine, 3-hydroxyanthranilic acid, and carboxymuconic aldehyde intermediate) and byproducts (including xanthurenic acid, picolinic acid, quinolinic acid, and niacin) (Birdsall, 1998).

The chief urinary metabolites in humans, dogs, and rats are kynurenine and kynurenic acid. Xanthurenic acid is a major metabolite in humans and rats, but not in dogs or cats (Brown and Price, 1956). *N*-methyl-2-pyridone-5-carboxamide, the main metabolite of nicotinamide (Moore et al., 2000), is a chief urinary tryptophan metabolite in humans, but not in rats, dogs, or cats (Brown and Price, 1956). Such interspecies comparisons have implications in the study of L-tryptophan's role in bladder cancer (*see Carcinogenesis* section).

Whereas indoleamine 2,3-dioxygenase appears to be inhibited by prednisone (Hisatomi et al., 1997), tryptophan pyrrolase is induced by cortisol (Pakes, 1979) and by increasing concentrations of tryptophan in animals (Green et al., 1985). Administration of L-tryptophan to human volunteers at a dose of 50 mg/kg twice daily for 1 wk is sufficient to increase trytpophan clearance, suggesting that tryptophan pyrrolase is inducible in humans as well as animals (Green et al., 1985).

Pyridoxine is a cofactor necessary in the hepatic metabolism of kynurenine by kynureninase and kynurenine aminotransferase, but not by kynurenine hydroxylase (Martinsons et al., 1999). Pyridoxine supplementation has been shown to prevent the accumulation of kynurenine, which can occur with L-tryptophan supplementation (Green et al., 1985). Elevated serum levels of kynurenine inhibit transport of L-tryptophan into the brain, thus reducing central nervous system serotonin levels (Birdsall, 1998). Kynurenine may also be involved in the development of EMS (*see Eosinophilia-Myalgia Syndrone* section).

Nicotinamide is thought to be an inhibitor of tryptophan pyrrolase (Pakes, 1979) and has been coadministered along with L-tryptophan in some clinical trials (e.g., MacSweeney, 1975); however, a pharmacokinetic study showed that pretreament with nicotinamide 500 mg twice daily for 1 wk did not affect the pharmacokinetics of L-tryptophan (Green et al., 1985).

Tryptophan is transported into the brain by an active transport mechanism. This carrier is not specific for tryptophan; it also transports other amino acids, including phenylalanine, tyrosine, methionine (Pakes, 1979), valine, leucine, and isoleucine (Birdsall, 1998) into the central nervous system. Each of these amino acids can thus inhibit the others' transport into the brain, explaining the fall in tryptophan brain concentrations after a high-protein meal. Conversely, a high-carbohydrate meal or administration of insulin increases tryptophan in the brain, perhaps by lowering plasma concentrations of other amino acids (Pakes, 1979). Once in the brain, tryptophan is hydroxylated to 5-hydroxytryptophan (5-HTP) by tryptophan 5-hydroxylase, a step that may require ascorbic acid (vitamin C) as a cofactor. This is the rate-limiting enzyme in the conversion of tryptophan to serotonin (Birdsall, 1998). 5-HTP is then decarboxylated to 5-hydroxytryptamine (serotonin, 5-HT), a step that is thought to require pyridoxine as a cofactor. Serotonin is further metabolized by monoamine oxidase to 5-hydroxyindole acetic acid (Pakes, 1979). The biotransoformation of L-tryptophan into serotonin also occurs in the intestine, platelets, and mast cells as well as in the brain (Sidransky, 1997).

Because of their role as cofactors in the conversion of L-tryptophan to serotonin, pyridoxine and ascorbic acid have been coadministered with L-tryptophan in clinical trials (e.g., Coppen et al., 1972; Murphy et al., 1974; Prange et al., 1974; Dunner and Fieve, 1975; Rao and Broadhurst, 1976). Comparison of L-tryptophan supplementation in unipolar depression with or without pyridoxine 10 mg/g L-tryptophan and ascorbic acid 20 mg/g L-tryptophan failed to reveal a statistically significant difference between the two groups based on the HAM-D; however, there was a trend favoring pyridoxine and ascorbic acid supplementation (Coppen, 1976).

22.9. ADVERSE EFFECTS AND TOXICITY

22.9.1. Adverse Effects Noted in Clinical Trials

In the Herrington et al. study (1974) described previously, in which L-tryptophan 6–8 g/d was compared with ECT, serum electrolytes, hematologic values, plasma protein, and liver function tests (alanine aminotransferase and aspartate aminotransferae) were measured before treatment and after 4 wk of supplementation with L-tryptophan 6–8 g/d. Compared with baseline, both liver function tests were significantly higher ($p < 0.01$, ANOVA) in the ECT group, and aspartate aminotransferase rose significantly in the L-tryptophan group ($p < 0.01$), with 3 of 22 L-tryptophan patients having values above the upper limit of normal. The authors noted that occasionally some of the hematologic values were outside normal limits, but no consistent effect was noted with either treatment. In a subsequent study by these same investigators (Herrington et al., 1976) comparing L-tryptophan up to 8 g/d with amitriptyline, red blood cell count dropped significantly from baseline in both treatment groups ($p < 0.05$). As in their previous study, the investigators noted that some hematologic values were occasionally abnormal, but no consistent or definite association with either treatment was noted.

In the study by D'Elia et al. (1977) in which L-tryptophan 6 g/d plus ECT was compared with placebo plus ECT, 30 subjects were asked to rate the following adverse effects on a scale of 0 to 3: tremor, dizziness, palpitations, sweating, dry mouth, urinary difficulty, taste disturbance, nausea, constipation, diarrhea, flatulence, abdominal pain, blurred vision, speech disturbance, and nystagmus. The investigators compiled this list based on side effects reported in other studies of L-tryptophan. Blurred vision, speech disturbance, and nystagmus were not experienced by patients in this study, and the other side effects were rated as no greater than 1 in severity.

In the investigation previously discussed comparing chlorpromazine 400 mg with L-tryptophan 6 g in acute mania (Prange et al., 1974), patients completed a side effect check list three times a week for 2 wk. The most common side effect of L-tryptophan was drowsiness, occurring in 36.8% of 30 observations (five patients taking L-tryptophan were asked about side effects six times). Patients in the D'Elia et al. study (1977) were not asked about drowsiness. Other adverse effects that occurred in this small ($n = 10$) study that were not addressed in the D'Elia study included paresthesia (26.3% of 30 observations), palpitations (20%), excitation (15.8%), confusion (15%), headache (10.5%), poor concentration (10.5%), insomnia (10.5%), tinnitus (5.3%), and agitation (4.8%). Blurred vision was reported in 20% of observations. Although D'Elia and colleagues (1977) inquired about blurred vision, no patients reported it. Conversely, dry mouth and urinary difficulty were not reported by subjects in this study. As in the D'Elia et al. study, constipation (25%), dizziness (10.5%), sweating (10%), tremor (10%), and nausea (5%) were reported. The differences in reported side effects in these two studies suggest that adverse effects may depend upon the population being studied. In addition, the only adverse effect that was seen significantly more frequently in the L-tryptophan group than in the placebo group in a study of PMDD was dizziness ($p = 0.03$; Fisher's exact test) (Steinbert et al., 1999). Many of the side effects reproted in these studies might therefore actually be symptoms of the patient's underlying psychiatric condition.

In the study by Mendels and colleagues (1975), which involved both unipolar and bipolar patients, subjects were asked about side effects each morning. As in the D'Elia et al. study (1977), patients were asked to choose from a list of symptoms. The symptoms were associated not only with ingestion of amino acid precursors but also with depression itself. Side effects reported in L-tryptophan patients included increased sleep difficulty in one of two bipolar and in one of four unipolar patients given L-tryptophan. One of the six L-tryptophan patients became more irritable and angry.

Coppen and associates (1972), in their study comparing L-tryptophan with imipramine with and without liothyronine, interviewed subjects at the end of the study about side effects they had experienced. Subjects were asked to rate 21 symptoms on a scale from 0 to 4. Considering only the eight subjects who received L-tryptophan alone, dry mouth and trembling hands were the most bothersome adverse effects, with mean intensity scores of 2. In addition to many of the same adverse effects already discussed (i.e., blurred vision, dizziness, drowsiness, headache, metallic taste, nausea, palpitations, sweating, urinary difficulty), the eight subjects also reported unsteady walk, feelings of unreality, giddiness, muscle stiffness, stuffy nose, and urticaria. The mean intensity rating was no greater than 1.3 for any of these symptoms. Patients were also asked about diarrhea, faintness, flushing, and indigestion, but no patient admitted to experiencing these side effects.

22.9.2. LD_{50}

The median lethal dose (LD_{50}) for L-tryptophan in rats has been reported to be 1.6 g/kg, which would be equivalent to a dose of greater than 100 g in a 70-kg human (Sidransky, 1997). In one study (Gullino et al., 1956) of rats injected with the LD_{50} dose, death occurred within 5 h to 3 d. Symptoms of toxicity appearing 10 min to 2 h after injection included dyspnea, which was constant in the final moments before death; hypothermia, with rectal temperature as much as 4°C below normal; and extreme prostration, often accompanied by uncoordinated movement. Violent, spastic contraction of the skeletal muscles occurred in a few animals. At the time of death, rectal temperature was commonly 35°C. Autopsy of these animals revealed that the kidney and liver were the organs most affected, with both the renal tubules and liver parenchyma cells showing diffuse degeneration and vacuolization. Degeneration of the brain and spinal cord were noted. Congestion of the lungs was evident, and the spleen was decreased in size. Autopsy of rats surviving 10 d after injection showed no evidence of either gross or microscopic pathology.

The rate-limiting enzyme in the hepatic metabolism of L-tryptophan, tryptophan pyrrolase, is regulated by adrenal corticosteroids. In a rat study (Trulson and Ulissey, 1987), adrenalectomy decreased the L-tryptophan LD_{50} from more than 1 g/kg to 11.4 mg/kg, and administration of metyrapone, inhibitor of adrenal steroid sysnthesis, decreased the LD_{50} to 24.9 mg/kg. Hormone replacement with corticosterone in adrenalectomized rats restored the LD_{50} to normal. Adrenalectomized rats that died after receiving L-tryptophan at a dose of at least 25 mg/kg died within 2–6 h, and those that died after receiving doses of 2.5–12.5 mg/kg died within 18–24 h. In adrenalecto-mized rats, tissue concentrations of tryptamine were more than doubled, and plasma and liver tryptophan concentrations were elevated. These findings were explained by a decrease in tryptophan pyrrolase acivity of more than 50%. The excess tryptophan that could not be metabolized by tryptophan pyrrolase was decarboxylated to tryptamine, which can cause elevated blood pressure and other adverse cardiovascular effects. The death of the animals was attributed to an acute increase in tryptamine effects to which they could not adjust rapidly. These findings have potential implica-tions for humans with adrenal insufficiency, who could theoretically experience tox-icity at doses normally tolerated. The authors of this study suggest that adrenal function be tested prior to prescription of L-tryptophan.

22.9.3. Eosinophilia-Myalgia Syndrome

L-Tryptophan ingestion has been associated with eosiniphilia-myalgia syndrome (EMS). EMS is defined by the Centers for Disease Control and Prevention (CDC) as an eosinophil count of 1000 cells/mm^3 or more, myalgia severe enough to limit usual daily activity, and no evidence of infection or neoplasm that could explain either find-ing (Daniels et al., 1995). The syndrome was first reported on October 30, 1989, when the CDC and the New Mexico Health and Environment Department (Swygert et al., 1990) were notified of three patients taking L-tryptphan supplements who had pre-sented with myalgias, weakness, skin rash, and eosinophilia (Daniels et al., 1995). By November 17, 1989, 287 cases, including 1 death, had been identified in 37 states and the District of Columbia (Swygert et al., 1990). In total, more than 1500 cases, includ-ing at least 37 deaths, have been reported to the CDC (FDA, 2001), with most people developing symptoms between July 1989 and February 1990 (Varga et al., 1992). Almost all the cases had taken L-tryptophan. The median dose of L-tryptophan ingested was 1.5 g/d—approximately twice the usual dietary intake. The duration of ingestion varied from weeks to years, and in a few patients symptoms appeared after they had stopped taking L-tryptophan (Medsger, 1990).

Insomnia, L-tryptophan use as a hypnotic, L-tryptophan dose, and older age have been identified as independent risk factors for EMS (Back et al., 1993). EMS symp-toms generally evolve over approximately 1 wk and include severe muscle pain and subjective weakness. Arthralgia was reported in 73% of the cases that had been reported to the CDC as of July 10, 1990 (Swygert et al., 1990). Although muscle pain is a defining symptom of EMS, muscle biopsy reveals minimal evidence of myofibrillar degeneration. There can be, however, inflammation and fibrosis in the connective tissue surrounding the muscle (Varga et al., 1992). Creatine kinase is elevated in only 10% of patients (Swygert et al., 1990). Muscle pain and weakness, which in some cases persists or worsens after product discontinuation, might actually be secondary to neuropathy, suggested by itching, paresthesia, and electrophysiologic evidence of axonal degeneration (Medsger, 1990). Muscle and nerve biopsy reveals collagen depo-sition and perivascular inflammation with accumulation of lymphocytes, plasma cells, and eosinophils (Medsger, 1990) causing thickening of the vessel walls and endothe-lial swelling (Medsger, 1990; Varga et al., 1992). Epineural and perineural infiltration with mononuclear cells and eosinophils, loss of myelinated nerve fibers, and axonal degeneration are seen (Varga et al., 1992).

Clinically, ascending polyneuropathy resembling Guillain-Barré syndrome has occurred, leading to respiratory failure and death. Elevated serum and urine levels of kynurenine and eosinophil-derived neurotoxin have been noted and may be involved in the pathogenesis of EMS-associated neurotoxicity (Medsger, 1990), which was reported in 27% of patients (Swygert et al., 1990). Independent of respiratory failure caused by neuropathy, some cases reported to the CDC had dyspnea and mild hypoxemia secondary to pulmonary vascular disease, supported by findings of right ventricular strain, tricuspid insufficiency, and pulmonary hypertension (documented by cardiac catheterization). Sudden death occurred in a patient with reduced carbon monoxide diffusion capacity and normal chest X-ray (Medsger, 1990). Of 718 cases reported to the CDC for whom chest X-ray results were available, 17% had pulmonary infiltrates, 12% had pleural effusions, and 8% had both. Cough, dyspnea, and peripheral edema were reported in 59% of patients (Swygert et al., 1990). Induration of the subcutaneous tissues and fascia of the extremities and trunk resembling findings in localized forms of scleroderma (Medsger, 1990) were reported in 32–50% of cases (Swygert et al., 1990; Varga et al., 1992). Skin biopsy revealed thickening of the fascia and dermis caused by an inflammatory infiltrate with mucopolysaccharide and collagen deposition (Varga et al., 1992).

Morphea-like lesions resembling those seen in carcinoid syndrome (in which patients have elevated levels of serotonin, a metabolite of tryptophan) may appear late in the course of the disease (Medsger, 1990). A maculopapular or urticarial rash may occur early in the course of illness, and was reported in 60% of 1075 cases reported to the CDC. Alopecia was noted in 28% and fever in 36%. Hepatomegaly was reported in 5% of cases, and elevation of one or more liver function tests (i.e., bilirubin, aminotransferase enzymes, alkaline phosphatase, or γ-glutamyl transferase) was found in 43%. Other abnormal laboratory tests of note included leukocytosis (85% of patients) and elevated erythrocyte sedementation rate (33% of patients) (Swygert et al., 1990). Maximal eosinophil counts have ranged from 1000 to 36,000/mm^3 (mean 4800/mm^3), with bone marrow biopsy revealing eosinophilic hyperplasia and normal precursors (Varga et al., 1992).

Treatment of EMS with glucocorticoids may cause a rapid decrease in eosinophil count, but skin induration, myopathy, and neuropathy respond poorly. The long-term outcome of patients treated with prednisone does not differ from that of untreated patients. In the absence of controlled trials, no specific treatment for EMS can be recommended (Varga et al., 1992).

The epidemiologic studies suggesting a relationship between L-tryptophan ingestion and EMS have been critiqued by Shapiro (1996) and by Daniels and colleagues (1995), who have served as paid consultants to Showa Denko (Belongia and Gleich, 1996; Clauw and Pincus, 1996). The first two studies identifying an association between L-tryptophan and EMS were case-control studies in which patients with EMS in New Mexico (Eidson et al., 1990) and Minnesota (Anonymous, 1989) were matched with controls who did not have EMS. Subjects were asked about exposure to various substances. Eidson and colleagues (1990) found that 100% of patients with EMS had consumed L-tryptophan, compared with 9% of matched controls; the Minnesota study found that 100% of EMS patients had consumed L-tryptophan, compared with none of the controls. Daniels and colleagues (1995) point to problems with identification of cases in the New Mexico study, such as use of hospital laboratory records as opposed to physician office records to identify cases, thus potentially selecting more seriously ill patients who might be of generally worse health than controls and therefore more likely to use a dietary supplement such as L-tryptophan. Of the patients identified with eosinophil counts of 2000/mm^3 or higher, 50 had incapacitating myalgia according to hospital records. Eleven cases were identified after excluding those patients with 1 of 30 conditions known to be associated with eosinophilia. Cases with diseases known to be associated with myalgias were not excluded. Two controls, matched by age and gender, were chosen from neighbors of each identified case. The eosinophil count of the control patients was not checked, and no exclusion criteria were applied to the control patients. Data analysis revealed an association between EMS and consumption of pork sausage as well as L-tryptophan.

Daniels and colleagues (1995) also had concerns that exclusion criteria applied to the cases were not applied to the controls, such that those patients excluded as cases might have been from a population with a lower prevalence of exposure to L-tryptophan than controls. For example, cases (but not controls) with allergies were excluded. Such patients might be less likely than the population at large to use supplements because of fear of an allergic reaction to such products. These differences could bias the results in favor of an association between L-tryptophan and EMS. An additional potential bias identified by Daniels and associates (1995) was that the cases and controls were not matched for ethnicity, and the control group contained more Hispanic persons. This difference would be important if there are cultural differences in dietary supplement use or in propensity to complain about aches and pains. Another potential problem with the study was the failure of the investigators to determine the onset of symptoms in relationship to L-tryptophan exposure (Daniels et al., 1995). This problem—counting an exposure although the exposure occurred after the onset of symptoms—is known as temporal-precedence bias.

Of the Minnesota study (Anonymous, 1989), Daniels and colleagues (1995) had additional concerns. Patients were identified through interviews with local physicians from November 9 through 12. Because the physicians might have already heard about the suspected association between L-tryptophan and EMS, they might have been more apt to identify and refer patients taking L-tryptophan. This problem is known as selection bias. Awareness of the suspected association might also have led physicians to give patients with eosinophilia and myalgias who were not taking L-tryptophan a diagnosis other than EMS. This theory is supported by Wagner and colleagues' (1996) study of L-tryptophan and diagnostic bias, in which physicians were more likely to make the diagnosis of EMS in patients with a history of L-tryptophan use. In response to such concerns, Belongia and Gleich (1996) explained that media coverage did not begin until a press release was issued on November 12, 1989, after the data had been collected and data analysis was under way. Physicians were notified of the association through an advisory letter shortly thereafter.

According to Daniels and colleagues (1995), in neither study were the interviewers blinded to the study hypothesis or to whether a patient was a case or a control, perhaps causing interviewers to look harder for a possible exposure to L-tryptophan in cases than in controls. Investigators were, however, blinded to subjects' history of L-tryptophan exposure (Belongia and Gleich, 1996).

Despite these criticisms, these studies independently showed a strong association between a specific exposure and a specific set of symptoms. The consistent conclusions of these two studies—that there was a statistically significant association between L-tryptophan and EMS—led the FDA to request a voluntary recall of L-tryptophan from the market on November 17, 1989 (Archer, 1991).

After the recall, studies were undertaken to elucidate whether a particular L-tryptophan manufacturer or product ingredient was associated with EMS. Three studies (Slutsker et al., 1990; Belongia et al., 1990; Kamb et al., 1992) found a statistically significant relationship between L-tryptophan manufactured by Showa Denko and EMS. Daniels and colleagues (1995) identified several potential sources of bias in these studies. In one case-control study, performed in Oregon (Slutsker et al., 1990), cases were identified by physician referral from the entire state of Oregon, whereas controls (asymptomatic L-tryptophan users) came only from the Portland area. If the brand of L-tryptophan predominantly available in the Portland area differed from the predominant brand in the state as a whole, the results could favor one brand over another. It is also possible that the controls, who were self-referred, had different buying patterns than the cases, who were physician-referred. The fact that only 41% of the controls used the Showa Denko brand, although this company had 60–70% of the market share, supports this concern. In addition, unpublished data collected by Belongia and colleagues (1990) showed that 55% of the self-referred controls and only 26% of the cases purchased L-tryptophan at a health food store, whereas 57% of the cases and 11% of controls purchased L-tryptophan at a department store, which may have carried different products. Of the 380 self-referred controls, 347 were excluded owing to "illness." If the excluded control patients had purchasing habits similar to those of the case subjects, exclusion of "ill" controls could have biased the results to favor a particular brand, when in fact the prevalence of use of a particular brand in cases and controls might have been similar.

Another exclusion criterion that could have biased the study results was the exclusion of subjects who could not identify the manufacturer of the product they had taken (Daniels et al., 1995). In the study by Slutsker and colleagues (1990), 79% of cases, but only 44% of controls could identify the manufacturer of the product taken. In addition, Belongia and colleagues (1990) found that 58% of the cases but only 38% of the randomly selected controls could identify the manufacturer of the product they had taken. This difference was not statistically significant $p = 0.10$; Belongia and Gleich, 1996). This finding is the opposite of what one might predict given that controls were asked to identify the product they had taken most recently, whereas cases were asked about the product taken prior to onset of symptoms, which could have occurred months earlier. Bias in favor of the Showa Denko products may have resulted if there were differences in brand availability during the different time periods. Belongia and Gleich (1996) explained that because the median month of symptom onset in cases was September, and most controls stopped using the product in mid-November, there was only a 2–3-mo difference in the period of use for most cases and controls. Market share would be unlikely to change in such a short time. They also explained that cases were more likely to keep their product in hopes that it would provide an explanation for their symptoms, whereas controls would have simply discarded their L-tryptophan after the recall, thus leading to manufacturer identification in a higher number of cases than controls. This tendency for case subjects, compared with controls, to have more detailed or more accurate information about their exposure is known as recall bias.

Daniels and colleagues (1995) felt that because self-referred cases were more likely to purchase their products in a department store (Belongia et al., 1990), bias could result if there was a difference in the ability to identify the manufacturer based on where the product was purchased. In fact, one distributor of L-tryptophan manufactured by Showa Denko that sold its product primarily in department stores cooperated extensively with investigators to help identify the product manufacturer, perhaps leading to a disproportionately larger number of cases being linked to the Showa Denko product (Daniels et al., 1995). Subsequently, the Minnesota Department of Health conducted an aggressive traceback in which all United States distributors cooperated. Their findings supported the data of Belongia and colleagues (1990), with only one traceback error identified: a product originally identified as a non-Showa Denko product was found to have been manufactured by Showa Denko, thus further strengthening the association between the Showa Denko product and EMS (Belongia and Gleich, 1996).

Kamb and colleagues (1992) reviewed the charts of a psychiatrist in South Carolina who routinely recommended or prescribed L-tryptophan to his patients. Four hundred eighteen patients who had taken at least 5 doses of L-tryptophan between January 1 and October 31, 1989 were identified. Although 39% of these patients had used a product manufacturered by Showa Denko, only 11% met the CDC definition of EMS, and another 16% had symptoms that suggested EMS but did not meet the CDC definition. All the patients with EMS or EMS-like symptoms had used a Showa Denko product; thus, 52% of the patients who had used a Showa Denko experienced EMS or EMS-like symptoms. Problems identified in this study were inclusion of products that were purchased after the onset of symptoms, complaint of "cramps" counting as myalgia in a subject who had taken the Showa Denko product but not counting as myalgia in a subject who had taken another brand, and questionable ability to identify product manufacturers definitively.

The authors of the South Carolina study (Kamb et al., 1992) subsequently followed up in August 1992 with 242 of the original 418 patients or their proxies (Sullivan et al., 1996). The participants were similar to nonparticipants (who were either unable to be contacted or apparently did not choose to participate) in demographics and dose of L-tryptophan taken in 1989. Seventy-six percent had a history of depression, and 77% were using at least one medication. Benzodiazepines were used by 49% of the participants between January 1989 and August 1992. Nineteen percent of patients were taking a corticosteroid, and two (<1%) were taking methotrexate.

Of the 418 original patients, 23 (5.5%) had died. Among all patients who took Showa Denko L-trytophan, 14 of 161 (9%) had died, which was approximately twice the expected number (6.5 deaths). Nine of the 14 deaths were in EMS patients, although the expected mortality for the EMS group based on age and sex was 2.5 persons. Of the additional deaths, three were in patients with EMS-like symptoms, and two were in asymptomatic patients. When all 418 patients were considered, the death rate was three times higher in patients with EMS. Of the nine deaths in EMS patients, EMS was listed as the cause of death on the death certificates of two patients and was listed as a significant condition on one other. Significant conditions listed in the hospital charts of the two patients whose deaths were attributed to EMS were polyneuropathy and respiratory arrest, and polyneuropathy and arrhythmias. EMS was listed as a significant condition on the death certificate or in the hospital chart of five other patients. Causes of death in these patients included renal failure, myeloproliferative disorder, atherosclerosis, coronary artery disease, and poor nutrition. Six of the nine deaths in EMS patients occurred within 18 mo of symptom onset.

Of the surviving patients who had experienced EMS or EMS-like symptoms in 1990, myalgia was the most common symptom still experienced, although the prevalence had decreased compared with the previous study. Sclerodermiform skin changes, arthralgia, rashes, and neuropathy had also improved in the interim. Of the six EMS patients who had progressive ascending neuropathy in 1990, two had died, two were seriously disabled, and two were functioning well. Patients with EMS who had taken relatively lower L-tryptophan doses were more likely to report resolution of sclerodermiform skin changes. Two patients with EMS and one with EMS-like symptoms were subsequently diagnosed with fibromyositis or fibromyalgia. Between 1990 and 1992, 4% of these patients developed new onset of neurologic disorders, 4% developed new-onset depression, and 12% developed Sjogren's syndrome. In contrast, the prevalence of myalgias increased in patients who were not reportedly ill in 1989 from 6% in 1990 to 30% in 1992. Increased symptoms might have been caused by publicity surrounding EMS, advancing age, somatization, error associated with self-report of symptoms, or higher participation among symptomatic individuals. Neuralgias also increased in this group from 8% in 1990 to 23% in 1992. Prior use of Showa Denko L-tryptophan was not associated with the presence of symptoms in 1992. None of the patients who were asymptomatic in 1990 developed symptoms matching the CDC definition of EMS, and none with an EMS-like symptoms in 1989 went on to develop EMS. Lab results (eosinophils, hemoglobin, complete white blood cell count, platelets, liver function tests, and electrolytes) were within normal limits for all patients in 1992. These findings suggest that delayed onset of EMS is unlikely to occur and that EMS symptoms improve over time.

Belongia and colleagues (1990) identified three manufacturing changes (use of a new strain of bacteria in the fermentation process, a decrease in the amount of powdered carbon used in the purification process, and bypass of a filtration step) at Showa Denko that may have been associated with EMS, based on lot numbers on products consumed by cases vs controls. These changes occurred in late 1988 or early 1989; however, the investigators of this study, as well as Slutsker and colleagues (1990), excluded patients whose symptoms began prior to the summer of 1989 in order to provide a more homogenous study group in regard to timing of L-tryptophan exposure. Daniels and colleagues (1995) felt that exclusion of these cases could bias the results in favor of an association between the new manufacturing process and EMS; however, inclusion of such cases would have further strengthened the association between Showa Denko L-tryptophan and EMS. It is possible that the 1988 cases were caused by a toxic contaminant present in sporadic lots, or that it was present in a lower concentration than in 1989 (Belongia and Gleich, 1996).

Belongia and colleagues (1990), using high-performance liquid chromatography (HPLC), identified an absorbance peak that they called *peak E* in 9 of 12 lots used by case subjects and 3 of 11 lots used by controls. There was a statistically significant association between the presence of this chemical and case lots. It was concluded that this peak may be the cause of or contribute to EMS, or that it may be a marker for another chemical constituent involved in the pathogenesis of the disorder. It was later determined that the chemical represented by peak E, 1,1'-ethylidenebis-L-tryptophan (EBT) was present to some degree in all case and control lots of L-tryptophan and that there was a statistically significant association between an additional chemical, 3-(phenylamino)alanine (PAA), and case lots (Daniels et al., 1995).

The association between EMS and L-tryptophan or a product contaminant remains unclear. Administration of EBT to rats causes some but not all of the pathology associated with EMS, and even uncontaminated L-tryptophan caused myofascial thickening and pancreatic fibrosis in these studies (FDA, 2001). Furthermore, neither PAA or the case lots themselves have been shown to cause EMS in animal studies (Simat et al., 1999). Although there is no animal model that definitively demonstrates that L-tryptophan or any identified contaminant causes EMS (Clauw, 1996), EBT has been shown to cause inflammation and fibrosis in dermal and subcutaneous tissue of C57BL/6 mice, as well as increased expression of genes that encode for collagen. In addition, EBT stimulates collagen production in vitro. Pure L-tryptophan appears to affect dermal collagen gene expression as well, but to a lesser extent than EBT (Suzuki et al., 1996). Consistent with these findings, fascia, subcutaneous adipose tissue, dermis, and fibroblasts from EMS patients show increased type I collagen gene expression (Varga et al., 1990).

Eight years prior to the EMS epidemic, an epidemic referred to as toxic oil syndrome (TOS) was identified in Spain. Although EMS and TOS were similar in regard to symptomatology, TOS was associated with rapeseed oil containing 3-(phenylamino)-1,2-propanediol (PAP). PAP has been shown to be metabolized in vitro by both rats and humans to the tryptophan contaminant PAA. This suggests a common etiologic agent for both syndromes (Mayeno et al., 1995). PAA is also known as peak UV-B. Other case-associated contaminants include peak 200 [2-(3-indolylmethyl)-L-tryptophan], peak C, also known as 3α-hydroxy-1,2,3,3a,8,8a-hexahydropyrrolo-[2-3b]-indole-2-carboxylic acid, and peak FF [2-(2-hydroxy- indoline)-tryptophan]. The presence of an indole ring in these compounds may facilitate formation of protein adducts upon ingestion of the contaminated product (Naylor et al., 1999).

L-Tryptophan supplements had been available in the United States since approximately 1974 (Medsger, 1990). Interestingly, the following year a syndrome of diffuse fasciitis with eosinophilia was first described (Shulman, 1975). It is important to note that many people who consumed L-tryptophan, even the Showa Denko product, did not develop EMS (FDA, 2001), and 3% of the cases reported to the CDC did not have a history of L-tryptophan consumption (Swygert et al., 1990). In one study case-control study (Flockhart et al., 1994), a higher percentage of patients with EMS lacked the hepatic drug-metabolizing enzyme CYP2D6 than controls $p = 0.007$; Mantel-Haenszel chi-squared). In addition, a higher percentage of EMS cases were deficient in CYP2C19 activity (p 0.005). It is possible that EMS is caused by an abnormality of L-tryptophan metabolism. An interaction between a prescription medication and enzymes that metabolize L-tryptophan could also be responsible.

As already discussed, skin lesions resembling those seen in carcinoid syndrome may appear in EMS sufferers (Medsger, 1990). Patients with carcinoid syndrome have elevated levels of the tryptophan metabolite serotonin. Serotonin stimulates the synthesis of collagen by cultured lung fibroblasts and causes dermal and synovial fibrosis in experimental animals (Varga et al., 1992).

As mentioned previously, some patients with EMS were noted to have elevated serum and urine levels of kynurenine, a tryptophan metabolite, which may be involved in the pathogenesis of EMS. Serum kynurenine levels were highest in untreated patients with the most active disease. It should be noted, however, that elevated kynurenine is a nonspecific finding common to several inflammatory conditions, including systemic sclerosis and eosinophilic fasciitis (Varga et al., 1992). This is because indolamine 2,3 dioxygenase, an enzyme involved in the production of kynurenine, is induced by interferon-γ during bacterial, viral, and autoimmune disorders (Martinsons et al., 1999). Kynureninase and kynurenine aminotransferase are pyridoxyl-5-phosphate-dependent enzymes involved in the metabolism of kynurenine; thus, pyridoxine (vitamin B6) deficiency can also increase kynurenine levels. The kidney is one location for the formation of pyridoxine-5-phosphate, as well as elimination of kynurenine (Martinsons et al., 1999). Renal failure, autoimmune disorders, infectious disease, and dietary vitamin B6 deficiency could theoretically be risk factors for development of EMS if kynurenine is, indeed, involved in the pathogenesis of EMS.

A case of EMS in which the kynurenine level was approximately three times normal and the L-tryptophan level was unusually low supports an abnormality of L-tryptophan metabolism as the cause of EMS. In this report (Hisatomi et al., 1997), a Japanese woman taking 1 g L-tryptophan daily presented with painful swelling of the extremities and an elevated eosinophil count. Both L-tryptophan and kynurenine levels normalized after 42 d of treatment with prednisone 40 mg/d, presumably because prednisone inhibits indoleamine 2,3-dioxygenase, the rate-limiting enzyme in the kynurenine pathway of L-tryptophan metabolism. Interestingly, serotonin levels were unchanged throughout the course of illness.

Another L-tryptophan metabolite, quinolinic acid, is a dicarboxylic acid that acts as a potent neurotoxin. It has been implicated in the pathogenesis of Huntington's disease, hepatic encephalopathy, and HIV-associated encephalopathy. Increased plasma levels of L-tryptophan induce enzymes involved in the production of kynurenines, and extracellular fluid concentrations of quinolinic acid following L-tryptophan loading equal or exceed those that have been shown to be neurotoxic in vitro. In addition, patients with severe EMS-associated neuropathy have increased cerebrospinal fluid levels of quinolinic acid. However, in contrast to the histologic findings in EMS, quinolinic acid-associated neurologic lesions are axon-sparing (Varga et al., 1992).

In light of the possibility that accumulation of L-tryptophan metabolites may have been involved in the pathogenesis of EMS, additional information from both cases and controls about concomitant disease states or use of medications that alter L-tryptophan metabolism would be potentially informative. Corticosteroids, adrenocorticotropic hormone, alcohol, antidepressants, and some cytokines can all influence the activity of enzymes involved in L-tryptophan metabolism (Varga et al., 1992). In the study by Kamb and colleagues (1992), all patients came from a psychiatric practice and were on many medications, including naproxen, trimipramine, and clonazepam, all of which are associated with both eosinophilia and myalgia. Although the investigators did not find an association between any class of prescription medication and EMS, perhaps analyzing the data separately for those drugs known to cause EMS-like symptoms would have revealed such an association.

Although the number of cases of EMS declined after the recall of L-tryptophan, this decline actually began prior to the recall of L-trypophan and may represent a decrease in publicity about EMS. In Canada, where L-tryptophan is available by prescription, Spitzer and colleagues (1994) identified 12 cases fitting the CDC's definition of EMS between July 1992 and June 1993; however, none of these patients had a history of L-tryptophan use. This information suggests that EMS is a collection of symptoms caused by other disorders observed in patients who were coincidentally taking L-tryptophan. For example, other disorders resembling EMS include eosinophilic fascitis and idiopathic hypereosinophilic syndrome (Varga et al., 1992). It has also been suggested that because L-tryptophan was promoted for the treatment of insomnia and depression, the EMS patients reported during the 1989 epidemic might have in fact been suffering from fibromyalgia, which is associated with depression, insomia, and several of the symptoms reported in EMS cases, including myalgias, arthralgias, and paresthesia. Although fibromyalgia does not cause eosinophilia, the eosinophilia might have been caused by L-tryptophan taken to treat symptoms of undiagnosed fibromyalgia (Hudson et al., 1996).

An explanation of the pathogenesis of EMS that would explain its similarity to other eosinophilic disorders is the ability of eosinophils to participate in the development of fibrosis. In vitro, eosinophil extracts are capable of causing fibroblast proliferation. Major basic protein secreted by eosinophils can cause release of fibrogenic cytokines such as transforming growth factor-β, which is associated with several fibrotic conditions. Eosinophils themselves can also produce transforming growth factor-α, which can cause fibroblast proliferation and connective tissue deposition. Eosinophils are known to participate in systemic sclerosis, another fibrotic human disease (Varga et al., 1992).

22.9.4. Sexual Dysfunction

Decreased sexual function has also been reported as a side effect of L-tryptophan ingestion (Sicuteri and Del Bene, 1975). The first case was a 42-yr-old university professor who was treated with L-tryptophan for intense and persistent headache. The patient reported partial improvement of headache, but because of anorgasmia, ejaculatory failure, and decreased libido, the patient discontinued L-tryptophan. Within 1–2 d, sexual activity returned to normal. The patient was rechallenged and dechallenged from L-tryptophan four additional times, each time with normalization of sexual function after L-tryptophan withdrawal. Another case involved a 48-yr-old physician who complained of intense, throbbing headaches at the nape of the neck and temple. The headaches occurred daily, were accompanied by nausea and vomiting, and were unresponsive to analgesics and ergotamine. The patient also reported a history of hypersexuality since adolescence. This sexual preoccupation had increased over the previous 2 yr, coinciding with onset of the headaches. The patient was admitted to the hospital for workup, but no cause for his symptoms was revealed. L-Tryptophan 4 g/d was prescribed. After beginning L-tryptophan, both the headaches and hypersexuality improved within the first week. The headaches eventually disappeared, and the sexual compulsions occurred only two to three times a week, as compared with several times daily prior to beginning L-tryptophan. After 2 mo of treatment, L-tryptophan was discontinued. Within a few weeks the headaches and hypersexuality returned to baseline. Placebo was administered, with no improvement of either problem. L-Tryptophan was readministered, with dramatic improvement of both problems.

22.9.5. Pregnancy

Beginning in the fourth month of pregnancy and continuing until delivery, a 27-yr-old woman ingested L-tryptophan 1000 mg/d for treatment of insomnia and hyperemesis gravidarum. Two weeks after starting L-tryptophan, the woman complained of a blistering rash after brief sun exposure, as well as severe leg cramps and myalgias, which resolved spontaneously after several weeks despite continuation of L-tryptophan. On the first day of life, her infant was found to have a white blood cell count of 22,200/mm^3 with 4% eosinophils, 33% polymorphonuclear leukocytes, 51% lymphocytes, and 8% monocytes. The infant was discharged but was readmitted on day 22 to rule out infection. White blood cell count was again elevated, at 29,700/mm^3, with 11% eosinophils and 65% lymphocytes. Platelet count was slightly elevated at 587,000/mm^3. Infection was ruled out. Eosinophilia, leukocytosis, thrombocytosis, and low-grade fever persisted for several months. At 6 mo, the infant was again hospitalized to rule out apnea. During hospitalization, one episode of apnea was documented, and the infant was discharged with an apnea monitor. The infant did not meet the case definition of EMS because myalgias could not be diagnosed. The authors concluded that one of the more likely causes of the infant's eosinophilia was transplacental transfer of contaminated L-tryptophan (Hatch et al., 1991).

22.9.6. Carcinogenesis

Sidransky (1997) has reviewed studies relating tryptophan to carcinogenesis. The results of several studies suggest that L-tryptophan is a promoter (a substance that does not itself cause cancer without the prior application of an initiating substance). Actions of L-tryptophan linking it to the neoplastic process include its ability to stimulate transcription and translation of enzymes that can biotransform various chemicals to carcinogenic substances (or, conversely, to deactivate other carcinogens) and its ability to increase activity of ornithine decarboxylase, the activity of which correlates with cell proliferation.

The results of animal studies on tryptophan's action as a bladder cancer promoter, as well as the structural similarity between known bladder carcinogens and the aromatic ring structure of tryptophan and its metabolites, led to studies of urine concentrations of tryptophan metabolites in patients with bladder cancer, who were found to have relatively high urinary concentrations of kynurenine. Interestingly, bladder cancer occurs only rarely in cats, which excrete tryptophan metabolites in very low concentrations (Brown and Price, 1956).

The mutagenicity of urinary tryptophan metabolites has been investigated. The L-tryptophan metabolites 3-hydroxy-L-kynurenine and 3-hydroxyanthranilic acid are mutagenic in mammalian cells (Bryan, 1971). Pyrrolysis products of tryptophan, such as those isolated from burnt meat, are metabolized to mutagenic substances by monooxygenase systems in the rat intestine, liver, and bladder epithelial cells. L-Tryptophan itself is not mutagenic (Sidransky, 1997). This does not rule out L-tryptophan as a tumor promoter, because promoters are generally not mutagenic or have only weak mutagenic activity. In contrast, most initiators are mutagenic in in vitro assays and may be complete carcinogens if applied in sufficient doses (Cohen et al., 1979). Several L-tryptophan metabolites, including L-kynurenine, acetyl-L-kynurenine, 3-hydroxy-d,L-kynurenine, 3-hydroxy-L-kynurenine, 3-hydroxyanthranilic acid, 3-methoxyanthranilic acid, 3-ethoxyanthranilic acid, 8-methyl ether of xanthurenic acid, xanthurenic acid, 8-hydroxyquinaldic acid, and quinaldic acid, are carcinogenic if applied directly to the bladder in experimental animals (Bryan, 1971). It should be noted that dietary administration of L-tryptophan or its metabolites, as opposed to direct application to the bladder, is unable to cause bladder tumors without prior application of an initiator.

The promoting effect of D,L-tryptophan on breast and liver cancer has been demonstrated in rats, but results are inconsistent, with some studies actually showing a protective effect. The reason for these discrepant results is not apparent, but they could be caused by a protective effect of loss of body weight in the tryptophan-supplemented rats, other dietary factors, stimulation of hepatic microsomal enzymes that inactivate chemical carcinogens, or antioxidant activity of L-tryptophan metabolites (Sidransky, 1997).

22.9.7. Bladder Tumors

Much study has been done on the association between tryptophan and bladder tumors in experimental animals. Dunning and coworkers (1950) were the first to report that tryptophan might play a role in bladder carcinogenesis. In this study, female Fisher rats fed a diet supplemented with 1.4 or 4.3% D,L-tryptophan and 0.06% 2-acetylaminofluorene exhibited a high incidence (100 and 92%, respectively) of bladder carcinomas. Bladder cancer did not develop in rats receiving 2-acetylaminofluorene without tryptophan supplementation. The investigators noted that despite consuming an isocaloric diet, these rats lost 20 and 40%, respectively, of their body weight, perhaps owing to amino acid imbalance. The investigators suggested that this imbalance, or D,L-tryptophan itself, was a factor in initiation of bladder cancer.

Eight purebred beagle dogs were fed a diet supplemented with D,L-tryptophan 6 g/d for 1 1/2 mo (Dog 5), 3 1/2 mo (dog 6), 14 mo (dog 7), 15 1/2 mo (dog 8), 55 mo (dog 1), 60 mo (dog 2), 81 mo (dog 3), and 83 mo (dog 4) to evaluate tryptophan's tumorigenic potential (Radomski et al., 1971). No bladder tumors were produced. However, in dogs 1, 2, and 4, the bladder mucosa was found to be darkened and covered with circular grey-white areas 1–2 cm in diameter. These gray-white areas observed grossly were thought to be caused by lymphocytic and macrophagic infiltration of the submucosa. There was also marked focal hyperplasia of the transitional epithelium of the bladder, accompanied by stromal edema. The cytoplasm of the transitional cells was frequently observed to contain vesicles surrounding the nucleus, which was described as having a clear or slightly hemophilic cast. In dog 1, large areas of the bladder were denuded of transitional cells; however, the bladder of dog 3 appeared almost normal grossly. Histologically, there was only slight hyperplasia, but as in the other three dogs, cytoplasmic vesicles were seen surrounding the nucleus. Dog 5 had no bladder pathology, but examination of the bladder of dog 6 revealed marked hyperplasia and the presence of hemosiderin-laden macrophages. These changes are consistent with a picture of chronic irritation occurring in the mucosa and submucosa in response to the administration of the D,L-tryptophan. The bladders of dogs 6 and 7 were also markedly hyperplastic, with lymphocytic and macrophagic infiltration and hyperemia of the submucosa. In dog 7, squamous metaplasia of the transitional epithelium and a microscopic hyperplastic papillary projection were noted. These changes were consistent with chronic irritation of the bladder.

Although no bladder tumors were produced, the investigators could not exclude the possibility that tryptophan may play a role in the induction of bladder tumors. It should be noted that D,L-tryptophan rather than L-tryptophan was used in this study because of its comparatively low cost. Even though the effect of the D-isomer could not be ruled out, the investigators felt that because the D-isomer of amino acids is frequently converted to the L-isomer, the observed effects were probably caused by L-tryptophan.

Other investigators (Miyakawa and Yoshida, 1973) studied the effects of a pyridoxine-deficient diet containing 1.4% D,L-tryptophan on 16 male Wistar rats. The control group was fed a regular pellet diet. After 56 wk, the rats were sacrificed. One hour prior to sacrifice, the rats were injected with tritiated thymidine, and autoradiograms of the bladder revealed increased labeling of [^{3}H]thymidine in bladder epithelial cells in comparison with controls ($p < 0.01$). Histologic examination revealed normal transitional epithelium with no mitotic figures, hyperplasia, or tumors. The investigators explained that although the D-isomer of tryptophan converts to the L-isomer and enters the normal metabolic pathway in rats, it was noted that large amounts of the D-isomer were excreted in the urine in the experimental rats. Therefore, the effects on the bladder epithelium could have been caused, at least in part, by D-tryptophan. In addition, because pyridoxine deficiency blocks purine biosynthesis, causing a relative increase in thymidine uptake, the observed increase in [^{3}H]thymidine uptake may have been caused by the effect of pyridoxine deficiency on DNA synthesis. The investigators concluded that because Radomski and colleagues (1971) showed that long-term administration of D,L-tryptophan in dogs caused hyperplasia of the bladder epithelium, the ability of tryptophan metabolites to stimulate DNA synthesis in the bladder epithelium could not be ruled out.

Recall that Radomski and colleagues (1971) concluded that L-tryptophan might play a role in bladder cancer via chronic irritation of the mucosa, a common action of tumor promoters. Cohen and colleagues (1979) designed an experiment to explore the promotion phase of bladder carcinogeneis. *N*-[4-(5-nitro-2-furyl)-2-thiazolyl]formamide (FANFT) is a known bladder carcinogen. These investigators had demonstrated in a previous study that FANFT acts as an initiator when administered at a low dose for a short period. In this study, FANFT was used as an initiator, and L-tryptophan was used as a promoter. Experimental rats were fed a chow diet containing 0.2% FANFT for 6 weeks, a dose and duration of therapy known not to produce bladder tumors if followed by a control diet. This was followed by a chow diet containing 2% D,L-tryptophan for 98 wk, or by 6 wk of control diet followed by 92 wk of D,L-tryptophan. Control animals received control diet alone; FANFT alone; control diet followed by d,L-tryptophan; control diet followed by FANFT; or FANFT followed by control.

Ten of 19 rats given FANFT followed by D,L-tryptophan, and 10 of 20 rats given FANFT followed by control diet for 6 wk and D,L-tryptophan for 92 wk developed bladder tumors. None of the remaining rats exposed to both FANFT and D,L-tryptophan had normal bladders; eight had simple hyperplasia, six had nodular or papillary hyperplasia, and 6 were found to have papilloma. Although only 4 of 20 rats given FANFT for 6 wk followed by control diet developed bladder cancer, the development of tumors in this group was unexpected in light of the investigators' previous study. All rats given FANFT for more than 6 wk developed bladder cancer. Although none of the 42 rats given the control diet alone developed bladder cancer, 4 had simple hyperplasia of the bladder epithelium, and 1 had nodular or papillary hyperplasia. Similar results were seen in the rats that received the control diet followed by D,L-tryptophan. The investigators concluded that D,L-tryptophan demonstated tumor-promoting acitivity but that it did not itself induce tumors.

The results of a subsequent study by Birt and colleagues (1987) did not support the hypothesis that excess dietary L-tryptophan promotes FANFT-induced bladder carcinogenesis. In this study, rats were fed FANFT for 4 wk, followed by control diet, L-tryptophan excess (2% dietary L-tryptophan), pyridoxine-deficient diet, or pyridoxine-deficient diet with L-tryptophan excess. The highest incidence of bladder tumors (40%) occurred in rats fed FANFT for 4 wk followed by a control diet. Twenty-nine percent of rats supplemented with 2% L-tryptophan developed bladder tumors, whereas 28% of those fed a pyridoxine-deficient diet with 2% L-tryptophan developed bladder tumors. Only 13% of rats fed a pyridoxine-deficient diet without excess L-tryptophan developed bladder tumors. Tumors at sites other than the bladder were highest in rats fed a pyridoxine-deficient diet with excess L-tryptophan. These results suggest that the amount of dietary pyridoxine relative to L-tryptophan might influence the development of tumors following FANFT initiation. The decrease in body weight noted in the rats fed excess L-tryptophan might also have had a protective effect against carcinogeneisis, as suggested by other investigators.

Despite the experimental data implicating L-tryptophan as a carcinogen, the association between L-tryptophan and human malignancy is unclear. There is a single case report (Bohme et al., 1998) of a patient taking L-tryptophan who presented with chronic B-cell leukemia (CLL) and EMS. Treatment with cyclophosphamide and prednisone led to resolution of both disorders, although the CLL returned several years later without EMS. Although malignant fibrous histiocytoma has been reported following EMS, this is the only report of EMS or L-tryptophan ingestion associated with a lymphocytic malignancy. Because some malignancies can present with eosinophilic syndromes, EMS must be differentiated from malignancy-associated eosinophilic syndromes.

22.10. INTERACTIONS

In a placebo-controlled study evaluating D,L-tryptophan's ability to augment the efficacy of monoamine oxidase inhibitors (MAOIs) in depressive illness, the hypotensive effect of phenelzine (Parnate®) was potentiated by tryptophan. Many patients taking combination therapy also reported feeling drowsy or drunk, and two patients complained of ataxia. The symptoms were not reported in the control group (Coppen et al., 1963).

In a subsequent placeo-controlled study of D,L-tryptophan in combination with the MAOI tranylcypromine (Glassman and Platman, 1969), side effects were described as "not frequent." No study patients experienced significant blood pressure fluctuations. The investigators do report that in a previous study, one patient receiving a MAOI took a single dose of tryptophan 18–20 g and experienced increased deep tendon reflexes, muscle twitching, and clonus of the masseter muscles. These symptoms resolved spontaneously in approximately 12 h. They also describe a patient not included in their study taking phenelzine who developed orthostasis and generalized tremor the day after the final dose of tryptophan. Tryptophan was restarted and tapered over 5 d, with a return of symptoms when the taper was complete. Phenelzine was discontinued, and symptoms resolved over the following 3 d. Whether these symptoms were caused by a drug interaction between L-tryptophan and phenelzine, a tryptophan withdrawal syndrome, or phenelzine itself is unclear.

Brotman and Rosenbaum (1984) described insomnia, profuse sweating, jerking of the extremities, ataxia, and polyuria in a 36-yr-old woman after a single dose of tryptophan 2 g. Tryptophan had been prescribed to augment the effects of phenelzine 60 mg/d, which she had been taking for atypical depression for 6 mo. Twelve hours after taking tryptophan, the patient had difficulty driving, was anxious, and had difficulty concentrating at work. Her blood pressure was checked by a nurse at work, who noted that it was somewhat labile, with diastolic pressures ranging from 95 to 105 mmHg over several h. Blood pressure normalized within 3–4 h. The patient was sent home from work, and her symptoms resolved approximately 24 h after taking tryptophan. She was not rechallenged with tryptophan but continued to take phenelzine without incident.

Levy and colleagues (1985) reported three similar cases in which patients who were taking a MAOI developed a transient syndrome of myoclonus, hyperreflexia, jaw quivering, teeth chattering, and diaphoresis after L-tryptophan ingestion. Each of the three patients had been tapered off a high dose of a tricyclic (imipramine 250 mg, doxepin 300 mg) or tetracyclic antidepressant (maprotiline 300 mg) over 2 d and switched to phenelzine. In one case, the reason for the switch was development of tremors and myoclonic jerks while on imipramine. The other two patients were switched because of treatment failure. In all three cases, L-tryptophan 2 g was added for treatment of insomnia. Within 3 h of taking L-tryptophan, one patient, who had been taking phenelzine 60 mg daily for 2 wk, awoke with myoclonic jerking, unsteady gait, and a "drunken" feeling that persisted for 8–10 h. The patient was rechallenged the next night and again developed myoclonus, teeth chattering, hyperreflexia, and diaphoresis within 2 h of the dose. Symptoms persisted for approximately 12 h. In the additional two cases, the use of a single dose of L-tryptophan within 3 d of beginning phenelzine resulted in no adverse reaction. The patients' phenelzine dosages were increased from 60 mg daily to 105 and 90 mg by week 2 and day 4, respectively. Within 2 h of taking L-tryptophan, the patient taking phenelzine 105 mg and lithium (blood level 0.9 mEq/L) experienced myoclonus, teeth chattering, jaw quivering, hyperreflexia, and diphoresis, which lasted approximately 12 h. The other patient awoke feeling restless and exhibited teeth chattering. Both symptoms subsided within 1 h. She was rechallenged with L-tryptophan the following night and experienced more pronounced teeth chattering, jaw quivering, hyerreflexia, and diaphoresis, which lasted approximately 8 h.

Other authors have reported mental status changes with the combination of L-tryptophan and a MAOI. A 20-yr-old woman with depression and anorexia nervosa requiring hospitalization experienced partial response to a 5-wk course of tranylcypromine 50 mg/d. L-Tryptophan 1 g was added at bedtime. The dose was increased to 2 g the second night. Within hours, she became confused and disoriented and was unable to remember familiar nurses' names or locate her room. Symptoms resolved overnight. Another patient, a 33-yr-old woman who had been taking tranylcypromine 40 mg/d for depression, experienced myoclonic jerking, shivering, confusion, agitation, and disorientation within hours of taking L-tryptophan 6 g, despite being titrated upward to this dose over a 2-wk period. Her symptoms required hospitalization and restraints. She became oriented by the next morning, but her movement disorders did not resolve for 2–3 d (Pope et al., 1985).

Two case reports have described fatal malignant hyperthermia occurring after combination therapy with L-tryptophan, lithium, and phenelzine. In one report, malignant hyperthermia was diagnosed in a 42-yr-old woman taking phenelzine 15 mg three times daily, lithium carbonate 800 mg/d, L-tryptophan 1 g/d, diazepam 2 mg three times daily, and triazolam 0.25 mg/d (Brennan et al., 1988). She presented to the emergency room with restlessness, sweating, confusion, and a temperature of 38.5°C. Within 3 h of presentation, she was comatose, with nonreactive pupils, absent corneal reflexes, and brisk tendon reflexes with flexor plantar response. Trunk and extremities were hypertonic and held in rigid hyperextension. One hour later, her temperature was 42.5°C, and she was tachycardic and hypotensive. She was treated with dantrolene within 4 h, and temperature returned to normal within 14 h. Blood pressure and temperature returned to normal with treatment with dopamine and practolol (a β-blocker).

The patient experienced severe disseminated intravascular coagulation (DIC) requiring infusion of blood products, as well as acute renal failure necessitating peritoneal dialysis. Mechanical ventilation was also required. Cerebrospinal fluid was normal, and blood and urine cultures were negative. A lithium serum level drawn on admission was 0.38 mmol/L (normal 0.5–1 mmol/L). Diazepam and its metabolite nordiazepam were also detected in the serum, but no tricyclic antidepressants were detected. An assay for MOAIs could not be performed. Abnormal lab values included mild leukocytosis, a peak creatine phosphokinase of 41,355 U/L (normal 24–175 U/L), elevated liver transaminases and alkaline phosphatase, and sudden severe hypoglycemia. On hospital day 6, the patient expired after repeated episodes of asystole. Autopsy revealed centilobular hepatocellular necrosis and glomerular thrombi.

In a second published case (Staufenberg and Tantam, 1989), a patient had, in the 6 mo prior to developing malignant hyperthermia, taken chlorpromazine 325–600 mg/d, trazodone 300 mg/d, L-tryptophan 3–6 g/d, and lithium 800 mg/d in combination without incident. At the time of her death, the patient was taking chlorpromazine 300 mg/d, lithum 800 mg/d, L-tryptophan 6 g/d, and phenelzine 45 mg/d. Approximately 1 1/2 mo after phenelzine was added to the patient's medication regimen, she was found lying on the floor, incontinent. She was transported to the hospital, where she was incoherent and was noted to have cogwheel muscle rigidity, nystagmus, hyperreflexia, Babinski sign, and a temperature of 38.8°C. Blood glucose, electrolytes, and complete blood cell count were normal. Blood cultures were negative. Chest X-ray was clear, and lumbar puncture revealed no cells or protein. A diagnosis of neuroleptic malignant syndrome was made, and procyclidine 10 mg was given. Her temperature increased to 42°C, and cardiac and respiratory arrest followed. Despite pacing and other resuscitatory efforts for over 1 h, the patient expired. The only significant autopsy findings were a small amount of hemorrhagic fluid in the right pleural cavity and pulmonary edema, attributed to cardiopulmonary resuscitation efforts and cardiac arrest, respectively. The syndrome was attributed to an increase in brain serotonin owing to the combination of the serotonergic drugs lithium, phenelzine, and L-tryptophan. Although the patient had a history of drug overdose, the authors did not comment on whether drug overdose was ruled out.

Another report (Thomas and Rubin, 1984) described several neuromuscular adverse effects 2 h after administration of L-tryptophan 6 g to a 21-yr-old man taking phenelzine 90 mg/d for depression. He exhibited shivering of the jaw, trunk, and limbs, diaphoresis, jocularity, fearfulness, moderate mood lability, and mild sexual suggestiveness. Horizontal nystagmus, bilateral Babinski signs, and ataxia were noted. With medication discontinuation, mental status changes and neurologic abnormalities resolved over 24 h.

As previously discussed, L-tryptophan may have efficacy in treating manic symptoms (Prange et al., 1974; Murphy et al., 1974); however, it has also been implicated as a cause of hypomania. Goff (1985) described two cases of hypomania following the addition of L-tryptophan to phenelzine and to tranylcypromine. It is possible that these were spontaneous switches. However, the rapidity of onset following L-tryptophan administration after a prolonged course of treatment with phenelzine and tranylcypromine, and the absence of prior history of bipolar illness, make it unlikely that the switches were spontaneous or were induced by the MAOI alone. One patient, who had been taking phenelzine 60 mg/d for 3 mo, was prescribed L-tryptophan 500 mg for insomnia. After a single dose, she reported being more talkative and less inhibited at work. The dose was increased to 1 g, and the next day the patient awoke feeling elated and displayed hyperkinesis, pressured speech, hypersexuality, and disinhibition. L-Tryptophan was discontinued 5 d later, with resolution of hypomanic symptoms over the following week. Another patient described by these same authors had been taking tranylcypromine 50–60 mg/d for over 3 mo when L-tryptophan was prescribed for insomnia and worsening depressive symptoms. The dose was increased to 2 g over 3 d; on day 4 the patient awoke feeling intoxicated and displayed hyperkinesis, disinhibition, and talkativeness. She also went on a financially disastrous shopping spree. Both medications were discontinued, with return of depressive symptoms within 3 d. The authors point out that euphoric mood was reported in five of seven normal subjects administered L-tryptophan 30-90 mg/kg in one study (Smith and Prockop, 1967).

Because concomitant use of MAOIs and tryptophan is associated with the various neurologic and psychiatric adverse effects described above, tryptophan use is contraindicated in patients taking the MAOIs tranylcypromine (Parnate®) and phenelzine (Nardil®), according to the products' package inserts.

Central nervous system symptoms were reported in five patients who were given L-tryptophan as an adjunct to fluoxetine in an attempt to augment the patients' response to fluoxetine (Steiner and Fontaine, 1986). The patients, three men and two women ranging in age from 34 to 58 yr (mean 44.6 yr), met the DSM-III criteria for obsessive-compulsive disorder (OCD) and had experienced at least a moderate response to fluoxetine. All patients had been taking fluoxetine for at least 3 mo (range 3–9 mo). Fluoxetine dosages were 50, 60, 80 mg (2 patients) and 100 mg. L-Tryptophan 2 g was added at bedtime, with the intention of increasing the dose by 2 g every 5 d to a maximum of 10 g/d. No patient was able to tolerate more than 4 g/d, with all patients requiring L-tryptophan discontinuation 7–22 d after it was started. Symptoms included agitation (five patients), anxiety (two patients), restlessness (three patients), insomnia, aggressive behavior, incoordination, headache, chills, nausea (two patients), abdominal cramps, diarrhea, incoordination, agitation, poor concentration (two patients), paresthesia, worsening OCD (two patients), palpitations, and development of mild depressive symptoms. All five patients had tolerated fluoxetine when it was used alone, and two patients had been previously treated with L-tryptophan alone, at twice the dosage used in conjunction with fluoxetine, without side effects. Based on this report, tryptophan use is listed as a precaution in the fluoxetine package insert.

22.11. REPRODUCTION

In rats, the rate-limiting enzyme in the metabolism of L-tryptophan, tryptophan pyrrolase, is absent in the fetus and is present in low amounts in neonates. This deficiency is apparently owing to a deficiency of adrenal steroids, which have been shown to induce production of tryptophan pyrolase in neonatal animals. L-Tryptophan has been shown to be lethal to 3-d-old rat pups, and human fetuses and neonates may also be at increased risk for toxicity. It is recommended that L-tryptophan supplements be avoided during pregnancy (Trulson and Ulissey, 1987).

L-Tryptophan was found to have teratogenic potential in a study investigating the effect of tryptophan on the development of chick embryos (Naidu, 1974). Twenty freshly laid fertile eggs comprised the control group, and a set of 30 eggs formed the experimental group. After 72 h of incubation, eggs in the experimental group were innoculated with 2 mg of tryptophan in 0.5 ml of saline, half of the control group received 0.5 mL of saline, and half were allowed to develop normally. One of the control embryos that had received saline died, and four of the experimental embryos died. After 8 d, the embryos were removed from the eggs. The experimental group displayed dysmorphogenetic effects such as limb deformities, rumplessness, and visceral abnormalities including exposed intestines and other organs. All the experimental embryos were smaller in size than the control group. The investigators attributed these effects to an amino acid imbalance resulting from excess L-tryptophan causing a relative deficiency of other amino acids.

A study was performed to determine the impact of supplemental L-tryptophan on pregnancy course and outcome in rats (Funk et al., 1991). From day 0 to day 20 of pregnancy, rats in the experimental group received a diet supplemented with L-tryptophan 500% (T-500), 1000% (T-1000), or 2500% (T-2500) excess over controls. The diet fed to controls had been shown to be satisfactory for reproduction and lactation and provided L-tryptophan 1.11 g/100 g. Pilot studies showed that the L-tryptophan-supplemented diet was associated with lower food consumption than the control diet. To control for the effects of reduced food consumption, each experimental rat was matched with a control animal fed the same amount of food that the experimental rat consumed. An additional group of 11 animals was fed the control diet *ad libitum*.

Statistical analysis was done using one-way ANOVA and Duncan's multiple comparison procdure, with statistical significance accepted at the $p < 0.05$ level. The only malformation observed was a fetus in the T-1000 group with a missing left kidney. The T-1000 group also had significantly more late resorptions than any other tryptophan group. The total fetal weight per litter was significantly less in the T-2500 group compared with the T-500 group, which consumed significantly more food than all other groups except the *ad libitum* control group. The average fetal weight was also significantly less in the T-2500 group than in the T-1000 group. The T-2500 group had a significantly lower maternal weight gain than any group. The investigators concluded that maternal and fetal weight might be compromised by diets highly supplemented with L-tryptophan. For comparison, the L-tryptophan supplementation in the T-2500 group is comparable to 38 g of L-tryptophan consumption in humans.

A report describes female rats fed a tryptophan-enriched diet from mating throughout pregnancy and lactation. Decreased serotonin content, decreased activity of tryptophan hydroxylase, and a reduced synaptosomal serotonin uptake was noted in the cortex and brainstem of 5-d-old rat pups of mothers fed the enriched diet. This was interpreted to reflect a delay in the development of serotonergic neurons. Serotonin is thought to act as a neurotrophic signal during fetal development. It has been hypothesized that increased maternal tryptophan increases serotonin synthesis in the fetus. The increased serotonin may stimulate serotonin 1A (HT_{1A}) receptors, inhibiting axonal outgrowth (Huether et al., 1992).

22.12. CHEMICAL AND BIOFLUID ANALYSIS

Several techniques exist for the measurement of tryptophan. The traditional fluorometric method for the measurement of tryptophan in biologic materials was developed based on the formation of the fluorophore norharman. The reaction involves the formation of the fluorophore norharman from tryptophan by condensation with formaldehyde and then oxidation with $FeCl_3$. The product is read at excitation and emission wavelengths of 373 nm and 452 nm in a quartz cuvette. The sensitivity and range permit the measurement of 0.04–20 nanomole of tryptophan in standard 1-cm cuvettes (Denckla and Dewey, 1967). A revision of the Denckla and Dewey method uses the same reagents and procedure with the exception of omitting $FeCl_3$ from the deproteinizing reagent and adding it at the last moment before the heating step. It was determined that $FeCl_3$ in the presence of trichloroacetic acid (TCA) causes the breakdown of tryptophan to a substance which does not subsequently produce fluorescence (Bloxam and Warren, 1974). A rapid fully automated method for the determination of amino acids is based on HPLC and precolumn *o*-phthaldialdehyde derivatization. Using a 150 × 4.6 mm i.d. HPLC column filled with 2–3 μm Spherisorb ODS II packing material, 30 physiologic amino acids can be determined within 28 min (van Eijk et al., 1993).

Analysis of indoleamines such as tryptophan and hydroxytryptophan frequently can be performed in a manner analogous to that of the catecholamines. In general, HPLC is the method of choice for separation of components, with various detection methods being employed such as ultraviolet (Widner et al., 1999), fluorescence detection (Kai et al., 1998; Mattivi et al., 1999; Wood and Hall, 2000), colorometric detection (Alvarez et al., 1999), and mass spectrometric detection (Williamson et al., 1998). Each detection method has advantages and disadvantages. Although it is sensitive and selective, coulometric detection can require lengthy column equilibration times and extensive mobile phase degassing to ensure the desired results. Mass spectrometry is generally highly sensitive and specific but requires equipment that may not be available in all laboratories. Fluorescent detection equipment is generally more readily available but is dependent on the native ability of the analyte or a chemical derivative to fluoresce. Recently, a simple and sensitive assay was developed for the detection of tryptophan and hydroxytryptophan (as well as other indoleamines and catecholamines) using HPLC and the native fluorescence of the analytes (Wood and Hall, 2000).

In the method of Wood and Hall (2000), approximately 250 µL of blood is placed in a cold 1.5-mL centrifuge tube. A 200-µL aliquot is then combined with ice-cold 2% EDTA. The blood-EDTA samples can then either be stored at –70°C or centrifuged at 5000g for 50 min in prewashed Ultrafree MC filters with a 10,000 mol wt cutoff. The filtrate can then be stored at –70°C until analysis. Chromatography is conducted using a 5-µm Alltima C_{18} column (150 × 4.6 mm i.d.) where mobile phase A is 0.05% trifluoroacetic acid-methanol (97.5:2.5, v/v) and mobile phase B is 0.05% trifluoroacetic acid-methanol (40:60, v/v). The flow rate is 1 mL/min, and a linear gradient is performed over 20 min under the following conditions: 0.00 min, 100% A; 1.00 min, 100% A; 16.00 min, 50% A and 50% B. At 16.05 min, the mobile phase is switched to 100% A for 4 minutes to return the column to initial conditions. Injection volume is 10 µL of the filtrate. The fluorescence detector is set to an excitation wavelength of 220 nm and an excitation wavelength of 340 nm. The retention time of hydroxytryptophan is approximately 11.9 min, and for tryptophan it is approximately 17.6 min. Linear calibration curves can be achieved to as low as 12.5 pmol/mL.

An EMS associated with contaminants in a batch of tryptophan led to more than 30 deaths and affected 1500 others. In an effort to identify the contaminants, a number of methods were developed. One of the most exact methods for identifying these contaminants has been published by Williamson and colleagues (1998). This method uses on-line HPLC-tandem mass spectrometry (MS) to identify contaminants positively, including both mass and structural identification. By using MS-MS analysis, combined with exact mass determination analysis, these researchers have identified two novel contaminants possessing an indoline ring that is potentially reactive chemically. Although it requires specialized equipment and expertise, this method has allowed researchers to identify trace quantities (quantities too small for nuclear magnetic resonance analysis and structural determination) of contaminants in the affected tryptophan formulation.

22.13. REGULATORY STATUS

In November of 1989, the FDA ordered a recall of all manufactured L-tryptophan (Nightingale, 1990). It is currently unavailable as a dietary supplement. However, the FDA has provided for the use of manufactured L-tryptophan for special dietary purposes. L-Tryptophan is considered a lawful and essential compoment of infant formulas, enteral products, parenteral drug products, and special dietary foods intended for use under medical supervision in compliance with Title 21 of the Code of Federal Regulations, Part 172.320. In addition, although the FDA has concerns about the safety of L-tryptophan as a dietary supplement, it does not explicitly prohibit the marketing of L-tryptophan as a dietary supplement. In fact, a manufacturer could market a supplement containing L-tryptophan if done so according to the provisions of the Dietary Supplement Health and Education Act (DSHEA). Because, according to the DSHEA, the burden of responsibility for the safety of the product falls on the manufacturer, it would be prudent for a manufacturer to have data supporting the safety of the product when it is used as a dietary supplement. Such data do not currently exist; therefore, no firm is marketing L-tryptophan as a dietary supplement (FDA, 2001). Some "compounding pharmacies" will dispense L-tryptophan pursuant to a doctor's prescription (California Pharmacy, 2000). This activity is permissible because there is a monograph for L-tryptophan in the USP24-NF19, and substances for which such a monograph exists can be compounded by prescription (Food and Drug Administration Modernization Act, 1997).

L-Tryptophan's availability is limited in some other countries as well. For example, in the United Kingdom, L-tryptophan's use is restricted to use by hospital specialists as an adjunct to antidepressants in patients with severe, disabling depression of more than 2 yr duration that has not responded to an adequate trial of conventional antidepressants (Parfitt, 1999). In Germany, L-tryptophan reentered the market in 1995. Its production is now regulated by Good Manufacturing Practices set by the Bundesministerium fur Arzneimittel und Medizinalprodukte to ensure the absence of impurities (Faurie and Fries, 1999).

22.14. SUMMARY

- L-Tryptophan was once a popular dietary supplement used in the treatment of insomnia, depression, and prementrual syndrome. Although it is no longer available as a dietary supplement, it is available by prescription from compounding pharmacies.
- Small studies have shown L-tryptophan to have moderate efficacy in the treatment of insomnia, depression, and seasonal affective disorder. It may aid in smoking cessation, and it may decrease perception of physical fatigue.

REFERENCES

Alvarez JC, Bothua D, Collignon I, Advenier C, Spreux-Varoquaux O. Simultaneous measurement of dopamine, serotonin, their metabolites and tryptophan in mouse brain homogenates by high-performance liquid chromatography with dual coulometric detection. Biomed Chromatogr 1999;13:293–8.

Anonymous. Eosinophilia-myalgia syndrome and L-tryptophan-containing products—New Mexico, Minnesota, Oregon and New York. MMWR 1989;38:785–8.

Archer DL. Testimony before the Subcommittee on Human Resources and Intergovernmental Relations Committee. United States Food and Drug Administration. Center for Food Safety and Applied Nutrition. July 18, 1991. Available from: http://cfsan.fda.gov/approx dms/dstryp2.html. Accessed September 23, 2000.

Back EE, Henning KJ, Kallenbach LR, et al. Risk factors for developing eosinophila myalgia syndrome among L-tryptophan users in New York. J Rheumatol 1993;20:666–72.

Belongia EA, Gleich GJ. The eosinophilia-myalgia syndrome revisited. J Rheumatol 1996;23:1682–5.

Belongia EA, Hedberg CW, Gleich GJ, et al. An investigation of the cause of the eosinophilia-myalgia syndrome associated with tryptophan use. N Engl J Med 1990;323:357–65.

Birdsall TC. 5-Hydroxytryptophan: a clinically-effective serotonin precursor. Alt Med Rev 1998;3:271–80.

Birt DF, Julius AD, Hasegawa R, St. John M, Cohe SM. Effect of L-tryptophan excess and vitamin B_6 deficiency on rat urinary bladder cancer promotion. Cancer Res 1987;47:1244–50.

Bloxam DL, Warren WH. Error in the determination of tryptophan by the method of Denckla and Dewey. A revised procedure. Anal Biochem 1974;60:621–5.

Bohme A, Wolter M, Hoelzer D. L-Tryptophan-related eosinophilia-myalgia syndrome possibly associated with a chronic B-lymphocytic leukemia. Ann Hematol 1998;77:235–8.

Bowen DJ, Spring B, Fox E. Tryptophan and high-carbohydrate diets as adjuncts to smoking cessation therapy. J Behav Med 1991;14:97–110.

Brennan D, MacManus M, Howe J, McLoughlin J. 'Neuroleptic malignant syndrome' without neuroleptics. Br J Psychiatry 1988;152:578–9.

Broadhurst AD. L-Tryptophan versus ECT. Lancet 1972;1:1392–3.

Brody T. Nutritional biochemistry, 2nd ed. San Diego, CA: Academic; 1999. p. 602.

Brotman AW, Rosenbaum JF. MAOIs plus tryptophan: a cause of the serotonin syndrome? Biol Ther Psychiatry 1984;7:45–6.

Brown RR, Price JM. Quantitative studies on metabolites of tryptophan in the urine of the dog, cat, rat, and man. J Biol Chem 1956;219:985–97.

Bryan GT. The role of urinary tryptophan metabolites in the etiology of bladder cancer. Am J Clin Nutr 1971;24:841–7.

Bunney WE Jr, Brodie HKH, Murphy DL, Goodwin FK. Studies of alpha-methyl-para-tyrosine, L-dopa, and L-tryptophan in depression and mania. Amer J Psychiat 1971;127:872–81.

California pharmacy. L-Tryptophan. Available from: URL:www.californiapharmacy.com/trypophan.html. Accessed December 17, 2000.

Carroll BJ, Mowbray RM, Davies B. Sequential comparison of L-tryptophan with ECT in severe depression. Lancet 1970;1:967–9.

Clauw DJ. Animal models of the eosinophilia-myalgia syndrome. J Rheumatol 1996;23(suppl 46):93–8.

Clauw DJ, Pincus T. The eosinophilia-myalgia syndrome: what we know, what we think we know, and what we need to know. J Rheumatol 1996;46(suppl):2–6.

Cohen SM, Masayuki A, Jacobs JB, Friedell GH. Promoting effect of saccharin and D,L-tryptophan in urinary bladder carcinogenesis. Cancer Res 1979;39:1207–17.

Coppen A. Treatment of unipolar depression. Lancet 1976;1:90–1.

Coppen A, Shaw DM, Farrell JP. Potentiation of the antidepressive effect of a monoamine-oxidase inhibitor by tryptophan. Lancet 1963;i:79–81.

Coppen A, Shaw DM, Herzberg B, Maggs R. Tryptophan in the treatment of depression. Lancet 1967;2:1178–80.

Coppen A, Whybrow PC, Noguera R, Maggs R, Prange AJ. The comparative antidepressant value of L-tryptophan and imipramine with and without attempted potentiation by liothyronine. Arch Gen Psychiatry 1972;26:234–41.

Cunliffe A, Obeid OA, Powell-Tuck J. A placebo controlled investigation of the effect of tryptophan or placebo on subjective and objective measures of fatigue. Eur J Clin Nutr 1988;52:425–30.

Daniels SR, Hudson JI, Horwitz RI. Epidemiology of potential association between L-tryptophan ingestion and eosinophilia-myalgia syndrome. J Clin Epidemiol 1995;48:1413–27.

D'Elia G, Lehmann J, Raotma H. Evaluation of the combination of tryptophan and ECT in the treatment of depression. Acta Psychiatr Scand 1977;56:303–18.

Denckla WD, Dewey HK. The determination of tryptophan in plasma, liver, and urine. J Lab Clin Med 1967;69:160–9.

Dunner DL, Fieve RR. Affective disorders: studies with amine precursors. Am J Psychiatry 1975;132:180–3.

Dunning WF, Curtis MR, Maun ME. The effect of added tryptophane on the occurrence of 2-acetylaminofluorene-induced liver and bladder cancer in rats. Cancer Res 1950;10:454–9.

Eidson M, Philen RM, Sewell CM, Voorhees R, Kilbourne EM. L-Tryptophan and eosinophilia-mylagia syndrome in New Mexico. Lancet 1990;335:645–8.

Faurie R, Fries G. From sugar beet to molasses to Lyphan®. Integrated quality management from the raw material to the drug. Adv Exp Med Biol 1999;467:443–52.

FDA. Information paper on L-tryptophan and 5-hydroxy-L-tryptophan. United States Food and Drug Administration. Center for Food Safety and Applied Nutrition. Office of Special Nutritionals. February, 2001. Available from: http://vm.cfsan.fda.gov/~dms/ds-tryp1.html. Accessed November 11, 2001.

Flockhart DA, Clauw DJ, Sale EB, Hewett J, Woosley RL. Pharmacogenetic characteristics of the eosinophilia-myalgia syndrome. Clin Pharmacol Ther 1994;56:398–405.

Food and Drug Administration Modernization Act of 1997, Pub. L. No. 105-115, 111 Stat. 2296 (Nov. 21,1997).

Funk DN, Worthington-Roberts B, Fantel A. Impact of supplemental lysine or tryptophan on pregnancy course and outcome in rats. Nutr Res 1991;11:501–12.

Ghadirian AM, Murphy BEP, Gendron MJ. Efficacy of light versus tryptophan therapy in seasonal affective disorder. J Affect Disord 1998;50:23–7.

Glassman AH, Platman SR. Potentiation of a monoamine oxidase inhibitor by tryptophan. J Psychiat Res 1969;7:83–8.

Goff DC. Two cases of hypomania following the addition of L-tryptophan to a monoamine oxidase inhibitor. Am J Psychiatry 1985;142:1487–8.

Green AR, Aronson JK, Cowen PJ. The pharmacokinetics of L-tryptophan following its intravenous and oral administration. Br J Clin Pharmacol 1985;20:317–21.

Gullino P, Winitz M, Birnbaum SM, et al. Studies on the metabolism of amino acids and related compounds in vivo. I. Toxicity of essential amino acids, individually and in mixtures, and the protective effect of L-arginine. Arch Biochem Biophys 1956;64:319–32.

Halkerston IDK. Biochemistry, 2nd ed. New York: John Wiley and Sons, 1988.

Hartmann E, Cravens J, List S. Hypnotic effects of L-tryptophan. Arch Gen Psychiatry 1974;31:394–7.

Hatch DL, Garona JE, Goldman LR, Waller KO. Persistent eosinophilia in an infant with probable intrauterine exposure to L-tryptophan-containing supplements. Pediatrics 1991;88:810–3.

Herrington RN, Bruce A, Johnstone EC, Lader MH. Comparative trial of L-tryptophan and ECT in severe depressive illness. Lancet 1974:ii:731–4.

Herrington RN, Bruce A, Johnstone EC, Lader MH. Comparative trial of L-tryptophan and amitriptyline in depressive illness. Psychol Med 1976;6:673–8.

Hisatomi A, Kubota A, Ohashi M, et al. Elevated L-kynurenine level and its normalization by prednisolone in a patient with eosinophila-myalgia syndrome. Fukuoka Igaku Zasshi 1997;88:11–7.

Huether G, Thomke F, Adler L. Administration of tryptophan-enriched diets to pregnant rats retards the development of the serotonergic system in their offspring. Dev Brain Res 1992;68:175–81.

Hudson JI, Pope HG, Carter WP, Daniels SR. Fibromyalgia, psychiatric disorders, and assessment of the longterm outcome of eosinophilia-myalgia syndrome. J Rheumatol 1996;23(suppl 46):37–43.

Jensen K, Fruensgaard K, Ahlfors U-G, et al. Tryptophan/imipramine in depression [letter]. Lancet 1975;2:920.

Kai M, Iida H, Nohta H, Lee MK, Ohta K. Fluorescence derivatizing procedure for 5-hydroxytryptamine and 5-hydroxyindoleacetic acid using 1,2-diphenylethylenediamine reagent and their sensitive liquid chromatographic determination. J Chromatogr B Biomed Sci Appl 1998;720:25–31.

Kamb ML, Murphy JJ, Jones JL, et al. Eosinophilia-myalgia syndrome in L-tryptophan-exposed patients. JAMA 1992;267:77–82.

Kline NS, Shah BK. Comparable therapeutic efficacy of tryptophan and imipramine. Average therapeutic ratings versus "true" equivalence: an important difference. Curr Ther Res 1973;15:484–7.

Lam RW, Levitan RD, Tam EM, et al. L-Tryptophan augmentation of light therapy in patients with seasonal affective disorder. Can J Psychiatry 1997;42:303–6.

Levy AB, Bucher P, Votolato N. Myoclonus, hyperreflexia and diaphoresis in patients on phenelzine-tryptophan combination treatment. Can J Psychiatry 1985;30:434–6.

MacSweeney, DA. Treatment of unipolar depression [letter]. Lancet 1975;2:510–1.

Marken PA, Schneiderhan ME. Assessment of psychiatric illness. In: DiPiro JT, Talbert RL, Yee GC, et al., eds. Pharmacotherapy: a pathophysiologic approach. 3rd ed. Stamford, CT: Appleton and Lange, 1997. p. 1293–1300.

Martinsons A, Rudzite V, Groma V, et al. Kynurenine and neopterin in chronic glomerulonephritis. Adv Exp Med Biol 1999;467:579–86.

Mattivi F, Vrhovsek U, Versini G. Determination of indole-3-acetic acid, tryptophan and other indoles in must and wine by high-performance liquid chromatography with fluorescence detection. J Chromatogr A 1999;855:227–35.

Mayeno AN, Benson LM, Naylor S, et al. Biotransformation of 3-(phenylamino)-1,2-propanediol to 3-(phenylamino)alanine: a chemical link between toxic oil syndrome and eosinophila-myalgia syndrome. Chem Res Toxicol 1995;8:911–6.

McCormick DB. Niacin, riboflavin, and thiamine. In: Stipanuk MH, ed. Biochemical and physiological aspects of human nutrition. Philadelphia: WB Saunders, 2000.

Medsger TA Jr. Tryptophan-induced eosinophilia-myalgia syndrome. N Engl J Med 1990;322:926–8.

Mendels J, Stinnet JL, Burns D, et al. Amine precursors and depression. Arch Gen Psychiatry 1975;32:22–30.

Miyakawa M, Yoshida O. DNA synthesis of the urinary bladder epithelium in rats with long-term feeding of D,L-tryptophan-added and pyridoxine-defecient diet. Gann 1973;64:411–3.

Moore WP, Bolton CH, Downs L, Gilmor HA, Gale EA. Measurement of N-methyl-2-pyridone-5-carboxamide in urine by high performance liqiuid chromatography. Biomed Chromatogr 2000;14:69–71.

Murphy DL, Baker M, Goodwin FK, et al. L-Tryptophan in affective disorders: indoleamine changes and differential clinical effects. Psychopharmacologia 1974;34:11–20.

Murty CN, Sidransky H. The effect of tryptophan on messenger RNA of the livers of fasted mice. Biochim Biophys Acta 1972;262:328–35.

Murty CN, Verney E, Sidransky H. In vivo and in vitro studies on the effect of tryptophan on translocation of RNA form nuclei of rat liver. Biochem Med 1979;22:98–109.

Naidu RCM. Teratogenic effects of tryptophane on the development of chick embryo. Experientia 1974;30:1462–3.

Naylor S, Williamson BL, Johnson KL, Gleich GJ. Structural characterization of case-associated contaminants peak C and FF in L-tryptophan implicated in eosinophilia-myalgia syndrome. Adv Exp Med Biol 1999;467:453–60.

Nightingale SL. "Dear colleague" letter on legal and regulatory background on L-tryptophan.

United States Food and Drug Administration. Office of Health Affairs. February 2, 1990. Available from: http://vm.cfsan.fda.gov/dms/~ds-ltr2.html. Accessed November 11, 2001.

Pakes GE. L-Tryptophan in psychiatric practice. Drug Intell Clin Pharm 1979;13:391–6.

Parfitt K, ed. Martindale: the complete drug reference, 32nd ed. London: Pharmaceutical Press, 1999. p. 310–1.

Pope HG, Jonas JM, Hudson JI, Kafka MP. Toxic reactions to the combination of monoamine oxidase inhibitors and tryptophan. Am J Psychiatry 1985;142:491–2.

Prange AJ Jr, Wilson IC, Lynn CW, et al. L-Tryptophan in mania. Arch Gen Psychiatry 1974;30:56–62.

Radomski JL, Glass EM, Deichmann WB. Transitional cell hyperplasia in the bladders of dogs fed D,L-tryptophan. Cancer Res 1971;31:1690–4.

Rao B, Broadhurst AD. Tryptophan and depression [letter]. BMJ 1976;21:460.

Sarma DSR, Verney E, Bongiorno M, Sidransky H. Influence of tryptophan on hepatic polyribosomes and protein synthesis in non-fasted and fasted mice. Nutr Rep Int 1971;4:1–7.

Segura R, Ventura JL. Effect of L-tryptophan supplementation on exercise performance. Int J Sports Med 1988;9:301–5.

Shapiro S. Epidemiologic studies of the association of L-tryptophan with the eosinophilia-myalgia syndrome: a critique. J Rheumatol 1996;23(suppl 46):44–59.

Shaw K, Turner J, Del Mar C. Tryptophan and 5-hydroxytryptophan for depression (Cochrane Review). In: The Cochrane Library, Issue 3. Oxford: Update Software, 2001.

Shulman LE. Diffuse fasciitis with eosinophilia: a new syndrome? Trans Assoc Am Physicians 1975;88:70–86.

Sicuteri F, Del Bene E. The influence of tryptophan and parachlorophenylalanine on the sexual activity in man. Acta Vitamin Enzymol 1975;29:100–2.

Sidransky H. Tryptophan and carcinogenesis: review and update on how tryptophan may act. Nutr Cancer 1997;29:181–94.

Sidransky H, Verney E, Sarma DSR. Effect of tryptophan on polyribosomes and protein synthesis in liver. Am J Clin Nutr 1971;24:779–85.

Simat TJ, Kleeberg KK, Muller B, Sierts A. Synthesis, formation, and occurrence of contaminants in biotechnologically manufacturerd L-tryptophan. Adv Exp Med Biol 1999;467:469–80.

Smith B, Prockop DJ. Central-nervous-system effect of ingestion of L-tryptophan by normal subjects. N Engl J Med 1967;267:1338–41.

Slutsker L, Hoesly FC, Miller L, et al. Eosinophilia-myalgia syndrome associated with exposure to tryptophan from a single manufacturer. JAMA 1990;264:213–7.

Spitzer WO, Haggerty J, Tamblyn R, et al. Continuing occurrence of eosinophilia myalgia syndrome. Clin Res 1994;42:292A.

Staufenberg EF, Tantam D. Malignant hyperpyrexia syndrome in combined treatment. Br J Psychiatry 1989;154:577–8.

Steinberg S, Annable L, Young SN, Liyanage N. A placebo-controlled study of the effects of L-tryptophan in patients with premenstrual dysphoria. Adv Exp Med Biol 1999;467:85–8.

Steiner W, Fontaine R. Toxic reaction following the combined administration of fluoxetine and L-tryptophan: five case reports. Biol Psychiatry 1986;21:1067–71.

Stensrud T, Ingier F, Holm H, Stromme SB. L-Tryptophan supplementation does not improve running performance. Int J Sports Med 1992;13:481–5.

Stockstill JW, McCall WD Jr, Gross AJ, Piniewski B. The effect of L-tryptophan supplementation and dietary instruction on chronic myofascial pain. J Am Dent Assoc 1989;118:457–60.

Sullivan EA, Kamb ML, Jones JL, et al. The natural history of eosinophilia-myalgia syndrome in a tryptophan-exposed cohort in South Carolina. Arch Intern Med 1995;156:973–9.

Suzuki S, Tourkina E, Ludwicka A, et al. A contaminant of L-tryptophan enhances expression of dermal collagen in a murine model of eosinophilia myalgia syndrome. Proc Assoc Am Physicians 1996;108:315–22.

Swygert LA, Maes EF, Sewell LE, et al. Eosinophilia-myalgia syndrome. JAMA 1990;264:1698–703.

Thomas JM, Rubin EH. Case report of a toxic reaction from a combination of tryptophan and phenelzine. Am J Psychiatry 1984;141:281–3.

Thomson J, Rankin H, Ashcroft G, et al. The treatment of depression in general practice: a comparison of L-tryptophan, amitriptyline, and a combination of L-tryptophan and amitriptyline with placebo. Psychol Med 1982;12:741–51.

Trulson ME, Ulissey MJ. Low doses of L-tryptophan are lethal in rats with adrenal insufficiency. Life Sci 1987;41:349–53.

Van Eijk HM, Rooyakkers DR, Deutz NE. Rapid routine determination of amino acids in plasma by high-performance liquid chromatography with 2-3 microns Spherisorb ODS II column. J Chromatogr 1993;620:143–8.

Varga J, Peltonen J, Uitto J, Jimenez S. Development of diffuse fasciitis with eosinophilia during L-tryptophan treatment: demonstration of elevated type I collagen gene expression in affected tissues. Ann Intern Med 1990;112:344–51.

Varga J, Uitto J, Jimenez SA. The cause and pathogenesis of the eosinophilia-myalgia syndrome. Ann Intern Med 1992;116:140–7.

Wagner KR, Elmore JG, Horwitz RI. Diagnostic bias in clinical decision making: an example of L-tryptophan and the diagnosis of eosinophilia-myalgia syndrome. J Rheumatol 1996;23:2079–85.

Widner B, Werner ER, Schennach H, Fuchs D. An HPLC method to determine tryptophan and kynurenine in serum simultaneously. Adv Exp Med Biol 1999; 467:827–32.

Wildman REC, Medeiros DM. Advanced human nutrition. Boca Raton, FL: CRC, 2000. p. 146.

Williamson BL, Johnson KL, Tomlinson AJ, Gleich GJ, Naylor S. On-line HPLC-tandem mass spectrometry structural characterization of case-associated contaminants of L-tryptophan implicated with the onset of eosinophilia myalgia syndrome. Toxicol Lett 1998;99:139–50.

Wood AT, Hall MR. Reversed-phase high-performance liquid chromatography of catecholamines and indoleamines using a simple gradient solvent system and native fluorescence detection. J Chromatogr B Biomed Sci Appl 2000;744:221–5.

Chapter 23

Vanadyl Sulfate

Timothy S. Tracy

23.1. HISTORY

Vanadium was first discovered by the Spanish mineralogist del Rio in 1813, who called the element panchromium because of the color changes it undergoes during the transition to various oxidation states. Nils Sefstrom purified vanadium oxide in 1831 and named it after the goddess Vanadis (Barceloux, 1999). Vanadium is a trace metal that exists in oxidation states from −1 to +5, but the most common valence states are +3, +4, and +5. Within extracellular body fluids it most commonly exists in the VO^{-3} (pentavalent) form, whereas it typically exists in the VO^{+2} (quadrivalent) form in intracellular fluids (Barceloux, 1999). Food is the primary source of vanadium exposure, although amounts in food are low. Occupational exposure to vanadium can also occur. Vanadium is most commonly administered as vanadyl sulfate oral formulations when used to treat various diseases.

Vanadium is thought to be important for normal cell function and development. Because of its hardness, it has historically been used primarily as a component of metal alloys. Vanadyl sulfate is used as a mordant in dyeing and printing textiles, colored glass, and pottery (The Merck Index, 1996).

23.2. CHEMICAL STRUCTURE

See Fig. 23-1 for the chemical structure of vanadyl sulfate.

23.3. CURRENT PROMOTED USES

Vanadyl sulfate is primarily promoted as a treatment for non-insulin-dependent diabetes. However, it has also been used for hyperlipidemia, heart disease, improving athletic performance in weight training, chemoprevention, syphilis, and tuberculosis (Natural Medicines Database, 2002). Since vanadium is considered an essential mineral, the National Institute of Medicine has set the upper intake level (UL) of vana-

From: *Forensic Science: Dietary Supplements: Toxicology and Clinical Pharmacology*
Edited by: M. J. Cupp and T. S. Tracy © Humana Press Inc., Totowa, New Jersey

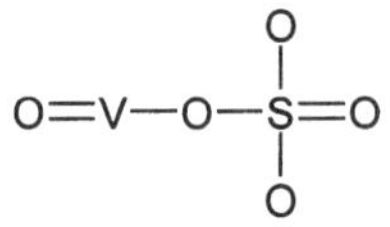

$$O=V-O-\overset{\displaystyle O}{\underset{\displaystyle O}{\overset{|}{\underset{|}{S}}}}=O$$

Fig. 1. Chemical structure of vanadyl sulfate.

dium at 1.8 mg/d for adults (Institute of Medicine, 2002). No UL has been established for infants, children, or pregnant or lactating women. In these groups, vanadium intake should be limited to that contained in normal dietary food or infant formula (a typical diet contains 6–18 µg of vanadium per day). Vanadyl sulfate contains 31% elemental vanadium, whereas sodium metavanadate contains 42% elemental vanadium.

23.4. PRODUCTS AVAILABLE

Some currently available products containing vanadyl sulfate include vanadyl sulfate (generic), Vanadyl Sulfate with Niacin®, VS-10 Vanadyl Sulfate®, Vanadyl Factors®, Vanadyl pH®, Vanadyl Plus with Chromium®, and Super Vanadyl Fuel®.

23.5. ANIMAL STUDIES

A number of studies have been published on the effects of vanadyl sulfate on diabetes in laboratory animals. For example, Yao et al. (1997) evaluated the response of streptozotocin-induced diabetic rats to both acute and chronic treatment with vanadyl sulfate. These investigators found that chronic administration of vanadyl sulfate produced sustained and significant decreases in plasma glucose over the 4 wk study period compared with control animals. Additionally, acute (1–3 d) treatment with vanadyl sulfate returned diabetic rats to a euglycemic state. Reul and colleagues (1999) studied the effects of vanadyl sulfate (and several other forms of vanadium) in streptozotocin-induced diabetic rats. Over the 12-wk study period, vanadyl sulfate produced an approximately 25% decrease in plasma glucose while having a minimal effect on body weight or plasma insulin concentrations. Administration of vanadyl sulfate also substantially decreased fluid intake, urine volume, glucosuria, and food intake compared with diabetic rats that did not receive vanadium treatment. Finally, during oral glucose tolerance test, animals receiving vanadyl sulfate exhibited substantially less increase in plasma glucose compared with diabetic animals. Similar positive results have also been reported by a number of investigators (e.g., Brichard et al., 1989, 1990; Blondel et al., 1990; Battell et al., 1992).

23.6. CLINICAL STUDIES

Virtually all the clinical studies with vanadyl sulfate have focused on its role in the treatment of diabetes mellitus. Cohen and colleagues (1995) studied the effects of vanadyl sulfate (100 mg/d for 3 wk) on insulin sensitivity in patients with non-insulin-dependent diabetes mellitus. These investigators found an approximately 15% decrease in fasting plasma glucose and an approximately 10% decrease in hemoglobin A_{1c} but insulin levels were unchanged. However, during glucose clamp studies, an almost twofold greater glucose infusion rate was required to maintain euglycemia in patients receiving vanadyl sulfate compared with those receiving placebo. Furthermore, glucose output was decreased almost 75%, whereas glucose uptake was increased. Five of the six subjects experienced mild gastrointestinal symptoms including nausea, diarrhea, and abdominal cramps. It was concluded that vanadyl sulfate increased insulin sensitivity (both hepatic and peripheral) in non-insulin-dependent diabetes mellitus patients.

In a study of longer duration (6 wk) and a higher dose of vanadyl sulfate (150 mg/d), Cusi et al. (2001) also studied the ability of vanadyl sulfate to improve insulin sensitivity in 11 patients with type 2 diabetes. Observed was an approx 20% decrease in plasma glucose levels but only a 5% decrease in hemoglobin A_{1c}. Additionally, a modest decrease in low-density lipoprotein (LDL) cholesterol was observed. Diarrhea was noted in four patients, and abdominal discomfort was noted in two patients. In one of the patients with diarrhea, the condition persisted and subsequently required a dose reduction to 75 mg/d. It was concluded that vanadyl sulfate at maximum tolerated doses for 6 wk improves insulin sensitivity.

Goldfine et al. (2000) have also studied the effects of vanadyl sulfate on patients with non-insulin-dependent diabetes mellitus. Patients received either 75, 150, or 300 mg of vanadyl sulfate per day for 6 wk. No change in glucose metabolism was noted at the 75-mg dose, but three of five subjects experienced an increase in glucose metabolism at the 150-mg dose and four of eight patients at the 300-mg dose (presumably owing to increased insulin sensitivity). No change in basal hepatic glucose production was noted at any of the doses. However, fasting glucose and hemoglobin A_{1c} decreased significantly at the 150- and 300-mg doses, and high-density lipoprotein (HDL) lipoprotein was significantly decreased with the 300-mg dose. Notably, the 150- and 300-mg doses caused gastrointestinal disturbances (cramping, abdominal discomfort, and/or diarrhea) and at the 300-mg dose, all subjects required treatment for their gastrointestinal symptoms. These investigators concluded that at tolerated doses (75 mg), there did not appear to be any substantial benefit of vanadyl sulfate on insulin sensitivity or glycemic control.

These same investigators also studied the effects of sodium metavanadate ($NaVO_3$) 125 mg/d in both insulin-dependent and non-insulin-dependent diabetes mellitus patients (Goldfine et al., 1995). Sodium metavanadate did not alter glucose metabolism in insulin-dependent diabetes patients but did alter glucose metabolism in non-insulin-dependent diabetes patients. No change in basal hepatic glucose production or suppression of hepatic glucose production by insulin was noted. However, sodium metavanadate did result in a significant decrease in insulin requirements in patients with insulin-dependent diabetes as well as a significant decrease in cholesterol levels in both patient groups. Mild nausea was the only reported side effect of therapy, and this was reported to have dissipated rapidly. The investigators concluded that sodium metavanadate may be a useful adjunct in non-insulin-dependent diabetes mellitus antidiabetic therapy. A lack of effect of vanadyl sulfate on insulin-dependent diabetes mellitus patients has also been noted by Aharon et al. (1998).

Boden et al. (1996) studied the effects of vanadyl sulfate (100 mg/d) over 4 wk in non-insulin-dependent diabetes mellitus patients. A 20% decrease in fasting glucose concentrations was noted in the vanadyl sulfate treatment group, and a decrease in hepatic glucose output during hyperinsulinemia was also observed. Vanadyl sulfate had no effect on total-body glucose uptake, glycogen synthesis, glycolysis, carbohydrate oxidation, or lipolysis during euglycemic-hyperinsulinemic clamp studies. Six of the eight patients experienced gastrointestinal side effects during the first week of therapy, but these subsequently subsided.

Halberstam and colleagues (1996) compared the effects of vanadyl sufate (100 mg/d) in moderately obese non-insulin-dependent diabetes mellitus patients and non-diabetic subjects. Following 3 wk of vanadyl sulfate therapy, significant decreases in fasting plasma glucose (approx 14%) and hemoglobin A_{1c} (approx 6%) were noted in the diabetic subjects but not in the moderately obese control subjects. Greater suppression of plasma free fatty acids and lipid oxidation was also noted in diabetic subjects. It was concluded that vanadyl sulfate increases insulin sensitivity in diabetic subjects but has no effect on normal subjects.

There are currently no reliable clinical studies on the use of vanadyl sulfate for the treatment of other conditions.

23.7. PHARMACOKINETICS

The only published study of vanadium pharmacokinetics upon administration to humans used ammonium vanadyl tartrate as the vanadium formulation (Dimond et al., 1963). The degree to which these results correlate to kinetic parameters achieved after the administration of vanadyl sulfate are unknown. Dimond and colleagues (1963) administered ammonium vanadyl tartrate tablets (25 mg) one to four times daily (most patients received 50–75 mg/d) for 45–68 d. All patients reported gastrointestinal distress exhibiting as black, loosened stools and increased intestinal cramping. No toxicities resulting in alteration of biochemical parameters were noted. Total amount of vanadium excreted in the urine was measured on various days throughout the study period. In the four patients for whom excretion of vanadium was reported, the intra- and intersubject variability in amount excreted in 24 h was substantial. Interestingly, in no case was more than 1.4% of the dose recovered in the urine in 24 h, and in some cases the 24-h recovery was as low as 0.07%. Also of note, in the two cases in which vanadium sampling was continued for a period of time after discontinuation of dosing, excretion of vanadium in the urine could be noted as long as 28 d post dosing. It appears that vanadium accumulates in the body following repeated dosing and that elimination may continue for a substantial period following stopping therapy.

23.8. ADVERSE EFFECTS AND TOXICITY

Most of the toxicology studies involving vanadyl sulfate administration have involved the use of laboratory animals. Pepato et al. (1999) studied the effect of oral vanadyl sulfate treatment on serum enzymes and lipids in diabetic rats. These investigators found that a concentration of 1 mg/mL placed in the drinking water for 4 wk resulted in a statistically significant decrease in total cholesterol and triglycerides. Additionally, the liver enzymes aspartate aminotransferase and alanine aminotransferase (ALT) were significantly decreased compared with the water-alone controls. Llobet and Domingo (1984) assessed the median lethal dose (LD_{50}) of vanadyl sulfate in both rats and mice. Upon oral administration, the LD_{50} in rats was 448 mg/kg, and in mice it was 467 mg/kg. After intraperitoneal administration, the LD_{50}s for rats and mice were 74 and 113 mg/kg, respectively. Most deaths were observed in the first 24 h. The most commonly noted effects were irregular respiration, diarrhea, ataxia, and hind limb paralysis. In those animals in which death did not occur, these signs usually disappeared within the first 48 h. In a 1-yr study of oral vanadyl sulfate administration to rats (34–155 mg/kg/d), Dai and McNeill (1994) found no effect of vanadyl sulfate on systolic blood pressure, hematocrit, hemoglobin, erythrocyte count, or platelet count. However, they did find that vanadyl sulfate alleviated the decreased leukocyte count typically observed in diabetic animals.

Few data exist on the adverse effects and toxicity of vanadyl sulfate in humans. Fawcett and colleagues (1997) found that vanadyl sulfate (0.5 mg/kg/d) had no effect on red cell count, white cell count, platelet count, red cell mean cell volume, or hemoglobin levels. No changes in hematocrit, plasma viscosity, or blood viscosity were noted. Blood pressure (systolic and diastolic) did not differ between the treatment group and the control group. Additionally, no changes were noted in liver and biochemical enzymes (albumin, protein, bilirubin, ALT, alkaline phosphatase, cholesterol, HDL, triglycerides, urea or creatinine) in those subjects receiving vanadyl sulfate. As stated above (*see* Clinical Studies section), the most commonly observed side effects of vanadyl sulfate are gastrointestinal symptoms such as cramping, abdominal discomfort and/or diarrhea (Cohen et al., 1995; Goldfine et al., 1995, 2000; Boden et al., 1996; Cusi et al., 2001).

23.9. INTERACTIONS

No documented information is currently available concerning drug interactions involving vanadyl sulfate. Vanadyl sulfate can potentially enhance the hypoglycemic effect observed with oral antidiabetic agents such as glyburide, glipizide, and so on. Funakoshi et al. (1992) have reported that sodium orthovanadate prolonged clotting time in human plasma, but vanadyl sulfate was not studied. In theory, this could result in an enhancement of the anticoagulant effect of agents such as warfarin.

23.10. REPRODUCTION

Insufficient reliable information exists to determine whether vanadyl sulfate, in amounts greater than those typically found in foods, is safe in pregnant or lactating women. Thus, it probably should not be taken in amounts exceeding the upper intake limit.

23.11. BIOFLUID ANALYSIS

Vanadium, the product resulting from the administration of vanadyl sulfate, can be measured in blood using atomic absorption spectrophotometry (Mongold et al., 1990). Twenty microliters of blood is diluted 1:1 with a 0.25 *M* sodium citrate solution containing 1% Triton, mixed, and used directly for analysis. A vanadium hollow cathode lamp is operated at 7 mA, with a wavelength of 318.5 nm and a 0.5 nm slit width. A deuterium lamp is used for background correction. A temperature program is used for sample analysis. Samples are first dried in two steps (at 120°C for 60 s and again at 450°C for 20 s), then ashing is conducted at 1400°C for 40 s, and finally the sample is atomized at 2850°C for 3.1 s. Samples are compared with a calibration curve prepared in a manner analogous to that for the blood samples. The limit of detection for this assay is 10 ng/mL vanadium.

23.12. REGULATORY STATUS

Vanadyl sulfate is regulated under the Dietary Supplement Health Education Act as a dietary supplement.

23.13. SUMMARY

- Vanadium (from vanadyl sulfate) is an essential mineral and is a component of most diets.
- Vanadyl sulfate has been shown to be modestly effective in reducing insulin resistance and lowering blood glucose levels in non-insulin-dependent diabetics. However, it does not appear to produce the same effect in insulin-dependent diabetics.
- The most commonly reported adverse effects of vanadyl sulfate administration are gastrointestinal symptoms, and these effects increase with increasing dose.
- The pharmacokinetic properties of vanadyl sulfate are not well understood, but it appears that after continued dosing above the upper intake level, vanadium accumulates in the body and is excreted for several weeks following discontinuation of therapy.
- Vanadium (from vanadyl sulfate) is regulated as a dietary supplement.

REFERENCES

Aharon Y, Mevorach M, Shamoon H. Vanadyl sulfate does not enhance insulin action in patients with type 1 diabetes. Diabetes Care 1998;21:2194–5.

Barceloux DG. Vanadium. J Toxicol Clin Toxicol 1999;37:265–78.

Battell ML, Yuen VG, McNeill JH. Treatment of BB rats with vanadyl sulfate. Pharmacol Commun 1992;1:291–302.

Blondel O, Simon J, Chevalier B, Portha B. Impaired insulin action but normal insulin receptor activity in diabetic rat liver: effect of vanadate. Am J Physiol 1990;258:E459–67.

Boden G, Chen X, Ruiz J, van Rossum GD, Turco S. Effects of vanadyl sulfate on carbohydrate and lipid metabolism in patients with non-insulin-dependent diabetes mellitus. Metabolism 1996;45:1130–5.

Brichard SM, Pottier AM, Henquin JC. Long term improvement of glucose homeostasis by vanadate in obese hyperinsulinemic fa/fa rats. Endocrinology 1989;125:2510–6.

Brichard SM, Bailey CJ, Henquin JC. Marked improvement of glucose homeostasis in diabetic ob/ob mice given oral vanadate. Diabetes 1990;39:1326–32.

Cohen N, Halberstam M, Shlimovich P, et al.. Oral vanadyl sulfate improves hepatic and peripheral insulin sensitivity in patients with non-insulin-dependent diabetes mellitus. J Clin Invest 1995;95:2501–9.

Cusi K, Cukier S, DeFronzo RA, et al. Vanadyl sulfate improves hepatic and muscle insulin sensitivity in type 2 diabetes. J Clin Endocrinol Metab 2001;86:1410–7.

Dai S, McNeill JH. One-year treatment of non-diabetic and streptozotocin-diabetic rats with vanadyl sulphate did not alter blood pressure or haematological indices. Pharmacol Toxicol 1994;74:110–5.

Dimond EG, Caravaca J, Benchimol A. Vanadium: excretion, toxicity, lipid effect in man. Am J Clin Nutr 1963;12:49–53.

Fawcett JP, Farquhar SJ, Thou T, Shand BI. Oral vanadyl sulphate does not affect blood cells, viscosity or biochemistry in humans. Pharmacol Toxicol 1997;80:202–6.

Funakoshi T, Shimada H, Kojima S, et al. Anticoagulant action of vanadate. Chem Pharm Bull (Tokyo) 1992;40:174–6.

Goldfine AB, Patti ME, Zuberi L, et al. Metabolic effects of vanadyl sulfate in humans with non-insulin-dependent diabetes mellitus: in vivo and in vitro studies. Metabolism 2000;49:400–10.

Goldfine AB, Simonson DC, Folli F, Patti ME, Kahn CR. Metabolic effects of sodium metavanadate in humans with insulin-dependent and noninsulin-dependent diabetes mellitus in vivo and in vitro studies. J Clin Endocrinol Metab 1995;80:3311–20.

Halberstam M, Cohen N, Shlimovich P, Rossetti L, Shamoon H. Oral vanadyl sulfate improves insulin sensitivity in NIDDM but not in obese nondiabetic subjects. Diabetes 1996;45:659–66.

Institute of Medicine. Dietary reference intakes for vitamin A, vitamin K, arsenic, boron, chromium, copper, iodine, iron, manganese, molybdenum, nickel, silicon, vanadium, and zinc. 2002, http://www.nap.edu/books/0309072794/html/. Accessed January 21, 0002.

Llobet JM, Domingo JL. Acute toxicity of vanadium compounds in rats and mice. Toxicol Lett 1984;23:227–31.

Mongold JJ, Cros GH, Vian L, et al. Toxicological aspects of vanadyl sulphate on diabetic rats: effects on vanadium levels and pancreatic B-cell morphology. Pharmacol Toxicol 1990;67:192–8.

Natural Medicines Database. Vanadyl sulfate. In: Jellin JM, ed. Natural medicines comprehensive database, 2002, Therapeutic Research Faculty. Available from : http://www.naturaldatabase.com/monograph.asp?mono_id=749&hilite=1. Accessed January 21, 2002.

Pepato MT, Magnani MR, Kettelhut IC, Brunetti IL. Effect of oral vanadyl sulfate treatment on serum enzymes and lipids of streptozotocin-diabetic young rats. Mol Cell Biochem 1999;198:157–61.

Reul BA, Amin SS, Buchet JP, et al. Effects of vanadium complexes with organic ligands on glucose metabolism: a comparison study in diabetic rats. Br J Pharmacol 1999;126:467–77.

The Merck Index, 12th ed. Whitehouse Station, NJ: Merck Research Laboratories, 1996.

Yao J, Battell ML, McNeill JH. Acute and chronic response to vanadium following two methods of streptozotocin-diabetes induction. Can J Physiol Pharmacol 1997;75:83–90.

Appendix
Summary Data on Dietary Supplements[a]

	Toxicities	Interactions	Elimination	Reproduction
Androstenedione	Priapism (C), decreased HDL (S)	Finasteride may increase levels (V)	Hepatic, peripheral	Premature labor, elevated CRH Levels (A
Chitosan	Gastrointestinal (S)	Decreased warfarin effect (T)	Metabolized, eliminated in urine	No data
Chondroitin	Gastrointestinal (S)	No data	Metabolized in liver, eliminated in urine	No data, theoretically may cross placenta and may distribute into breast milk (T)
Chromium piolinate	Renal failure, cognitive impairment, rhabdomyolysis (C)	None reported or suspected	Renal	Avoid (T)
Coenzyme Q10	Generally well tolerated (s) nephrotoxicity (?) (S), gastrointestinal side effects (S), headache (S), bodyache (S)	Statins, β-blockers, and gemfibrozil decrease endogenous levels (S); may antagonize radiation therapy (A)	Used by cells throughout body in energy production	No data
Creatine	Nephrotoxicity (C, A)	Caffeine may decrease creatine's effect on exercise performance (S); NSAIDs, ACE inhibitors (T), and cyclosporine (C) may enhance nephrotoxicity; cimetidine, trimethoprim, and probencid may inhibit creatine excretion (T)	Renal	No data

(continued)

	Toxicities	Interactions	Elimination	Reproduction
Dehydroiepian-drosterone (DHEA)	In women; acneform rash, hirsutism, weight gain, emotional changes, abnormal menses, impaired glucose tolerance (S) Mania (C) In men; decreased HDL (S), prostate cancer (T), benign prostatic hypertrophy (T), pancreatic cancer (T)	Certain drugs may affect endogenous DHEA or DHEA-Sulfate (S) production; DHEA inhibits triazolam metabolism through the enxyme CYP3A4 (S); levels of other drugs eliminated by this enzyme (e.g., calcium channel blockers, some benzodiazepines, certain antilipemics, the HIV protease inhibitors, certain macrolide antibiotics, some synthetic narcotics, several immunosupressants, some antifungals, certain antidepressants, and several antineoplastics may also be affected (T)	Hepatic peripheral metabolism	No evidence of harm (S)

	Toxicities	Interactions	Elimination	Reproduction
Dimethylglycine	Well tolerated (S)	No data	Hepatic	No data
Fish oil	Fishy taste and odor, prolonged bleeding time, increased LDL cholesterol (S), mood elevation, hypervitaminosis A (C), cancer (A, C), exposure to mercury, dioxins, PCBs (T)	Aspirin (S) clopidogrel NSAIDS, warfarin (T)	Standard fatty acid metabolism pathways	May be beneficial (S)
γ-hydroxybutyric acid, (GHB) γ-butyrolactone, and 1,4-butanediol (BD)	Central nervous system depression, impaired gag reflex, vomiting (S, C), respiratory arrest (C); dependence and withdrawal (C)	Protease inhibitors may inhibit GHB metabolism (C); other drugs that inhibit CYP450 isoenzymes may prolong GHB action or enhance its effects (T)	Hepatic and peripheral metabolism	No data
Germanium	Nephrotoxicity, central and peripheral neurotoxicity, myopathy, bone marrow suppression nausea, vomiting, anorexia, anemia (C)	Diuretic resistance (C), aluminum toxicity (T)	Renal	Avoid in pregnancy (A); no data on lactation
Glucosamine	Gatrointestinal disturbances (S), dematologic reactions (S, C), headache, dizziness, drowsiness, edema (S), insulin resistance (S, C), manganese toxicity (T), angioedema (C)	None reported; used in patients taking other medications in clinical studies with no obvious interaction, may antagozine effects of antidiabetic agents (T)	Metabolized in liver and eliminated in urine	No data; may cross placenta and be excreted in breast milk (T)

(continued)

	Toxicities	Interactions	Elimination	Reproduction
Huperizine	Nausea (S), vomiting (S), diarrhea (S), hyperactivity (S), dizziness (S), anorexia (S)	Anticholinergics (T), β-blockers (T)	No data	No data
Hydrazine	Hepatorenal failure (C), elevated liver enzymes (C), paresthesias (S), nausea (S), vomiting (S), drowsiness (S)	MAOIS (A) benzodiazepines (A), tyramine-containing foods (C)	Metabolism	Avoid (A)
5-Hydroxytryptophan	EMS (C), nausea (S), vomiting (S), diarrhea (S)	Carbidopa (C), reserpine (T) MAOIS (T)	Metabolism by several organs	Avoid
Melatonin	Sleep disturbances (S,C), headache (S), disorientation (S), nausea (S), gastrointestinal symptoms (S), allergic reactions (C), cardiac stimultion (C), seizures (C), eosinophilia (C)	Nifedipine (S), warfarin (C), fluoxetine (C), fluvoxamine (S)	Hepatic metabolism (S)	No data for pregnancy, may have a contraceptive effect? (T)
Methylsulfonyl-methane	Nausea, diarrhea, headache	None reported	Metabolism (probably liver)	No data
Pyruvate	Gastrointestinal complaints (S)	None reported	Metabolized throughout body	No data
Red yeast rice	Rhabdomyolysis, myopathy, hepatotoxicity (T)	CYP3A inhibitors (T)	Hepatic metabolism	Avoid in preganancy (T)
S-adenosyl-L-methionine	Hyperhomocysteinemia (T), dizziness, drowsiness, headache, insomnia, mania, mood elevation, gastrointestinal complaints (S)	Antidepressants (serotonin syndrome) (C)	Metabolized throughout body	No adverse outcomes in small studies (S)

	Toxicities	Interactions	Elimination	Reproduction
Shark cartilage	Nausea, vomiting, constipation, hyperglycemia, decreased motor strength, decreased sensation, decreased performance (S), hepatotoxicity (C)	None reported	Metabolized in liver, eliminated renally (chondroitin sulfate (S)	Avoid (T)
L–Tryptophan	EMS (C), bladder, tumors ? (A), sexual dysfunction (C)	MAOIS (S), lithium (C), phenelzine (C), Chlorpromazine (C), fluoxetine	Hepatic and peripheral metabolism (S)	Avoid (A, V)
Vanadyl sulfate	Cramping (S), abdominal discomfort (S), diarrhea (S)	Antidiabetic agents (T)	Renal	No data

[a]Data were compiled by Melanie Johns Cupp and Timothy S. Tracy. See pertinent sections in individual chapters for more detailed information. C, case report; A, animal data; T, theoretical concern based on mechanism of action or information on closely related products; S, study; V, in vitro data; ACE, angiotensin-converting enzyme; CRH, corticotropin-releasing hormone; EMS, eosinophilia-myalgia syndrome; HDL, high-density lipoprotein; LDL, low-density lipoprotein; MAOI, monoamine oxidase inhibitor; NSAID, nonsteroidal antiinflammatory drug.

Index